AF606415

1993
YEAR BOOK OF
OBSTETRICS AND GYNECOLOGY®

Statement of Purpose

The YEAR BOOK Service

The YEAR BOOK series was devised in 1901 by practicing health professionals who observed that the literature of medicine and related disciplines had become so voluminous that no one individual could read and place in perspective every potential advance in a major specialty. In the final decade of the 20th century, this recognition is more acutely true than it was in 1901.

More than merely a series of books, YEAR BOOK volumes are the tangible results of a unique service designed to accomplish the following:

- to *survey* a wide range of journals of proven value
- to *select* from those journals papers representing significant advances and statements of important clinical principles
- to provide *abstracts* of those articles that are readable, convenient summaries of their key points
- to provide *commentary* about those articles to place them in perspective

These publications grow out of a unique process that calls on the talents of outstanding authorities in clinical and fundamental disciplines, trained literature specialists, and professional writers, all supported by the resources of Mosby, the world's preeminent publisher for the health professions.

The Literature Base

Mosby subscribes to nearly 1,000 journals published worldwide, covering the full range of the health professions. On an annual basis, the publisher examines usage patterns and polls its expert authorities to add new journals to the literature base and to delete journals that are no longer useful as potential YEAR BOOK sources.

The Literature Survey

The publisher's team of literature specialists, all of whom are trained and experienced health professionals, examines every original, peer-reviewed article in each journal issue. More than 250,000 articles per year are scanned systematically, including title, text, illustrations, tables, and references. Each scan is compared, article by article, to the search strategies that the publisher has developed in consultation with the 270 outside experts who form the pool of YEAR BOOK editors. A given article may be reviewed by any number of editors, from one to a dozen or more, regardless of the discipline for which the paper was originally published. In turn, each editor who receives the article reviews it to determine whether or not the article should be included in the YEAR BOOK. This decision is based on the article's inherent quality, its probable usefulness to readers of that YEAR BOOK, and the editor's goal to represent a balanced picture of a given field in each volume of the YEAR BOOK. In addition, the editor indicates when to include figures and tables from the article to help the YEAR BOOK reader better understand the information.

Of the quarter million articles scanned each year, only 5% are selected for detailed analysis within the YEAR BOOK series, thereby assuring readers of the high value of every selection.

The Abstract

The publisher's abstracting staff is headed by a physician-writer and includes individuals with training in the life sciences, medicine, and other areas, plus extensive experience in writing for the health professions and related industries. Each selected article is assigned to a specific writer on this abstracting staff. The abstracter, guided in many cases by notations supplied by the expert editor, writes a structured, condensed summary designed so that the reader can rapidly acquire the essential information contained in the article.

The Commentary

The YEAR BOOK editorial boards, sometimes assisted by guest commentators, write comments that place each article in perspective for the reader. This provides the reader with the equivalent of a personal consultation with a leading international authority—an opportunity to better understand the value of the article and to benefit from the authority's thought processes in assessing the article.

Additional Editorial Features

The editorial boards of each YEAR BOOK organize the abstracts and comments to provide a logical and satisfying sequence of information. To enhance the organization, editors also provide introductions to sections or individual chapters, comments linking a number of abstracts, citations to additional literature, and other features.

The published YEAR BOOK contains enhanced bibliographic citations for each selected article, including extended listings of multiple authors and identification of author affiliations. Each YEAR BOOK contains a Table of Contents specific to that year's volume. From year to year, the Table of Contents for a given YEAR BOOK will vary depending on developments within the field.

Every YEAR BOOK contains a list of the journals from which papers have been selected. This list represents a subset of the nearly 1,000 journals surveyed by the publisher, and occasionally reflects a particularly pertinent article from a journal that is not surveyed on a routine basis.

Finally, each volume contains a comprehensive subject index and an index to authors of each selected paper.

The 1993 Year Book Series

Year Book of Anesthesia and Pain Management: Drs. Miller, Abram, Kirby, Ostheimer, Roizen, and Stoelting

Year Book of Cardiology®: Drs. Schlant, Collins, Engle, Gersh, Kaplan, and Waldo

Year Book of Chiropractic: Drs. Phillips and Adams

Year Book of Critical Care Medicine®: Drs. Rogers and Parrillo

Year Book of Dentistry®: Drs. Meskin, Currier, Kennedy, Leinfelder, Berry, Roser, and Zakariasen

Year Book of Dermatologic Surgery: Drs. Swanson, Salasche, and Glogau

Year Book of Dermatology®: Drs. Sober and Fitzpatrick

Year Book of Diagnostic Radiology®: Drs. Federle, Clark, Gross, Madewell, Maynard, Sackett, and Young

Year Book of Digestive Diseases®: Drs. Greenberger and Moody

Year Book of Drug Therapy®: Drs. Lasagna and Weintraub

Year Book of Emergency Medicine®: Drs. Wagner, Burdick, Davidson, Roberts, and Spivey

Year Book of Endocrinology®: Drs. Bagdade, Braverman, Horton, Kannan, Landsberg, Molitch, Morley, Odell, Rogol, Ryan, and Sherwin

Year Book of Family Practice®: Drs. Berg, Bowman, Davidson, Dietrich, and Scherger

Year Book of Geriatrics and Gerontology®: Drs. Beck, Reuben, Burton, Small, Whitehouse, and Goldstein

Year Book of Hand Surgery®: Drs. Amadio and Hentz

Year Book of Health Care Management: Drs. Heyssel, Brock, Moses, and Steinberg, Ms. Avakian, and Messrs. Berman, Kues, and Rosenberg

Year Book of Hematology®: Drs. Spivak, Bell, Ness, Quesenberry, and Wiernik

Year Book of Infectious Diseases®: Drs. Wolff, Barza, Keusch, Klempner, and Snydman

Year Book of Infertility: Drs. Mishell, Paulsen, and Lobo

Year Book of Medicine®: Drs. Rogers, Bone, Cline, O'Rourke, Greenberger, Utiger, Epstein, and Malawista

Year Book of Neonatal and Perinatal Medicine®: Drs. Klaus and Fanaroff

Year Book of Nephrology: Drs. Coe, Favus, Henderson, Kashgarian, Luke, Myers, and Curtis

Year Book of Neurology and Neurosurgery®: Drs. Bradley and Crowell

Year Book of Neuroradiology: Drs. Osborn, Eskridge, Harnsberger, and Grossman

Year Book of Nuclear Medicine®: Drs. Hoffer, Gore, Gottschalk, Zaret, and Zubal

Year Book of Obstetrics and Gynecology®: Drs. Mishell, Kirschbaum, and Morrow

Year Book of Occupational and Environmental Medicine: Drs. Emmett, Brooks, Frank, and Hammad

Year Book of Oncology®: Drs. Young, Longo, Ozols, Simone, Steele, and Glatstein

Year Book of Ophthalmology®: Drs. Laibson, Adams, Augsburger, Benson, Cohen, Eagle, Flanagan, Nelson, Rapuano, Reinecke, Sergott, and Wilson

Year Book of Orthopedics®: Drs. Sledge, Poss, Cofield, Frymoyer, Griffin, Hansen, Johnson, Simmons, and Springfield

Year Book of Otolaryngology-Head and Neck Surgery®: Drs. Holt and Paparella

Year Book of Pathology and Clinical Pathology®: Drs. Gardner, Bennett, Cousar, Garvin, and Worsham

Year Book of Pediatrics®: Dr. Stockman

Year Book of Plastic, Reconstructive, and Aesthetic Surgery: Drs. Miller, Cohen, McKinney, Robson, Ruberg, and Whitaker

Year Book of Podiatric Medicine and Surgery®: Dr. Kominsky

Year Book of Psychiatry and Applied Mental Health®: Drs. Talbott, Frances, Freedman, Meltzer, Perry, Schowalter, and Yudofsky

Year Book of Pulmonary Disease®: Drs. Bone and Petty

Year Book of Sports Medicine®: Drs. Shephard, Eichner, Sutton, and Torg, Col. Anderson, and Mr. George

Year Book of Surgery®: Drs. Copeland, Deitch, Eberlein, Howard, Ritchie, Robson, Souba, and Sugarbaker

Year Book of Transplantation®: Drs. Ascher, Hansen, and Strom

Year Book of Ultrasound: Drs. Merritt, Mittelstaedt, Carroll, Babcock, and Goldstein

Year Book of Urology®: Drs. Gillenwater and Howards

Year Book of Vascular Surgery®: Dr. Porter

Roundsmanship® '93–'94: A Student's Survival Guide to Clinical Medicine Using Current Literature: Drs. Dan, Feigin, Quilligan, Schrock, Stein, and Talbott

1993

The Year Book of OBSTETRICS AND GYNECOLOGY®

Editors

Daniel R. Mishell, Jr., M.D.

Lyle G. McNeile Professor and Chairman, Department of Obstetrics and Gynecology, University of Southern California School of Medicine, Los Angeles

Thomas H. Kirschbaum, M.D.

Professor, Department of Obstetrics and Gynecology, Albert Einstein College of Medicine, Bronx, New York

C. Paul Morrow, M.D.

Professor, Department of Obstetrics and Gynecology; Director of Gynecologic Oncology, University of Southern California School of Medicine, Los Angeles

Contributing Editors

Arieh Bergman, M.D.

Professor, Department of Obstetrics and Gynecology, University of Southern California School of Medicine, Los Angeles

William H. Hindle, M.D.

Professor of Clinical Obstetrics and Gynecology, University of Southern California School of Medicine; Director, Breast Diagnostic Center, Women's Hospital LAC/USC Medical Center, Los Angeles, California

Editorial Assistant

Shirley J. Davenport

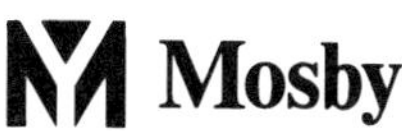

St. Louis Baltimore Boston Chicago London Philadelphia Sydney Toronto

Mosby, Inc.
11830 Westline Industrial Drive
St. Louis, MO 63146

Editorial Office:
Mosby, Inc.
200 North LaSalle St.
Chicago, IL 60601

International Standard Serial Number: 0084-3911
International Standard Book Number: 0-8151-6015-1

Table of Contents

Journals Represented xi
Publisher's Preface xv
Introduction xvii

Controversial Issues in Menopausal Management by Leon Speroff, M.D. xix

OBSTETRICS
1. Maternal and Fetal Physiology 3
2. Maternal Complications of Pregnancy 31
3. Maternal Abnormalities of Pregnancy 71
4. Medical Complications of Pregnancy 73
5. Fetal Diagnosis 117
6. Fetal Complications of Pregnancy 119
7. Fetal Surveillance 141
8. Labor, Surgery, and Delivery 163
9. Genetics. 185
10. The Puerperium 203
11. The Newborn 211
12. Fetal Therapy 235

GYNECOLOGY
13. Operative Gynecology 245
14. Gynecologic Urology 263
15. Tumors 293
Cervix: Benign 293
Cervix: Malignant 305
Uterus 309
Ovary 323
Gestational Trophoblastic Disease 345
Vulva/Vagina 348
16. Infections 357

17. ENDOCRINOLOGY 383
18. MENOPAUSE 409
19. INFERTILITY 433
20. CONTRACEPTION 479
21. ABORTION 505
22. ECTOPIC PREGNANCY 517
23. PREMENSTRUAL SYNDROME 529
24. BREAST DISEASES 537
Subject Index 603
Author Index 641

Journals Represented

Mosby subscribes to and surveys nearly 1,000 U.S. and foreign medical and allied health journals. From these journals, the Editors select the articles to be abstracted. Journals represented in this YEAR BOOK are listed below.

Acta Cytologica
Acta Endocrinologica
Acta Neurologica Scandinavica
Acta Obstetricia et Gynecologica Scandinavica
American Journal of Cardiology
American Journal of Clinical Nutrition
American Journal of Clinical Oncology
American Journal of Diseases of Children
American Journal of Epidemiology
American Journal of Hypertension
American Journal of Kidney Diseases
American Journal of Medicine
American Journal of Neuroradiology
American Journal of Obstetrics and Gynecology
American Journal of Perinatology
American Journal of Physiology
American Journal of Preventive Medicine
American Journal of Public Health
American Journal of Roentgenology
American Journal of Surgery
American Journal of Surgical Pathology
Anaesthesia and Intensive Care
Anesthesia and Analgesia
Anesthesiology
Annals of Internal Medicine
Annals of Surgery
Archives of Disease in Childhood
Archives of Internal Medicine
Archives of Pathology and Laboratory Medicine
Archives of Physical Medicine and Rehabilitation
Archives of Surgery
Arthritis and Rheumatism
Australian and New Zealand Journal of Obstetrics and Gynaecology
Breast Disease
British Heart Journal
British Journal of Cancer
British Journal of Family Planning
British Journal of Obstetrics and Gynaecology
British Journal of Radiology
British Journal of Surgery
British Journal of Urology
British Medical Journal
Canadian Family Physician
Canadian Journal of Surgery
Cancer
Cancer Research
Cardiovascular Research
Cell
Clinical Endocrinology
Clinical Nephrology

Contraception
Epilepsia
European Heart Journal
European Journal of Cancer
European Journal of Obstetrics, Gynecology and Reproductive Biology
Fertility and Sterility
Gut
Gynecologic Oncology
Gynecological Endocrinology
Health Services Research
Human Reproduction
Hypertension
Intensive Care Medicine
International Journal of Cancer
International Journal of Epidemiology
International Journal of Gynecological Pathology
International Journal of Radiation, Oncology, Biology, and Physics
Journal of Acquired Immune Deficiency Syndromes
Journal of Applied Physiology: Respiratory, Environmental and Exercise Physiology
Journal of Clinical Endocrinology and Metabolism
Journal of Clinical Epidemiology
Journal of Clinical Microbiology
Journal of Clinical Oncology
Journal of Clinical Pathology
Journal of Clinical Psychiatry
Journal of Epidemiology and Community Health
Journal of Family Practice
Journal of Health and Social Behavior
Journal of Medical Genetics
Journal of Reproductive Medicine
Journal of Ultrasound in Medicine
Journal of Urology
Journal of the American Geriatrics Society
Journal of the American Medical Association
Journal of the National Cancer Institute
Journal of the Royal Society of Medicine
Lancet
Maturitas
Medical Journal of Australia
Metabolism
Neurosurgery
New England Journal of Medicine
New York State Journal of Medicine
Nursing Research
Obstetrics and Gynecology
Paediatric and Perinatal Epidemiology
Pediatric Neurology
Pediatric Research
Pediatrics
Plastic and Reconstructive Surgery
Postgraduate Medical Journal
Prenatal Diagnosis
Radiology

Surgery, Gynecology and Obstetrics
Ultrasound in Medicine and Biology
Urology
Yale Journal of Biology and Medicine

Standard Abbreviations

The following terms are abbreviated in this edition: acquired immunodeficiency syndrome (AIDS), the central nervous system (CNS), cerebrospinal fluid (CSF), computed tomography (CT), electrocardiography (ECG), human immunodeficiency virus (HIV), and magnetic resonance (MR) imaging (MRI).

Publisher's Preface

As publishers, we feel challenged to seek ways of presenting complex information in a clear and readable manner. To this end, the 1993 YEAR BOOK OF OBSTETRICS AND GYNECOLOGY now provides structured abstracts in which the various components of a study can easily be identified through headings. These headings are not the same in all abstracts but, rather, are those that most accurately designate the content of each particular journal article. We are confident that our readers will find the information contained in our abstracts to be more accessible than ever before. We welcome your comments.

Introduction

Staying current with the medical literature in the specialty of Obstetrics and Gynecology has become increasingly more difficult for practitioners of the specialty. Time contraints prevent busy practitioners from reviewing more than a few publications each month. To provide clinicians with a convenient but efficient method of reviewing the entire worldwide literature in 1 publication, the editors of the YEAR BOOK OF OBSTETRICS AND GYNECOLOGY perform periodic reviews not only of the journals relevant to the specialty, but also of those articles in other journals that are pertinent to obstetrical and gynecologic practice. After the review, the editors select those articles believed to have the most pertinent clinical relevance. The articles are then abstracted, and the editor writes a short comment regarding the relevance of the article for the practicing clinician.

During the past year, after reviewing hundreds of scientific journals, the authors have selected 435 articles from 107 journals to appear in the 1993 YEAR BOOK OF OBSTETRICS AND GYNECOLOGY. My co-editors, Dr. Thomas H. Kirschbaum and Dr. C. Paul Morrow, reviewed and selected articles in the field of maternal fetal medicine and gynecologic oncology, respectively, whereas I reviewed articles in the fields of reproductive endocrinology and infertility and gynecologic infection. Our contributing editors, Dr. Arieh Bergman and Dr. William H. Hindle, reviewed articles in the fields of gynecologic urology and breast disease, respectively.

This year, because of the controversy regarding the perception of the risks and benefits of postmenopausal hormone replacement, one of the world's experts in this area, Dr. Leon Speroff, graciously accepted an invitation to write a comprehensive review article on the subject. We believe that clinicians will derive substantial benefit regarding treatment of their patients from reading Dr. Speroff's article, as well as the abstracts and comments in this volume.

Suggestions from readers are solicited in an effort to improve this YEAR BOOK'S relevance to clinical practice.

Daniel R. Mishell, Jr., M.D.

Controversial Issues in Menopausal Management

LEON SPEROFF, M.D.
Professor of Obstetrics and Gynecology, Oregon Health Sciences University, Portland, Oregon

I like to define medical judgment as making a decision when you don't have all the facts needed to make that decision. Clinicians make medical judgments every day, and this is certainly true when dealing with the controversial issues surrounding menopause. The clinical needs of our patients force us to make decisions without the comfort of full scientific support. I would like to share my own personal medical judgments in providing answers to some important and common clinical questions regarding postmenopausal hormonal therapy.

In general, 3 indications exist for the use of postmenopausal hormone therapy: (1) symptoms related to estrogen deficiency, such as vasomotor symptoms or atrophy of the genitourinary tissues; (2) osteoporosis prophylaxis and treatment; and (3) prevention of cardiovascular morbidity and mortality.

Treatment with estrogen and, usually, progesterone should be offered to most women with evidence of estrogen deprivation. This includes women with gonadal dysgenesis, women with ovarian failure (premature menopause), some perimenopausal women, and women in both the menopausal and postmenopausal periods of life. The duration of hormone treatment is not well defined. Existing data indicate that estrogen's preventive health benefits persist as long as use continues. Thus, postmenopausal women should consider the use of hormone treatment for a relatively long duration, perhaps lifelong.

What Hormonal Agent or Route of Administration is Best?

There is no evidence that one form of estrogen is superior to another. More important are the duration, dose, and presence or absence of progestin. Studies have demonstrated that a dose of either .625 mg of conjugated estrogens or 1 mg of micronized estradiol is necessary to preserve bone density (1). A small nonrandomized study in women who had not undergone oophorectomy showed that a lower dose of conjugated estrogens, .3 mg/day, prevented loss of vertebral trabecular bone when combined with calcium supplementation (2). A study of 66 women randomized to treatment either with continuous transdermal delivery of estradiol, .05 mg/day, or oral estrogen demonstrated that both equally prevented postmenopausal bone loss (3). Whether fracture protection with either the lower dose oral regimen or the transdermal route of administration is equal to the standard oral program awaits further epidemiological study.

The effect of steroids on lipids and lipoproteins is determined by the type of steroid, the dose, and the route of administration. An obstacle to the use of transdermal hormone therapy has been the lack of data indicating a beneficial impact on the lipoprotein profile. There has been concern that delivery of estrogen through the skin yields a blood level that might be too low to provide this important benefit. English data now indicate that the transdermal administration of 50 μg of estradiol twice a week is as effective as .625 mg of oral conjugated estrogen on bone density and lipids over 1 year (3, 4). Nevertheless, the concentration of estrogen in the portal system after oral administration is 4–5 times higher than that in the periphery (5). The estradiol/estrone ratio differs in the portal system; therefore, the first-pass effect is either significant for the lipoprotein effects, or it is important only in the short term. For example, a short-term study (6 weeks) documented increased catabolism of low-density lipoprotein with oral estrogen, but it could not find any effect when transdermal estrogen was used (6).

Until data are available documenting the degree of the various routes of administration on actual clinical events (fractures and cardiovascular disease), the prudent clinical decision is to select the method (an oral program) that has epidemiological support. The argument that the transdermal route is safer is specious. Because the proper oral dose of estrogen has no impact on hypertension or the clotting cascade, how can a method be safer than safe?

What is the Best Regimen, Sequential or Continuous?

Several regimens for oral administration are currently used. The 2 most common sequential methods involve administration of .625 mg of conjugated estrogen or 1 mg of micronized estradiol, given either daily or from the 1st through the 25th day of each month. A daily dose of 10 mg of medroxyprogesterone acetate (MPA) is added for the first 14 days of the month or for the final 10 days of estrogen administration, respectively. Problems with this sequential regimen include adverse symptoms related to the dose of progestin, such as breast tenderness, bloating, fluid retention, and depression. A lower dose (5 mg) usually resolves these complaints. However, the lowest effective dose of MPA required for endometrial protection in a sequential program has not been established, and the standard dose remains at 10 mg. Unfortunately, bleeding resulting from progesterone withdrawal occurs in 90% of women.

The continuous/combined method of treatment evolved to improve patient compliance in the presence of bleeding and other symptoms (7–14). The continuous presence of progesterone allows the use of lower doses. This approach involves the continuous daily use of the following estrogen-progesterone combinations: daily estrogen (.625 mg of conjugated estrogen or 1 mg of micronized estradiol) and daily progesterone (2.5 mg of MPA or .35 mg of norethindrone). After 4–6 months of such continuous treatment, 80% to 90% of women experience no bleeding, and essentially all biopsy specimens show atrophic endometrium. In my experience, in the first year of use, this continuous approach maintains a beneficial lipoprotein pattern and increases the bone density in the spinal column to a level which is then maintained. Others have noted an increasing bone density for a least 18 months. It also is of note that no adverse effects on blood pressure are encountered.

Compliance with hormone therapy programs is notoriously poor. The 2 most common reasons why women discontinue or fail to start hormone treatment are fear of cancer and vaginal bleeding (15). The current data on breast cancer are reassuring, and the addition of a progestational agent has effectively prevented endometrial cancer. However, the persistence of bleeding when the traditional sequential regimen is used continues to be a barrier to good compliance. The continuous approach allows patients with 80% to 90% withdrawal bleeding to experience 80% to 90% no bleeding, a significant advantage over traditional methods. I would argue that the decision to provide continuous therapy before full scientific support was available was justified, because by solving an important compliance problem, even more women have been able to gain from the preventive health benefits of hormone replacement therapy.

How to Treat Breakthrough Bleeding With Continuous Therapy?

The most aggravating and worrisome problem associated with daily, continuous therapy is breakthrough bleeding. One can expect 30% to 40% of patients to experience breakthrough bleeding during the first 4 months of treatment; however, this percentage decreases to only 10% after 1 year (12). Although this rate of incidence of amenorrhea is a gratifying accomplishment, the number of women who experience breakthrough bleeding is considerable and presents a difficult management problem.

Such breakthrough bleeding is similar to that seen with oral contraceptives. It originates from an endometrium dominated by progestational influence; hence, the endometrium is usually atrophic and yields little, if anything, to the exploring biopsy instrument. It takes confidence and experience with this method to withstand the urge to perform a biopsy. In this circumstance, the endometrial biopsy—no matter what instrument or method is used—is not cost effective. I would urge clinicians to support their patients through the early months of continuous therapy. If bleeding persists for 6 months, consider an office hysteroscopy; an impressive number of polyps and intrauterine fibroids will be discovered.

I have tried every method of drug alteration and substitution to manage this breakthrough bleeding, and nothing works! I am convinced that the best approach is to gain time, because most patients will cease bleeding. This requires good educational preparation of the patient beforehand and frequent telephone contact to allay anxiety and encourage persistence. It is appropriate to perform an endometrial aspiration biopsy when the patient's anxiety over the possibility of pathology requires this response. It is also appropriate to perform a biopsy when the physician is concerned, although, with increasing experience with this method, it takes more and more to build concern.

Nevertheless, we are left with a core of patients who continue to bleed. The closer a patient is to having bled recently (close either to her premenopausal state or to having undergone a sequential method with withdrawal bleeding), the more likely it is that the patient will experience breakthrough bleeding. Some clinicians, therefore, prefer to start patients near menopause with the sequential method and then convert to the continuous method some years later. For the small number of patients who persist in having breakthrough bleeding, it is better to return to the sequential program to have expected and orderly withdrawal bleeding instead of the irregularity of breakthrough bleeding.

Does Progesterone Subtract From the Cardiovascular Benefit of Estrogen?

Postmenopausal hormone therapy deserves consideration as a legitimate component of preventive health care for older women. One can argue convincingly that protection against cardiovascular disease is the major benefit of postmenopausal estrogen treatment, and that the magnitude of this benefit is considerable. There is a sound rationale for this protection in the link between cardiovascular disease and the sex hormones.

During the reproductive years, women are "protected" from coronary heart disease. Women lag behind men in the incidence of coronary heart disease by 10 years, and for myocardial infarction and sudden death, women have a 20-year advantage (16). The reasons for this advantage are complex, but a significant contribution to this protection can be assigned to the higher high-density lipoprotein (HDL) cholesterol levels in younger women, which is an effect of estrogen. Throughout adulthood, the blood HDL cholesterol level is approximately 10 mg/dL higher in women, and this difference continues through the postmenopausal years. Total and low-density (LDL) cholesterol levels are lower in premenopausal women than in men, but after menopause they increase rapidly. After menopause, the risk of coronary heart disease doubles for women, because the atherogenic lipids increase until about 60 years of age and then decrease. At all ages, HDL cholesterol values in women are 10 mg/dL higher than those in men.

Cross-sectional studies indicate a shift to an atherogenic lipid and lipoprotein profile after menopause (17). This is confirmed by longitudinal surveillance which reveals a decline in HDL and an increase in LDL during menopause which exceed that caused by aging alone (18). This is reflected by the increasing incidence of cardiovascular disease in the years after menopause.

The gender difference in the cholesterol-lipoprotein profile is probably one reason for both female protection against atherosclerosis before menopause and the acceleration that occurs after menopause. The higher HDL levels in women compared with men represent the net effect of estrogen (HDL-increasing) in women and androgens (HDL-reducing) in men. In women, data from 2 large, prospective studies indicate that HDL cholesterol is more closely related to cardiovascular disease than is LDL cholesterol (19, 20).

The pharmacological effects of estrogen as used postmenopausally are just beginning to be understood. Estrogen increases LDL catabolism as well as lipoprotein receptor activity, resulting in decreased LDL levels and increased HDL levels (21). In addition, animal studies have indicated that estrogen inhibits the development of atherosclerotic lesions by means of 1 or more mechanisms, independently of any effects on lipids and lipoproteins. This is supported by the significant presence of estrogen and progesterone receptors in the endothelium and smooth muscles of human arterial vessels (22). Many studies indicate that these receptors are physiologically active, effecting cholesterol changes, platelet aggregation, smooth muscle cell proliferation, and changes in the prostaglandin system. Thus, there is a biological and plausible rationale supporting a protective role for the use of estrogen against cardiovascular disease.

A review of the literature finds overwhelming support for a reduced risk of cardiovascular disease in estrogen users. Only 1 of 12 case-control studies failed to show a decreased relative risk of cardiovascular disease (23–34). Of 11 cohort studies, 9 showed a reduced risk of coronary heart disease in estrogen users; the 2 other studies produced conflicting data (35–47). In its first report, the Walnut Creek Study, which initially had conflicting data, revealed 26 women with infarctions, only 9 of whom were estrogen users (39). An update of the Walnut Creek data now documents a 50% reduction in death from diseases of the circulatory system when adjusted for all other factors (47).

The Framingham Study, which presented data in 1978 and in 1985, argued that there was a 50% increased risk for cardiovascular disease among estrogen users, although there was no difference in fatality rates between users and nonusers (37, 41). Because of the respect the Framingham Study carries, its impact was significant. The Framingham reports adjusted the data for total and HDL cholesterol levels; this is an inappropriate adjustment, because an impact on these variables is a major effect of estrogen. Re analysis of the Framingham data (excluding angina as an endpoint) indicated a protective effect among women 50–59 years of age, with too few estrogen users to estimate risk among older women (48). Because this analysis still adjusted for HDL, it probably underestimated the benefit of postmenopausal use of estrogen. Therefore, the early reports from the Framingham Study (now reversed), stand in lonely opposition to overwhelming evidence that appropriately low doses of estrogen protect postmenopausal women against cardiovascular disease.

There has been one randomized, clinical trial of estrogen (49). Although the numbers were very small, the results indicated that postmenopausal estrogen treatment protects against cardiovascular disease.

A case-control study found no evidence for a protective effect of estrogen against stroke (50). However, only 16% of the women in the study had filled more than 1 prescription, only 1% were current users, and average use was only 15 months. In a prospective cohort study, estrogen therapy was associated with a 46% overall reduction in the risk of death from stroke, with a 79% reduction in recent users (51). This protection was present both in women with hypertension and in those without; it was also present in smokers and nonsmokers. This level of protection was similar to that observed in this same Leisure World population for estrogen protection against deaths resulting from myocardial infarction (45). The failure to observe protection against stroke in the Nurses' Health Study cohort is in striking contrast to the Leisure World cohort. This difference may be the result of an older population in the Leisure World cohort than in the Nurses' Health Study. Perhaps an effect against stroke will be demonstrated in the Nurses' Health Study as the cohort reaches older age when stroke is more common.

Hypertension is both a risk factor for cardiovascular mortality and a common problem in older individuals. It is important, therefore, to know that no relationship has been established between hypertension and the doses of estrogen used for postmenopausal therapy. Studies have either demonstrated no effect or a small, but statistically significant decrease in blood pressure resulting from estrogen treatment (52–56). This has been the case in both normotensive and hypertensive women. Women with hypertension need estrogen's protection against cardiovascular disease. The very rare cases of increased blood pressure caused by estrogen therapy truly represent idiosyncratic reactions.

An important question to ask is whether estrogen treatment is a marker for variables (e.g., better diet and improved health care) that place postmenopausal estrogen users in a low-risk group for cardiovascular disease. This question has been directly addressed by the Lipid Research Clinics study, as well as by the Nurses's Health Study (42, 43). Both groups of epidemiologists have concluded that women receiving estrogen treatment are slightly healthier, but not to a degree that would explain the difference between estrogen users and nonusers.

Difficulties may arise when a woman wishes to use hormonal therapy but has a cardiovascular event, such as a myocardial infarction, stroke, or embolism, in her history. It is known that the doses of estrogen used for postmenopausal therapy have no significant impact on the clotting mechanism, and no increased risks for thrombotic clinical events have been demonstrated (57). The woman with a previous arterial event may be the very woman who needs the protection of estrogen against cardiovascular disease. There is evidence to support this contention. In the Leisure World cohort study, women with previous myocardial infarctions, strokes, or hypertension had a 50% reduction in risk of death from a subsequent stroke or myocardial infarction. In the Lipids Research Clinics study, the cardiovascular mortality in women with increased lipid levels was reduced by 79%. Finally, and very impressively, in women with severe coronary disease (documented by arteriography), estrogen users had a 97% survival rate at 10 years, compared with a significantly lower rate of 60% in nonusers (58). In women with mild-to-moderate disease, there was no difference at 5 years; however, at 10 years, estrogen users had a 96% survival rate compared with 85% in nonusers. Again, women with existing cardiovascular disease need the beneficial impact of estrogen. I am also willing to prescribe appropriate doses of estrogen for women who have a history of venous thrombosis.

The impact of estrogen therapy on the lipid profile is maintained as long as women continue to take the estrogen. A higher HDL choloesterol and lower LDL cholesterol have been documented to persist through at least 10 years of postmenopausal treatment. However, the degree of protection is greater than that which can be statistically attributed to the impact on the lipoprotein profile (43). Thus, protection that is not mediated by lipoproteins is growing in importance.

In monkey colony studies at Bowman-Gray, treatment with either estrogen alone or estrogen with a progesterone given in a sequential manner significantly reduced atherosclerosis compared with no hormone treatment. This reduction occurred independently of the circulating lipid and lipoprotein profile (59). A direct inhibition of LDL accumulation could be demonstrated in these monkeys being fed a highly atherogenic diet (60). Therefore, estrogen exerts a protective effect directly on the arterial wall independently of its effects on circulating lipoproteins.

Estrogen (with or without progesterone) also prevents the tendency to increase central body fat with aging (61). This inhibits the interaction among abdominal adiposity, hormones, and an atherogenic lipid profile, making yet another positive contribution to protection against cardiovascular disease.

Because the public health benefit of postmenopausal estrogen therapy on cardiovascular disease is of such enormous impact, it is vital that we know whether the addition of monthly progesterone has an adverse effect on the lipid profile and, ultimately, on cardiovascular disease. A review of the literature concerning this question suggests a dose-response relationship (13, 62–68).

A decrease in HDL cholesterol has been noted with 10-day monthly treatment with norethindrone (5 mg), megestrol acetate (5 mg), levonorgestrel (250 μg), and even MPA (10 mg). A lack of an effect was noted when micronized progesterone was used in a daily dose of 200 mg, which yields a normal luteal phase blood level of progesterone. A similar "physiological" dose of synthetic progesterone may be free of an adverse impact on HDL cholesterol. In a study of the adult residents of Rancho Bernardo, California, those women using both estrogen and progesterone demonstrated the same favorable impact on cardiovascular risk factors as did users of estrogen only compared with the nonusers (69). On the other hand, a well-designed study indicated that, although the sequential estrogen-plus-progesterone program had a favorable impact on lipids and the lipoprotein profile, the impact was less than that achieved by estrogen alone (70).

Conclusions regarding the impact of progestational agents on cardiovascular disease are heavily influenced by dose and the duration of administration of the progestational agent involved. Although short-term studies suggest a negative impact of progesterone (i.e., subtracting from the beneficial effect of estrogen), long-term studies indicate that this short-term effect disappears.

Studies using a combination of an estrogen and a low dose of a progestational agent administered continuously (every day without a break) are emerging and documenting a favorable impact on lipids and lipoproteins. The various formulations include estradiol and levonorgestrel (7), estradiol and 1 mg of norethindrone acetate (8), ethinyl estradiol and 5–1 mg of norethindrone acetate (9), and .625 of conjugated estrogen and 2.5–5 mg of MPA (10, 12). Christiansen has documented the maintenance of a favorable lipid profile during a 5-year treatment program with continuous combined estradiol and 1 mg of norethindrone acetate (8).

The administration of a daily dose of 2.5 mg of MPA in a combined estrogen-progesterone program has been demonstrated to have a favorable impact on the lipoprotein profile. In Spain, 8 months of uninterrupted treatment produced an effect that was not substantially different than that achieved with estrogen alone (11). During a 12-month period, large multicenter trial in the United States produced a favorable lipoprotein profile in women receiving daily doses of .625 mg of conjugated estrogen and 2.5 mg of MPA; the positive effect was more pronounced in women with lower baseline HDL levels (12).

A preliminary report from the ongoing cohort study from Uppsala, Sweden, is now available (71). This study provides information from a follow-up evaluation of approximately 23,000 women who were prescribed hormone therapy. Overall, there was a 30% reduction in myocardial infarction in women prescribed estradiol valerate or conjugated estrogens. What is especially noteworthy is the 50% reduced risk of myocardial infarction in women exposed to a sequential estrogen-progesterone regimen consisting of 2 mg of estradiol valerate and 10 days of administration of levonorgestrel, 250 μg, each month. These data do not support the contention that exposure to a progesterone (even the most androgenic of progesterone) counteracts the cardiovascular benefit of estrogen.

Studies of the Doppler ultrasound flow patterns in women with arterial vascular resistance have indicated no detrimental effects of exogenous progesterone on the beneficial decrease in resistance produced by estrogen administration (72). Similarly, the monkey studies could detect no difference in the favorable direct impact on atherosclerosis when progesterone was added to estrogen treatment (59). Thus, the growing importance of estrogen's direct action on blood vessels further minimizes the impact of progestational agents.

I believe we have witnessed a major clinical achievement through medical decision-making: the determination of a dose and regimen of progestin treatment that can protect the endometrium against cancer, while not subtracting from the cardiovascular protection of estrogen. Scientific, epidemiological support for this contention is now emerging.

When Should Progesterone be Administered to Hysterectomized Women?

There are least 3 clinical examples of special conditions that, in my view, warrant the use of a combined estrogen-progesterone regimen in women who have undergone hysterectomy. It has been demonstrated that patients who have had stage I adenocarcinoma of the endometrium can take estrogen without fear of recurrence (73, 74); however, the combination of estrogen and progesterone is recommended because of the potential protective action of the progestational agent. A similar approach makes sense for patients who have previously been treated for endometrioid tumors of the ovary. Finally, because adenocarcinoma has been reported in patients with pelvic endometriosis who were treated with unopposed estrogen (75), the combined estrogen-progesterone program is advised for patients with a history of endometriosis.

There is evidence that the combination of estrogen and progesterone has a greater positive impact on bone density than estrogen alone. Thus, in women who have undergone hysterectomy and are at high risk for osteoporosis, the combined estrogen-progesterone program offers an important potential advantage.

I believe it is legitimate to discuss with patients who have had hysterectomy the present state-of-the-art concerning combined estrogen-progesterone treatment. Some patients and physicians will believe that it is appropriate to add progesterone in appropriately low doses to hormone therapy. Only time and epidemiological studies will bring us closer to the facts, and by then, we will be making medical judgments on the cutting edge in other clinical issues.

When is it Appropriate to Add Androgens to the Hormonal Regimen?

After menopause, the circulating level of androstenedione is nearly half that seen before menopause (76). Most of this postmenopausal androstenedione is derived from the adrenal gland, with only a small amount secreted from the ovary. Testosterone levels do not decrease appreciably, and in most women, the postmenopausal ovary, for a few years, actually secretes more testosterone than the premenopausal ovary. The remaining active stromal tissue in the ovary is stimulated by the increased gonadotropins to this level of increased testosterone secretion. However, the total amount of testosterone produced is decreased, because the primary source, the peripheral conversion of androstenedione, is reduced. Because of this decrease, some argue that androgen treatment is indicated in the postmenopausal period.

The potential benefits of androgen treatment include improvement in psychological well-being and an increase in sexually motivated behavior (77, 78). This effect, however, follows the administration of relatively large doses of androgen. In a well-designed, placebo-controlled study, lower doses of androgen contributed little to actual sexual behavior, although an increase in sexual fantasies and masturbation was documented. (79).

Any benefit must be balanced by the unwanted effects, in particular, a negative impact on the cholesterol-lipoprotein profile. Unfortunately, data are scant on this issue. We recently completed a short-term study comparing a product with estrogen and a relatively low dose of testosterone (1.25 mg of methyltestosterone) with estrogen alone; a negative impact on the lipid profile was apparent within 3 months (80). It should also be remembered that the addition of androgen does not protect the endometrium, and the addition of a progestin is still necessary. It is uncertain (and unstudied) to what extent aromatization of the administered testosterone increases the estrogen impact, and whether this might further increase the risk of endometrial and/or breast cancer are uncertain (and unstudied).

In my view, there is no doubt that pharmacological amounts of androgen can increase libido; however, these same doses produce unwanted effects (81). In addition, patients given high doses of androgens are often somewhat addicted to this therapy. I provide small amounts of androgen supplementation (Estratest-HS) in situations in which the patient and I are convinced that a depressed libido cannot be explained by psychosocial circumstances. In these cases, I carefully monitor the lipid profile, and I am aware that any positive clinical response may well be a placebo effect. After some months or a few years, conversion to a standard hormone replacement therapy program is recommended.

Is Calcium Supplementation Necessary?

Calcium absorption decreases with age and becomes significantly impaired after menopause. A positive calcium balance is mandatory to achieve adequate prevention against osteoporosis. However, without estrogen, calcium—even in supplemental doses of 2,000 mg/day—has little impact on trabecular bone (82). Estrogen improves calcium absorption and makes it possible to use effective supplemental calcium in a dose of 500 mg per day to achieve the daily requirement of approximately 1,000—1,500 mg of elemental calcium per day. Therefore, most women receiving postmenopausal hormone treatment should supplement their diet with an extra 500 mg of calcium daily.

The addition of vitamin D or its active metabolite has no impact on the osteoporosis fracture rate, and it may cause hypercalcemia and renal stone formation. The addition of fluoride, a potent stimulator of bone formation, does offer some benefit, but with a high rate of side effects.

A further concern is that this therapy may lead to more brittle bones, which are subject to fracture. Calcitonin acts to prevent bone resorption, and it eventually might be used in patients for whom hormone therapy is contraindicated. Given by injection to women soon after menopause, it is as effective as estrogen in conserving bone density (83). Studies of intranasal delivery of calcitonin suggest that it may be similarly effective (84).

Etidronate disodium is an oral diphosphonate compound that is known to reduce bone resorption by inhibiting osteoclastic activity. A recent study (in which 66 postmenopausal women with osteoporosis were randomized to intermittent cyclical etidronate or placebo) demonstrated a significant increase in vertebral bone mineral content and a significant decrease in fracture rate in the treatment group (85). Etidronate may prove to be an effective addition to osteoporotic prevention, because it is well tolerated and has no discernible side effects. However, unlike estrogens, etidronate has no effect on the cardiovascular disease, hot flushes, or the atrophic changes seen in menopause. Further studies must be performed to evaluate its efficacy and value in the prevention of osteoporosis.

Finally, life-style can have a beneficial effect on bone density. Physicial activity (as little a 30 minutes a day for 3 days a week) will increase the mineral content of bone in older women (86). Adverse habits, such as cigarette smoking or excessive alcohol consumption, are associated with an increased risk of osteoporosis. The lower blood levels of estrogen in smokers have been correlated with earlier menopause and reduced bone density; therefore, estrogen will not totally counteract the predisposition of smoking toward osteoporosis. The titration of estrogen dosage with circulating blood levels in smokers has not been reported in the literature, but such an approach makes clinical sense. Finally, a healthy balanced diet is required to provide an adequate allowance of elemental calcium to maintain a positive calcium balance.

Patients with osteoporosis or a history of osteoporotic fracture should be treated more vigorously. Although hormone therapy will significantly increase bone mass, agents such as fluoride, calcitonin, and perhaps etidronate should also be considered.

Should Very Old Women be Started on HRT?

The positive impact of hormone therapy on bone has been demonstrated to take place even in women older than 65 years of age (87). This is a strong argument in favor of treating very old women who have never been given estrogen. Estrogen use between the ages of 65 and 74 years has been documented to protect against hip fractures. (88). Whether estrogen's cardiovascular protection has anything significant to contribute in the elderly has not been addressed. It makes clinical sense, however, that some positive contribution can be expected. Adding a pharmacological regimen to an old woman's daily life is not a trivial consideration.

This judgment requires the conclusion that a relatively youthful and vigorous elderly woman has something to gain from such treatment.

Does HRT Increase the Risk of Breast Cancer?

The Cancer and Steroid Hormone Study (CASH) of the Centers for Disease Control is a large, population-based, case-control study from 8 geographic locations. The CASH study has not detected an overall increased risk of breast cancer with postmenopausal use of estrogen, nor has it discovered any relationship with duration of use as much as 20 years or longer (89). There were positive findings in certain subgroups, most notably in women with menopause because of bilateral oophorectomy. However, the confidence intervals in these subgroup analyses include 1; therefore, the conclusions did not reach statistical significance.

This study is large enough to have reliable results in various subcategories, and an absence of an effect was evident in all of the following: parity, age at first pregnancy, early or late menopause, monopause by hysterectomy or oophorectomy, family history of breast cancer, presence of benign breast disease, use for many years (20 years or longer), and use of high doses. Therefore, this absence of an increase in relative risk was not modified by the other known breast cancer risk factors.

The latest report from the Nurses' Health Study represents 12 years of follow-up (1976–1988) (90). During that period, 1,050 cases of breast cancer were identified among more than 20,000 women. The analysis revealed that women who had used estrogen in the past (even for 10 or more years) were not at an increased risk of breast cancer, and that the risk was not influenced by a family history of breast cancer in mother or sister, or by a personal history of benign breast disease. However, the relative risk for current users was 1.33 (confidence interval, 1.12–1.57). Compared with those who had never used estrogen, current users were slightly more likely to have certain risk factors (e.g., history of benign breast disease, nulliparity, use of alcohol). However, adjustment for several of these risk factors only minimally reduced the relative risk for current use. The one confounding variable that appeared to play a prominent role was alcohol intake. Among women who did not consume alcohol, the risk of breast cancer was not increased by current use of postmenopausal estrogen.

By virtue of the large numbers in the Nurses' Health Study and the careful analyses by the investigators, reports from this study must be given great credibility. The 12-year follow-up report is disturbing because of its finding of an increased risk in current users. Because estrogen users may be examined more frequently, detection bias is a major concern. The investigators analyzed various factors that might be affected by detection bias (e.g., tumor size, lymph node metastasis at diagnosis), and they found no difference between current users and "never-users." It is noteworthy, however, that a higher percentage of current users had a mammogram during the previous 2 years, and that current users had a lower odds ratio for death (.75) compared with never-users. The investigators argue that if the association between breast cancer and current use of estrogen were the result of increased detection, past users would show evidence of protection. Overall, they believe that increased surveillance for breast cancer among current users of estrogen cannot, by itself, explain the apparent increased relative risk. They suggest that the lack of association between duration of estrogen use and increased risk of breast cancer among past users suggests that estrogen therapy may promote or accelerate development of breast cancer that was present during the early years of use. However, the finding of an increased relative risk in current users is not definitive and is not free of all confounding variables. Both the reduced odds ratio for death from breast cancer in current users and the absence of a statistically significant increased overall risk of fatal breast cancer among current users in the total cohort support the possibility of surveillance and detection bias. The size of the statistical risk is not outside the range of influence by this bias.

A case-control study from Australia, which attempted to control for secular trends in estrogen use, type of menopause, and duration of estrogen use, concluded that there was no evidence for an association between estrogen use and the risk of breast cancer in postmenopausal women (91).

There is a very helpful study that specifically addressed the relationship between the use of estrogen and benign breast disease (92). This study is impressive in that it is based on 10,366 consecutive breast biopsy specimens, with follow-up information on 4,227 biopsy specimens in 3,303 women (mean follow-up, 17 years). Analysis indicated that the use of estrogen was associated with a reduced risk of breast cancer developing. Most importantly, in patients with atypical hyperplasia on their biopsies specimens, the use of estrogen reduced the risk of breast cancer. Although the protective effect may indicate surveillance bias, this is certainly strong evidence that estrogen use does not increase the risk of breast cancer in women with surgically proven benign breast disease.

In September 1991, the Royal Society of Medicine sponsored a conference on postmenopausal hormone therapy and breast cancer risk in London. Several case-control studies were updated, and preliminary data were reported from 5 new studies. Not a single report from the London meeting indicated an increased risk of breast cancer associated with unopposed estrogen of sufficient magnitude to be free of potential biases and/or a confidence interval tight enough to be statistically significant (93–97). Furthermore, these reports failed to support the conclusion of the Nurses' Health Study indicating that current users are associated with an increased risk.

Meta-analysis is an increasingly popular statistical method in which many studies are combined and rigorously analyzed. Simply put, the purpose of a meta-analysis is to gain the statistical power lacking in individual studies. An Australian meta-analysis of 23 studies of estrogen use and breast cancer concluded "unequivocally" that estrogen use did not alter the risk of breast cancer (98).

In the meta-analysis by Dupont and Page (Nashville, Tennessee), the authors concluded that "considerable and consistent" evidence exists that a daily dose of .625 mg of conjugated estrogens, taken for several years, does not appreciably increase the risk of breast cancer (99). They found no evidence of an association between the duration of treatment and the risk of breast cancer at this dosage. On the other hand, the bulk of the data suggests that a daily dose of at least 1.25 mg of conjugated estrogens may increase the risk of breast cancer. This analysis failed to reveal an increased risk in patients with a history of benign breast disease.

A third meta-analysis is from the Centers for Disease Control (CDC) (100). This meta-analysis was conducted using what the authors called a "dose-response curve" for duration of use. The curve for each study analyzed was calculated by plotting breast cancer risk against duration of estrogen use. The combined dose-response slope represented the average change in risk associated with estrogen use over time. The analysis concluded that duration of estrogen use was associated with an increased risk of breast cancer, regardless of whether menopause was natural or surgical. No increase in risk was noted in the first 5 years of use, but the risk was increased by 30% after 15 years of use. The effect was present irrespective of other risk factors, such as family history, parity, or history of benign breast disease. The effect of estrogen therapy on risk of breast cancer was enhanced in women with a positive family history of breast cancer.

The latest meta-analysis, which is from Spain, concludes that estrogen therapy is associated with a very small, but statistically significant, increased relative risk of breast cancer, and that the increased risk is higher among current users (101). Confining their analysis to a dose of .625 mg of conjugated estrogens, the Spanish epidemiologists could not detect a statistically significant increased risk. Indeed, this meta-analysis concludes that an estrogen dose of .625 mg of conjugated estrogens is safe.

In contrast to the CDC report, the other meta-analyses did not find an increased risk of breast cancer with increasing duration of estrogen use. The conclusion of the CDC meta-analysis may reflect the impact of high doses of estrogen. The other 3 meta-analyses indicated an increased risk with a daily dose of conjugated estrogens greater than .625 mg (or its equivalent). The Nashville and CDC analyses did not find an enhanced risk in women with a history of benign breast disease. In contrast to the CDC report, the Australian study found no link between positive family history and estrogen use. The Nashville investigators did not consider family history.

The conclusions of the CDC meta-analysis are heavily influenced by a European study that had limited statistical meaning, as well as by other studies in which high doses of estrogen were administered. In addition, this meta-analysis contains a strong element of author-induced selection bias of studies favoring increased risk. Cohort and case-control studies with a decreased relative risk were excluded. The results of a meta-analysis should not be accepted in a sacrosanct fashion. A meta-analysis can have the same problems encountered by individual epidemiological studies. Selection bias is a major confounding variable.

Where does that leave clinicians and patients? My impression is that the positive conclusions are strongly influenced by statistical limitations or by dose. The largest case-control study (from the CDC) and the largest cohort follow-up study (the Nurses' Health Study) failed to find a link between breast cancer and duration of use of estrogen for up to 20 years. If estrogen use were associated with an increased risk of breast cancer, wouldn't you expect to see an impact on mortality? In the Leisure World follow-up study in California, the risk of breast cancer mortality was .81 (102). This lower relative risk is probably influenced by an element of surveillance bias, but there certainly is no evidence that women using estrogen for a long time are dying of breast cancer at a greater rate.

Doses of estrogen known to protect against osteoporosis and cardiovascular disease (.625 mg of conjugated estrogens and 1 mg of estradiol) are not known to be associated with any clear-cut increased risk of breast cancer. There is reason to be concerned over the use of higher doses. Patients who use higher doses of oral estrogen or who receive estrogen by injection or in pellet form might be at greater risk. For patients who are receiving estrogen by methods other than the standard oral route, monitoring blood estradiol levels is a useful precaution. The blood estradiol level should be in the range of 40–100 pg/mL; levels within this range are known to be associated with the benefits of estrogen. Estrogen dosage cannot be titered by follicle-stimulating hormone levels. Follicle-stimulating hormone (FSH) is regulated by both estrogen and peptides from the ovarian follicle. When the follicles are gone, the peptide influence is lost, and the usual postmenopausal dose of estrogen cannot suppress FSH to reproductive age levels.

Only 2 reports have claimed that the addition of a progestational agent protects against breast cancer; the first, although it is the only randomized, placebo-controlled trial, was hampered by small numbers, and the second was limited by bias in treatment selection (49,103). The report from Uppsala, Sweden, is the first to *suggest* that the estrogen-progesterone combination has an unfavorable impact on the risk of breast cancer, however, this conclusion has little statistical power (104). The Nurses' Health Study found no evidence for protection against breast cancer by the combined use of estrogen and progesterone, and the increased relative risk (1.54) in current users was associated with a wide, nonsignificant confidence interval (.99–2.39) (90).

There are several arguments indicating that exposure to progestational agents may protect against breast cancer. The risk of breast cancer is increased in women who have an earlier menarche and in women who have a later menopause. Both situations are associated with periods of anovulation, exposure to unopposed estrogen. During the reproductive years, anovulation has been demonstrated to be associated with an increased relative risk of breast cancer. According to data from Minnesota, 2% of all women 11–40 years of age are anovulatory, and they have a threefold to fourfold increased risk of postmenopausal breast cancer (105). Former users of birth control pills in whom breast cancer develops have a better overall survival rate. There also is evidence that progestins inhibit the multiplication of human breast cancer cells in vitro.

The argument that adding progesterone might actually be risky is based on the observation that mitosis in the breast reaches a peak level during the luteal phase (106). It is by no means certain that this cyclic and physiological event portrays the performance of the breast under the pharmacological influence of an estrogen-progesterone program.

Conclusions in this area cannot be accepted as definitive; nevertheless, there is some logic to the contention that progestational exposure may protect against breast cancer. Only future epidemiological studies will reveal the facts. Until then, the clinician must make a medical judgment on this issue, and that judgment will influence the position the clinician takes on this question.

Will sequential estrogen-progesterone have a different impact on the breast than the daily exposure to combined estrogen-progesterone? Perhaps, in keeping with the hypothesis stated by Key and Pike (106), cyclic estrogen and progesterone as seen in the normal menstrual cycle are more stressful for breast tissue. A daily exposure to a relatively stable environment may prove to be beneficial. Only time will tell.

How to Treat the Perimenopausal Woman?

Not all climacteric women have symptoms or signs of estrogen deprivation. Some actually manifest estrogen excess via the presence of uterine bleeding (dysfunctional uterine bleeding). Although the greatest concern provoked by this symptom is endometrial neoplasia, the usual finding is non-neoplastic tissue displaying estrogen effects unopposed by progesterone. This results from anovulation in premenopausal women and from extragonadal endogenous estrogen production or estrogen administration in postmenopausal women.

In all women, whether premenopausal or postmenopausal, whether receiving or not receiving hormone therapy, specific organic causes (neoplasia, complications of unexpected pregnancy, or bleeding from extrauterine sites) must be ruled out. In addition to careful history and physical examination, dysfunctional uterine bleeding should be evaluated by aspiration endometrial biopsy. If the uterus is found to be normal by pelvic examination, for reasons of both accuracy and cost-effectiveness, the method of biopsy should be an office aspiration curettage—*not* the traditional, more costly and risky, in-hospital dilatation and curettage (D & C).

Fewer than 10% of menopausal women cannot be adequately evaluated by office biopsy. Most commonly, the reason is an inability to enter the uterine cavity. In such instances, an in-hospital D & C is in order.

Furthermore, if the uterus is not normal on pelvic examination, the office endometrial biopsy must yield to an in-hospital D & C to achieve accuracy of diagnosis.

If the vulva, vagina, and cervix appear normal on inspection, perimenopausal bleeding can be assumed to be intrauterine in origin. Confirmation requires the absence of abnormal cytology on the Pap smear. The principal symptom of endometrial cancer is abnormal vaginal bleeding, but carcinoma will be encountered in only approximately 2% of endometrial biopsies specimens (107). Normal endometrium is found more than half the time, polyps approximately 3% of the time, and endometrial hyperplasia almost 15% of the time.

In the absence of organic disease, appropriate management depends on the age of the woman and the endometrial tissue findings. In the perimenopausal woman who has dysfunctional uterine bleeding associated with proliferative or hyperplastic endometrium (uncomplicated by atypia or dysplastic constituents), periodic oral progestin therapy, e.g., 10 mg of medroxyprogesterone acetate given daily the first 10 days of each month, is mandatory. If hyperplasia is present, follow-up aspiration curettage after 3–4 months is required, and if periodic progesterone is ineffective and histological regression is not observed, then more intensive progesterone treatment (in dose and duration) is indicated.

When monthly progesterone therapy reverses hyperplastic changes (which it does in 95%–98% of cases) and controls irregular bleeding, treatment should be continued until withdrawal bleeding ceases. This is a reliable sign (in effect, a bioassay), which indicates the onset of estrogen deprivation and the need for the addition of estrogen. If vasomotor disturbances begin before the cessation of menstrual bleeding, then the combined estrogen-progesterone program can be initiated, as needed, to control the flushes.

If contraception is required, the clinician and healthy, nonsmoking patient should seriously consider the use of oral contraception. The anovulatory woman cannot be guaranteed the spontaneous ovulation and pregnancy will not occur. At the same time, the use of a low-dose oral contraceptive will provide contraception and prophylaxis against irregular, heavy anovulatory bleeding and the risk of endometrial hyperplasia and neoplasia.

Clinicians have been made so wary of providing oral contraceptives to older women that a traditional hormone regimen is often used to treat a woman with the kind of irregular cycles usually experienced in the perimenopausal years. This addition of exogenous estrogen when a woman is not amenorrheic or experiencing menopausal symptoms is inappropriate—even risky—because it exposes the endometrium to excessively high levels of estrogen. The appropriate response is to regulate anovulatory cycles with monthly progestational treatment or to use low-dose oral contraception.

Knowing when to change from oral contraception to postmenopausal hormone therapy is a common clinical dilemma. It is important to change therapy because, even with the lowest estrogen dose oral contraceptive available, the estrogen dose is fourfold greater than the standard postmenopausal dose, and with increasing age, the dose-related risks associated with estrogen become significant. One approach to establish the onset of the postmenopausal years is to measure the FSH level, beginning at 50 years of age, on an annual basis, being careful to obtain the blood sample on day 6 or 7 of the pill-free week (when steroid levels have decreased sufficiently to allow the FSH level to increase. When the FSH level is greater than 30 mIU/mL, it is time to change to a postmenopausal hormone program.

Are Hot Flushes Always Caused By Estrogen Deficiency?

The physiology of the postmenopausal hot flush is still not understood, but it apparently originates in the hypothalamus and is brought about by a decrease in estrogen. However, not all hot flushes are the result of estrogen deficiency. In a massive review of hot flushes, exact estimates on prevalence were hampered by inconsistencies and differences in methodologies, cultures, and definitions (108). In the longitudinal follow-up of a large number of American women, 10% of the women experienced hot flushes before menopause, whereas in other studies, as many as 25% of premenopausal women report hot flushes (108, 110). Unfortunately, the hot flush is a relatively common psychosomatic symptom, and women often are unnecessarily treated with estrogen. When the clinical situation is not clear and obvious, menopause as the cause of hot flushes should be documented by increased levels of FSH. In my opinion, hot flushes in the presence of normal levels of FSH are not the result of estrogen deficiency; therefore, estrogen treatment is not indicated.

What Is Normal About Menopause?

The symptoms and implications of menopause can often result in a decreased sense of well-being. The menopausal syndrome refers to a group of additional symptoms, including fatigue, anxiety, headaches, depression, palpitations, insomnia, myalgias, and irritability. There is controversy, however, as to which of these symptoms are directly related to estrogen. Cross-sectional data and 1 short-term, double-blind, randomized study indicated that estrogen improved or prevented depressive symptoms (111, 112). A prospective, double-blind crossover study suggested that, whereas many symptoms demonstrated improvement with estrogen therapy, these findings could be ascribed secondarily to relief of hot flushes (113). Estrogen therapy certainly improves the quality of sleep, decreases the time to onset of sleep, and increases rapid eye movement sleep time (114). Perhaps the improvement in sleep patterns diminishes symptoms that may have been considered problems of menopause before therapy. There is good reason to believe that, apart from an inefficiency of behavior caused by hot flush-induced sleep disturbances, psychological problems are the result of psychosocial and situational issues.

The belief that behavioral disturbances are related to manifestations of the female reproductive system, although an ancient one, has persisted to contemporary times. This belief is not totally illogical; there is reason to assume that, for many, the middle years of life are largely filled with negative experiences. The events that come to mind are impressive: onset of a major illness or disability (and even death) in a spouse, relative, or friend; retirement from employment; financial insecurity; the need to provide care for very old parents and relatives; and separation from children. It is not surprising that a middle age event, menopause, may share in this negative outlook.

On the other hand, menopause should and *can* mark the beginning of a positive and promising period of life, one that is relatively free from previous obligations and which may involve for new career choices, more education, and new ventures. The concerned clinician should support menopausal patients in a positive outlook and, with scientific justification, should avoid the promotion of outdated, negative notions.

The scientific study of all aspects of menstruation has been hampered by the overpowering influence of social and cultural beliefs and traditions. Problems arising from life circumstances often have been erroneously attributed to menopause. However, data (especially more reliable longitudinal data) now indicate that the increase in most symptoms and problems in middle-aged women reflects social and personal circumstances, not the endocrine events of menopause (115, 116). The view that menopause has a deleterious effect on mental health is not supported in the psychiatric literature, nor is it supported in surveys of the general population (117). The concept of a specific psychiatric disorder (involutional melancholia) has been abandoned. Indeed, depression is *less* common, not more common, among middle-aged women (118–121). A negative view of mental health at the time of menopause is not justified; many of the problems reported at menopause are caused by the vicissitudes of life.

The Massachusetts Women's Health Study, the largest and most comprehensive prospective, longitudinal study of middle-aged women, provides a powerful argument that menopause is not and should not be viewed as a negative experience by the vast majority of women (109, 120). The cessation of menses was perceived by these women to have almost no impact on subsequent physical and mental health. This is reflected by women expressing either positive or neutral feelings about menopause. An exception is the group of women who experienced surgical menopause; however, there is good reason to believe that the reasons for the surgical procedure are most important than the cessation of menses.

It can be further argued that physicians have had a biased (negative) point of view, because the majority of women, being healthy and happy, do not seek contact physicians. It is important, therefore, that clinicians not ony are familiar with the facts relative to menopause, but also have an appropriate attitude and philosophy regarding this period of life. Medical intervention at menopause should be regarded as an opportunity to provide and reinforce a program of preventive health care. The issues of preventive health care for women are familiar ones. They include family planning, cessation of smoking, control of body weight and alcohol consumption, prevention of heart disease and osteoporosis, maintenance of mental well-being (including sexuality), cancer screening, and treatment of urological problems.

I believe that menopausal women do not suffer from a disease (specifically, a hormone deficiency disease). Postmenopausal hormone therapy should be viewed as a specific treatment for symptoms in the short term and as preventive pharmacology in the long term. It is time to stress the normalcy of this life event. It also is important to educate women and clinicians about the normal events of this time period. Changes in menstrual function are not symbols of some ominous "change." There are good physiological reasons for changing menstrual function, and understanding the physiology will do much to reinforce a healthy, normal attitude.

References

1. Lindsay R, Hart DM, Clark DM: The minimum effective dose of estrogen for postmenopausal bone loss. *Obstet Gynecol* 63:759, 1984.
2. Ettinger B, Gerrant HK, Cann CE: Postmenopausal bone loss is prevented by treatment with low-dosage estrogen with calcium. *Ann Intern Med* 106:40, 1987.
3. Stevenson JC, Cust MP, Gangar KF, et al: Effects of transdermal versus oral hormone replacement therapy on bone density in spine and proximal femur in postmenopausal women. *Lancet* 336:1327, 1990.
4. Cust MP, Gangar KF, Crri D, et al: Lipid effect of oral versus transdermal oestrogen/progestogen regimens in postmenopausal women. Annual Meeting of the American Fertility Society, 1989, Abstract P-065.
5. Pasetto N, Piccione E, Pasetto, et al: Treatment of patients at risk. Cross-over study between natural estrogens, in Passetto N (ed): *The Menopause and Postmenopause.* Lancaster, England, MTP Press, 1980, pp 141–151.
6. Colvin PL Jr, Auerbach BJ, Koritnik DR, et al: Differential effects of oral estrogen versus 17B-estradiol on lipoproteins in postmenopausal women. *J Clin Endocrinol Metab* 70:1568, 1990.
7. Wolfe BM, Huff MW: Effects of combined estrogen and progestin administration on plasma lipoprotein metabolism in postmenopausal women. *J Clin Invest* 83:40, 1989.
8. Christiansen C, Riis BJ: Five years with continuous combined oestrogen/progestogen therapy. Effects on calcium metabolism, lipoproteins, and bleeding pattern. *Br J Obstet Gynaecol* 97:1087, 1990.
9. Williams SR, Frenchek B, Speroff T, et al: A study of combined continuous ethinyl estradiol and norethindrone acetate for postmenopausal hormone replacement. *Am J Obstet Gynecol* 162:438, 1990.
10. Weinstein L, Bewtra C, Gallagher JC: Evaluation of a continuous combined

low-dose regimen of estrogen-progestin for treatment of the menopausal patient. *Am J Obstet Gynecol* 162:1534, 1990.
11. Cano A, Fernandes H, Serrano S, et al: Effect of continuous oestradiol-medroxyprogesterone administration on plasma lipids and lipoproteins. *Maturitas* 13:35, 1991.
12. Gibbons WE, Judd HL, Luciano AA, et al: Comparison of sequential versus continuous estrogen/progestin replacement therapy on serum lipid patterns. Annual Meeting of the Society for Gynecological Investigation, 1991, Abstract 491.
13. Mattsson L, Cullberg G, Samsioe G: A continuous estrogen-progestogen regimen for climacteric complaints. *Acta Obstet Gynecol Scand* 63:673, 1984.
14. Magos AL, Brincat M, Studd JWW, et al: Amenorrhea and endometrial atrophy with continuous oral estrogen and progestogen therapy in postmenopausal women. *Obstet Gynecol* 65:496, 1985.
15. Ravnikar VA: Compliance with hormonal therapy. *Am J Obstet Gynecol* 156:1332, 1987.
16. Kannel WB: Metabolic risk factors for coronary heart disease in women: Perspective from the Framingham Study. *Am Heart J* 114:413, 1987.
17. Campos H, McNamara JR, Wilson PW, et al: Differences in low density lipoprotein subfractions and apolipoproteins in premenopausal and postmenopausal women. *J Clin Endocrinol Metab* 67:30, 1988.
18. Matthews KA, Meilahn E, Kuller LH, et al: Menopause and risk factors for coronary heart disease. *N Engl J Med* 321:641, 1989.
19. Jacobs DR Jr, Mebane IL, Bangdiwala SI, et al: High density lipoprotein cholesterol as a predictor of cardiovascular disease mortality in men and women: The follow-up study of the Lipid Research Clinics Prevalence Study. *Am J Epidemiol* 131:32, 1990.
20. Wilson PW, Garrison RJ, Castelli WP, et al: Prevalence of coronary heart disease in the Framingham offspring study: Role of lipoprotein cholesterols. *Am J Cardiol* 46:649, 1980.
21. Walsh BW, Schiff I, Rosner B, et al: Effects of postmenopausal estrogen replacement on the concentrations and metabolism of plasma lipoproteins. *N Engl J Med* 325:1196, 1991.
22. Ingegno MD, Money SR, Thelmo W, et al: Progesterone receptors in the human heart and great vessels. *Lab Invest* 59:353, 1988.
23. Mant D, Villard Mackintosh L, Vessey MP, et al: Myocardial infarction and angina pectoris in young women. *J Epidemiol Comm Health* 41:215, 1987.
24. Rosenberg L, Armstrong B, Jick H: Myocardial infarction and estrogen therapy in postmenopausal women. *N Engl J Med* 294:1256, 1976.
25. Pfeffer RI, Whipple GH, Kurosake TT, et al: Coronary risk and estrogen use in postmenopausal women. *Am J Epidemiol* 107:479, 1978.
26. Jick H, Dinan B, Rothman KJ: Noncontraceptive estrogens and non-fatal myocardial infarction. *JAMA* 239:1407, 1978.
27. Rosenberg L, Sloane D, Shapiro S, et al: Noncontraceptive estrogens and myocardial infarction in young women. *JAMA* 224:339, 1980.
28. Ross RK, Paganini-Hill A, Mack TM, et al: Menopausal oestrogen therapy and protection from death from ischaemic heart disease. *Lancet* i:585, 1981.
29. Bain C, Willett W, Hennekens CH, et al: Use of postmenopausal hormones and risk of myocardial infarction. *Circulation* 64:42, 1981.
30. Adam S, Williams V, Vessey MP: Cardiovascular disease and hormone replacement treatment: A pilot case-control study. *BMJ* 282:1277, 1981.
31. Szklo M, Tonascia J, Gordis L, et al: Estrogen use and myocardial infarction risk: A case-control study. *Prevent Med* 13:510, 1984.
32. Sullivan JM, Vander Zwagg R, Lemp GF, et al: Postmenopausal estrogen use and coronary atherosclerosis. *Ann Intern Med* 108:358, 1988.
33. Gruchow HW, Anderson AJ, Barboriak JJ, et al: Postmenopausal use of estrogen and occlusion of coronary arteries. *Am Heart J* 115:954, 1988.
34. McFarland KF, Boniface ME, Hornung CA, et al: Risk factors and noncon-

traceptive estrogen use in women with and without coronary disease. *Am Heart J* 117:1209, 1989.

35. Beard CM, Kottke TE, Annegers JF, et al: The Rochester Coronary Heart Disease Project: Effect of cigarette smoking, hypertension, diabetes, and steroidal estrogen use on coronary heart disease among 40- to 59-year-old women, 1960 through 1982. *Mayo Clin Proc* 64:1471, 1989.
36. Burch JC, Byrd BF, Vaughn WK: The effects of long-term estrogen on hysterectomized women. *Am J Obstet Gynecol* 118:778, 1974.
37. Gordon T, Kannel WB, Hjortland MC, et al: Menopause and coronary heart disease: The Framingham Study. *Ann Intern Med* 89:157, 1978.
38. Hammond CB, Jelovsek FR, Lee KL, et al: Effects of long-term estrogen replacement therapy: I. Metabolic effects. *Am J Obstet Gynecol* 133:525, 1979.
39. Petitti DB, Wingerd J, Pellegrin F, et al: Risk of vascular disease in women: Smoking, oral contraceptives, non-contraceptive estrogens, and other factors. *JAMA* 242:1150, 1979.
40. Lafferty FW, Helmuth DO: Postmenopausal estrogen replacement: The prevention of osteoporosis and systemic effects. *Maturitas* 7:147, 1985.
41. Wilson PWF, Garrison RJ, Castelli WP: Postmenopausal estrogen use, cigarette smoking, and cardiovascular morbidity in women over 50. The Framingham Study. *N Engl J Med* 313:1038, 1985.
42. Stampfer MJ, Colditz GA, Willett WC, et al: Postmenopausal estrogen therapy and cardiovascular disease: Ten-year follow-up from the Nurses' Health Study. *N Engl J Med* 325:756, 1991.
43. Bush TL, Barrett-Connor E, Cowan DK, et al: Cardiovascular mortality and noncontraceptive use of estrogen in women: Results from the Lipid Research Clinics Program Follow-up Study. *Circulation* 75:1102, 1987.
44. Criqui MH, Suarez L, Barrett-Connor E, et al: Postmenopausal estrogen use and mortality. *Am J Epidemiol* 128:606, 1988.
45. Henderson BE, Paganini-Hill A, Ross RK: Estrogen replacement therapy and protection from acute myocardial infarction. *Am J Obstet Gynecol* 159:312, 1988.
46. Perlman J, Wolf P, Finucane F, et al: Menopause and the epidemiology of cardiovascular disease in women, in *Menopause: Evaluation, Treatment, and Health Concerns.* Alan R. Liss, Inc, 1989, pp 283–312.
47. Petitti DB, Perlman JA, Sidney S: Noncontraceptive estrogens and mortality: Long-term follow-up of women in the Walnut Creek study. *Obstet Gynecol* 70:289, 1987.
48. Eaker ED, Castelli WP: Coronary heart disease and its risk factors among women in the Framingham Study, in Eaker ED, Packard B, Wenger NG, (eds): *Coronary Heart Disease in Women.* New York, Haymarket Doyma Inc, 1987, pp 122–130.
49. Nachtigal LE, Nachtigall RH, Nachtigall RD, et al: Estrogen replacement therapy: II. A prospective study in the relationship to carcinoma and cardiovascular and metabolic problems. *Obstet Gynecol* 54:74, 1979.
50. Thompson SG, Meade TW, Greenberg G: The use of hormonal replacement therapy and the risk of stroke and myocardial infarction in women. *J Epidemiol Comm Health* 43:173, 1989.
51. Paganini-Hill A, Ross RK, Henderson BE: Postmenopausal oestrogen treatment and stroke: a prospective study. *BMJ* 297:519, 1988.
52. Lind T, Cameron EC, Hunter WM, et al: A prospective, controlled trial of six forms of hormone replacement therapy given to postmenopausal women. *Br J Obstet Gynaecol* (Suppl 3) 86:1, 1979.
53. Pfeffer RI, Kurosaki TT, Charlton SK: Estrogen use and blood pressure in later life. *Am J Epidemiol* 110:469, 1979.
54. Lutola H: Blood pressure and hemodynamics in postmenopausal women during estradiol-178 substitution. *Ann Clin Res* 15 (Suppl 38):9, 1983.
55. Wren BG, Routledge AD: The effect of type and dose of oestrogen on the blood pressure of postmenopausal women. *Maturitas* 5:135, 1983.

56. Hassager C, Christiansen C: Blood pressure during oestrogen/progestogen substitution therapy in healthy post-menopausal women. *Maturitas* 9:315, 1988.
57. Devor M, Barrett-Connor E, Renvall M, et al: Estrogen replacement therapy and the risk of venous thrombosis. *Am J Med* 92:275, 1992.
58. Sullivan JM, Vander Zwagg R, Hughes JP, et al: Estrogen replacement and coronary artery disease: Effect on survival in postmenopausal women. *Arch Intern Med* 150:2557, 1990.
59. Adams MP, Kaplan JR, Manuck SB, et al: Inhibition of coronary artery atherosclerosis by 17-beta estradiol in ovariectomized monkeys. Lack of an effect of added progesterone. *Arteriosclerosis* 10:1051, 1990.
60. Wagner JD, Clarkson TB, St Clair RW, et al: Estrogen and progesterone replacement therapy reduces low density lipoprotein accumulation in the coronary arteries of surgically postmenopausal cynomolgus monkeys. *J Clin Invest* 88:1955, 1991.
61. Hassager C, Riis BJ, Christiansen C: Relation of body fat distribution to serum lipids and lipoproteins in elderly women. *Atherosclerosis* 80:57, 1989.
62. Hirvonen E, Malkonen M, Manninen V: Effects of different progestogens on lipoproteins during postmenopausal therapy. *N Engl J Med* 304:560, 1981.
63. Mattsson L, Cullberg LG, Samsioe G: Influence of esterified estrogens and medroxyprogesterone on lipid metabolism and sex steroids. A study in oophorectomized women. *Hormone Metab Res* 14:602, 1982.
64. Silferstolpe G, Gustafsson A, Samsioe G, et al: Lipid metabolic studies in oophorectomized women: Effects on serum lipids and lipoproteins of three synthetic progestogens. *Maturitas* 4:103, 1983.
65. Ylostalo P, Kauppila A, Kivinen S, et al: Endocrine and metabolic effects of low-dose estrogen-progestin treatment in climacteric women. *Obstet Gynecol* 62:682, 1983.
66. Ottosson UB, Carlstrom K, Damber JE, et al: Serum levels of progesterone and some of its metabolites including deoxycorticosterone after oral and parenteral administration. *Br J Obstet Gynecol* 91:1111, 1984.
67. Wren B, Garrett D: The effect of low-dose piperazine oestrogen sulphate and low-dose levonorgestrel on blood lipid levels in postmenopausal women. *Maturitas* 7:141, 1985.
68. Ottosson UB, Johansson BG, von Schoultz B: Subfractions of high-density lipoprotein cholesterol during estrogen replacement therapy: A comparison between progestogens and natural progesterone. *Am J Obstet Gynecol* 151:746, 1985.
69. Barrett-Connor E, Wingard DL, Criqui MH: Postmenopausal estrogen use and heart disease risk factors in the 1980s. *JAMA* 261:2095, 1989.
70. Sherwin BB, Gelfand MM: A prospective one-year study of estrogen and progestin in postmenopausal women: Effects on clinical symptoms and lipoprotein lipids. *Obstet Gynecol* 73:759, 1989.
71. Persson I, Falkeborn M, Lithell H, et al: HRT and cardiovascular disease, with special emphasis on combined therapy. XIII World Congress of Gynaecology and Obstetrics (FIGO), Singapore, 1991, Abstract 0710.
72. de Ziegler D, Bessis R, Frydman R: Vascular resistance of uterine arteries: Physiological effects of estradiol and progesterone. *Fertil Steril* 55:775, 1991.
73. Creasman WT: Estrogen replacement therapy: Is previously treated cancer a contraindication? *Obstet Gynecol* 77:308, 1991.
74. Lee RB, Burke TW, Park RC: Estrogen replacement therapy following treatment for stage 1 endometrial carcinoma. *Gynecol Oncol* 36:189, 1990.
75. Heaps JM, Nieberg RK, Berek JS: Malignant neoplasms arising in endometriosis. *Obstet Gynecol* 75:1023, 1990.
76. Meldrum DR, Davidson BJ, Tataryn IV, et al: Changes in circulating steroids with aging in postmenopausal women. *Obstet Gynecol* 57:624, 1981.
77. Sherwin BB, Gelfand MM: The role of androgen in the maintenance of sexual functioning in oophorectomized women. *Psychosom Med* 49:397, 1987.

78. Sherwin BB: Affective changes with estrogen and androgen replacement therapy in surgically menopausal women. *J Affective Disord* 14:177, 1988.
79. Myers LS, Dixen J, Morrissette D, et al: Effects of estrogen, androgen, and progestin on sexual psychophysiology and behavior in postmenopausal women. *J Clin Endocrinol Metab* 70:1124, 1990.
80. Hickok LR, Toomey C, Speroff L: A comparison of esterified estrogens with and without methyltestosterone: Effects on endometrial histology and serum lipoproteins in postmenopausal women. In press.
81. Urman B, Pride SM, Ho Yuen B: Elevated serum testosterone, hirsutism, and virilism associated with combined androgen-estrogen hormone replacement therapy. *Obstet Gynecol* 77:595, 1991.
82. Riis B, Thomsen K, Christiansen C: Does calcium supplementation prevent postmenopausal bone loss? *N Engl J Med* 316:173, 1987.
83. MacIntyre I, Stevenson JC, Whitehead MI, et al: Calcitonin for prevention of postmenopausal bone loss. *Lancet* i:900, 1988.
84. Reginster JY, Denis D, Albart A, et al: One year controlled randomized trial of prevention of early postmenopausal bone loss by intranasal calcitonin. *Lancet* ii:1481, 1987.
85. Store T, Thamsborg G, Steiniche T, et al: Effect of intermittent cyclical etidronate therapy on bone mass and fracture rate in women with postmenopausal osteoporosis. *New Engl J Med* 322:1265, 1990.
86. Chow RK, Harrison JE, Brown CF, et al: Physical fitness effect on bone mass in postmenopausal women. *Arch Phys Med Rehabil* 67:231, 1986.
87. Quigley MET, Martin PL, Burnier AM, et al: Estrogen therapy arrests bone loss in elderly women. *Am J Obstet Gynecol* 156:1516, 1987.
88. Kiel DP, Felson DT, Anderson JJ, et al: Hip fracture and the use of estrogens in postmenopausal women: The Framingham Study. N Engl J Med 317:1169, 1987.
89. Wingo PA, Layde PM, Lee NC, et al: The risk of breast cancer in postmenopausal women who have used estrogen replacement therapy. *JAMA* 257:209, 1987.
90. Colditz GA, Stampfer MJ, Willett WC, et al: Type of postmenopausal hormone use and risk of breast cancer: 12-year follow-up from the Nurses' Health Study. In press.
91. Rohan TE, McMichael AJ: Non-contraceptive exogenous oestrogen therapy and breast cancer. *Med J Aust* 1988;148:217, 1988.
92. Dupont WD, Page DL, Rogers LW, et al: Influence of exogenous estrogens, proliferative breast disease, and other variables on breast cancer risk. *Cancer* 1989;63:948, 1989.
93. La Vecchia C: Non-contraceptive oestrogens and breast cancer: Update of an Italian case-control study. The Royal Society of Medicine, London, September 24–26, 1991.
94. Kaufman DW, Palmer JR, de Mouzon J, et al: Oestrogen replacement therapy and breast cancer: New results from the Slone Epidemiology Unit's Case Control Surveillance Study. *Am J Epidemiol* 134:1375, 1991.
95. Rohan T: Hormone replacement therapy and risk of breast cancer: A population-based case-control study in Australia. The Royal Society of Medicine, London, September 24–26, 1991.
96. Palmer JR, Rosenberg L, Clarke EA, et al: Oestrogen replacement therapy and breast cancer: Results from the Slone Epidemiology Unit's Toronto Breast Cancer Study. *Am J Epidemiol* 134:1386, 1991.
97. Ross RK, Bernstein L: Why can't we prove that HRT causes breast cancer? Methodologic and biologic challenges. The Royal Society of Medicine, London, September 24-26, 1991.
98. Armstrong BK: Oestrogen therapy after the menopause — boon or bane? *Med J Aust* 148:213, 1988.
99. Dupont WD, Page DL: Menopausal estrogen replacement therapy and breast cancer. *Arch Intern Med* 151:67, 1991.

100. Steinberg KK, Thacker SB, Smith SJ, et al: A meta-analysis of the effect of estrogen replacement therapy on the risk of breast cancer. *JAMA* 265:1985, 1991.
101. Sillero-Arenas M, Delgado-Rodriguez M, Rodriguez-Canteras R, et al: Menopausal hormone replacement therapy and breast cancer: A meta-analysis. *Obstet Gynecol* 79:286, 1992.
102. Henderson BE, Paganini-Hill A, Ross RK: Decreased mortality in users of estrogen replacement therapy. *Arch Intern Med* 151:75, 1991.
103. Gambrell RD Jr, Maier RC, Sanders BI: Decreased incidence of breast cancer in postmenopausal estrogen-progestogen users. *Obstet Gynecol* 62:435, 1983.
104. Bergkvist L, Adami H-O, Persson I, et al: The risk of breast cancer after estrogen and estrogen-progestin replacement. *New Engl J Med* 321:293, 1989
105. Coulam CB, Annegers JF: Chronic anovulation may increase post-menopausal breast cancer risk. *JAMA* 249:445, 1983.
106. Key TJA, Pike MC: The role of oestrogens and progestogens in the epidemiology and prevention of breast cancer. *Eur J Cancer Clin Oncol* 24:29, 1988.
107. Einerth Y: Vacuum curettage by the Vabra method. A simple procedure for endometrial diagnosis. *Acta Obstet Gynecol Scand* 61:373, 1982.
108. Kronnenberg F: Hot flashes: Epidemiology and physiology. *Ann NY Acad Sci* 592:52–133, 1990.
109. McKinlay SM, Brambilla DJ, Posner JG: The normal menopause transition. *Maturitas* 14:102–115, 1992.
110. Hunter M: The South-East England longitudinal study of the climacteric and postmenopause. *Maturitas* 14:117–126, 1992.
111. Palinkas LA, Barrett-Connor E: Estrogen use and depressive symptoms in postmenopausal women. *Obstet Gynecol* 80:30, 1992.
112. Ditkoff EC, Crary WG, Cristo M, et al: Estrogen improves psychological function in asymptomatic postmenopausal women. *Obstet Gynecol* 78:991, 1991.
113. Campbell S, Whitehead M: Estrogen therapy and the menopausal syndrome. *Clin Obstet Gynecol* 4:31, 1977.
114. Schiff I, Regestein Q, Tulchinsky D, et al: Effects of estrogens on sleep and psychological state of hypogonadal women. *JAMA* 2442:2405, 1979.
115. Matthews KA, Wing RR, Kuller LH, et al: Influences of natural menopause on psychological characteristics and symptoms of middle-aged healthy women. *J Consult Clin Psych* 58:345–351, 1990.
116. Koster A: Change-of-life anticipations, attitudes, and experiences among middle-aged Danish women. *Health Care Women Internatl* 12:1–13, 1991.
117. Ballinger CB: Psychiatric aspects of the menopause. *Br J Psych* 156:773–781, 1990.
118. Hallstrom T, Samuelsson S: Mental health in the climacteric. The longitudinal study of women in Gothenburg. *Acta Obstet Gynecol Scand* 130(suppl):13–18, 1985.
119. Gath D, Osborn M, Bungay G, et al: Psychiatric disorder and gynaecological symptoms in middle aged women: A community survey. *BMJ* 294:213–218, 1987.
120. McKinlay JB, McKinlay SM, Brambila D: The relative contributions of endocrine changes and social circumstances to depression in middle-aged women. *J Health Soc Behav* 28:345, 1987.
121. Kaufert PA, Gilbert P, Hassaret T: Researching the symptoms of menopause; An exercise in methodology. *Maturitas* 10:117–131, 1988.

OBSTETRICS

1 Maternal and Fetal Physiology

Elevated Maternal Plasma Corticotropin-Releasing Hormone Levels in Pregnancies Complicated by Preterm Labor

Warren WB, Patrick SL, Goland RS (Columbia Univ, New York)

Am J Obstet Gynecol 166:1198–1207, 1992 1–1

Background.—Evidence suggests that placental corticotropin-releasing hormone (CRH) is biologically active and stimulates the pituitary-adrenal axis in pregnancy. The increase in maternal plasma CRH levels that

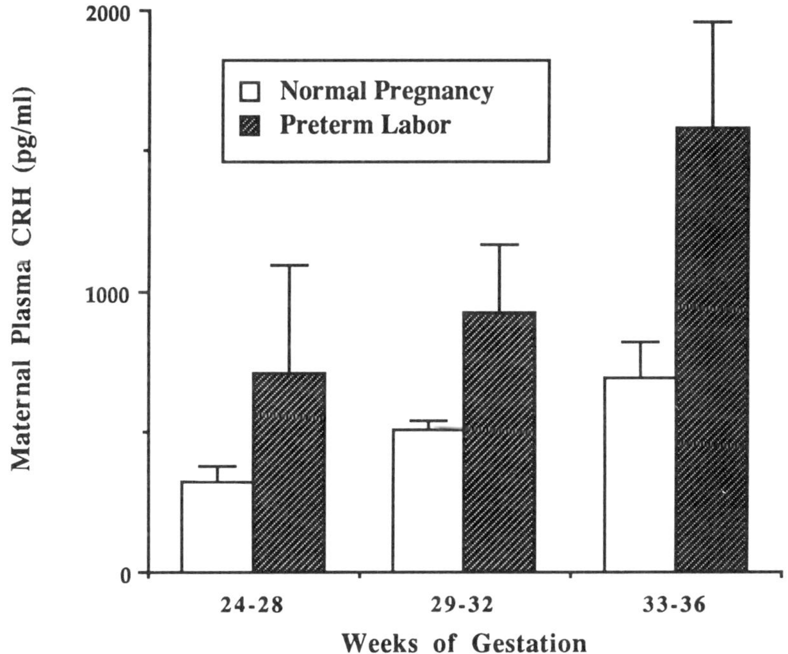

Fig 1–1.—The mean maternal plasma CRH levels (pg/mL) in 2 study groups: women admitted for preterm labor and women with normal pregnancies not in labor in 3 gestational age groups. By 2-way analysis of variance, there was a significant main effect of study group on the mean maternal plasma CRH levels ($F_{5.21}$ [1, 69], $P < .05$), with higher mean maternal plasma CRH levels in women with preterm labor. (Courtesy of Warren WB, Patrick SL, Goland RS: *Am J Obstet Gynecol* 166:1198–1207, 1992.)

precedes normal parturition at term was hypothesized to occur early in pregnancies complicated by preterm labor.

Methods.—Single venous blood samples were obtained from 39 women between 24 and 36 weeks of gestation who were admitted to 1 labor and delivery suite. The samples were obtained before any medications were given in 34 cases. The mean maternal CRH levels were assessed. Levels of corticotropin-releasing hormone in the latent and active phases in term labor also were studied.

Findings.—The maternal CRH levels were higher in pregnancies complicated by preterm labor than in normal pregnancies. This increase occurred before labor was diagnosed clinically. The mean CRH levels were not elevated in cases of preterm labor associated with infection. During labor at term, the mean plasma levels were comparable in the latent and active phases (Fig 1–1).

Conclusion.—Maternal plasma CRH levels are increased in association with preterm labor. This increase does not appear to result from labor itself. It may reflect an early activation of the placenta before preterm labor begins.

▶ The increase in concentration of placental corticotropin-releasing hormone (PCRH) during pregnancy offers some interesting possibilities regarding the onset of labor that make investigation of this sort particularly interesting. Unlike hypothalamic CRH, PCRH is stimulated by glucocorticoids, which are, in turn, produced in larger amounts by the adrenal in response to the releasing hormone, thereby resulting in a positive extrapituitary feedback loop. In addition, PCRH is active in vitro, both in stimulating prostaglandin E_2 and prostaglandin $F_{2\alpha}$ by the placenta and in potentiating the effects of oxytocin on uterine contractions. Therefore, it is possible that the role of PCRH is to remove control of glucocorticoid production from the hypothalamus to the placenta, where, if glucocorticoids and fetal cuing are as important in the human as in other species in initiating labor, the placenta serves as an important initiator.

In the 39 cases of preterm labor reviewed in this study (all but 5 of the 39 maternal blood samples were obtained before magnesium sulfate administration), the results suggest long-term modulation by PCRH in some cases of preterm labor. In such cases, PCRH existed in higher concentrations than were found at specified gestational ages in normal pregnancies, were unaffected by tocolysis, and did not differ in concentration in 9 cases of preterm labor caused by intrauterine infection. Placental corticotropin-releasing hormone, as measured by maternal blood concentrations, did not appear to play a role in the transition from normal latent to active phase labor at term. The small number of cases forms only part of my reservations concerning this study, regardless of how intriguing its results are. If glucocorticoids are important in the onset of human labor, increased hormone receptor binding must be posited because, unlike ungulates, the corticol concentration in maternal blood does not increase with the onset of labor. If this is true, there is no reason to assume that PCRH adrenal receptor density and affinity, which were not measured in this study, might not be equally important in understanding what's happening. Nevertheless, as predicted earlier (see the 1990 YEAR BOOK OF OBSTETRICS AND GYNECOLOGY, pp 4–5) this is proving to be a most interesting investigative direction.—T.H. Kirschbaum, M.D.

Adrenocorticotropin and Cortisol Responses to Vasopressin During Pregnancy

Goland RS, Wardlaw SL, MacCarter G, Warren WB, Stark RI (Columbia Univ, New York)

J Clin Endocrinol Metab 73:257–261, 1991 1–2

Introduction.—During pregnancy, the placentas of humans and nonhuman primates secrete large amounts of corticotropin-releasing hormone (CRH) into the maternal and fetal circulation. A recent study in pregnant baboons reported that exogenous placental CRH blunts the pituitary adrenocorticotropic hormone (ACTH) and cortisol responses. The diminished ACTH and cortisol production was attributed to down-regulation by the pituitary CRH receptors in response to chronic placental CRH production. The role of placental CRH in the regulation of maternal pituitary-adrenal function during primate gestation was further defined.

Methods.—Both the ACTH and cortisol responses to .3-unit and 3-unit vasopressin infusions were measured in chronically catheterized pregnant and nonpregnant female baboons. Thirteen studies were done in 4 pregnant animals, and 8 were done in 6 nonpregnant animals.

Results.—The baseline plasma CRH concentration was unmeasurable in nonpregnant animals, and it was 240 pmol/L in pregnant animals. The plasma levels of CRH did not change in response to vasopressin infusion. Vasopressin at both doses elicited an ACTH response in both pregnant and nonpregnant animals, but the mean peak ACTH response to vasopressin was significantly higher in the pregnant animals than in those that were not pregnant. The ACTH responses to vasopressin increased as pregnancy progressed and then diminished in the postpartum period. Vasopressin at the higher dose also caused cortisol levels to increase significantly in both pregnant and nonpregnant animals. However, the lower dose significantly increased cortisol levels only in pregnant animals.

Conclusion.—In baboons, both ACTH and cortisol responses to exogenous vasopressin are enhanced during gestation, although responses to exogenous CRH are blunted. The chronic placental CRH stimulation of the pituitary-adrenal axis during pregnancy results in an enhanced response to vasopression and a down regulation of the pituitary response to exogenous CRH.

▶ This is a further step in understanding the role of CRH production in the human placenta, using the remarkable chronic catheterized pregnant baboon preparations of Dr. Raymond Stark of Columbia University. Placental CRH (as does the hypothalamic product) acts to stimulate gene expression of the 31 KD protein gene product proopiomelanocortin (POMC) (see the 1990 YEAR BOOK OF OBSTETRICS AND GYNECOLOGY, pp 4–5). By peptide cleavage, this huge molecule yields melanocyte-stimulating hormone, ACTH, and beta lipotropin, the latter of which is a precursor to the endorphins and met-enkephalin. This research group has previously demonstrated an increased ACTH response to the increased CRH levels in baboons, the same finding which has been described by others in human pregnancy. In the baboon, the presence and, indeed, augmentation of the ACTH response to vasopressin proves that downregulation of the CRH response does not reflect downregulation by increased cortisol concentration in pregnancy. The increased vasopressin sensitivity may stem from the increased amount of unsecreted pituitary ACTH that is available for release by vasopressin. This finding has the same general thrust that has been seen in other work, and it has possible relevance to the onset of labor (see the 1991 YEAR BOOK OF OBSTETRICS AND GYNECOLOGY, pp 16–17). An effect of placental CRH may be to shift trophic control from the hypothalamic-anterior pituitary focus to other sites—in this case, the placenta and posterior pituitary. This raises the possibility that the onset of labor may be associated with the role that placental CRH has in altering endocrine cybernetics to allow direct influence from the placenta to supersede the regulatory mechanisms present in the nonpregnant state.—T.H. Kirschbaum, M.D.

Plasma Immunoreactive Endothelin-1 Concentration in Human Fetal Blood: Its Relation to Asphyxia

Isozaki-Fukuda Y, Kojima T, Hirata Y, Ono A, Sawaragi S, Sawaragi I, Kobayashi Y (Kansai Med Univ, Osaka, Japan; Tokyo Med and Dental Univ, Japan)

Pediatr Res 30:244–247, 1991 1–3

Introduction.—Endothelin-1 (ET-1) is a potent vasoconstrictor peptide produced by vascular endothelial cells, and it may have an important role in the control of blood pressure and/or local blood flow. Recent studies have demonstrated high levels of circulating ET-1 in fetal blood. However, it is not known whether the ET-1 levels in the umbilical cord plasma change under physiological and pathophysiological states during delivery. The effects of birth stress on the ET-1 levels in human umbilical cord plasma were examined.

Patients.—Cord blood was drawn just after birth from the cord artery and vein of 14 preterm and 21 term infants. Maternal venous blood was drawn during delivery from 10 mothers with uncomplicated deliveries.

An ET-1 radioimmunoassay was performed using a new polyclonal antibody specific for ET-1. Venous and arterial cord blood samples from all asphyxiated infants were analyzed for concentrations of blood gas.

Results.—Concentrations of plasma immunoreactive ET-1 (irET-1) in both the umbilical artery and the vein were significantly higher than those in maternal venous blood at delivery. There was no difference in the irET-1 levels between preterm and term infants; however, the plasma irET-1 levels of healthy infants born by vaginal delivery were significantly higher than those in infants born by cesarean section without labor. Furthermore, the irET-1 levels in vaginally delivered infants with asphyxia were significantly higher than those in nonasphyxiated infants.

Conclusion.—Birth stress, especially asphyxia, may contribute to the increase in fetal circulating irET-1 levels.

▶ Set aside for a moment the apparent unresolved question as to whether the differing antibodies used to measure fetal ET-1 by various investigators are comparable. This study shows that the cord blood endothelin concentration is 3 to 4 times greater than the maternal uterine vein concentration independent of premature delivery and is slightly greater in normal infants delivered vaginally compared with those delivered abdominally. This latter small difference likely reflects the role of endothelin in umbilical cord vessel constriction after delivery (see the 1989 YEAR BOOK OF OBSTETRICS AND GYNECOLOGY, p 26). In the 6 infants born with severe metabolic acidosis, the endothelin concentrations were very large, as was a simultaneous series of indicators of organ and cell injury. These observations confirm both in vitro evidence that endothelin production by the endothelium is stimulated by catecholamines and the in vivo evidence for the same effect from surgical trauma, ischemia, and hemorrhage. There is more to learn about the economy of this peptide; the multiple stimulants to its production and release will, of course, complicate analysis of its role in pregnancy hypertension.—T.H. Kirschbaum, M.D.

Regulation of Corticotropin Responsiveness in Human Fetal Adrenal Cells

Rainey WE, McAllister JM, Byrd EW, Mason JI, Carr BR (Univ of Texas Southwestern, Dallas)

Am J Obstet Gynecol 165:1649–1654, 1991 1–4

Background.—In the human fetus, the adrenal gland provides most of the steroids used in estrogen synthesis by the placenta. Although corticotropin appears to be the main regulator of fetal adrenal steroidogenesis, little is known about the regulation of corticotropin receptors. The effects of chronic treatment with corticotropin and forskolin on corticotropin responsiveness were studied.

Methods.—Adrenal glands were obtained from fetuses aborted in the second trimester. Tissues from the definitive and fetal zones of the gland were separated and dispersed mechanically. These cells were then treated for 3 hours with corticotropin, after which their ability to produce cyclic adenosine monophosphate (cAMP) was measured. In addition, corticotropin receptor regulation was evaluated through iodine-125-labeled corticotropin binding to fetal adrenal cells.

Results.—Corticotropin induced a sevenfold to tenfold increase in production of cAMP, suggesting a functional corticotropin receptor-adenylate cyclase coupling. This decreased to a twofold increase when cells from either zone were grown and passed in monolayer culture. This was accompanied by a loss of the steroid metabolizing enzyme 17α-hydroxylase ($P\text{-}450_{17\alpha}$), which can be stimulated by treatment of fetal adrenal cells with corticotropin or forskolin. Therefore, cells were pretreated with corticotropin or forskolin for 4 days, and their ability to produce cAMP in response to corticotropin was measured. There was a dose-dependent increase in the ability of corticotropin to produce cAMP. Forskolin pretreatment increased production of cAMP by 35- to 50-fold. The effect was not as great with corticotropin pretreatment, and $P\text{-}450_{17\alpha}$ enzyme levels were also induced. Iodine-125-labeled corticotropin binding to definitive zone cells was increased 2.8 times by corticotropin pretreatment and 7 times by forskolin pretreatment.

Conclusion.—Corticotropin appears to be a positive regulator of its own responsiveness. The mechanism of corticotropin responsiveness and corticotropin receptors in human fetal adrenal cells appears to depend on cAMP. This agrees with studies of bovine and ovine adrenal cells, in which corticotropin or cAMP treatment increased the number of corticotropin receptors.

▶ This study demonstrates the capacity for adrenocorticotropic hormone (ACTH) to upregulate its own receptor in vitro in cell preparations from both fetal and definitive zones of the human fetal adrenal system. This is part of an interesting story in terms of adrenal developmental change in the fetus. In the sheep and some primates, the fetal adrenal appears to approach maximal function in early pregnancy. There then appears to be an interval of relative quiescense in midpregnancy, which is followed by an apparent increase in adrenal production of ACTH in the face of increasing fetal serum concentrations of corticosteroids; this process is exactly the reverse of the expected downregulation. Such an increase seems important in view of the increased concentration of fetal dehydroepiandrosterone sulfate (DHEAS), which is useful as a precursor to augment estrogen production and appears at approximately this time in development.

Estrogen obviously plays a role in the initiation of labor in ungulates and, perhaps, in primates, including man. These findings mean that the ability of corticosteroids to downregulate ACTH must be diminished, perhaps by a reduction in adrenal glucocorticoid receptors in late pregnancy before the onset of labor. Whether the ability of ACTH to upregulate its receptor exists or is augmented in late pregnancy as well as in the second trimester becomes an important question with implications for understanding and, possibly, manipulating the onset of labor. If so, then increased ACTH receptors may set the stage for increased DHEAS production and, for that source, increased estrogen production, which, undetected in blood concentration, may play a role at a cellular level in the onset of labor.—T.H. Kirschbaum, M.D.

The Presence of Platelet-Activating Factor Binding Sites in Human Myometrium and Their Role in Uterine Contraction

Zhu Y-p, Word RA, Johnston JM (Univ of Texas, Dallas)

Am J Obstet Gynecol 166:1222–1228, 1992 1–5

Background.—Recent research has suggested that platelet-activating factor (PAF) is involved in many processes associated with reproduction. A critical role for this autacoid in initiating and maintaining parturition in animals and humans has been demonstrated. Therefore, the presence of PAF receptors in human myometrium was examined.

Methods.—Uterine specimens were obtained from premenopausal women who were undergoing hysterectomy for reasons other than endometrial or myometrial disease. Membrane fractions were prepared for PAF binding studies. Intracellular Ca^{2+} concentrations were quantified, and phosphorylation of light chain of myosin was determined.

Results.—Platelet-activating factor affected contraction in strips of human myometrium at concentrations as low as 10^{-10} mol/L. A PAF receptor was identified and characterized. The platelet-activating factors cause

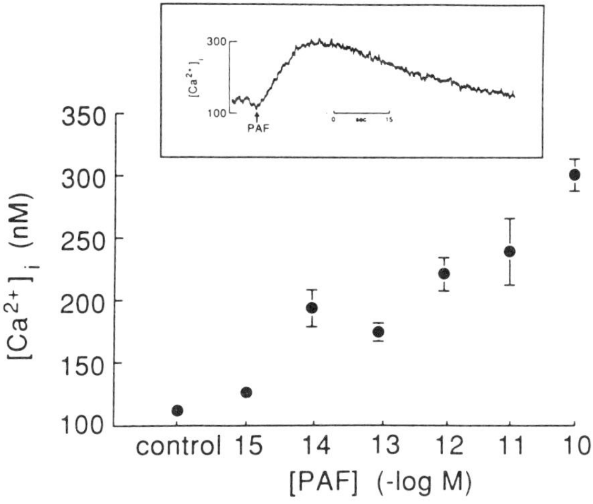

Fig 1–2.—Effect of PAF in intracellular Ca^{2+} in human myometrial smooth muscle cells. The data are expressed as mean ± SEM for 3–10 samples. **Inset**, recording of fluorescence (340 nm) of fura-2-containing myometrial cells treated with PAF (10^{-10} mol/L). Data are represented as mean ± SEM. (Courtesy of Zhu Y-p, Word RA, Johnston JM: *Am J Obstet Gynecol* 166:1222–1228, 1992.)

an increase in the intracellular Ca^{2+} concentration of isolated myometrial smooth muscle cells in culture and an increase in the phosphorylation of the 20-kd light chain of myosin in a concentration-dependent manner (Fig 1–2).

Conclusion.—A PAF receptor was demonstrated in human myometrium. Human myometrial smooth muscle cells in culture respond to PAF with an increase in intracellular Ca^{2+} concentration and myosin light chain phosphorylation. A PAF receptor antagonist blocks PAF binding to the membrane fraction. Platelet-activating factor may have an important part, along with other autacoids, in initiating and maintaining parturition.

▶ This peptide, which is found in platelets and is produced by type 2 pneumatocytes and unknown cells in the fetal kidney, has a probable role both in pulmonary maturation of the fetus and in facilitation of prostaglandin E_2 production by human amnion (see the 1988 YEAR BOOK OF OBSTETRICS AND GYNECOLOGY, pp 28–29). This study provides new information regarding the maternal regulation of PAF activity in pregnancy, and it also illustrates a possible direct myometrial cell relationship in vitro. Enzyme activity capable of degrading PAF is reduced in human maternal blood in late pregnancy, thereby increasing PAF effectiveness and tissue response. Prepregnancy enzyme activity returns within 24 hours after delivery. This work demonstrates both the presence of PAF receptors in human myometrial cell membranes in vitro and the effect of receptor complexing in increasing the intracellular calcium concentration (as measured by fluorescent spectoscopy). The resulting chemical alteration of myosin light chains, which are essential intermediates in the role of PAF as strong initiators of myometrial contractuity, are also seen. It is an interesting possibility that fetal lungs and kidneys indicate their functional maturity at term by secreting PAF into the amniotic fluid, where it functions to ripen in the cervix via its effect on amnion prostaglandin E_2 production and to increase myometrial contractility through a direct effect on the myometrium as PAF diffuses through the chorion into the uterus.—T.H. Kirschbaum, M.D.

Oxytocin Secretion and Human Parturition: Pulse Frequency and Duration Increase During Spontaneous Labor in Women

Fuchs A-R, Romero R, Keefe D, Parra M, Oyarzun E, Behnke E (Cornell Univ, New York; Yale Univ, New Haven, Conn; Hospital Sotero del Rio, Santiago, Chile)

Am J Obstet Gynecol 165:1515–1523, 1991 1–6

Background.—Disagreement persists as to the changes in maternal oxytocin secretion during labor. Great variability is noted between individual values, even in patients who are not in labor. Measurement would be further confounded if oxytocin were secreted in a pulsatile manner in women, as it is in cows and sheep. Oxytocin secretion was studied in pregnancy, both before and during labor, using a highly specific and sensitive antibody and frequent sampling.

Methods.—The subjects were 32 women in week 38–42 of gestation. Blood was sampled every minute for 30 minutes. The samples were taken so as to minimize degradation by plasma oxytocinase. The antibody used for radioimmunoassay was sensitive and specific, and it did not react with estrogen-induced peptide. Women were studied before labor, in the first stage of labor, or in the second stage of labor. Eighteen women at term were studied after intravenous injection of 4–16 mU of oxytocin.

Findings.—Oxytocin appeared to be secreted in short, discrete pulses. The pulses were significantly more frequent during spontaneous labor than before labor began. Before labor, the mean pulse frequency was 1.2 per 30 minutes; in the first stage, 4.2 per 30 minutes; and in the second and third stages, 6.7 per 30 minutes. These pulses lasted a mean of 1.2, 1.9, and 2 minutes, respectively. They varied in amplitude, but most were approximately 1 mμ/mL, with no significant differences between the groups. Pulses of similar magnitude were noted on oxytocin injection.

Conclusion.—Oxytocin pulses occur with increasing frequency in women undergoing spontaneous labor. These pulses are physiologically significant and suggest that oxytocin plays a role in the onset and maintenance of labor. The increase in myometrial oxytocin receptor concentrations in early labor correlates well with the increase in uterine responsiveness to oxytocin during the last days of gestation.

▶ This is one of the nicest reviews of oxytocin secretion in relation to labor to appear in a long time. It is not surprising that oxytocin, like other pituitary peptides hormones, is released in pulsatile fashion. This is important in understanding previous conflicting reports of changes in oxytocin secretion in labor, because the increased frequency of pulses does little to increase the overall basal concentrations of oxytocin in blood. One needs to remember that signal froquency is often more important than baseline signal intensity. A nice example is the way the frequency of electrical signals from the arcuate nucleus of the hypothalamus regulates secretion of gonadotropin-releasing hormone, even to determining the ratios of follicle-stimulating hormone and luteinizing hormone released by the pituitary. What's still a puzzle is the irregularity of oxytocin pulsativity and the variability noted from woman to woman. Part of this variability surely comes from differences in receptor activity and in rates of degradation by oxytocinase action. Thorton et al. (1) noted a sharp increase in plasma oxytocin levels in the third trimester of pregnancy in 40% of gravidas, a finding which makes teleologic sense in preventing postpartum hemorrhage. Fuchs et al. failed to see it regularly, although 2 cases in Figure 3 in the original article suggest third trimester increases. There is still much that is uncertain in the oxytocin story, but this very nice work advances our knowledge a great deal.—T.H. Kirschbaum, M.D.

Reference

1. Thornton S, et al: *BMJ* 297:167, 1988.

The Effects of Glycemia on Breathing Movements and Plasma Prostaglandin E Concentrations in the Sheep Fetus

Fowden AL, Thian S, Silver M, Ralph MM, Harding R (Physiological Lab, Cambridge, England; Monash Univ, Clayton, Australia)

Am J Obstet Gynecol 166:713–719, 1992 1–7

Background.—Glucose concentration has an important effect on fetal breathing movements. The low incidence of such movements during fetal hypoglycemia may result in part from a concomitant increase in the fetal concentration of prostaglandin E_2 (PGE_2). The functions of fetal plasma glucose and concentration of PGE_2 in breathing movements were studied in sheep.

Methods.—Twin fetuses of 5 late pregnant ewes were catheterized, and the ewes were fasted for 48 hours. During this time, 1 fetus was kept normoglycemic by glucose infusion, and the other was allowed to become hypoglycemic. Fetal breathing movements and fetal and maternal concentrations of plasma PGE_2 and glucose were monitored throughout the study period.

Findings.—At both 24 and 48 hours, plasma concentrations of glucose were significantly decreased in both the mother and the uninfused fetus.

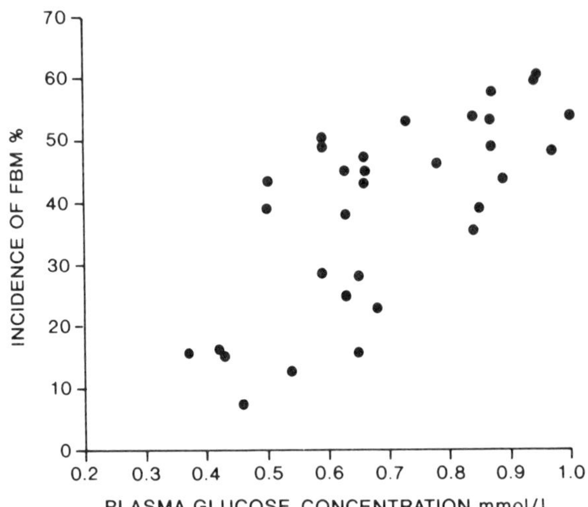

Fig 1–3.—Relationship between incidence of fetal breathing movement (FBM) and arterial concentration of plasma glucose in individual fetuses, irrespective of their nutritional state. (Courtesy of Fowden AL, Thian S, Silver M, et al: *Am J Obstet Gynecol* 166:713–719, 1992.)

The infused fetus had no significant changes in the plasma concentration of glucose from prefasting values. At the end of the fasting period, the mean incidence of fetal breathing movements were significantly greater in normoglycemic fetuses than in hypoglycemic fetuses (Fig 1-3). However, both groups of fetuses had significant and similar increases in levels of PGE_2.

Conclusion.—In pregnant, fasting ewes the reduced incidence of fetal breathing movements appears to result mainly from fetal hypoglycemia, with no direct effect of fetal PGE_2. The effect of hypoglycemia may result from changes in the chemical environment of the central chemoreceptors. Prostaglandin synthesis by the mother appears to be stimulated by either maternal or fetal hypoglycemia.

▶ The mechanisms for the inhibition of fetal breathing movements in relation to the onset of labor, which often are attributed to increased prostaglandin production by the placenta and its membranes, have always been uncertain. To be sure, this study attacks a somewhat different problem—reduced breathing in maternal fasting. In this study, the role of PGE is seen to be small in determining the respiratory activity of the fetus compared with fetal plasma glucose concentration, and its role is abolished by coincident administration of PGE and glucose. This sets the stage for investigating changes in glucose metabolism near the time of the onset of labor, in hopes of determining—at least in experimental animals—whether the same inverse relationship between PGE and fetal glucose concentration is operative in humans as well.—T.H. Kirschbaum, M.D.

Relationship Between Inspiratory Effort and Breathlessness in Pregnancy

Field SK, Bell SG, Cenaiko DF, Whitelaw WA (Foothills Hosp, Calgary, Alta)
J Appl Physiol 71:1897–1902, 1991 1–8

Objective.—Breathlessness is a common but poorly understood complaint during pregnancy. Using open magnitude scaling, breathlessness was quantified during a progressive exercise test in the last trimester of pregnancy and post partum; it was then correlated with respiratory mechanics previously shown to correspond with breathlessness in normal subjects breathing against mechanical loads.

Methods.—Thirteen healthy women performed progressive cycle exercise tests at 33 weeks' gestation and at 12 weeks post partum. The relationships between breathlessness, inspiratory esophageal pressure swing (ΔPes), and minute ventilation were studied.

Results.—There were no significant changes in pulmonary function and maximal transdiaphragmatic pressure in the third trimester and postpartum periods. Minute ventilation was greater in the third trimester, and this was entirely caused by the increase in tidal volume (Vt). The inspiratory esophageal pressure swing was greater in the third trimester, but the relationship between ΔPes and Vt was the same in the third trimester and post partum. Likewise, despite the rapid increase in breathlessness in the third trimester, the relationship between ΔPes and breathlessness was the same in the 2 conditions. The relationships between Vt and tidal abdominal volume and between tidal abdominal volume and tidal gastric pressure swing were the same in the 2 conditions.

Conclusion.—The relationship between ΔPes and breathlessness is the same in the third trimester of pregnancy and post partum, and the breathlessness that most pregnant women experience is the normal awareness of their greater minute ventilation. Despite the enlarging uterus and consequent chest wall distortion, the tidal abdominal volume contribution is maintained, suggesting that the abdominal wall accommodates these changes.

▶ The origin of dyspnea in pregnancy, or the sense of difficult respiration, has always been a puzzle; however, this study clarifies things considerably. A comparison between the first and third trimesters of ventilatory mechanics might have made the results a bit clearer than comparing the third trimester of pregnancy with the postpartum period; nevertheless, the conclusions seem relatively firm. Pregnancy imposes an increment of roughly 15% oxygen consumption by the time the third trimester is reached. This increment is necessary to provide respiratory gas exchange to the fetus and the placenta. This increased demand is met by an increase in minute volume of respiration, largely through an increase in tidal volume. Increased tidal volume comes about to the extent of 35% by enhanced abdominal volume excursion, and to 65% from greater rib cage expansion. The differences between maximum and minimum pressure recorded in the esophagus seem to be related to a sense of awareness of respiratory effort in pregnant women. This study shows the relationship between that range and tidal volume to be the same in late pregnancy and the postpartum state. That idea forms the basis for the contention that the dyspnea of pregnancy is simply an awareness of the increased minute volume of respiration imposed by the augmented metabolic demands of pregnancy, arising primarily from the augmented expansion of the rib cage that becomes necessary.—T.H. Kirschbaum, M.D.

Natural Killer Cell Activity From Pregnant Subjects is Modulated by RU 486

Hansen KA, Opsahl MS, Nieman LK, Baker JR Jr, Klein TA (Walter Reed Army Med Ctr, Washington, DC; Natl Naval Med Ctr; Natl Inst of Child Health and Development, Bethesda, Md)

Am J Obstet Gynecol 166:87–90, 1992 1–9

Introduction.—The influence of the human fetus on allogeneic immune responses in the woman remains unknown. Although natural-killer cell activity decreases during pregnancy, the mechanism of this immunosuppressive response has not been delineated. The RU 486 is a synthetic steroid hormone with antiprogesterone and antiglucocorticoid actions.

Methods.—To determine whether progesterone receptor inhibition of lymphocytes changes the effects of the natural killer cells in pregnant women, the effects of RU 486 were studied in 49 women, aged 17–43 years. The women had a mean gestational age of 30 weeks. Whole blood was drawn from target cell (K562 cells) culture and was harvested for further experiments. The RU 486 hormone, progesterone, and hydrocortisone were dissolved into RPMI medium for an 18-hour incubation.

Results.—The RU 486 increased the natural killer cell action 3–5 times greater than the normal levels for each lymphocyte:target cell ratio tested. The specified lysis activity increased significantly compared with control samples. The RU 486 plus lymphocyte solution from 9 women served as the medium for the progesterone and hydrocortisone assays. Both the progesterone and the hydrocortisone additions reduced Ru 486-increased lysis activity, with progesterone showing a significant effect.

Conclusion.—Progesterone may serve as the immunomodulating factor that allows a woman's system to accept the fetal allograft. Theoretically, this hormone could increase lymphokine secretion by the T-suppressor cells, thereby reducing natural killer-cell activity.

▶ Natural immunity is comprised of a series of reactions to foreign host invaders, none of which require prior exposure to the host or show enhancement of the reaction after prior exposure. The components of such a response include blood- and tissue-borne phagocytes, natural-killer lymphocytes (NK), and tissue interfaces that serve as barriers to foreign invaders. These mechanisms are distinct from specific or acquired immunity, the components of which are lymphocyte and antibody responses to specific antigens. This study shows that RU 486, a competitive inhibitor for progesterone and glucocorticoid receptors, enhances NK cell activity in vitro. At least it is clear that progesterone functions to downregulate natural immunity just as it does acquired immunity. Although the role of progesterone in both these systems is well known, this is the first study to suggest that loss of humorally modified natural immunity may be part of the abortifacient defects of RU 486. Conversely, it raises the likelihood that immunosuppression of natural immunity may be part of the immune tolerance to the fetal allograft, which is part of normal pregnancy. Works such as this one demonstrate the importance of research on both the use of this agent and the short-sightedness (seen at several levels of government) in interdicting its presence in this country.—T.H. Kirschbaum, M.D.

Maternal and Fetal Haemodynamics in Hypertensive Pregnancies During Maternal Treatment With Intravenous Hydralazine or Labetalol

Harper A, Murnaghan GA (Queen's Univ of Belfast)

Br J Obstet Gynaecol 98:453–459, 1991 1–10

Introduction.—Hydralazine is the most commonly used antihypertensive agent in the treatment of preeclampsia and eclampsia; however, labetalol is a newer and effective alternative in the treatment of acute maternal hypertension. A pulsed Doppler ultrasound study was used to examine whether hydralazine or labetalol given to treat maternal hypertension causes any detectable changes in fetal heart rate (FHR) or umbilical artery flow velocity waveform (FVW) characteristics.

Patients.—Among 30 pregnant women with acutely increased or labile blood pressure (BP) that had not responded to bed rest, 15 were randomly allocated to receive a single intravenous injection of 10 mg of hydralazine, and 15 received a single intravenous injection of 100 mg of labetalol. All women had singleton pregnancies. Umbilical artery FVWs were recorded by using a pulsed Doppler duplex scanner. The umbilical artery pulsatility index (PI) and the FHR were derived from these recordings. The measurements were obtained before the injection over 3 minutes of the antihypertensive drug and at regular intervals up to 120 minutes after the start of the injection.

Results.—Maternal BP decreased significantly after administration of hydralazine and labetalol, but the decreases in systolic BP and mean arterial pressure were smaller after receiving hydralazine than after receiving labetalol. The maternal pulse rate increased after hydralazine but not after labetalol. The FHR did not change significantly after hydralazine, but it decreased significantly after labetalol. However, the FHR remained within normal range after injection of labetalol. The umbilical artery PI

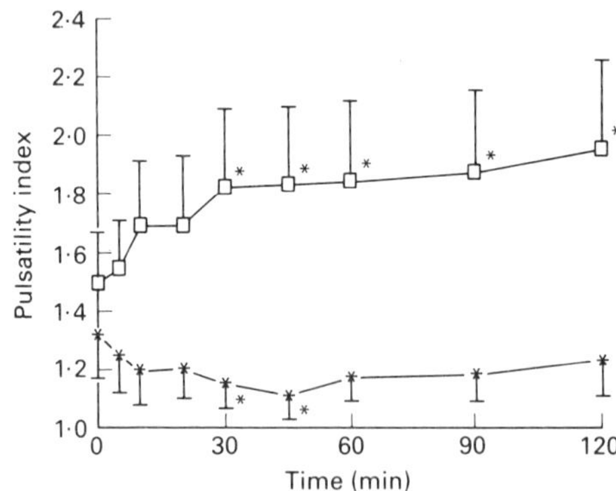

Fig 1–4.—The mean (± SE) of umbilical artery pulsatility index after 10 mg of hydralazine in 15 patients (*stars*) or 100 mg of labetalol in 15 patients (*squares*). *Asterisk* denotes significant difference from baseline. (Courtesy of Harper A, Murnaghan GA: *Br J Obstet Gynaecol* 98:453–459, 1991.)

decreased after hydralazine and increased after labetalol (Fig 1–4). The decrease in PI in some fetuses after administration of hydralazine was attributed to vasodilation, and the increase in PI after labetalol was attributed to vasoconstriction in the fetoplacental circulation, which suggests that fetal β-blockade may occur after maternal treatment with labetalol. However, in most fetuses, the changes were statistically not significant. Both drugs were generally well tolerated, and minor side effects were usually transient.

Conclusion.—Labetalol used in the treatment of maternal hypertension may cause β-blockade in the fetus, and it should be used with caution if fetal compromise is suspected.

▶ Using umbilical artery Doppler signals as a dependent variable in this study introduces some problems of interpretation, but the observations are interesting. Labetalol, a β-blocker with some β2 agonist activity, has come into increasing use in the past few years in the treatment of pregnancy-induced hypertension. Like hydralazine, the agent crosses the placenta and has been reported to produce fetal plasma concentrations that are roughly comparable to maternal plasma concentrations, at least transiently. In experimental animals, the agent has proven capable of reducing umbilical blood flow, especially with preexistent hypoxia. Perhaps this is the reason for the increase in PI that was noted within 10 minutes after administration of maternal labetalol in this study. This is the opposite of what is seen with administration of hydralazine, as far as fetal effects are concerned. Because Doppler-induced potentials measure blood velocity, they cannot be transformed to bulk flow and to vascular resistance measurements. Nonetheless, these data suggest something deleterious may ensue in the fetus after administration of labetalol. It's an observation worth keeping in mind.—T.H. Kirschbaum, M.D.

Suppression of Thromboxane A_2 But Not of Systemic Prostacyclin by Controlled-Release Aspirin

Clarke RJ, Mayo G, Price P, FitzGerald GA (Vanderbilt Univ, Nashville)

N Engl J Med 325:1137–1141, 1991 1 11

Background.—Aspirin reduces the risk of death from unstable coronary artery disease, presumably through inhibiting the production of thromboxane A_2. Its efficacy, however, may be limited by inhibition of prostacyclin, which has effects on vascular tone and platelet function opposite those of thromboxane A_2. If the rate of drug delivery is below the hepatic threshold for extraction of aspirin, it may be possible to inhibit the production of thromboxane A_2 while limiting exposure of the systemic vascular endothelium to aspirin.

Methods.—A controlled-release preparation containing 75 mg of aspirin, desiged to release 10 mg per hour, was developed to inhibit platelet prostaglandin synthase activity in the prehepatic circulation. Its effects were compared with those of immediate-release aspirin (162.5 mg, followed by 75 mg daily) in 45 normal male volunteers.

Results.—The serum level of thromboxane B_2 was suppressed more rapidly with immediate-release aspirin; however, over a 28-day period, controlled-release aspirin suppressed thromboxane A_2 as effectively as intermediate-release aspirin (given in a dose of either 162.5 mg daily or 325 mg every other day). All regimens increased bleeding time to a similar degree. Only immediate-release aspirin prevented the increase in prostacyclin metabolite induced by bradykinin.

Conclusion.—Controlled-release aspirin may allow a controlled assessment of the clinical value of preserving the synthesis of prostacyclin during platelet inhibition.

▶ In the studies of aspirin's effectiveness in preventing preeclampsia, there is a growing concern with the assumption that 60–80 mg of aspirin suffices to inhibit platelet production of thromboxane A_2 without parallel inhibition of endothelium-produced prostocycline. Aspirin acts by irreversible acetylation of cyclooxygenase enzyme activity in platelets (see the 1991 YEAR BOOK OF OBSTETRICS AND GYNECOLOGY, pp 29–30), but whether the same irreversibility applies to reduction of enzyme activity in the endothelium is uncertain. It is an important concern because of the opposite effects of thromboxane and prostacyclin on platelet aggregation and vasoconstriction. If both of these eicosanoids are inhibited, any possible benefit proceeding from the reduction of the thromboxane may be abolished by the failure of the beneficial effects of prostacyclin. Already, small groups of subjects have demonstrated that the validity of the dosage assumption must be proven by measurement of metabolites to evaluate properly aspirin's effectiveness in prophylaxis. Two alternatives are to reduce the aspirin dose or to use alternate day dosage, possibly to allow repair of endothelium prostaglandin synthetase activity and to rely on the irreversible effect of the drug on platelets. This study demonstrates that 75 mg of controlled release aspirin in 10 male subjects sufficed to spare prostacyclin production while inhibiting thromboxane production. More such studies in pregnant women are needed to clarify this important issue.—T.H. Kirschbaum, M.D.

Attenuation of the Vasoconstrictor Effects of Thromboxane and Endothelin by Nitric Oxide in the Human Fetal-Placental Circulation

Myatt L, Brewer AS, Langdon G, Brockman DE (Univ of Cincinnati)

Am J Obstet Gynecol 166:224–230, 1992 1–12

Background.—Many researchers are currently studying the production and mechanism of action of endothelial-derived vasoactive agents that may act to regulate vascular tone in an autocrine or paracrine manner. The hypothesis that the endothelial-derived relaxing factor nitric oxide might contribute to low resting vascular tone and attenuate vasoconstrictor action in human fetal-placental circulation was tested.

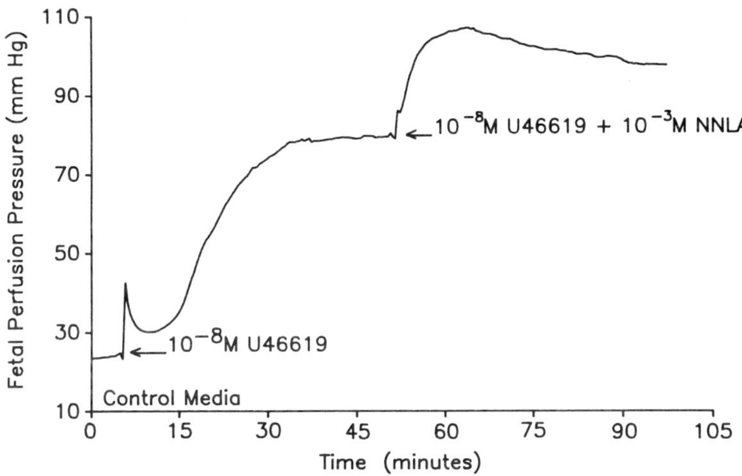

Fig 1–5.—Representative tracing of the effect of infusion of NNLA on perfusion pressure in fetal-placental vasculature preconstricted by constant infusion of U46619 (10^{-8} mol/L). (Courtesy of Myatt L, Brewer AS, Langdon G, et al: *Am J Obstet Gynecol* 166:224–230, 1992.)

Methods.—Isolated human placental cotyledons were perfused dually in vitro. The effects of N-monomethyl-L-arginine (NMLA) and N-nitro-L-arginine (NNLA) (3×10^{-4} mol/L), which are nonmetabolizable analogues of L-arginine, the substrate for nitric oxide synthase, on resting perfusion pressure and on the fetal-placental circulation preconstricted with U46619 or endothelin-1 were determined. Responses before and after inhibition were compared. Also determined were the effects of glyceryl trinitrate, acetylcholine, the calcium ionophore A23187, and histamine in the preconstricted fetal-placental circulation.

Results.—Both NMLA and NNLA increased resting perfusion pressure, and NNLA promptly and significantly increased perfusion pressure in the fetal-placental circulation preconstricted with U46619 or endothelin-1. Glyceryl trinitrate-generated nitric oxide attenuated the vasoconstrictor effects of U46619 or endothelin-1. Neither acetylcholine nor A23187 affected the fetal-placental circulation. Bradykinin further increased perfusion pressure. Histamine only relaxed the preconstricted preparations at levels above those that released nitric oxide in other systems (Fig 1–5).

Conclusion.—In fetal-placental circulation, the stimulus to generation of nitric oxide may be hydrodynamic. Nitric oxide seems to contribute to the maintenance of basal vascular tone and to attenuate vasoconstrictor actions in fetal-placental circulation.

▶ Using an exotic perfused human placental cotyledon preparation, these authors explored the regulation of vasomotor tone and, therefore, blood flow by substances produced in vessel walls and cells. The placenta was the target of investigational opportunity, and the vasoregulatory principles are probably valid for most perfused tissues. These studies suggest that vasoregulation is ultimately the balance between vasoconstrictive endothelin and vasodilating endothelial relaxing factor (nitric oxide). The infusion of endothelin 1 (the porcine and human product) produces vasoconstriction and increased NO_2 production to modulate the effect, as was demonstrated by inhibitors of NO_2 synthesis in this experiment. General infusion of the inhibitor demonstrated that tonic vasodilatory effects from NO_2 exist as well. These opposed substances, like other second messengers resulting from agonist-receptor coupling (cyclic adenosine monophosphate, cyclic guanosine monophosphate, calcium, phospholipids, etc.) may be the medium through which other vasoreactive agents ultimately exert their effects on blood vessels.—T.H. Kirschbaum, M.D.

Venous Drainage of the Human Uterus: Respiratory Gas Studies in Normal and Fetal Growth-Retarded Pregnancies

Pardi G, Cetin I, Marconi AM, Bozzetti P, Buscaglia M, Makowski EL, Battaglia FC (Univ of Milan, Italy; Univ of Colorado, Denver)

Am J Obstet Gynecol 166:699–706, 1992 1–13

Objective.—There is little information on the physiology of venous drainage in the human uterus. The location of the placenta may cause constant differences in respiratory gas concentrations between the right and left sides. Animal studies have suggested that the maternal and fetal circulations may form a relatively ineffective "venous equilibrator." Respiratory gas relationships between the uterine and umbilical veins both in

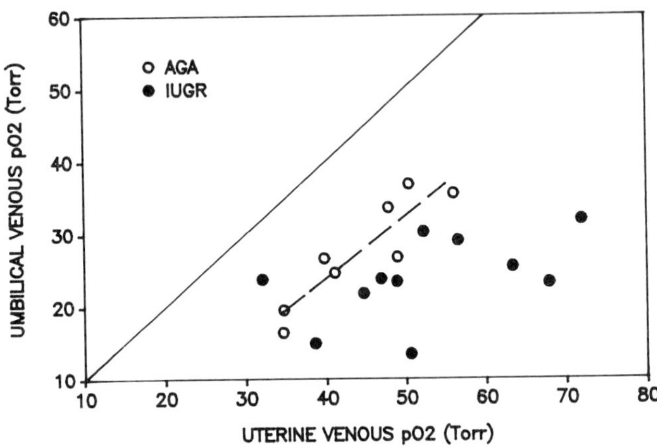

Fig 1–6.—The relationship between uterine venous and umbilical venous Po_2 in appropriate-for-gestational age (AGA) (*open circles*) and IUGR (*filled circles*) pregnancies. For AGA pregnancies, the regression line is presented. For IUGR pregnancies, the relationship is not significant. The *solid line* represents the identity line. (Courtesy of Pardi G, Cetin I, Marconi AM, et al: *Am J Obstet Gynecol* 166:699-706, 1992.)

normal pregnancies and in those with intrauterine growth retardation (IUGR) were examined.

Methods.—The study subjects were 21 patients who had elective cesarean section. Eight of these pregnancies were normal, and 13 were complicated by IUGR. Respiratory gases were measured in both uterine veins and in the umbilical vein immediately after induction of anesthesia.

Findings.—None of the study parameters were significantly different between the placental and nonplacental uterine veins. Umbilical and uterine venous values of partial pressure of oxygen (Po_2) and partial pressure of carbon dioxide (Pco_2) were significantly correlated in the normal pregnancies. In the umbilical vein, Po_2 was always less than in the uterine vein, and Pco_2 was always greater in the umbilical vein. In IUGR pregnancies, the transplacental gradient was significantly higher for both Po_2 and Pco_2 (Fig 1–6). The IUGR pregnancies also had a lower uterine oxygen extraction. The relationship between placental venous drainage in each uterine vein and the location of the placenta was inconsistent.

Conclusion.—Analysis of the respiratory gas exchange pattern across the human placenta supports the concept of a relatively inefficient venous equilibrator. Larger transplacental gradients are noted in IUGR pregnancies, presumably reflecting the decreased surface area of these small placentas. The finding of hypoxia in fetuses with IUGR seems to be related to the placenta and its fetal perfusion rather than to decreased uterine blood flow.

▶ The term "uteroplacental insufficiency" has so little significance because the relationship between maternal and fetal respiratory gas partial pressures, for instance, are functions of so many variables that, to date, they are unmeasurable in the human. Included among them are ratios of total uterine to umbilical blood flow rates (which actually enter into placental exchange) compared with total measured blood flow, and patterns of the relationship between well-perfused maternal and fetal segments of cotyledons. Only when changes in these variables can be excluded as significant can one say anything about the diffusion capacity of the placenta as it functions as a complicated membrane. It is in this domain that this interesting study offers some contributions.

Lateralization of placental implantation confers no predictable relationship on uterine venous blood concentration, and variability is great between individuals. This means that uterine venous drainage is complex, with anastomoses from one side to the other that are sizable and unpredictable. Also, in appropriate-for-gestational-age pregnancy, there is evidence suggesting concurrent flow patterns between maternal and fetal circulations where uterine vein and umbilical vein Po_2 and Pco_2 tend to come into equilibrium. Because of placental metabolism and unequal flow patterns, they never reach equilibrium. For infants who are small for gestational age, the suggestion of the concurrent relationship is lost for reasons that can't be discerned. The net effect is a decrease in umbilical vein Po_2 and an increase in Pco_2, which may reflect changes in blood flow rates, quantities of shunted blood flow, or changes in patterns of blood flow on either the maternal or fetal side of the placenta. Because blood flow rates were not measured and patterns were not describable, one can only wonder about the role of those changes in contrast to changes in placenta permeability per se. For this reason, the authors' contention that these changes stem from altered permeability alone is not supported by their data.—T.H. Kirschbaum, M.D.

Incidence of Doppler Regurgitant Flow Velocities During Normal Pregnancy

Robson SC, Richley D, Boys RJ, Hunter S (Dryburn Hosp, Durham, England; Univ of Newcastle Upon Tyne; Freeman Hosp, Newcastle Upon Tyne, England)

Eur Heart J 13:84–87, 1992 1–14

Background.—The best way to study maternal cardiovascular changes, both in normal women and in those with heart disease, is echocardiography. Doppler ultrasound should be useful in studying flow disturbances, but normal flow patterns for pregnant women must first be established. Color flow mapping and pulsed Doppler were used to study the incidence of regurgitant flow velocities in pregnant women.

Methods.—A total of 107 pregnant women were studied, 55 of them before 28 weeks' gestation. Fifty-five nonpregnant women younger than 40 years of age were also studied as controls. All women underwent Doppler echocardiography with color flow imaging and pulsed Doppler interrogation.

Findings.—The control group had a 42% incidence of tricuspid regurgitant velocities vs. 67% for women at 28 weeks or more of gestation. The median peak regurgitant velocity was 1.7 ms^{-1}. For pulmonary regurgitant velocities, the incidence was 50% in controls vs. 96% in women at 28 weeks or more of gestation. The median peak regurgitant velocity was 1.1 ms^{-1}. The pregnant women showed no substantial increase in left-sided regurgitant velocities.

Conclusion.—Many healthy women have regurgitant flow velocities of the tricuspid, mitral, and pulmonary valves. Tricuspid and pulmonary regurgitant velocities increase in frequency during pregnancy, but they rarely go over 2 ms^{-1}. Dilation of valve orifices from volume loading may account for the increased incidence of right heart regurgitant velocities in pregnancy.

▶ These findings are astonishing, but they have been demonstrated independently by sufficient numbers of investigators to establish their validity. Regurgitation of flow through the pulmonary and tricuspid valves is present as often as not in normal women, and it is present in almost all pregnant women. Even when one restricts the finding to instances in which the regurgitation is holosystolic and of high velocity, the findings are common in pregnancy. It is likely that these changes, which account for the "hemic murmur" of pregnancy, are maximal over the left second to third intercostal space at the left sternal border. Similarly, mitral regurgitation stemming from the dilation of the atrioventricular annulus (resulting from increased stroke volume during pregnancy) is very common. Even aortic regurgitation, which is rare in the absence of pregnancy, is occasionally seen in gravidas. These changes underlie the reluctance of cardiologists to explore asymptomatic gravidas with murmurs until after delivery. The hazard of that approach is that ultrasonic findings of valve incompetence during pregnancy might be overinterrupted to suggest a false positive diagnosis of valvular heart disease in the pregnancy.—T.H. Kirschbaum, M.D.

The Greater Renin System: Its Prorenin-Directed Vasodilator Limb Relevance to Diabetes Mellitus, Pregnancy, and Hypertension

Sealey JE, von Lutterotti N, Rubattu S, Campbell WG Jr, Gahnem F, Halimi J-M, Laragh JH (Cornell Univ, New York)

Am J Hypertens 4:972–977, 1991 1–15

Background.—Much has been written about tissue renin systems and their link to high blood pressure and heart disease. However, a great deal of this research is at odds with studies of prorenin. As experimental evidence about prorenin accumulates, the existence of a tissue renin system seems more plausible. A new model of a greater renin system has been proposed.

Discussion.—The proposed model is based on evidence that both prorenin and renin can generate angiotensin, and that angiotensin causes vasodilation at high concentrations and vasoconstriction at low concentrations. Prorenin acts only at particular target sites in this model, but renin of renal origin acts through the general circulation. In this model, prorenin should more appropriately be called "renin I," and circulating active renin, "renin II." Renin I generates localized high levels of angiotensin II, causing renal dilation by rendering tissues insensitive to the vasoconstrictor effect of circulating angiotensin II or by releasing vasodilator substances. The role of renin II is to constrict resistance vessels and the renal efferent arteriole of the kidney, thereby increasing blood pressure, maintaining the glomerular filtration rate, and enabling more blood flow to the organs that selectively bind prorenin. Blood flow to vital organs is maintained in this twin control system. A lack of coordination between these 2 parts of the greater renin system with an excess of renin I would explain the relationship of high levels of prorenin to the hyperperfusion injury of diabetes mellitus and the devastating consequences of hypertension in pregnancy. A relative excess of renin II would result in the hypertension and ischemic vascular injury of high renin hypertensive disorders (Fig 1–7).

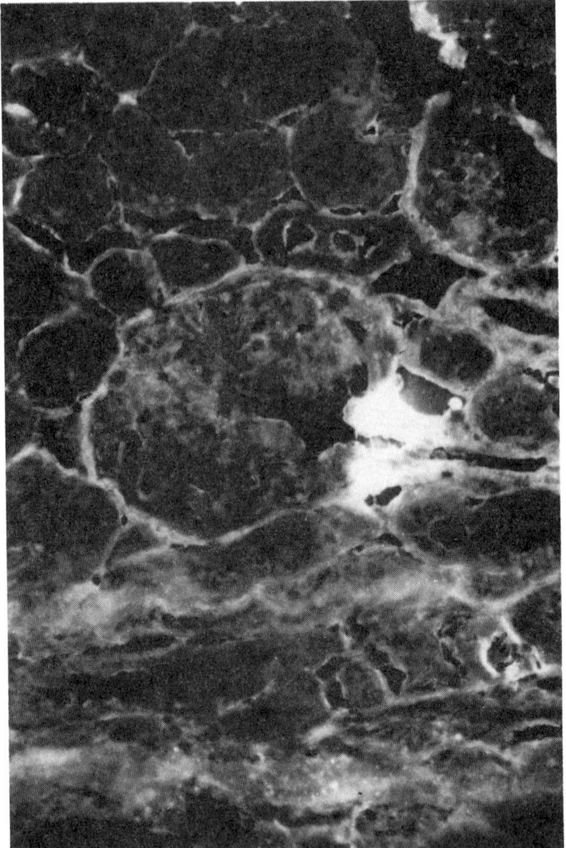

Fig 1–7.—Glomerulus with juxtaglomerular apparatus (JGA) of cynomolgus monkey kidney fresh frozen 6 hours after intravenous infusion of 20 Goldblatt units of recombinant human prorenin. Percentage of JGA reacting with antiserum directed against human renin was a mean of 28.5%, whereas kidneys of control monkeys showed mean staining of only 5.3%. Magnification; × 400. (Courtesy of Sealey JE, von Lutterotti N, Rubattu S, et al: *Am J Hypertens* 4:972–977, 1991.)

Conclusion.—New research will prove or disprove this concept of a greater renin system. In the meantime, it is consistent with the experimental evidence on tissue renin and the renal-endocrine circulating renin system.

▶ This construct nicely fits the existing data and helps to explain the high concentration of prorenin produced in the placenta and reproductive tract tissues, especially during pregnancy. If one conceives of prorenin acting as a precursor for renin (a potent vasoconstrictor and secretogogue for angiotensin, an agent that is in turn active in sodium retention), then the tenfold increase in prorenin concentrations during the first week of pregnancy and the increase up to 100,000 times in later pregnancy makes no sense at all. In the proposed model, renin produced solely in the juxta glomerular sites in the kidney from prorenin operates primarily on the general circulation, causing vasodilation at high concentrations and vasoconstriction at low concentrations. Its dominant effect in the kidney is to constrict renal arterioles and reduce glomerular filtration.

Prorenin, on the other hand, has focally protective actions that oppose the action of renal renin in the major resistance vessels in the kidney and efferent glomerular arteriole, a regulating glomerular pressure, and, therefore, an increasing glomerular filtration rate. In this view of a coupled antagonistic system, one substance (prorenin) serves as the precursor to another in selective organs and also provides the basis for protection from ischemia and hypertension in the uterus and placenta; however, it also allows a different set of interactions that takes place in the systemic circulation. What results is vascular stability in the changes of normal pregnancy and the kind of disturbance in organ perfusion and function that is seen in hypertensive pregnancy and diabetes. Hypotheses are the structures upon which new research is constructed. It will be interesting to see the results stimulated by this ingenious proposition.—T.H. Kirschbaum, M.D.

Relationship Between Placental Blood Flow and Combined Ventricular Output With Gastational Age in Normal Human Fetus

St John Sutton MG, Plappert T, Doubilet P (Brigham and Women's Hosp, Boston)

Cardiovasc Res 25:603–608, 1991 1–16

Introduction.—Although several studies have used Doppler ultrasound (US) in an attempt to assess placental perfusion in the human fetus, no systematic attempts have been made to quantitate the interrelationship between cardiac output and placental blood flow in the normal human fetus with increasing gestational age. The changes in placental blood flow and total cardiac output were quantified through the second and third trimesters of normal human pregnancy.

Methods.—Sixty-four normal human fetuses aged 20–42 weeks' gestation made up the study sample. All mothers were undergoing routine obstetric US examination for assessment of gestational age and placental location. High-quality, 2-dimensional echocardiographic images of the umbilical vein, proximal aorta, and proximal main pulmonary artery were obtained and transferred from videotape to a digital disc to obtain velocity-time integrals. The cross-sectional areas were calculated from vessel diameters. Placental blood flow per minute was calculated from the umbilical vein as the product of flow velocity integral per second and umbilical vein cross-sectional area. Combined ventricular output was the sum of right and left ventricular minute outputs.

Results.—Both placental blood flow and combined ventricular output increased exponentially with gestational age. There was a linear relationship between placental blood flow and combined ventricular output throughout the second and third trimesters. Placental blood flow comprised almost one third of the combined ventricular output. This proportion did not change with gestational age.

Conclusion.—Knowledge of the proportion of combined ventricular output that the placental flow comprises in the normal fetus may be helpful in the assessment of placental insufficiency, and, thus, enable early recognition of intrauterine growth retardation.

▶ The errors inherent in calculating blood flow rates from average velocity figures and vessel diameter have been discussed here frequently. In that sense, the absolute values presented in this study should not be taken seriously. Note, for instance, the regression line for the umbilical vein blood flow per unit of body weight vs. gestation indicates an umbilical vein blood flow of approximately 100 mL/K/minute at term, which is far below the previously reported values for the human and also is far below data from animal experimentation. Although that may explain all that is of apparent interest, some of the findings deserve further investigation. In this study, the data suggest placental blood flow is only one third of the cardiac output in humans compared with the 65% to 75% figure reported in experimental animals. In contrast, 40% of the biventricular output appears to go to the head and upper extremities compared with approximately 5% reported uniformly in experimental animals. If correct, these data suggest that the margin of safety regarding the effects of cord compromise is less in the human than animal data would suggest, because of increased protection conferred by the relatively larger fractional blood flow to the fetal brain. It is an observation worthy of more careful study.—T.H. Kirschbaum, M.D.

Human Decidua: A Source of Cachectin-Tumor Necrosis Factor

Romero R, Mazor M, Manogue K, Oyarzun E, Cerami A (Yale Univ, New Haven, Conn; Rockefeller Univ, New York)

Eur J Obstet Gynecol Reprod Biol 41:123–127, 1991 1–17

Background.—Cachectin-tumor necrosis factor (TNF-α) is a possible signal of the initiation of human parturition in infection. Whether human decidua can produce TNF-α in response to bacterial lipopolysaccharide was determined in decidual explants from 9 women undergoing elective cesarean sections at term.

Methods.—The explants were incubated with and without *Escherichia coli* lipopolysaccharide, 25 ng/mL, for 20 hours. An enzyme-linked immunoassay and bioassay, L929 bioassay, were used to measure TNF-α concentration in the conditioned media.

Results.—Conditioned media from unstimulated decidual explants contained either low or undetectable amounts of TNF-α. However, conditioned media from lipopolysaccharide-stimulated decidua contained a mean 2.6 pmol of TNF-α per mg. The immunoreactive and bioactive TNF-α were strongly correlated.

Conclusion.—Human decidua in vitro can produce TNF-α in response to lipopolysaccharide. A proposed mechanism involves control of the onset of labor by the host in the presence of infection. Systemic or localized intrauterine infection leads to the onset of parturition by activating the monocytemacrophage system to secrete cytokines. This, in turn, stimulates prostaglandin production. Preterm labor and delivery can be seen as an event that occurs when the intrauterine environment is hostile and threatening to the maternal-fetal pair. Thus, the initiation of parturition may have survival value.

▶ Here is another clarification in the pathophysiology of the infectious disease-mediated onset of preterm labor. Although phospholipases A_2 and C and lipopolysaccharide (LPS) are bacterial products capable of increasing substrate for prostaglandin synthesis and accelerating production of prostaglandin in E_2 and prostaglandin $F_{2\alpha}$ by placental membrane, the role of these products in the onset of preterm labor has always been arguable. The issues largely concern dosage. Bacteria may exist in the amniotic cavity without resulting in labor, and the concentrations of LPS needed to show effectiveness in labor are larger than those found in vivo.

This nice piece of work demonstrating decidual production of tumor necrotizing factor (TNF) from LPS to be an intermediate-to-enhanced production of prostaglandin provides an explanation which better fits the in vivo data. Choriodeciduitis is more effective than uncomplicated amnionitis in inducing labor. Abruptio placenta and even membrane stripping result in decidual inflammation, TNFα release, and labor with relative efficiency. Large doses of LPS produce decidual necrosis both in vivo and in vitro. What remains to be determined is whether TNF is a product of decidual macrophages, or whether decidua, a product of ondometrial stromal cell adaptation, retains the capacity to produce this potent cytokine.—T.M. Kirschbaum, M.D.

Acute Carbon Monoxide Intoxication and Hyperbaric Oxygen in Pregnancy

Elkharrat D, Raphael JC, Korach JM, Jars-Guincestre MC, Chastang C, Harboun C, Gajdos P (Hôpital Raymond Poincaré, Garches, France; Hôpital Saint Louis, Paris)

Intensive Care Med 17:289–292, 1991 1–18

Introduction.—Patients with acute carbon monoxide (CO) intoxication are commonly treated with either normobaric or hyperbaric oxygen (HBO). The use of HBO in pregnancy is controversial because it is thought to be hazardous to the fetus. However, the treatment of CO intoxication in pregnancy is poorly defined. Fetal and obstetric tolerance to HBO was assessed in pregnant women with acute CO intoxication.

Patients.—Forty-four pregnant women (mean age, 27.5 years) who sustained acute CO poisoning at home were treated with a combination of 2 hours of HBO at a pressure of 2 atmospheres absolute (ATA) and 4 hours of normobaric oxygen, irrespective of the clinicial severity of the intoxication or the age of pregnancy. The mean duration of CO intoxication was 2.6 hours, and the mean interval from the end of CO exposure to the initiation of HBO was 5.3 hours. Admission levels of carboxyhemoglobin ranged from 5% to 40%. The mean gestational age was 21 weeks.

Results.—At maternal follow-up 1 month after CO intoxication, 4 women were about to deliver or had just delivered, and 5 had moved away. Of the 35 remaining women, none had severe sequelae, 25 (70%) had completely recovered, and 10 (30%) had moderate sequelae. Six women were lost to obstetric follow-up. Of the 38 remaining women, 32 (85%) had a normal delivery of a normal infant, 1 had a premature delivery of a normal infant at 35 weeks' gestation, 1 required induction of labor at 36 weeks' gestation and gave birth to a normal infant, 2 sustained a spontaneous abortion, 1 underwent a medical abortion at 10 weeks' gestation for personal reasons, and 1 gave birth to a baby with Down's syndrome and major cardiopulmonary defects.

Conclusion.—Two hours of HBO at a pressure of 2 ATA in the treatment of acute CO intoxication in pregnant women is safe.

▶ Carbon monoxide poisoning produces histotoxic hypoxemia by virtue of both its stable binding to hemoglobin and the inability of carboxyhemoglobin (HbCO) to perform its normal oxidation reduction functions at physiologic Po_2. Hyperbaric oxygenation is useful in sufficiently increasing Po_2 so that the physically dissolved oxygen in the plasma, the amount of which is solely dependent on Po_2, suffices to meet the oxygen requirements of mother and fetus in transition from arterial to venous blood. At 2 ATA, 100% oxygen will result in arterial Po_2s as high as 1,400 mmHg. The impact on the fetus has been researched in sheep fetuses (1). As plasma-dissolved oxygen increases enough to meet the entire oxygen requirement of the gravid uterus, the ability of hemoglobin to maintain fetal blood Po_2 at the accustomed normal low values below approximately 60 mmHg is lost. The increase in fetal umbilical vein Po_2 to 100 mm Hg or more results in fetal pulmonary vasodilatation, even with unexpanded lungs; this reduces fetal cardiac output by as much as 50%, because the parallel connections of the ventricles, for which high fetal pulmonary resistance is required, are abolished. Evidence of reduced cardiac output should be scrutinized in judging the hazard of hyperbaric oxygenation to the human fetus.—T.H. Kirschbaum, M.D.

Reference

1. Assali NS, et al: *Circ Res* 22:573, 1968.

Effect of Birth-Related Events on Metabolism in Fetal Sheep

Iwamoto HS, Teitel DF, Rudolph AM (Univ of California, San Francisco)

Pediatr Res 30:158–164, 1991 1–19

Introduction.—At birth, the continuous nutrient supply from the placenta ceases, whereas the requirement for oxygen and exogenous substrates increases dramatically. The newborn mobilizes its fat and glycogen reserves, and the concentrations of blood glucose, lactate, and free fatty acid increase. The function and metabolic demands of several organs also change at birth. However, the events that initiate these changes at birth are not known. Whether the major metabolic changes that occur at birth are related to certain birth events was determined.

Methods.—The immediate effects of ventilation, oxygenation, and umbilical cord occlusion on oxygen, glucose, and lactate fluxes across the umbilical-placental, cerebral, myocardial, and hindlimb circulations were examined by measuring oxygen, glucose, and lactate uptake rates in the fetal hindlimb, myocardium, and brain of 15 chronically instrumented fetal sheep at 133–137 days' gestation. Blood flow was measured with the use of radionuclide-labeled microspheres. Measurements were obtained at rest, during in utero ventilation with 3% oxygen, and during in utero oxygenation and umbilical cord occlusion.

Results.—Ventilation of the fetal lungs with 3% oxygen decreased oxygen uptake by the fetus and by the cerebral circulation, but it did not produce any other significant changes in oxygen uptake. Ventilation with 3% or 100% oxygen dramatically reduced the glucose uptake by the fetus from the placental circulation to zero. In contrast, the blood glucose concentration increased, and the glucose uptake by the fetal brain, heart, and hindlimb were not altered significantly.

Conclusion.—Ventilation, oxygenation, and umbilical cord occlusion at birth do not have an effect on total fetal oxygen consumption or on oxygen uptake by individual fetal organs. However, these birth events have a significant effect on fetal glucose production, uptake, and use.

▶ This is an important study; however, several things need to be borne in mind in its interpretation. Nutrient delivery, a product of afferent blood concentration and blood flow rate, is not the same as nutrient uptake. The latter value is obtained by subtracting unabsorbed nutrients from delivered nutrients through the use of arteriovenous concentration differences. When delivery of nutrients to the organs studied comes via substrates that are not measured, total organ oxygen content (for instance) may correspond to far more glucose than is actually delivered. This results in a respiratory quotient less than 1 and is a clue to changes in metabolic accessibilities. Remember, too, that these fetuses were ventilated with 3% O_2, followed by 100 O_2 in utero, and that they are experiencing transient changes not seen in normal birth.

In the immediate neonatal period, oxygenation in utero reduces cardiac output and blood flow to most organs, whereas increased fetal blood Po_2

produces pulmonary vasodilatation and also changes ventricular coupling from the parallel arrangement of fetal life to the series pattern of the neonate. Therefore, the use of the sum of ventricular outputs to approximate cardiac output (such as these investigators have used) no longer becomes applicable. The placental oxygen uptake decreases with oxygenation, because the pulmonary circuit now meets a large part of the oxygen need. Total oxygen consumption does not increase, proving again that the normal fetus is not in a state of oxygen deprivation in utero. Glucose consumption is reduced, particularly in the myocardium where lactate takes on a role as primary metabolite. Nutrient stores are mobilized as fetal catecholamines produce glycogenolysis, and amino acid concentrations are increased in fetal blood. Free fatty acids, which are also likely mobilized from fetal stores but were not studied here, also probably contribute.

Within approximately 30 minutes after ventilation, the fetus is well on its way with adult metabolic patterns of nutrient use. It should be noted that the umbilical-placental blood flow rates during control were lower in this study than those usually reported using the labeled mircosphere method; the respiratory quotient of .3 during control indicates distinctly less fetal carbohydrate metabolism than is usually reported.—T.H. Kirschbaum, M.D.

2 Maternal Complications of Pregnancy

Erythromycin Therapy in Preterm Premature Rupture of the Membranes: A Prospective, Randomized Trial of 220 Patients

Mercer BM, Moretti ML, Prevost RR, Sibai BM (Univ of Tennessee, Memphis)

Am J Obstet Gynecol 166:794–802, 1992 2–1

Background.—Most studies on the use of antibiotics in preterm premature rupture of the membranes, a major cause of maternal, fetal, and neonatal morbidity, have been poorly designed. Two recent articles reported mezlocillin and ampicillin to be beneficial, but no randomized studies have examined the use of erythromycin. The efficacy of oral erythromycin therapy in increasing the latency period and reducing the incidence of maternal and neonatal infectious morbidity in patients with premature rupture of the membranes was evaluated in 220 women.

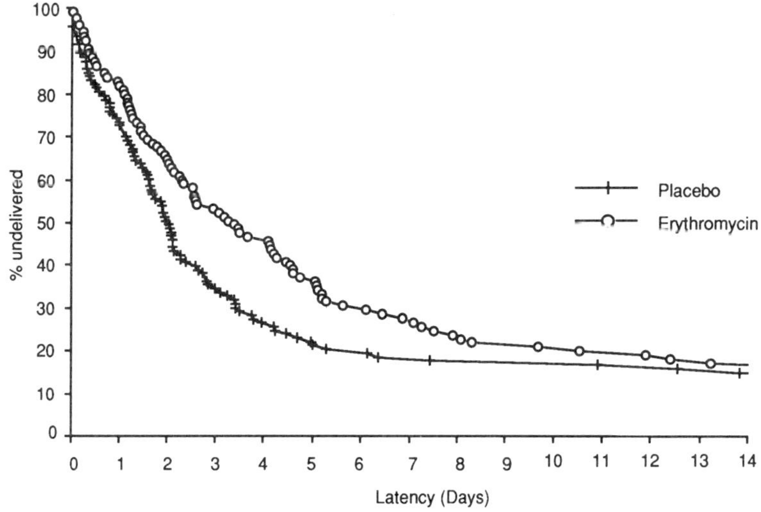

Fig 2–1.—Latency from randomization to delivery for patients receiving erythromycin base or placebo. (Courtesy of Mercer BM, Moretti ML, Prevost RR, et al: *Am J Obstet Gynecol* 166:794–802, 1992.)

Methods.—Eligible women who consented to take part in the study were between 20 weeks' and 34 weeks' 6 days' gestation. They were randomly assigned in a double-blind fashion to receive 333 mg of erythromycin (106 women) or placebo (114 women) every 8 hours until delivery. The women and neonates received whatever additional treatment and procedures were standard for their condition.

Results.—Both groups had a surprisingly high incidence of clinical abruptio placentae. No differences in the incidences of clinical chorioamnionitis or endometritis were observed. Positive amniotic fluid cultures were present in 17.9% of the placebo group and in 18.4% of the erythromycin group. Erythromycin therapy was associated with a significant prolongation of latency from randomization to delivery (Fig 2–1). particularly in those who would have chorioamnionitis and those with oligohydramnios. Subsequent to the first week after randomization, no differences in latency were seen. Infant morbidity and mortality and maternal morbidity were not reduced significantly by erythromycin therapy.

Conclusion.—Prophylactic oral erythromycin therapy significantly prolonged the latency period in patients with preterm premature rupture of the membranes. The combination of this drug with broader spectrum agents might be more effective in treating the organisms identified in the amniotic fluid.

▶ In 1988, a prospective study by Amon et al. from the University of Tennessee demonstrated that intravenous administration of ampicillin to patients with preterm rupture of membranes prolonged the latent period between rupture of membranes and delivery and also reduced infectious morbidity in the newborn (see the 1990 YEAR BOOK OF OBSTETRICS AND GYNECOLOGY, pp 33–34). This more recent experience, based on patients treated from 1989 to 1990, benefits by its larger number of cases, double-blind design, and the use of erythromycin, which quite probably deals better with the wide range of microbial species recovered. The authors' result confirms the delay in the onset of labor judged at 7 days after treatment compared with controls, but it shows no improvement in maternal or fetal outcome. This is the sixth study in this area to be reported since 1988. Prolongation of latency has been demonstrated in all but one study (1), and evidence of improved outcome was seen in nearly half the studies.

The 1990 YEAR BOOK comment is still valid. Latent chorioamnionitis causing preterm rupture of membranes vs. secondary infection of the membranes after aseptic rupture of membranes constitutes an uncontrolled determinant of outcome. In this study, positive amniotic fluid cultures were seen in 17.9% of placebo- and 18.4% of antibiotic-treated cases. Amniocentesis was completed in only 44.1% of the 220 cases in the study; therefore, we are unable to say anything definitive about the relative incidence of latent infection in the 2 groups. As long as this differential between cause and effect of infection and/or inflammation remains unclear, the therapeutic recommendations in this important area will also be unclear.—T.H. Kirschbaum, M.D.

Reference

1. Kurki T, et al: *Am J Perinatol* 9:11, 1992.

Mortality Among Infants of Black as Compared With White College-Educated Parents

Schoendorf KC, Hogue CJR, Kleinman JC, Rowley D (Natl Ctr for Health Statistics, Hyattsville, Md; Centers for Disease Control, Atlanta)

N Engl J Med 326:1522–1526, 1992 2–2

Background.—Black infants are twice as likely to die as are white infants in the United States. The difference reflects black infants' higher rates of low birth weight and the higher mortality among black infants of normal birth weight. Mortality in infants born to college-educated parents was studied to further investigate this mortality gap.

Methods.—The National Linked Birth and Infant Death Files for 1983 through 1985 were used to calculate infant death rates. Data on 865,128 white infants and 42,230 black infants were analyzed. The effect of birth weight was considered.

Findings.—The infant mortality was 10.2 per 1,000 live births for black infants and 5.4 per 1,000 live births for whites, the black infants' adjusted odds ratio for death was 1.82. A total of 7% of blacks and only 3% of whites had low birth weights, although the death rate in this group was not higher among the black infants compared with white infants. Black infants were 3 times as likely as whites to die of causes that could be attributed to perinatal events, such as prematurity. Black infants were no more likely to die of sudden infant death syndrome. The death rates among black and white infants were equal after low-birth-weight infants were excluded.

Conclusion.—Black infants born to college-educated parents have higher death rates than do white infants born to college-educated parents, only because they have higher rates of low birth weight. Mortality among black and white infants with normal birth weights is equivalent.

▶ This study of linked birth-death files from the National Center for Health Statistics provides important information concerning the social implications of being a black American as it affects premature birth and infant mortality. The selection of white and black college-educated parents for this study imposes the assumption that black-white differences in income, health care access, and health maintenance are reduced comparatively by that selective step. In that way, the resultant difference between infant mortality in blacks and whites is reduced and found to be solely attributable to the surplus of premature births in blacks. Infant mortality for birth weight equal to or greater than 2.5 kg becomes identical between the races, but the figure of 7.05% of black infants with birth weights less than 2.5 kg compared with the 3.08% figure for white infants makes a continuing difference. The lower black (compared with white) birth-weight-specific mortality rates failed to compensate for the 2.3 times greater number of preterm infants produced by blacks in this study. If surplus infant mortality for unselected cases is attributable to emotional and other socioeconomic variables, the basis for the increased prematurity rate that persists can only be a source of speculation.

Nationally, very-low-birth-weight rates increased in 1989 after decades of stability and previous decreases. Part of the increase is a result of the greater number of women younger than 20 years of age (increased by 1% in 1989) and older than 35 years of age (increased by 3%) for whom prematurity rates are higher. The lower rates of optimal prenatal care, increased incidence of unmarried birth status, and low parity in blacks, although not large enough to make a demonstrable difference in this sample, may combine to have an effect nationally. As the editorial comment in this issue points out, the stresses of living amidst constant discriminatory sociopolitical measures may be what plays an important role in the higher rate of premature births in socioeconomically favored blacks than in whites. Like all good studies, this one provides both some answers and some increasingly important further questions.—T.H. Kirshbaum, M.D.

Induction of Labor as Compared With Serial Antenatal Monitoring in Post-Term Pregnancy: A Randomized Controlled Trial

Hannah ME, Hannah WJ, Hellman J, Hewson S, Milner R, William A, Canadian Multicenter Post-Term Pregnancy Trial Group (Women's College Hosp, Univ of Toronto; Hosp for Sick Children, Toronto; McMaster Univ, Hamilton Ont

N Engl J Med 326:1587–1592, 1992 2–3

Background.—Post-term pregnancy rates of perinatal mortality and neonatal morbidity are higher than those for term pregnancies. Whether labor induction results in better outcomes than serial fetal monitoring while awaiting spontaneous labor is not known.

Methods.—A total of 3,407 women with uncomplicated pregnancies of 41 or more weeks' duration were studied. The women were assigned to labor induction or to serial antenatal monitoring and spontaneous labor. When there was evidence of fetal or maternal compromise, labor was induced or cesarean section done. The intracervical application of prostaglandin E_2 was used to induce labor. Monitoring consisted of counting fetal kicks, nonstress tests, and amniotic-fluid volume assessment.

Outcomes.—Of the 1,701 women in the induction group 21% underwent cesarean section compared with 25% of the 1,706 in the monitoring group. Fewer cesarean sections were done because of fetal distress in the induction group. Two infants with lethal congenital anomalies were excluded from the analysis. The perinatal deaths in the 2 groups did not differ significantly; there were none in the induction group and 2 in the monitoring group. The 2 groups had similar frequencies of neonatal morbidity.

Conclusion.—Inducing labor in post-term pregnancy results in a lower rate of cesarean section compared with serial antenatal monitoring. The rates of perinatal mortality and neonatal morbidity were comparable.

► This is the second recent attempt to rationalize the management of post-term pregnancy through a collaborative randomized trial comparison of labor induction vs. antenatal monitoring (1). In both trials, fetal and maternal outcomes were uninfluenced by assignment to monitored or induction groups. In this study, only the incidence of cesarean section and evidence of fetal distress were distributed inequitably, both being more common in the antenatal surveillance group. Perhaps the outcome reflected some errors in design. Approximately 90% of the entrants were selected at 41 completed weeks of pregnancy, and it is uncertain how many cases went to 42 completed weeks instead of the diagnostic requirement for post-term pregnancy. One third of those who were assigned randomly to the induction group did not undergo induction of labor, perhaps because many went into spontaneous labor in the 4 days after randomization during which interval induction was scheduled. Because one third of those randomized to the antenatal-monitored subset underwent induction of labor, presumably for abnormal test results, the role of induction of labor in managing this problem cannot be evaluated unquestionably. What's common to both trials is that there is no objective basis for deciding between these 2 options after 287 completed days of gestation.—T.H. Kirschbaum, M.D.

Reference

1. Medearis AL: *Proceedings of the 10th Annual Meeting of the Society of Perinatal Obstetricians,* Jan 23-27, 1990. Washington DC, Society of Perinatal Obstetricians, 1990, p 17.

Calcium Supplementation on Normotensive and Hypertensive Pregnant Women

Knight KB, Keith RE (Univ of Mississippi; Auburn Univ, Ala)

Am J Clin Nutr 55:891–895, 1992 2–4

Background.—Recent studies suggest that there is an inverse relationship between calcium intake and blood pressure. Relatively few clinical intervention studies have been done with hypertensive pregnant women. The effects of supplementing 1 g of calcium per day on blood pressure and ionic and total serum calcium values were studied in hypertensive and normotensive pregnant women.

Methods.—Thirty normotensive and 20 hypertensive pregnant women (aged 18-28 years) were investigated. Each woman was enrolled at approximately 12 weeks' gestation and was observed to term. By random assignment, the women were placed in control or supplemented groups. During the 20-week supplementation period, blood pressure and serum total and ionic calcium were measured.

Findings.—Calcium supplementation significantly reduced diastolic blood pressure over the course of the study in the hypertensive women only. The hypertensive women in the control group had a significant decrease in mean serum ionic calcium values during the study. Dietary calcium intake and blood pressure were significantly inversely related.

Conclusion.—Calcium supplementation appears to have a slight lowering effect on diastolic blood pressure in hypertensive pregnant women. At the dosage studied, calcium supplementation did not produce marked changes in blood pressure, total serum calcium, or ionic serum calcium during gestation. However, calcium still may play a role in hypertension during pregnancy.

▶ The authors appropriately decline to draw conclusions of clinical relevance from this study, which reflects the problems of establishing the effectiveness of calcium supplementation on pregnancy-induced hypertension. The study was confined to 50 primigravid women who entered at approximately 12 weeks' gestation; the group was predominantly black, and of the 50 women, 30 were normotensive and 20 were hypertensive at the time of entry (blood pressure greater than 140/85). The hypertensive group was comprised of women who failed the diagnosis of preeclampsia showing first trimester hypertension, most likely reflecting some form of chronic cardiovascular renal disease; mean patient age was 23.4 years. Calcium supplementation to the level of 1 g per day for 20 weeks resulted in no change in the aggregate total or free serum calcium concentration, but that does not entirely exclude the possibility of any benefit from the supplementation. In the hypertensive group, the mean blood pressure changed in the 20-week treatment period from 146.1/87.7 to 144/86.8. In the hypertensive control group, the final mean blood pressure was 146.7/86.3. Although the authors point to a statistical significance of the 5% level for a reduction in the mean diastolic blood pressure in supplemented hypertensives, for reasons that simply are inexplicable, that difference stems largely from a variance in the final mean diastolic blood pressure in the treated group, which is .1% to .5%, rather than from normotensive diastolic blood pressure values. These results have no bearing on preeclampsia, and they may pertain to chronic hypertension in pregnancy; however, they likely represent no changes of any significance.—T.H. Kirschbaum, M.D.

Fetal Fibronectin in Cervical and Vaginal Secretions as a Predictor of Preterm Delivery

Lockwood CJ, Senyei AE, Dische MR, Casal D, Shah KD, Thung SN, Jones L, Deligdisch L, Garite TJ (Mount Sinai School of Medicine, New York; Adeza

Biomedical, Sunnyvale, Calif; Univ of California at Irvine)
N Engl J Med 325:669–674, 1991 2–5

Background.—The leading cause of neonatal mortality in the United States is preterm delivery. However, efforts to address the problem are hindered because physicians cannot accurately predict which pregnancies are at risk. It has been hypothesized that damage to the fetal mem-

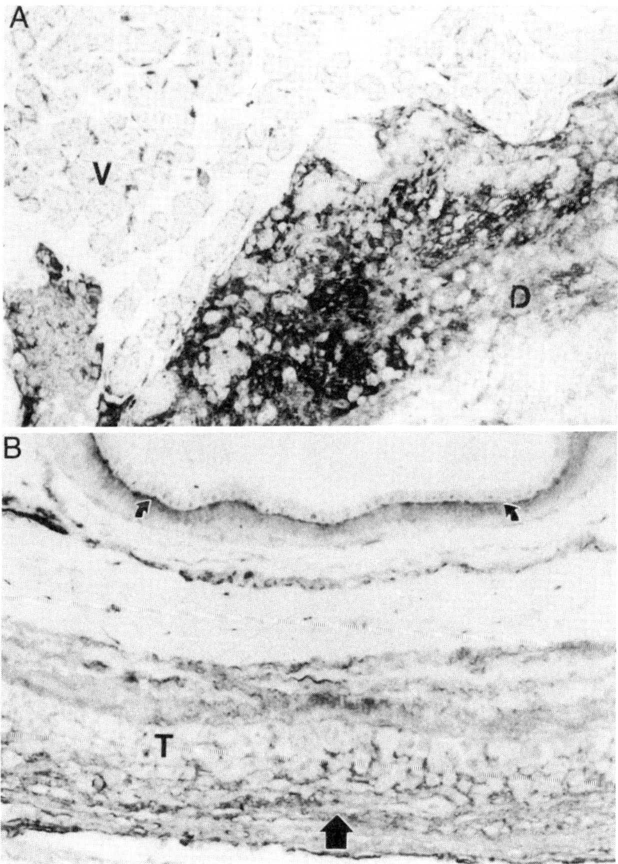

Fig 2–2.—Immunohistochemical studies of fetal fibronectin. Formalin-fixed paraffin-embedded tissue sections were immunohistochemically stained with fetal-fibronectin–specific monoclonal antibody FDC-6. **A,** uteroplacental junction in a woman with pregnancy at term has distinct band of brownish staining for fetal fibronectin in extracellular matrix of decidua basalis (*D*) adjacent to intervillous space, with progressively less decidual staining for fetal fibronectin distal to this site. Chorionic villous trophoblasts (*V*) did not stain for fetal fibronectin. There is no cytoplasmic staining for fetal fibronectin (×20). In **B,** amniochorionic membrane and adjacent decidua from a woman with uncomplicated pregnancy at term have brownish staining for fetal fibronectin from amniotic basement membrane (*arrows*) through the chorion to the adjacent attached decidua (*D*). The most intense staining for fetal fibronection is near the chorionic trophoblasts (*T*) (×200). (Courtesy of Lockwood CJ, Senyei AE, Dische MR, et al: *N Engl J Med* 325:669–674, 1991.)

branes may release fetal fibronectin into the cervix and vagina, giving rise to a biochemical marker for preterm delivery.

Methods.—A sensitive immunoassay using the monoclonal antibody FDC-6 was used to measure fetal levels of fibronectin in cervical and vaginal secretions, amniotic fluid, and maternal plasma. The distribution of fetal fibronectin in the placenta and amniochorionic membranes and its cell of origin were determined through immunohistochemical studies.

Results.—One hundred sixty-three women with uncomplicated pregnancies who delivered at term rarely had cervicovaginal fetal levels of fibronectin greater than .05 μg/mL between 21 and 37 weeks' gestation. Among 65 women with preterm rupture of the membranes, 93.8% had high levels of fetal fibronectin in the amniotic fluid and in the cervical or vaginal secretions. Cervical or vaginal fetal fibronectin was also found in 50.4% of 117 women with preterm uterine contractions and intact membranes. Its presence identified the women who delivered before term with a sensitivity of 81.7% and a specificity of 82.5%. Fetal fibronectin was detected at points of contact with the uterine wall in the placenta and membranes (Fig 2–2).

Conclusion.—A subgroup of women who are at high risk for preterm delivery can be identified by the presence of cervicovaginal fetal fibronectin in the second and third trimesters of pregnancy. This may reflect the separation of the chorion from the decidual layer of the uterus, with the release of intact or degraded chorionic components of the extracellular matrix into the cervical and vaginal secretions.

▶ Detection of higher-than-normal concentrations of this protein in cervical and vaginal secretions may serve to define with greater reliability a subset of women who are in threatened preterm labor and in whom the use of tocolytics or other therapeutics may be applied with greater possibility of discerned effectiveness. The problem is clearly seen when one looks at clinical evaluation of β-adrenergic tocolytics. When women with threatened preterm labor are treated with such agents, maintenance of pregnancy results in many of the experimental subjects; however, roughly the same "effectiveness" is seen in women who, as alternative controls, are not given tocolytics. An inescapable conclusion is that many women who present in preterm labor and are treated by these agents are not in prodomal labor and don't benefit from therapy. The sensitivity and specificity values in this study suggest that oncofetal fibronectin may be useful in excluding those women at low risk of progressing into labor without therapy.

Of equal importance is the possible role of this ground substance component in the attachment of trophoblastic epithelium to the decidua in the course of placentation. Note that histological distribution finds it maximally present in precisely such areas. It is understandable why, in early placental attachment, the material should be obtainable in the lower reproductive tract. Similarly, if the Liggens hypothesis is applicable to humans, some decidual-placental disruption likely precedes the onset of labor at term, resulting in the extraovular escape of this extracellular maxtrix protein. This is an excellent example of the immediate clinical promise of an item of basic research into the mechanisms of placentation.—T.H. Kirschbaum, M.D.

Endomyocardial Ultrastructural Findings in Preeclampsia

Barton JR, Hiett AK, O'Connor WN, Nissen SE, Greene JW Jr (Univ of Kentucky, Lexington)

Am J Obstet Gynecol 165:389–391, 1991 2–6

Background.—The exact cause of preeclampsia remains unknown; however, specific ultrastructural aspects consistently are found in tissue from patients with preeclampsia.

Case Report.—A 31-year-old, gravida 4, para 1, aborta 1 woman sought medical attention at nearly 36 weeks' gestation for a 4-day history of worsening shortness of breath. Pulmonary edema was diagnosed, but her condition did not improve with treatment. Invasive hemodynamic monitoring yielded results consistent with pulmonary edema. Within 12 hours of hospitalization, her clinical picture appeared more consistent with severe preeclampsia. A 2,640-g infant was delivered by cesarean section. Because of the patient's atypical presentation, she underwent cardiac catheterization and endomyocardial biopsies 7 days after surgery. Left ventricular dysfunction with anterolateral hypokinesis, but with preserved left ventricular systolic and diastolic function, was found. She had minimal coronary artery disease. Microscopic assessment of the endomyocardial biopsy specimen showed myocardial fiber hypertrophy with focal interstitial fibrosis. Electron micrographs showed a diffuse, extensive degenerative process. Prominent swelling of the endothelial cell cytoplasm with luminal narrowing, bleb formation, and red blood cell trapping were noted in small blood vessels

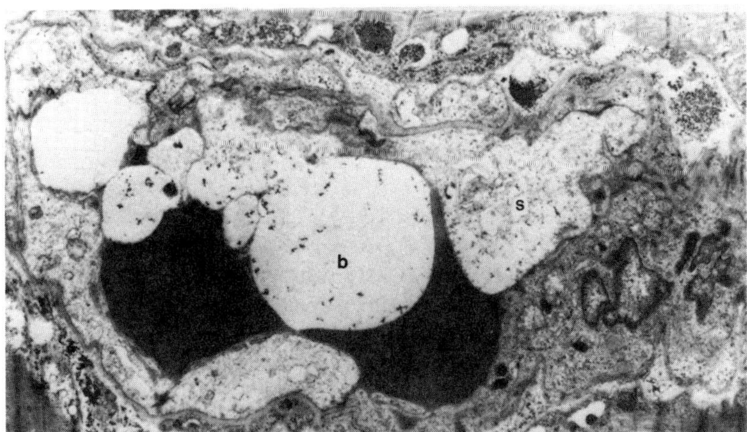

Fig 2–3.—Electron micrograph of intramyocardial vessel showing endothelial cell swelling (*s*), blebs of disrupted endothelial cell cytoplasm (*b*), and erythrocytes (*e*). Glutaraldehyde fixation and Epon embedment. Uranyl acetate-lead citrate; original magnification, ×6,000, reduced by 24%. (Courtesy of Barton JR, Hiett AK, O'Connor WN, et al: *Am J Obstet Gynecol* 165:389–391, 1991.)

(Fig 2-3). Cardiac myocyte mitochondria demonstrated swelling and clearing in the matrix. The intramyocardial cristae retracted against the lateral membrane.

Conclusion.—The ultrastructural changes described in the endothelium of the placental bed, uterine boundary vessels, and renal glomeruli from patients with preeclampsia may also occur in the microvasculature of the heart. Recently reported changes in the myometrial smooth muscle cell mitochondrial ultrastructure seen in patients with preeclampsia may also be found in the heart muscle cells.

▶ Following the suggestion of Gunner et al. that endocardial biopsy is useful in the diagnosis of peripartum cardiomyopathy (see the 1988 YEAR BOOK OF OBSTETRICS AND GYNECOLOGY, pp 49–51), these authors have provided us with new information regarding the effects of preeclampsia on the heart. Preeclampsia increasingly is becoming recognized as an endovasculitis with patchy and unpredictable distribution. The organ-referenced preponderance determines the individual characteristics of this broad ranging syndrome, affecting peripheral vascular resistance, renal or hepatic function, brain metabolism, or blood coagulation in all possible combinations, and apparently reflecting in the distribution of the endothelial lesions. In this study, the same endothelial cell swelling and injury with luminal narrowing and impairment of microvascular circulation that is seen most often in the decidual vessels is seen in the myocardial vessels. This case report also makes it clear that not all the pathophysiology of congestive failure in preeclampsia is caused by increased vascular resistance. Myocardial vascular injury is always a possible risk in preeclampsia, and it may be part of the increased sensitivity to volume overload that occurs in such patients.—T.H. Kirschbaum, M.D.

Prevention of Fetal Growth Retardation With Low-Dose Aspirin: Findings of the EPREDA Trial

Uzan S, Beaufils M, Breart G, Bazin B, Capitant C, Paris J (Hôpital Tenon, Paris; INSERM U 149, Paris; Laboratoires Théramex, Bagnolet, France)

Lancet 337:1429–1431, 1991 2–7

Background.—Aspirin has long been known to prevent arterial thrombosis. The results of several studies have suggested that low-dose aspirin can prevent preeclampsia and/or fetal growth retardation. A trial was designed to test the efficacy of this treatment and to determine whether the administration of dipyridamole improves the efficacy of aspirin.

Methods.—Twenty-five centers took part in the randomized, placebo-controlled trial conducted between 1985 and 1989. The women included in the study had had a previous pregnancy with fetal growth retardation and were seen at 15–18 weeks since the last menstrual period. In the first phase of the trial, treatment (aspirin or aspirin plus dipyridamole) was compared with placebo. In the second phase of the trial, the 2 treatment groups were compared.

Results.—Of 323 patients who entered the study, 284 conformed with all requirements of the protocol. In the first phase, mean birth weight was significantly higher in the treated group, and proteinuria was significantly more common in the placebo group. The frequency of poor outcomes in the treated group was about half that in the placebo group, a difference primarily attributable to the different rates of fetal growth retardation. Women with 2 or more pregnancies with poor outcome received the greatest benefit from treatment. The second phase of the trial showed no apparent advantage to the addition of dipyridamole (225 mg/day).

Conclusion.—Although the use of aspirin has been discouraged in pregnant women, there is as yet no evidence of a definite risk from the low dose (150 mg/day) used in this study. Use of low-dose aspirin for pregnant women at high risk is recommended, although the benefit vs. risk ratio should be weighed carefully in each case.

▶ This is another in a series of European trials of the prophylactic efficacy of aspirin in the prevention of cardiovascular complications of pregnancy (see the 1991 YEAR BOOK OF OBSTETRICS AND GYNECOLOGY, pp 27–30, for other studies and their rationale). In this study, the dosage was 150 mg of aspirin per day, with or without dipyridamole, 225 mg per day. The latter, which is an agent of possible use as a coronary vasodilator, was used as a possible potentiator of the effects of aspirin on cyclooxygenase activity. It appeared to have no effect. The results of the double-blind prospective comparison with placebo were not impressive. Only a lesser incidence of proteinuria met a test of statistical significance among the aspirin users, and only a subset of women with 2 prior poor pregnancy outcomes (the nature of those outcomes not defined) showed any apparent benefit in outcome from aspirin use. This 25-center study involving 156 treated patients and 73 controls must be characterized as failing to show an effect of low-dose aspirin administered for nearly the latter half of pregnancy. Many more such studies like this are on their way to press.—T.H. Kirschbaum, M.D.

Renal Vascular Hypertension During Pregnancy

Easterling TR, Brateng D, Goldman ML, Strandness DE, Zaccardi MJ (Univ of Washington, Seattle)

Obstet Gynecol 78:921–925, 1991 2–8

Introduction.—Although renal artery stenosis is a common cause of secondary hypertension, it is rarely diagnosed during pregnancy. Only 14 pregnancies complicated by renovascular hypertension have been reported in the literature. In 1 new case, transluminal angioplasty was performed during the pregnancy; in another, the procedure was performed postpartum.

Case 1.—Woman, 34, who was nulliparous, had a blood pressure of 180/120 mm Hg at 8 weeks' gestation. Methyldopa therapy for 10 weeks did not reduce her blood pressure, and she was referred at 19 weeks' gestation. Renal duplex ultrasound revealed a greater than 60% reduction in the diameter of the right main renal artery. Because the prognosis for the pregnancy seemed poor, the patient underwent angioplasty at 20 weeks' gestation. The angiographic findings were consistent with fibromuscular hyperplasia of the right renal artery. After angioplasty, the hypertension resolved and the vascular resistance decreased from 2,455 to 1,600 dyne/sec/cm^{-5}; however, it did not reach normal pregnant levels. The pregnancy was carried to term without complications, and the patient delivered a normal infant weighing 2,740 g.

Case 2.—Woman, 34, had a blood pressure of 132/88 mm Hg at 10 weeks' gestation. Renal duplex ultrasound examination revealed a greater than 60% reduction in the diameter of the right renal artery. She was followed expectantly, but at 39 weeks her blood pressure acutely increased to 138/100 mm Hg. Labor was induced, and she delivered a normal infant (weighing 3,490 g) without complications. At 8 weeks' post partum, her blood pressure was 128/68 mm Hg. At 12 weeks' post partum, it again increased to 145/115 mm Hg, and the patient underwent transluminal angioplasty, which resolved the hypertension. The results of renal angiography were consistent with fibromuscular hyperplasia.

Conclusion.—Women who are persistently hypertensive in the first half of pregnancy should be evaluated with duplex sonography of the renal artery. When maternal hypertension secondary to renal artery stenosis cannot be managed medically, transluminal angioplasty is an important alternative to pregnancy termination.

▶ Hypertension caused by unilateral renal artery stenosis is surely underdiagnosed in pregnancy, and these case reports are useful in 2 respects. Use of Doppler velocity readings from the renal arteries makes renal arteriography unnecessary, and x-ray exposures necessary to cannulate renal arteries via the aorta and to follow the dye injections are probably contraindicated. On the other hand, Bernoulli's principle assures exceptionally high velocity flow through a stenotic conduit vessel and makes it possible to diagnose the lesion with ultrasound. Note that in neither of these cases were plasma renin or urine aldosterone measurements reported in confirmation of the diagnosis. Second, the ability to make the diagnosis during pregnancy is enhanced in value by the ability to treat the arterial lesions transluminally at the cost (in case 1) of .1 Gy of radiation exposure. The authors' recommendation that renal artery velocimetry be used in women with first trimester hypertension seems sound.—T.H. Kirschbaum, M.D.

Calcium Supplementation to Prevent Hypertensive Disorders of Pregnancy

Belizán JM, Villar J, Gonzalez L, Campodonico L, Bergel E (Centro Rosarino

de Estudios Perinatales, Rosario, Argentina)
N Engl J Med 325:1399–1405, 1991 2–9

Introduction.—An inverse relationship between calcium intake and gestational hypertension and eclampsia has been described in previous studies. Further investigations have suggested that hypertensive disorders in pregnancy may be prevented by reducing blood pressure through changes in calcium metabolism.

Methods.—The results of a large, double-blind trial of the preventive effect of supplemental calcium in 1,194 nulliparous women in week 20 of gestation were reviewed. The entry criteria included blood pressure less than 140/90 mm Hg and no evidence of present or past disease. The women were randomly assigned to receive calcium carbonate, 2 g/day, or placebo.

Results.—There were 588 women in the placebo group and 579 in the calcium group who were available for final analyses. The risk of a diagnosis of a hypertensive disorder of pregnancy was significantly lower in the calcium group, particularly after week 28 of gestation. The overall rate of hypertensive disorders was 14.8% in the placebo group and 9.8% in the calcium group. Among the women who had low ratios of urinary calcium to urinary creatinine at study entry, those who received calcium had a lower risk of hypertensive disorders of pregnancy and less of an increase in diastolic and systolic blood pressure than those assigned to receive placebo.

Conclusion.—Calcium supplementation may be beneficial in reducing the risk of hypertension in men and nonpregnant women. Although the calcium treatment had no side effects, pregnant women should be screened for a history of renal disease and chronic urinary tract infections. The value of calcium supplementation in preventing preeclampsia and pregnancy-induced hypertension remains to be established.

▶ This is a most thorough investigation of the possible relationship between pregnancy hypertension and calcium intake. The daily dose of calcium carbonate (2 g) is very large, and it is likely to be tolerated by only the most highly motivated patients because of its gastrointestinal effects. The data support the contention that at least two thirds of the women receiving calcium supplementation increased their urinary calcium excretion. It is interesting that preeclampsia represented only approximately half the cases of hypertension noted in this group of primigravidas with a mean age of 20–20.8 years. Only the life-table data array purports to show the significant reduction of hypertension as a result of calcium supplementation.

For the most part, other comparative observations have a risk ratio in which the 95% confidence range includes unity and, therefore, they show no significant effect at the $P = .05$ level. This lack of significance was true for the risk ratios for the development of preeclampsia, the rates of occurrence of hypertension in both low and high baseline calcium excretion values, and the mean adjusted systolic and diastolic blood pressures and pulse pressures. Significant differences were seen only in blood pressure at follow-up exam after delivery and in the risk ratios for overall hypertension of pregnancy, combining preeclampsia and exogenous hypertension of pregnancy. No benefit appeared to accrue from the use of calcium supplementation in that regard. Therefore, the role of calcium in pregnancy preeclampsia cannot be assayed in this study. Data from other investigators purport to show a benefit from calcium supplementation in men and nonpregnant women. Perhaps it is the long-term benefit from calcium supplementation, independent of pregnancy, which results from what little benefit is seen here.—T.H. Kirschbaum, M.D.

Randomized Comparative Trial of Indomethacin and Ritodrine for the Long-Term Treatment of Preterm Labor

Besinger RE, Niebyl JR, Keyes WG, Johnson TRB (Johns Hopkins Hosp; Francis Scott Key Med Ctr, Baltimore)

Am J Obstet Gynecol 164:981–988, 1991 2–10

Introduction.—Indomethacin has been evaluated in several trials for its efficacy in inhibiting preterm labor, but some reports suggest that the agent may have adverse effects on the neonate. A randomized trial was designed to evaluate the efficacy and side effects of indomethacin compared with ritodrine, the only tocolytic agent currently approved by the Food and Drug Administration for treatment of preterm labor.

Patients.—Women recruited for the study were between 23 and 34 weeks' gestation and had preterm contractions and documented cervical change. They were randomly assigned to receive either ritodrine intravenously or indomethacin orally as the first-line tocolytic agent. Failure was defined as subsequent rupture of the membranes, cervical dilation greater than 5 cm, or clinical evidence of chorioamnionitis or oligohydramnios.

Results.—The 2 agents were equally successful in delaying preterm labor. The criteria for success included attainment of the 35th week of gestation, a delay of delivery greater than 7 days, infant birth weight, and the need for intravenous magnesium sulfate therapy. Clinical evidence of primary pulmonary hypertension appeared in 3 neonates in the indomethacin group. In 2 infants, a twin pregnancy, this complication may have been attributable to growth retardation. All 3 infants who experienced pulmonary hypertension are now alive and well.

Conclusion.—Indomethacin appears to be as effective as ritodrine in inhibiting preterm labor. However, prolonged treatment (longer than 48 hours) with indomethacin may carry an increased risk for primary pulmonary hypertension. The cost differential between the 2 agents is considerable: $560 for intravenous ritodrine therapy and $33 for short-term oral indomethacin therapy.

▶ This study reflects most of the problems that appear in the evaluation of pharmacological agents in the treatment of preterm labor. Indomethacin is shown to be equally effective as ritodrine, but no comparison with untreated controls is included. This is important, because the incidence of spontaneous cessation of uterine contractions in untreated women who meet these entry criteria is very large, and because, in this study, most women failed to show a significant impact of drug therapy. The authors refer to their own studies of 15 patients, in which patients given indomethacin therapy were compared with "untreated" controls, and in which prolongation of pregnancy was noted to be significantly more common in indomethacin-treated women than in controls for a period of 48 hours. This comparison suffered from small numbers of cases, successive withdrawal of cases and, therefore, decreasing numbers of subjects, because some went into labor during the 48-hour span. Also, 30% of the controls were treated with tocolytics as well. No one has been able to document any value in such prolongation in terms of reductions in perinatal morbidity/mortality or in the incidence of respiratory distress syndrome.

Using an agent that has been demonstrated to prolong pregnancy by, at most, 48 hours, one can only conclude that most of the 18 ritodrine-treated women with approximately 28 days' prolongation of pregnancy and the 23 women treated with indomethacin (average prolongation of pregnancy, 25.5 days) must have been instances of false labor at the time of treatment. The authors' evaluation of the potential of indomethacin to be associated with newborn pulmonary hypertension after prolonged use is valuable. However, this work proves nothing about the value of either agent in arresting preterm labor.—T.H. Kirschbaum, M.D.

Adjunctive Clindamycin Therapy for Preterm Labor: Results of a Double-Blind, Placebo-Controlled Trial

McGregor JA, French JI, Seo K (Univ of Colorado Health Sciences Ctr, Denver)

Am J Obstet Gynecol 165:867–875, 1991 2–11

Objective.—The efficacy, safety, and tolerance of clindamycin used as adjunctive antimicrobial therapy in hospitalized women with idiopathic preterm labor were evaluated in a double-blind, placebo-controlled, randomized trial.

Treatment.—A group of 103 women who were hospitalized at ≤ 34 weeks' gestation and were treated with parenteral tocolytic agents for idiopathic preterm labor received either 900 mg of intravenous clindamycin every 8 hours for 9 doses or an identical appearing lactose placebo. Intravenous therapy was followed by 300 mg of oral clindamycin administered 4 times daily for 4 days.

Results.—Preterm birth (< 37 weeks' gestation) occurred in 62% of the women. Univariate analysis showed the pregnancies continued significantly longer in women treated with clindamycin (mean, 35.3 days) than in women treated with placebo (mean, 25.4 days). Survival analysis showed the pregnancies continued at least 35.5 days in 50% of the women who were given clindamycin, compared with 20 days for 50% of the patients treated with placebo. When controlling for gestational age at enrollment, clindamycin treatment was associated with an increased interval to delivery only among those mothers enrolled before 33 weeks' gestation. Side effects, most commonly nausea and vomiting, were reported in 28% of the clindamycin-treated women and in 32% of the placebo-treated women. Analysis of obstetric and microbiological parameters in relation to treatment outcomes showed that preterm birth occurred significantly more often among women with bacterial vaginosis than among women without bacterial vaginosis. Clindamycin treatment in women with bacterial vaginosis was associated with trends for prolongation of pregnancy, increased birth weight, and an increased mean gestational age at delivery. Preterm premature rupture of membranes occurred more frequently in women with either group B streptococcus, *Chlamydia trachomatis, Trichomonas vaginalis*, or *Staphylococcus aureus* infection. Clindamycin treatment reduced the incidence of preterm premature rupture of membranes in these women to that found in uninfected women.

Conclusion.—Although adjunctive clindamycin therapy for preterm labor appears to be safe and effective, its benefits are limited to those women who are seen at or before 32 weeks' gestation.

▶ This is as close as anyone has come to proving the value of antibiotic therapy for preterm labor. The antibiotic chosen has general effectiveness against organisms for which a suggestive role in chorioamnionitis has been proposed. It is distributed in the amniotic fluid and, presumably, in the fetal membranes in relatively high concentrations; it appears to have a role in enhancing segments of general host immunity. Drug treatment proved effective in reducing—but not abolishing—mycoplasma, *Gardnerella vaginalis*, and the organisms associated with bacterial vaginosis. The principal finding was an average increase of 10 days from treatment to delivery. Despite this, the mean gestational age at enrollment for patients given clindamycin (30.5 weeks) and controls (31 weeks), and the mean gestational age at delivery (35.4 and 34.9, respectively) were not statistically significantly different. That can only indicate the presence of outliers that affect the mean values of the differences between entry and delivery dates. The basis for claiming an effect from antibiotics only in those patients enrolled at or before 32 weeks' gestation is not apparent in the data, and it may be a part of the distribution of outliers. In any event, there is more reason to support the antibiotic treatment of patients with preterm labor in the second trimester than was apparent earlier (see the 1991 YEAR BOOK OF OBSTETRICS AND GYNECOLOGY, pp 43–44).—T.H. Kirschbaum, M.D.

A Meta-Analysis of Low-Dose Aspirin for the Prevention of Pregnancy-Induced Hypertensive Disease

Imperiale TF, Petrulis AS (Case Western Reserve Univ, Cleveland; Metro-Health Med Ctr, Cleveland)

JAMA 266:261–265, 1991 2–12

Introduction.—Pregnancy-induced hypertension (PIH) occurs in 5% to 15% of pregnancies and is associated with maternal and neonatal morbidity. Six published controlled trials from 1980–1990 found that aspirin given in small doses during the second and third trimesters reduces the risk of PIH. A meta-analysis was conducted to determine the magnitude of protection of aspirin from PIH, the risk of adverse effects, and the effect of aspirin on infants with severe low birth weight (SLBW) and also on cesarean section and perinatal mortality.

Methods.—Meta-analysis is a relatively new research method that allows pooling of the results across trials to yield a more precise estimate of treatment effect. Study methods in the 6 trials were critically and independently evaluated and assigned a quality score, and the quantitative outcome data were abstracted. For each outcome, both relative risk (RR) and the number needed to be treated were calculated.

Results.—The outcomes of isolated hypertension and proteinuric hypertension were combined in the meta-analysis. The RR and PIH among 394 women who took aspirin in 6 trials was .35, and the number who needed to be treated was 4.4. The risk of SLBW, defined as less than the 10th percentile for gestational age, was reduced by 44%. The risk of cesarean section was reduced by 66% overall, with delivery by cesarean section occurring in 36% of the women in the control group. However, the specific indications for cesarean section were not described, and combining trials for this outcome may not be appropriate statistically. Aspirin had no effect on fetal and neonatal death. There were no maternal or fetal adverse effects associated with taking aspirin.

Conclusion.—Low-dose aspirin reduces the risk of PIH and SLBW with no maternal or neonatal adverse effects.

▶ This statistical device is useful in raising to statistical significance inferences from the results of several studies of usually small numbers and power, no single study of which is conclusive. The risks implicit in the method come from the many judgments that must be made by the analyst regarding the quality of the studies and their comparability before they are pooled for analysis. This report demonstrates some of the problems.

The 6 reports studied all concluded that aspirin was useful in preventing PIH. It is not surprising that this conclusion clearly emerges from meta-analysis; as always, the problems rest with the associated outcomes. With respect to reduction of the instances of cesarean section, the result is strongly influenced by the 4 studies deemed of high quality with respect to randomization, blinding, inclusion and exclusion characteristics, etc. For those 4 studies, the risk ratio for cesarean section was apparently reduced; in the other 2 studies, the risk was apparently uninfluenced by aspirin. Measurements of heterogeneity indicate that these 6 studies differ sufficiently, making pooling questionably appropriate. In the prevention of intrauterine growth retardation, a risk ratio significantly less than 1 is seen only from the 2 studies of lower quality, which casts doubts on the validity of pooled results. No effect on perinatal death rates is claimed. We are left with the conclusions which stem from reading the 6 papers individually. Aspirin appears to reduce the instance of PIH when given in the fashion described. Its effect on other outcomes remains arguable.—T.H. Kirschbaum, M.D.

The Imbalance Between Thromboxane and Prostacyclin in Preeclampsia Is Associated With an Imbalance Between Lipid Peroxides and Vitamin E in Maternal Blood

Wang Y, Walsh SW, Guo J, Zhang J (Med College of Virginia, Richmond; Harbin Med College, Harbin, People's Republic of China)

Am J Obstet Gynecol 165:1695–1700, 1991 2–13

Introduction.—The development of preeclampsia during pregnancy depends on the ratio of prostacyclin to thromboxane in the woman's serum, with the vasodilator prostacyclin increasing as the condition worsens. Throughout a normal pregnancy, the ratio of vitamin E to lipid peroxides in blood also changes so that vitamin E increases as time passes. Possible lipid peroxides and antioxidant activity imbalances in preeclampsia were assessed and compared with imbalances in the prostacyclin and thromboxane ratio.

Methods.—Twelve women donated blood samples during the 36–40 weeks of gestation. The results of serum analysis for postacyclin, thromboxane, lipid peroxides, and antioxidants from these normal subjects were compared with the test outcomes from 16 patients with mild preeclampsia and 19 patients with severe preeclampsia.

Results.—Figure 2–4 presents the lipid peroxide and vitamin E levels in all 3 groups of patients. Those patients with mild preeclampsia had significantly higher lipid peroxides compared with normal subjects, but peroxides increased still further in those with severe preeclampsia. The vitamin E concentrations remained unaltered in patients with mild preeclampsia, but they decreased significantly in those with severe preeclampsia. Thromboxane significantly increased in severe preeclampsia, but a metabolite of prostacyclin significantly decreased in both mild and severe disease. The ratios of thromboxane to prostacyclin and lipid peroxides to vitamin E both increased in mild preeclampsia and increased even further in the severe condition. The 2 ratios highly correlated with each other.

Conclusion.—Preeclampsia is related to imbalances between thromboxane and prostacyclin and lipid peroxides and vitamin E in the woman's blood. As the severity of the condition progresses, these imbal-

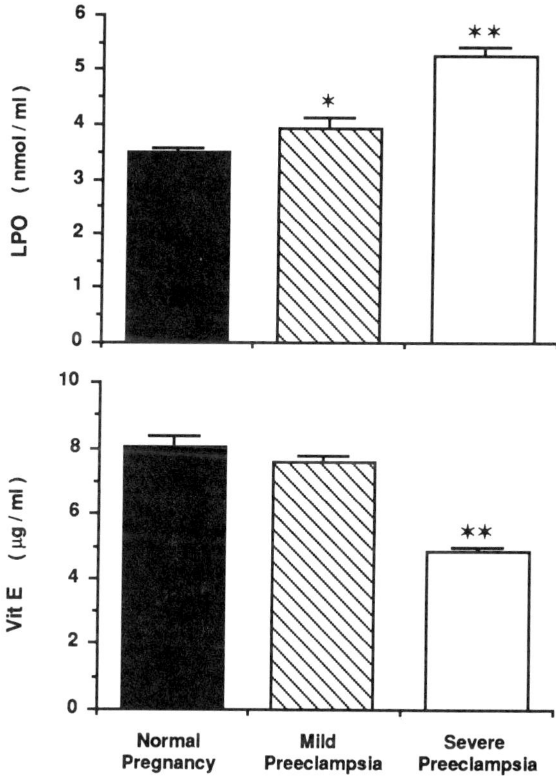

Fig 2–4.—The maternal serum concentrations of lipid peroxides (*LPO*) and vitamin E (*Vit E*) in normal pregnancy and in mild and severe preeclampsia between 36 and 40 weeks of gestation. The data represent mean ± SE. *Asterisk*, $P < .05$; *2 asterisks*, $P < .01$ (compared with normal pregnancy). (Courtesy of Wang Y, Walsh SW, Guo J, et al: *Am J Obstet Gynecol* 165:1695–1700, 1991.)

ances stress thromboxane and the lipid peroxides. The imbalance between the lipid peroxides and vitamin E may cause prostacyclin synthesis to be reduced and endothelial cell injury to occur.

▶ In preeclampsia, some mechanism produces endothelial cell injury in vivo and endothelial cell cultures in vitro (1). The 2 leading candidates for this function are maternal antibodies against fetal epitopes with cross-reactivity to human endothelium and increases in lipid peroxidases produced and acting in paracrine fashion, i.e., on cells immediately adjacent to the cells of origin. In this study, the serum concentrations of lipid peroxides seem to be increased in proportion to the severity of preeclampsia; vitamin E, which is a dietary-derived antioxidant, seem to be reduced correspondingly. Bear in mind that serum concentration provides a somewhat distorted view of what's happening at the tissue sites, because it represents bloodborne presence of a paracrine—not endocrine—agent. Remember also that the co-relationship of these changes cannot be used to differentiate between a causal relationship or an effect on both vitamin E and lipid peroxides by some other unrecognized agent.—T.H. Kirschbaum, M.D.

Reference

1. Roberts JM, et al: *Am J Obstet Gynecol* 161:1200, 1989.

High Risk of HIV-1 Infection for First-Born Twins

Goedert JJ, Duliège A-M, Amos CI, Felton S, Biggar RJ, and The International Registry of HIV-Exposed Twins (Natl Cancer Inst, Rockville, Md; Genentech Inc, South San Francisco; Research Triangle Inst, Washington, DC)

Lancet 338:1471–1475, 1991 2–14

Introduction.—The transmission of HIV-1 from mother to infant occurs only in 13% to 40% of cases assessed in prospective population studies. The mode of transmission, whether by free virus or through maternal cells, remains unknown. The epidemiology and natural history of mother-to-infant transmission of HIV-1 infection, particularly genetic and intrapartum exposure factors, were investigated in twins.

Methods.—Cases were recruited from a registry of physicians, obstetricians, and infectious disease personnel. Those participating in the study provided demographic, clinical, and epidemiological information about the female patients with HIV-1 and their children. Both infected and uninfected offspring underwent a series of laboratory tests specific for HIV-1 detection.

Results.—Information from 100 sets of twins and 1 set of triplets showed that HIV-1 infection occurred significantly more often in the twin who was born first (twin A) than in the twin who was born second (twin B). For vaginal deliveries, 16 of 32 firstborn twins and 10 of 26 second-born twins had HIV-1 infection, whereas in cesarean deliveries, 6 of 32 firstborn and 5 of 26 second-born twins had the infection. Data analysis demonstrated that the first twin born had a significantly greater chance of contracting HIV-1 infection than did twin B when both were delivered vaginally, but not when both were delivered by cesarean section. The infection occurred slightly more often in dizygotic than in monozygotic twins. Maternal race, gestational age, and AIDS status of the mother did not influence the HIV-1 transmission rates.

Conclusion.—The risk of HIV-1 transmission was the highest for the first twin delivered vaginally, second highest for the first twin delivered by cesarean section, and third highest for the second twin delivered by either method. A placebo-controlled, randomized clinical study is warranted to determine whether cleaning the birth canal could reduce the rate of HIV-1 infection in the newborns. Cesarean delivery should not be used routinely for all HIV-1-positive pregnant women.

▶ This collaborative collection of data from 9 countries has changed the views of many by increasing the evidence for fetal HIV infection from affected mothers via the birth canal as opposed to in utero hematogenous infection. Newborn infection was defined by the presence of characteristic findings of infection, or by persistence of newborn IgG past 15 months of age. The overall 51.5% incidence of fetal transmission is slightly higher than the reported 25% to 30% figure for singlet pregnancies. Of 32 sets of twins with evidence of infection, only 10 sets (31%) showed both fetuses to be infected. Although the risk of infecting either twin A or B was lower with abdominal birth than with vaginal delivery, the difference was not statistically significant. The risk for infection of twin B only among cases of discordant infection was approximately 15%. If that figure represents the occurrence of in utero hematogenous infection, then the effect of vaginal first birth is roughly to increase the risk to twin A by 6-fold. There remains the possibility that twin A is rendered increasingly susceptible to infection from viruses transmitted from the vagina and cervix through the intact chorlion levae in direct contact with the lower birth canal. This observation raises questions regarding both the advisability of abdominal birth and attempts of disinfection of the birth canal in hopes of decreasing the risk of fetal infection from HIV-1–infected mothers.—T.H. Kirschbaum, M.D.

Randomized Controlled Trial of Antenatal Social Support to Prevent Preterm Birth

Bryce RL, Stanley FJ, Garner JB (Finders Med Ctr, Bedford Park, Australia; Princess Margaret Hosp for Children, Subiaco, Australia)

Br J Obstet Gynaecol 98:1001–1008, 1991 2–15

Introduction.—Stress in pregnancy is associated with preterm birth and low birth weight. A randomized controlled trial was designed to test the effect of a program of additional antenatal social support in the home on the occurrence of preterm birth in a cohort of women at high risk of such an event.

Study Design.—Of 1,970 pregnant women with poor obstetric histories, 983 were randomly assigned to receive additional antenatal social support, and 987 were assigned to the control group. All women received normal antenatal care either at public hospital antenatal clinics or at the private offices of obstetricians and general practitioners. Five midwives received some training in providing expressive social support, concentrating on listening skills and personal interaction. Each study woman received home visits from a single midwife at 4- to 6-week intervals, with intervening telephone calls made as desired.

Results.—There were 126 (12.8%) preterm births in the special social support group and 147 (14.9%) preterm births in the control group. Thus, a clinically significant reduction in preterm births was not obtained.

Conclusion.—Antenatal social support interventions in the home are not effective in preventing preterm birth in a high-risk population of women.

▶ This subject was first reviewed in the YEAR BOOK in a report by Papieirnik et al. (see the 1987 YEAR BOOK OF OBSTETRICS AND GYNECOLOGY, pp 60–62); it was later reviewed in the form of the contradictory evidence by Main et al. (see the 1991 YEAR BOOK OF OBSTETRICS AND GYNECOLOGY, pp 131–133). This report constitutes the fourth subsequent, prospective, controlled trial that has failed to demonstrate a beneficial effect of social support on preterm labor. Reasonably enough, the augmented support is provided by midwives (who were trained for that function) in a country where their services are readily accepted by women. This study is uncommon in that it contains a clear discussion of power calculations. A difference resulting from this intervention would have to have a 60% effectiveness to be distinguishable on the basis of these data. That is why combining the results of 4 studies is most useful. An odds ratio of 1.06 for the confidence interval .82–1.36 results—and fairly convincingly refutes—the value of this approach used alone in the treatment of preterm labor.—T.H. Kirschbaum, M.D.

Evaluation of a Rapid Screening Test for Detecting Group B Streptococci in Pregnant Women

Granato PA, Petosa MT (State Univ New York Health Science Ctr, Syracuse; Community-Gen Hosp, Syracuse)

J Clin Microbiol 29:1536–1538, 1991 2–16

Background.—Group B streptococci (GBS) infection carries a mortality rate of 20% to 30% in newborns. Previous studies have shown that GBS-associated mortality can be significantly reduced by the intrapartum treatment of pregnant women colonized with GBS. Because routine culture is a time-consuming process, the accuracy of a rapid enzyme immunoassay (EIA) for the detection of GBS colonization in women in early labor was assessed in 331 pregnant women.

Methods.—Vaginal or cervical samples were prepared for culture and examined with the QUIDEL Group B Strep Test. A positive GBS control, included in the kit, was performed with each test assay. The culture plates were incubated for 48 hours and examined daily for the presence of bacterial growth. The entire EIA can be performed in less than 10 minutes.

Results.—Cultures detected GBS in 19 women. Compared with culture, the EIA had a sensitivity of 89%, a specificity of 99%, a positive predictive value of 89%, and a negative predictive value of 99%. Both of the 2 false negative EIA samples grew moderate numbers of GBS on culture. The overall test correlation of EIA with culture was 98.8%.

Conclusion.—Prophylactic administration of ampicillin to all women in labor is neither practical nor desirable. Because the time required for routine culture means that the results will not be available until after delivery, the speed and reliability of the QUIDEL EIA test make it a useful alternative to cultures.

▶ The key to effective prophylaxis of neonatal GBS infection is a screening method that will allow the detection of maternal colonization during labor, early enough to allow effective antibiotic treatment to preclude maternal to fetal transmission of the organism. For that reason, the reported results are interesting; however, interpretation is somewhat misleading. The use of a GBS-positive control incorporated as part of the test protocol is a fine contribution. The problem in interpretation comes from the manufacturer'contention that fewer than 10 colonies per plate should constitute a negative finding. Of course, some assumptions regarding desirable sensitivity must be made to strike a balance between false positive and false negative results, but the exclusion of 4 cases determined negative by this criterion, but which subsequently grew positive cultures, biases the reported results. Inclusion of those 4 cases as being infected reduces sensitivity to approximately 75%. The 99% specificity relates primarily to the low prevalence figure of 5.7%. All in all, this test appears to be worthy of further evaluation, but it probably is not as valuable as this report suggests.—T.H. Kirschbaum, M.D.

Lupus Anticoagulants, Anticardiolipin Antibodies, and Fetal Loss: A Case-Control Study

Infante-Rivard C, David M, Gauthier R, Rivard G-E (Univ of Montreal and McGill Univ, Montreal)

N Engl J Med 325:1063–1066, 1991 2–17

Background.—Both lupus anticoagulants and anticardiolipin antibodies are antibodies directed against negatively charged phospholipids. Although antiphospholipid antibodies often are present in healthy individuals, they also are associated with thrombosis, thrombocytopenia, and fetal loss.

Objective.—The risk of fetal loss in association with these antibodies was examined in a hospital-based case-control study of 331 women with a first spontaneous abortion or fetal death. The control group numbered 993 pregnant women without a history of spontaneous fetal loss.

Findings.—Lupus anticoagulant was identified in 5.1% of the case patients and in 3.8% of controls, for an odds ratio of 1.36. An IgG anticardiolipin level of 5 units or more was found in 1.2% of case patients and 1.5% of controls. The odds ratio for an association of IgG anticardiolipin antibody with fetal loss was .8.

Conclusion.—The results do not warrant considering lupus anticoagulant or IgG anticardiolipin antibody to be risk factors for fetal loss in women with a first spontaneous abortion or fetal death. It remains possible that an association exists for women who have repeated fetal losses.

▶ This case-controlled study forces us to look at the relationship between antiphospholipid antibodies and pregnancy wastage. The primary observation is that the incidence of lupus anticoagulant and anticardiolipin antibody is no greater in women suffering a first spontaneous abortion or mid trimester loss than in a control group chosen to match gestational age. Because approximately 75% of the patients had pregnancy loss equal to or less than 16 weeks' gestation, it would be useful to know the frequency distribution of cases in smaller intervals of gestational age, as well as the incidence of developmental anomaly in both the case and control groups. An interesting question is raised by this tudy: Why, if antiphospholipid antibody development is an important cause of pregnancy loss (as it appears to be when one takes the usual approach of evaluating antibodies in women with multiple losses), is it not in evidence with a first pregnancy loss? One possibility is that multiple pregnancy losses without evident cause might be a discriminator of the important role of these antibodies. Another is that there are important intermediate steps between the development of lupus and anticardiolipin antibody and pregnancy loss, of which so far we know nothing.—T.H. Kirschbaum, M.D.

Should Continuous Hydralazine Infusions Be Utilized in Severe Pregnancy-Induced Hypertension?

Kirshon B, Wasserstrum N, Cotton DB (Baylor College of Medicine, Houston)
Am J Perinatol 8:206–208, 1991 2–18

Introduction.—Intravenous hydralazine may be administered by intermittent bolus therapy or continuous intravenous infusion for blood pressure control in severe preeclampsia. The continuous intravenous infusion method has been associated with a high incidence of fetal distress. The maternal hemodynamic responses to a continuous hydralazine infusion regimen were studied to elucidate the causes of fetal distress.

Methods.—Seven patients with severe preeclampsia who were undergoing right heart catheterization were candidates for blood pressure reduction. After percutaneous catheterization of the right side of the heart, hydralazine was given by continuous intravenous infusion. The starting infusion dose of 5 mg/hr was increased every 15–20 minutes by 1–2 mg/hr to attain either a 20% reduction in the mean arterial blood pressure or a diastolic blood pressure of 90–100 mm Hg. Hemodynamic parameters were evaluated before and after therapy.

Results.—The initial mean systolic blood pressure of 208.3 ± 24.8 mm Hg was reduced to 144 ± 13.6 mm Hg after hydralazine therapy. The mean diastolic blood pressure of 124.3 ± 11.6 mm Hg was reduced to 87 ± 11.6 mm Hg. Although cardiac output increased, the sudden reduction in blood pressure during the continuous intravenous infusion of hydralazine was associated with fetal distress requiring cesarean delivery in 5 of 7 women. The mean hydralazine dose in this study was 16.04 ± 3.65 mg/hr. The prolonged and unpredictable duration and onset of action in association with this dosage schedule may have resulted in the high incidence of fetal distress.

Conclusion.—Continuous intravenous infusion of hydralazine at the dosage schedule described is contraindicated for the treatment of severe preeclampsia. Intermittent bolus therapy is more appropriate for treatment of severe preeclampsia-eclampsia.

▶ The key to this study is that, although a 20% reduction in the mean arterial blood pressure was an aim, an overall reduction of 30% was obtained. This apparently was the result of a secondary therapeutic goal, which was to reduce diastolic blood pressure into the range of 90–120 mm of mercury. This degree of acute blood pressure reduction likely caused the problems noted in the fetus. Hydralazine reduces systemic vascular resistance and increases cardiac output, in part by increasing the heart rate with either no change or a slight reduction in stroke volume. With a decrease of blood pressure and systemic vascular resistance in patients who are often hypovolemic, uteroplacental perfusion decreases, and fetal death with its premonitory signs can be seen. The authors are correct, of course, that both the cardiovascular instability of severe pregnancy-induced hypertension and the relatively long time span (more than 20 minutes) between changes in intravenous infusion rates of hydralazine and changes in systemic vascular resistance make the continuous intravenous route hazardous. To reduce the mean blood pressure by 30% or more makes it potentially lethal to the fetus.—T.H. Kirschbaum, M.D.

Plasma Antiepileptic Drug Concentrations During Pregnancy

Lander CM, Eadie MJ (Univ of Queensland, Herston, Brisbane, Australia)

Epilepsia 32:257–266, 1991 2–19

Introduction.—It has been reported that in epileptic pregnancy, plasma antiepileptic drug (AED) levels tend to decrease relative to AED dosage as pregnancy progresses, resulting in increased seizures and requiring AED dosage adjustments. However, most studies were based on small patient samples. A large group of epileptic women who carried their pregnancy to term were studied.

Patients.—During a 15-year period, 105 epileptic women with a mean age of 24.5 years underwent 134 pregnancies with steady-state plasma AED monitoring throughout the pregnancy and during the postnatal period. Twenty women had 2 pregnancies, 3 had 3 pregnancies, and 1 had 4 pregnancies. Forty-three women primarily had generalized seizures, 48 had partial seizures, and seizure type was not known in 14 women. Antiepileptic drug dosages were adjusted to keep the steady-state plasma AED levels within the accepted therapeutic ranges without waiting for seizure relapse. The dosages also were adjusted if seizures became more frequent, regardless of plasma levels.

Results.—The plasma AED levels decreased with the same AED dosage as taken before pregnancy in a majority of the patients. A decrease in plasma phenytoin (PHT) levels occurred in 58 of 65 pregnancies (89.2%) with PHT monotherapy and remained unchanged in the other 7. Plasma PHT levels were reduced in 35 of 41 pregnancies (85.4%) in which PHT was given in combination with other AEDs. A similar reduction occurred in 10 of 12 pregnancies (83.3%) treated with carbamazepine (CBZ) monotherapy, and in 15 of 31 pregnancies (48.4%) in which CBZ was given with other AEDs. The altered disposition of the AEDs usually began in the first 10 weeks of pregnancy. Complete seizure control data were available for 122 women. Despite AED dosage adjustments during pregnancy, seizure control worsened in 31 patients (25.4%), remained unchanged in 79 (64.8%), and improved in 10 (8.2%). However, 9 women whose seizure control worsened during pregnancy were untreated when they became pregnant. Considering only the 111 women who were receiving AED therapy when they became pregnant, the seizures worsened in 12.7% of those previously fully controlled and in 27.8% of those not previously controlled. Control remain full in 87.3% of those previously fully controlled and became full or improved in only 18.5% of those previously inadequately controlled. Thus, full seizure control before pregnancy was associated with a more favorable outcome for freedom from seizures during pregnancy.

Conclusion.—Seizure control in epileptic women should begin well before pregnancy. Optimal seizure control for a long period before pregnancy will give the best seizure control during pregnancy.

▶ This report of 134 gravidas with seizures provides substantiation of some important clinical perceptions. Experienced neurologists frequently find it necessary to increase medication dosage to hold the plasma concentration within reasonable therapeutic limits during pregnancy. The size of the increase varies with the agent from 11% to 40% of prepregnancy dosage. Despite a decrease of plasma phenobarbitol concentration in 81% of the 33 women receiving that drug, its dosage administration was not increased. Issues of comparability of duration and degree of seizure control before pregnancy cloud evaluation of the effectiveness of adjusting dosage using plasma concentration measurements. It may be that even larger-than-effective nonpregnancy maternal blood drug concentrations need to be maintained in pregnancies necessitating dosage increase beyond the customary 10% to 40% increase.—T.H. Kirschbaum, M.D.

Anaerobic Coverage for Intra-Amnionic Infection: Maternal and Perinatal Impact

Maberry MC, Gilstrap LC III , Bawdon R, Little BB, Dax J (Univ of Texas)

Am J Perinatol 8:338–341, 1991 2–20

Introduction.—There is no consensus on the most effective antibiotic regimen for the prevention of maternal and neonatal morbidity in intra-amniotic infection, particularly with regard to anaerobic organisms. To assess the impact of providing anaerobic coverage for the treatment of intra-amniotic infection, 133 women with intra-amniotic infection were randomly assigned to either dual agent therapy with ampicillin and gentamicin or triple agent therapy consisting of ampicillin, gentamicin, and clindamycin.

Results.—The frequency of intrapartum complications was similar in both groups, but the rate of induction and augmentation was high in both groups. The frequency of cesarean and vaginal delivery also was similar in both groups. Overall, the incidence of endometritis did not differ significantly between the 2 groups; however, the incidence of endometritis among women who delivered vaginally was significantly higher among women who received dual agent therapy (13%) than among those who received triple agent therapy (0%). Neonatal outcome was comparable in the 2 groups.

Conclusion.—There appears to be no therapeutic advantage in providing anaerobic coverage in the treatment of intra-amniotic infection in women who require cesarean section. The possible beneficial effects of providing anaerobic coverage in women delivering vaginally require further studies.

▶ There is growing evidence for fetal benefit with intrapartum antibiotic therapy vs. its postpartum application, especially in preterm labor (see the 1990 YEAR BOOK OF OBSTETRICS AND GYNECOLOGY, pp 209–210). This study deals with a peripheral issue seen predominantly (88%) in term labors with clinical amnioitis. What is being tested is not whether intrapartum antibiotics are of benefit, but whether adding clindamycin for anaerobic coverage provides benefit beyond the use of ampicillin and gentamicin. As in all similar well-conducted studies, there is a high exclusion rate resulting from the rigorous requirements for documented disease and interdiction of antibiotics before entry into the study. A comparison of the study and control groups verifies that true randomization took place past that point. In addition, the 15% overall incidence of endometritis produces case numbers available for study. The results suggest a benefit in prevention of endometritis only in those patients who delivered vaginally, not in the overall incidence of endometritis including patients who delivered abdominally. Evidence for newborn benefit was sought but was not found. Clearly, if there is a benefit from adding clindamycin to the drug regimen described, it is not large.—T.H. Kirshbaum, M.D.

Sonographic Visualization of the Ureter in Pregnancy

MacNeily AE, Goldenberg SL, Allen GJ, Ajzen SA, Cooperberg PL (St Paul's Hosp, Vancouver, BC; Univ of British Columbia, Vancouver)

J Urol 146:298–301, 1991 2–21

Background.—Hydronephrosis during pregnancy occurs in the absence of obstructive pathology. The pelvic ureters usually are not affected, and the dilation typically extends to the sacral promontory. Sonographic visualization of the ureter in pregnancy was assessed.

Methods.—A method was developed for differentiating physiological from pathological dilation of the renal collecting system in pregnant women. In 2 patients with distal ureteral stones, a dilated ureter was visualized past the vessels. The frequency and reliability of ureter visualization in pregnancy were determined in 105 consecutive asymptomatic patients.

Results.—Hydronephrosis was discovered in 83 kidneys of 59 patients. In 64 renal units, the dilated ureter was visualized. Color flow Doppler scanning demonstrated the anatomy well, and in all these cases, the dilated ureter tapered where it crossed the common iliac artery (Fig 2–5).

Conclusion.—The presence of high-grade left hydronephrosis or visualization of a dilated infrailiac ureter suggests a pathologic obstruction, not gestational hydronephrosis. Further study should be done when such findings are seen in antenatal ultrasound screening. In women with hydronephrosis that is symptomatic but only mild or moderate, and in

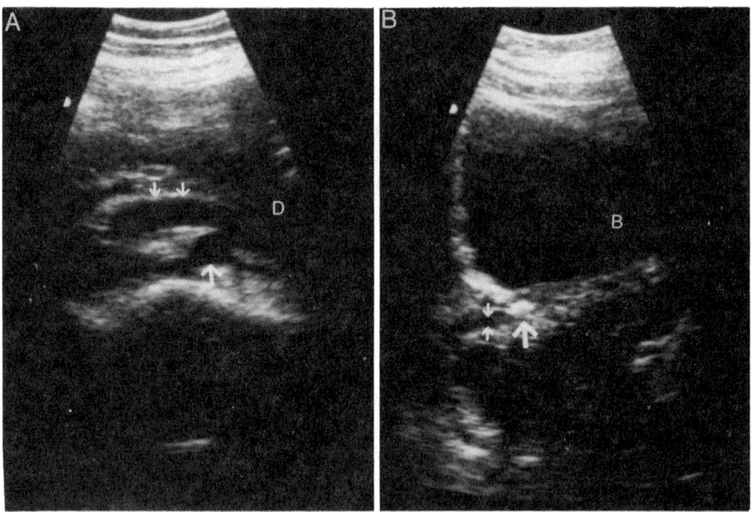

Fig 2–5.—A, real-time ultrasound (sagittal view) demonstrates dilated ureter (*small arrows*) over and beyond iliac vessels (*large arrow*). Distal ureter (*D*) runs toward right side of image. **B,** sagittal view of bladder (*B*) with stone (*large arrow*) at ureterovesical junction (ureter, *small arrows*). (Courtesy of MacNeily AE, Goldenberg SL, Allen GJ, et al: *J Urol* 146: 298–301, 1991.)

whom there is tapering of the ureter at the vessels, conventional contrast radiography is not needed.

▶ This paper deals with an issue that arises either when a gravida with urolithiasis has pain that cannot be explained by infection or apparent obstruction, or when one works with a urological consultant who is not familiar with the hydronephrosis of pregnancy. Because the gravid uterus and its contents displace bowel loops from the true pelvis, ultrasonic visualization of the distal ureter is facilitated. This is particularly true for the right ureter (seen 88% of the time in the asymptomatic cases in this study), where hydroureter is more common and more marked than the left ureter. Color flow Doppler enables one to focus on the ureter below the level of the iliac vessels, which can readily be seen because of their opposite flow directions and, therefore, contrasting image colorations. The authors found that asymptomatic normal women showed tapering of the ureter at the iliac artery with hydroureter predominantly proximal to that level. They reported 2 cases with distal ureteral stones in which hydroureter continued into the infra-iliac segment. There is not enough data with which to calculate a sensitivity figure for the detection of distal ureteral stones, but the study provides an approach worth remembering.—T.H. Kirschbaum, M.D.

Endothelin-1-Induced Vasoconstriction Is Not Mediated by Thromboxane Release and Action in the Human Fetal-Placental Circulation

Myatt L, Langdon G, Brewer AS, Brockman DE (Univ of Cincinnati)

Am J Obstet Gynecol 165:1717–1722, 1991 2–22

Background.—The contractile effect of endothelin-1 may be mediated by thromboxane release and action. It has a potent vasoconstrictive effect and causes an apparent release of thromboxane in perfused placenta. Thromboxane and prostacyclin release by the fetal-placental circulation were measured during endothelin-1-induced vasoconstriction in relation to perfusate flow rate.

Methods.—Experiments were performed in the perfusion laboratory on placentas collected immediately after delivery. Arteries were cannulated and perfused, and the effects of endothelin-1 on perfusion pressure and eicosanoid release in the fetal-placental circulation were studied. In addition, the effects of a thromboxane synthetase inhibitor and a thromboxane receptor antagonist of the action of endothelin-1 were examined.

Findings.—An 8×10^{-10}-to 1×10^{-8}-mol/L dose of endothelin-1 caused a cumulative increase in fetal-placental perfusion pressure from 30 to 123 mm Hg; it also caused a corresponding decrease in the flow rate of fetal-placental perfusate. When corrected for flow rate, the levels of thromboxane B_2 and 6-ketoprostaglandin $F_{1\alpha}$ in the perfusate were found to be reduced significantly. The vasoconstrictive action of endothelin-1 could not be blocked by the thromboxane synthesis inhibitor dazoxiben or by the thromboxane receptor antagonist SQ29548, both of which were given at doses of 10^{-6} mol/L.

Conclusion.—Thromboxane release or action does not appear to mediate the vasoconstrictor effect of endothelin-1. This action is probably mediated by calcium channels. Eicosanoid may be released in response to hydrodynamic factors, namely flow or shear stress.

▶ In this confusing domain of preeclampsia pathophysiology, the smallest simplification is useful. Endothelins are a family of 3-21 amino acid peptides that appear to play a role in endothelial-derived modification of vasomotor tone on a paracrine basis. Increased concentrations of endothelins have been reported in the blood of preeclamptics, apparently as a result of maternal endothelial cell injury. Alterations in the already abnormal patterns of vascular prostaglandin production (increased thromboxane A_2 and decreased prostaglandin GI_2) have been postulated as causing the endothelin-produced veno- and arterial vasoconstriction.

This in vitro study using perfused human placental cotyledons shows that this is not the case. Effluent blood shows an increased concentration in metabolites of thromboxane and prostacyclin; however, the increased concentration actually represents decreased production rates that are transported by the sharply decreased rates of blood flow caused by the resulting vasoconstriction. That is to say, production of the eicosanoids is decreased, but at a rate less than the rate of blood flow decreased through the cotyledon; therefore, the concentration in effluent blood appears to increase. Thus, blockage of the production of thromboxane would be expected to play no role in endothelium effects. This means that endothelial damage results in increased thromboxane A_2 metabolite (TxB_2) and decreased prostacyclin production by mechanisms that are wholly separate from the constrictive effects of endothelin on vessels where those peptides are produced in excess.—T.H. Kirschbaum, M.D.

Infection and Labor: VII. Microbial Invasion of the Amniotic Cavity in Spontaneous Rupture of Membranes at Term

Romero R, Mazor M, Morrotti R, Avila C, Oyarzun E, Insunza A, Parra M, Behnke E, Montiel F, Cassell GH (Yale Univ, New Haven, Conn; Univ of Alabama, Birmingham)

Am J Obstet Gynecol 166:129–133, 1992 2–23

Introduction.—Microbial infection has been reported to occur upon the premature rupture of membranes in preterm deliveries. However, no available data address the microbial status of the amniotic cavity when the membranes rupture at full gestation. In a retrospective study, the prevalence and characteristics of microbial invasion after spontaneous membrane rupture at term were studied.

Methods.—An obstetric database provided a retrospective patient sample of women who delivered infants weighing more than 2,500 grams 48 hours after membrane rupture and amniocentesis. The amniotic fluid from these patients was cultured for both aerobic and anaerobic bacteria by standard methods including the limulus amebocyte lysate assay. Patients received antibiotic therapy and induction of labor if they had a positive Gram stain. A search was also made for chorioamnionitis and puerperal endometritis.

Results.—Thirty-two patients were included in the study, 11 of whom had a positive amniotic fluid culture. The most frequently cultured organisms were *Ureaplasma urealyticum* (10 patients), *Peptostreptococcus* species (4 patients), and *Lactobacillus* species (2 patients). The prevalence of polymicrobial amnionitic fluid infection was 45.4%. One patient had clinical chorioamnionitis, and 3 (9.4%) had puerperal endometritis. Women delivering vaginally with a positive amniotic fluid culture had significantly more endometritis than did women with negative cultures. Three women, 2 with a positive amniotic fluid culture and 1 with a negative culture, underwent cesarean delivery.

Conclusion.—Microbial infection of the amniotic fluid of pregnant women who have had prematurely ruptured membranes can often occur without overt signs of maternal or fetal infection. Endometritis may result from this type of infection.

▶ This is a nice example of the uses of serendipity. The study is limited in the number of cases presented by a design that admits for study women delivering infants of birth weight ≥ 2.5 kg, despite the initial mistaken evaluation which led to the presumption of preterm rupture of membranes. Only with the mistaken diagnosis of prematurity would amniocentesis be done, and that is the basis of this important observation. The results are surprising. Approximately one third of the cases with a medium of 4.5 hours' duration from rupture of membranes to the time of amniocentesis showed positive cultures, and only 1 case (3% of the total) subsequently showed chorioamnionitis. The study derives further value from the author's fine discussion of the basis for presuming that a fair share of culture positive cases manifested rupture of the membranes caused by bacterial infection rather than membrane rupture-causing infection. This conclusion has long been held for instances of ruptured membranes occurring in infants weighing less than 2.5 kg. What's surprising is that roughly the same quantitative likelihood appears in these infants born at term.—T.H. Kirschbaum, M.D.

Effect of Gestational Age on Obstetric Performance: When Is "Term" Over?

Saunders N, Paterson C (St Mary's Hosp, Med School, London)
Lancet 338:1190–1192, 1991 2–24

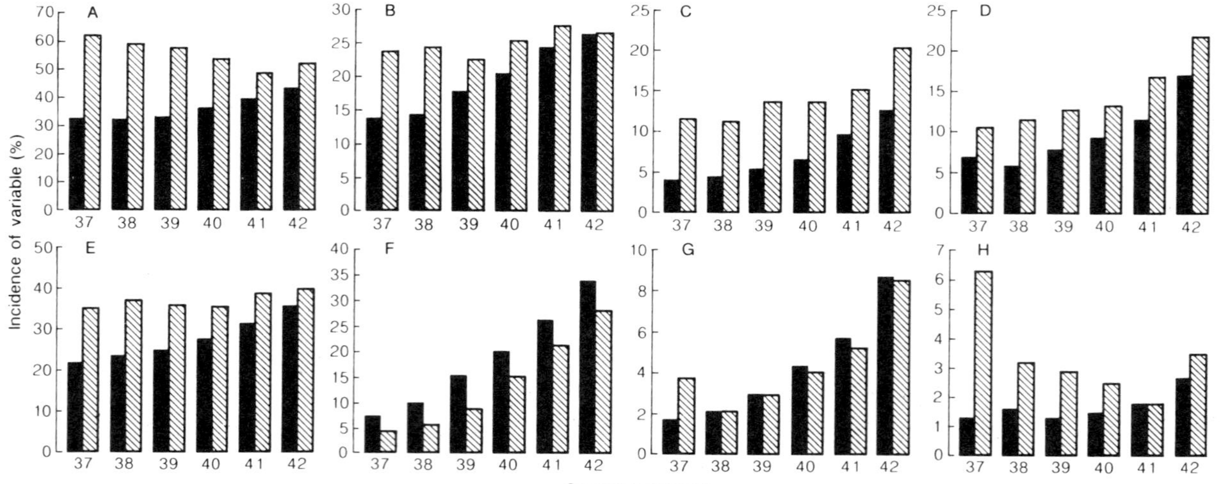

Fig 2–6.—Obstetric outcome variables in primigravidae by week of gestation during spontaneous (*filled bars*) and induced (*striped bars*) labor. **A,** oxytocin use; **B,** forceps delivery; **C,** cesarean secion; **D,** postpartum hemorrhage; **E,** abnormal cardiotocogram; **F,** meconium staining; **G,** neonatal intubation; **H,** Apgar score below 7 at 5 minutes. Number = 22,000. (Courtesy of Saunders N, Paterson C: *Lancet* 338:1190–1192, 1991.)

Background.—According to the World Health Organization, delivery that occurs from 37 to 42 completed weeks of pregnancy is "term." Inherent in this definition of term delivery is the assumption that delivery in this interval is associated with the best obstetric outcomes. However, 5 weeks is a long interval. A data analysis was used to determine whether outcomes vary with gestational age during this 5-week interval.

Data Collection.—Information on 75,974 consecutive deliveries was collected in London. Preterm deliveries were excluded, and 4 subgroups were analyzed: primiparae or multiparae in spontaneous or induced labor.

Findings.—Obstetric complications in labor were infrequent in multiparous women. The cesarean section and operative vaginal delivery rates in this group were 3% and 5%, respectively. Gestational age between 37 and 42 weeks seemed to have little effect on labor. However, among primigravidae in spontaneous labor, the rate of almost all variables studied increased progressively from 37 weeks' gestation (Fig 2–6). Compared with labor in the first week of term, labor at 41 weeks was associated with twice the rate of forceps delivery and cesarean section. The median duration of labor increased by more than 2 hours in these cases. The effect of gestational age on the rate of operative delivery remained significant after correcting for birth weight. Among primigravidae undergoing induced labor, such trends were seen only for cesarean section, postpartum hemorrhage, neonatal induction, and meconium staining. The indices of obstetric morbidity and intervention rates, except for neonatal intubation and meconium staining, were higher during induced than spontaneous labor by gestational week.

Conclusion.—For primigravidae, the incidence of obstetric complications associated with spontaneous labor increases progressively with each week of pregnancy after 37 weeks. Recognizing this risk gradient in "term" pregnancy may lead to a reassessment of problems traditionally attributed to induction of labor and post-term pregnancy.

▶ There are 2 fundamental implicit concepts introduced by this provocative review. The first is that post-term delivery is not a hazard to multigravid patients, because their rates of cesarean section and operative delivery are so low. This is a position that certainly is arguable, because it's the state of the neonate that is the measure of the successful management of postdatism—not the incidence of spontaneous birth. The second concept, that fetal and maternal hazard is a continuous incremental function past 37 weeks, is interesting. Many who have studied postdatism hold to this view intuitively, that a little fetal "reserve," the undefinable but so often used concept, is lost during the time after 37 weeks. That is not to say that interference past 37 weeks by induction or abdominal birth is better, only that those who deliver at term are for some reason favored compared with those who deliver after term. A troubling note here is the fourfold greater risk of an APGAR score less than 7 in induced vs. spontaneous labor at 37 weeks. It is hard to imagine how that result comes about, and it certainly is incompatible with the implicit assumption which underlies this work.—T.H. Kirschbaum, M.D.

Repeated Albumin Infusions Do Not Lower Blood Pressure in Preeclampsia

Stratta P, Canavese C, Dogliani M, Gurioli L, Porcu MC, Todros T, Fianchino O, Benedetto C, Massobrio M, Balbi L (Univ of Torino, Italy; St Anna-Hosp, Torino)

Clin Nephrol 36:234–239, 1991 2–25

Introduction.—Normal pregnancy usually includes an expansion of plasma volume in the woman. However, intravascular volume contraction can become pathologic when the woman experiences preeclampsia. Some have suggested the use of plasma volume expansion to offset these developments. To establish the basic parameters and volumes needed to conduct a randomized trial, the results of an open plot trial of albumin infusions in 10 patients with preeclampsia were examined.

Methods.—The 10 women (mean age, 36 years) had preeclampsia in the third trimester. The mean systolic blood pressure was 173 mm Hg, and the mean diastolic pressure was 103 mm Hg. On hospitalization antihypertensive therapy was administered, which maintained the mean blood pressure at 145/95 mg. The patients received .4–1 g of human serum albumin low in salt per day in a slow infusion. Blood chemistry and placental impedance were evaluated.

Results.—The 10 patients received a mean total of 352 g of infused albumin, administered for a minimum of 6 days to a maximum of 36. All 10 patients had cesarean sections, which resulted in 5 neonatal deaths within 3 days and 1 stillbirth. The patients had no further complications after delivery. In 50% of cases, the patients experienced a 175% increase in urine volume and a 285% and a 167% increase in sodium and potassium excretion, respectively. Creatinine and osmolar clearance also increased, but levels of aldosterone and renin decreased. These effects of albumin infusion where transient and weakened within 3 hours after the infusion was stopped. Renal clearance and urine electrolyte excretion did not change after albumin infusion. In the 6 patients who were followed up for 10 days, no long-term alterations were observed after the albumin infusion. No patient demonstrated a fall in blood pressure.

Conclusion.—A slow infusion of up to 1 g of albumin per kg per day did not cause any serious adverse effects in pregnant patients with preeclampsia. This expensive treatment protocol did not change the severity of fetal outcome.

▶ Volume expansion in women with preeclampsia has the effect of reducing systemic vascular resistance and increasing cardiac output. Because blood pressure is the product of these 2 values, there is little—if any—regular decrease in blood pressure noted with acute volume expansion. This report demonstrates the same failure of blood pressure change with volume expansion carried out from 6 to 36 days. Regrettably, there is little else to conclude, except for the presence of a transient diuresis at the start of albumin infusion. Neither cardiac output nor systemic vascular resistance was measured. Doppler velocity indices from "uterine" and umbilical vessels showed no change and an inexplicable increase in systolic to diastolic ratio, respectively. The parity of the experimental subjects is not listed, so even the certainty of the diagnosis of preeclampsia is in question. Nonetheless, this sort of data refutes the position of those who believe preeclampsia represents a vasoconstrictive response to hypovolemia as a primary cause.—T.H. Kirschbaum, M.D.

Risk Factors Associated With Preterm Deliveries Among Racial Groups in a National Sample of Married Mothers

Virji SK, Cottington E (Allegheny Gen Hosp, Pittsburgh; Allegheny Singer Research Inst, Pittsburgh)

Am J Perinatol 8:347–353, 1991 2–26

Introduction.—Preterm delivery is the most important cause of perinatal morbidity and perinatal death in the United States. Several sociodemographic and health behavior risk factors, including racial differences and lack of prenatal care, have been identified. Seven sociodemographic and behavioral factors that may explain the increased risk of preterm deliveries among black women were examined.

Methods.—A total of 5,823 women with children responded to a questionnaire in a 1980 survey conducted by the National Natality Survey (NNS) from the National Center for Health Statistics. The data were analyzed as case-control pairs. Birth certificates provided other basic maternal information.

Results.—Black women had nearly twice the percentage of preterm births that white women did. Black women had a mean gestational age 1 week shorter than did white women, for a significant difference. In general, for each risk factor reviewed, black women had a higher percentage of preterm infants than did white women. White women demonstrated a correlation between a low level of education and preterm deliveries, but black women did not. For both groups of patients, age (younger than 20 years and older than 35 years), smoking, weight gain of less than 20 pounds, heavy alcohol consumption, lack of prenatal care, and less than 9 prenatal visits correlated with an increased incidence of preterm births. Overall, black women with these risk factors had higher percentages of preterm deliveries than white women did.

For all subjects in the study, the odds ratio (OR) for each factor was greater than 1. The number of prenatal visits and weight gain had the greatest point estimates. The ORs appeared consistent for all race divisions, except for education and weight gain (greater risks for white women) and age (higher risk of preterm birth for black women). Multiple regression analysis showed that the OR for race with respect to preterm delivery remained higher than 1.

Conclusion.—Race is an independent risk factor for preterm births. Certain health behaviors that are amenable to change increase the odds of having a preterm delivery.

▶ This study is an attempt to determine whether the increased risk of preterm delivery among blacks is attributable solely to race or to a series of confounding variables distributed differentially by race. The data favors the former conclusion (but with some reservations) and the conclusion stems from multiple and logistic regression applied to a sample of 5,823 gravidas. The results show that heavy alcohol usage, no prenatal care, less than a high school education, and age younger than 20 years or older than 35 years at the time of pregnancy fail a test of significance as risk factors for preterm birth. On the other hand, smoking, fewer than 10 prenatal visits, and weight gain of 20 pounds or less are significant risk factors which, when applied to black/white differences fail to account completely for the racial difference in preterm birth incidence. The problems of this analysis are the exclusion of drug usage and unmarried gravidas, and the lower questionnaire response rates from blacks than from whites. Nonetheless, the results point to a possibility of an irremediable racial difference in the risk of preterm labor.—T.H. Kirschbaum, M.D.

The Association of Occult Amniotic Fluid Infection With Gestational Age and Neonatal Outcome Among Women in Preterm Labor

Watts DH, Krohn MA, Hillier SL, Eschenbach DA (Univ of Washington, Seattle)

Obstet Gynecol 79:351–357, 1992 2–27

Background.—Infections of the vagina, cervix, placenta, and amniotic fluid (AF) may be associated with preterm delivery. Previous studies of the effects of AF infection on the neonate have been inconclusive. The relationships among gestational age, neonatal outcome, and AF bacteria were studied.

Methods.—The subjects were 105 women with intact membranes who were undergoing amniocentesis for investigation of idiopathic preterm labor. All had completed 23 to 34 weeks of gestation and required tocolytic therapy. Amniotic fluid cultures were obtained for each woman, with split samples being studied at the hospital clinical laboratory and the research microbiology laboratory.

Findings.—There was an inverse relationship between the frequency of positive cultures and gestational age (Fig 2–7). The most common organisms were *Fusobacterium nucleatum*, *Bacteroids ureolyticus*, and *Ureaplasma urealyticum*. Women at less than 30 weeks' gestation more

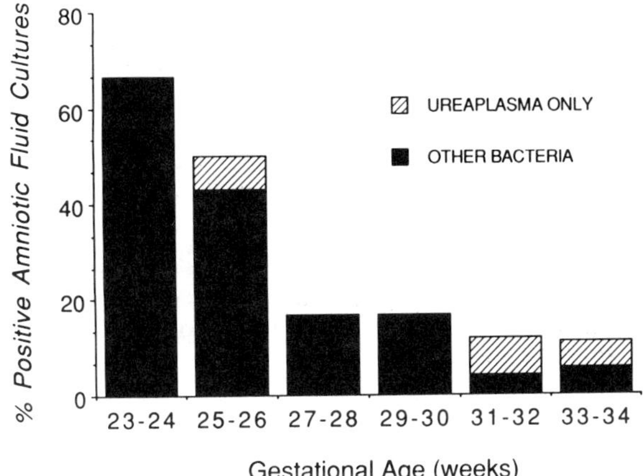

Fig 2–7.—Relationship of positive AF cultures to gestational age at amniocentesis among patients in preterm labor with intact membranes. *Striped bars*, ureaplasma only, *filled bars*, other bacteria. (Courtesy of Watts DH, Krohn MA, Hillier SL, et al: *Obstet Gynecol* 79:351–357, 1992.)

commonly showed facultative and anaerobic bacteria; those at greater than 30 weeks' gestation more commonly had *U. urealyticum*. Clinical laboratory cultures of AF were negative in 40% of the patients who had positive facultative and anaerobic cultures according to the research laboratory findings. There were no differences in clinical characteristics and maternal white blood cell and differential counts between women who did and did not have positive cultures. The most sensitive and specific predictors of positive cultures were increased levels of C-reactive protein and a positive AF Gram stain. Time to delivery was significantly shorter in women with positive cultures than in those with negative cultures, 1 vs. 28.5 days. Women with positive cultures had a median gestational age at delivery of 27.5 weeks and a median birth weight of 866 g. Neonatal outcomes were also significantly different: infants with positive cultures were more likely to die, and the survivors were more likely to have respiratory distress syndrome, and bronchopulmonary dysplasia and to remain hospitalized for a longer time.

Conclusion.—Treatment of occult AF infection in women with preterm labor can decrease perinatal morbidity and mortality. When amniocentesis is done after 30 weeks' gestation for evaluation of fetal lung maturity, cultures can be done as a secondary examination. This may be particularly important when multiagent tocolytic therapy or nonsteroidal anti-inflammatory drug treatment is considered.

▶ This is a direct attempt to estimate the risk of occult chorioamnionitis specific to gestational age, a problem discussed here previously (see the 1987 YEAR BOOK OF OBSTETRICS AND GYNECOLOGY, pp 113–115; the 1989 YEAR BOOK OF OBSTETRICS AND GYNECOLOGY, pp 151–152; and the 1991 YEAR BOOK OF OBSTETRICS AND GYNECOLOGY, pp 34–35). The relatively large number of cases and the technical expertise of this fine infectious disease study group at the University of Washington make it particularly valuable. The inverse relationship of occult infection to gestational age, which is often assumed without proof to be true, is very nicely demonstrated, as is the adverse fetal effect of blatant chorioamnionitis. The particularly strong evidence for amniotic fluid infected with pathogenic organisms before 30 completed weeks of gestation in 30% of the cases of preterm labor calls into question whether administration of steroids and tocolytics might be unwise before the week 31 of gestation in preterm labor. The authors' conclusion that amniocentesis done to exclude infected amniotic fluid might well be appropriate in patients with preterm labor and intact membranes before 30 completed weeks of gestation in population similar to this one seems well taken.—T.H. Kirschbaum, M.D.

Pregnancy in Patients With Cerebrospinal Fluid Shunts: Report of a Series and Review of the Literature

Wisoff JH, Kratzert KJ, Handwerker SM, Young BK, Epstein F (New York Univ; Booth Mem Med Ctr, Queens, NY)

Neurosurgery 29:827–831, 1991 2–28

Introduction.—Patients who are hydrocephalic at birth can now expect to live to adulthood, with 60% to 70% achieving nearly normal intelligence. Many hydrocephalic female patients with CSF shunts reach reproductive age and wish to have children. The results of 21 pregnancies in 18 hydrocephalic patients with cerebrospinal shunts were analyzed.

Methods.—Ten of the 21 pregnancy outcomes have been previously reported. In 4 of the other 11 patients, hydrocephalus was diagnosed during pregnancy and a shunt was placed. Fourteen women with 17 pregnancies had a ventricular shunt already in place.

Results.—The patients with newly diagnosed hydrocephalus all had increased intracranial pressure (ICP) symptoms, which occurred in 3 of the 4 women during the last 2 trimesters of pregnancy. Thirteen of the 17 women with preexisting shunts had neurological complications. Axial CT scans verified shunt patency. The shunts functioned normally in 7 of 11 pregnancies. Several women took anticonvulsants during their pregnancies. Five patients experienced complications during pregnancy and immediately after delivery, including preterm membrane rupture, premature labor and delivery, intrauterine growth retardation, and possible fetal macrosomia. Eight of the 11 patients in the later group underwent cesarean section, with 4 being second sections with tubal ligations. Four patients received epidural anesthesia, 5 had local anesthesia, 5 had general anesthesia, and 1 had narcotic anesthesia. All 11 patients had successful deliveries with no perinatal complications.

Conclusion.—As the number of pregnant patients with cerebral shunts to treat hydrocephalus increases, obstetricians must learn to manage these patients. These women should receive pregnancy counseling and careful clinical management (and also have cesarean deliveries if neurologically unstable) to ensure the best outcome for both the patient and the infant.

▶ This is one of very few accounts of the complications inherent in pregnancies in women with shunted hydrocephalus, but it conveys an impression of the daunting complications that exist. Eight such women with 10 pregnancies treated by the authors were added to 10 cases from 5 patients collected from the literature. Seventeen of these pregnancies occurred in 14 women with stable shunts, and they need to be considered separately from the 4 patients in whom shunts were performed only during pregnancy, thereby mixing the consequences of CSF shunting with the new diagnosis of hydrocephalus sufficiently severe to make bypass necessary. In 58% of the pregnancies with stable shunts, signs of increased intracranial fluid pressure occurred, and nearly three fourths showed symptoms of neurological abnormalities (nausea, vomiting, lethargy, atxia, and visual abnormality). These findings make the differential diagnosis of eclampsia in gravidas who are hypertensive with hydrocephalus a real problem. Although approximately half the pregnancies received prophylactis antibiotics, infection was not reported. Tests for shunt patency are commonplace. In almost 15%, an unstable neurological state made cesarean section necessary on that indication alone, and it also made avoidance of repeated Valsalva efforts through use of obstetrical forceps attractive, if not mandatory. Patients anticipating pregnancy with this preexisting problem require extensive preconceptional counseling to gain a clear understanding of the hazards they face.—T.H. Kirschbaum, M.D.

3 Maternal Abnormalities of Pregnancy

Placenta Accreta: Additional Sonographic Observations

Hoffman-Tretin JC, Koenigsberg M, Rabin A, Anyaegbunam A (Bronx Municipal Hosp Ctr, NY; Albert Einstein College of Medicine, Bronx, NY)

J Ultrasound Med 11:29–34, 1992 3–1

Background.—Placenta accreta, an abnormal attachment of the placenta to the uterine wall in pregnancy, is being recognized more frequently. Several reports have based the antenatal sonographic diagnosis of placenta accreta on the nonvisualization of a hypoechoic zone peripheral to the placenta. At least 2 new sonographic features of placenta accreta have recently been demonstrated.

Patients and Findings.—Seven patients aged 27–35 years were given a diagnosis of placenta accreta, a diagnosis established sonographically on the basis of a lack of a hypoechoic zone peripheral to the placenta. New observations included prominent large or multiple placental venous lakes and periuterine vascularity in 6 cases. In 2 cases, there was progressive thinning and a disappearance of the retroplacental hypoechoic zone on sequential assessments. Also of value was the loss of a normal venous

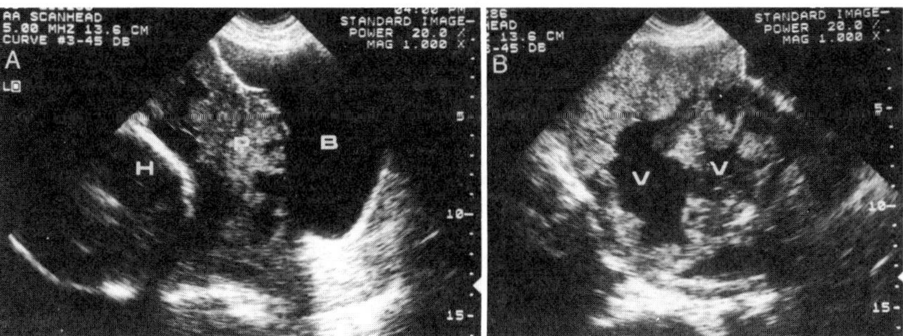

Fig 3–1.—Evolution of placenta percreta on sequential sonograms (case 1). **A,** a sagittal midline sonogram of the lower uterine segment at 35 to 37 weeks of fetal development reveals partial placenta previa and absence of the hypoechoic zone peripheral to the placenta (*P*), which abuts on the dome of the bladder (*B*). Invasion of the bladder wall may be suspected from this view. **B,** section depicting the bizarre intraplacental vascular spaces (V), confirmed by Doppler interrogation. (Courtesy of Hoffman-Tretin JC, Koenigsberg M, Rabin A, et al: *J Ultrasound Med* 11:29–34, 1992.)

flow pattern on Doppler interrogation of the peripheral placental margin in 2 cases. Histological correlates were suggested on the basis of the primary histopathological feature of placenta accreta, deficiency of the decidua basalis. Differential diagnostic considerations included abdominal pregnancy and trophoblastic disease (Fig 3–1).

Conclusion.—The progression of sonographic findings of placenta accreta in sequential studies supports the view that placenta accreta is an acquired abnormality. There are at least 2 differential diagnoses to be considered in cases suggesting placenta accreta.

► The increasing incidence of placenta accreta in contemporary obstetrics has lent urgency to the capacity of ultrasonic confirmation of the diagnosis before attempts of delivery. Fortunately, criteria for the diagnosis have been established (1); however, they are relatively subtle. In normal placentation, there is a junctional plane between the maternal and fetal tissue, a region comprised largely by decidualized maternal vessels subserving the intervillus space. The relative sparsity of connective tissue in these structures in the absence of villus tissue confers echolucency on this narrow region. The failure to visualize the hypoechoic zone beneath the placenta is suggestive of placenta previa. As these authors point out, the abnormal vascular adaptations within the placenta and in the adjoining uterine musculature help in confirmation. An additional observation of great interest is the initial demonstration of normal ultrasonic architecture in some cases that go on to have placenta accreta develop, which suggests that this abnormality is acquired in the course of fetal development from what begins as normal placentation.—T.H. Kirschbaum, M.D.

Reference

1. Mendonca LK: *J Ultrasound Med* 7:211, 1988.

4 Medical Complications of Pregnancy

A Prospective Study of Lymphocyte-Initiated Immunosuppression in Normal Pregnancy: Evidence of a T-Cell Etiology for Postpartum Thyroid Dysfunction

Stagnaro-Green A, Roman SH, Cobin RH, El-Harazy E, Wallenstein S, Davies TF (Mount Sinai School of Medicine, New York)

J Clin Endocrinol Metab 74:645–653, 1992 4–1

Background.—Immune function during normal pregnancy and the postpartum period is not well understood. A cohort of pregnant women at risk for having postpartum thyroid dysfunction (PPTD) and healthy pregnant women were compared.

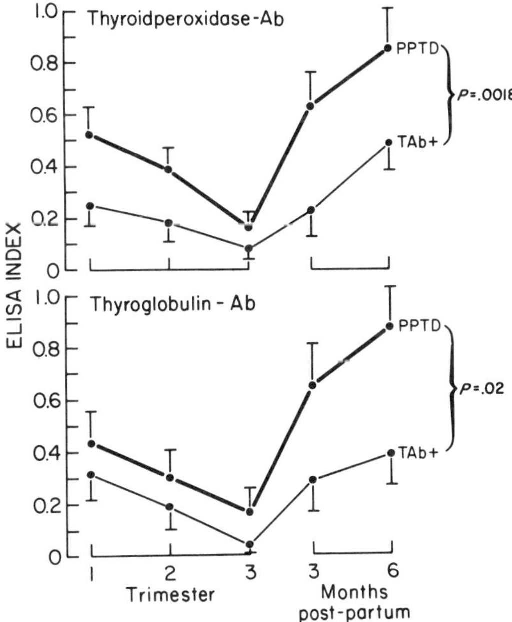

Fig 4–1.—Thyroid autoantibody titers for the (PPTD+) and thyroid autoantibody-positive (TAb+) groups, expressed as the mean and SEM at each time point of the study. The statistical test performed was a repeated measure-mean. (Courtesy of Stagnaro-Green A, Roman SH, Cobin RH, et al: *J Clin Endocrinol Metab* 74:645–653, 1992.)

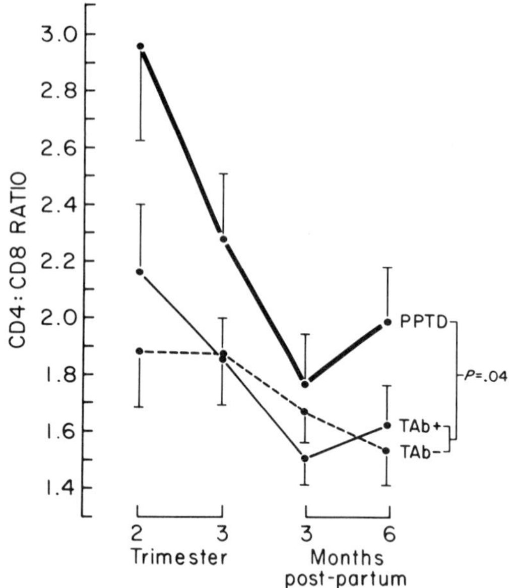

Fig 4–2.—Helper/suppressor ratio (CD4/CD8) for the PPTD+, thyroid autoantibody-positive (TAb+), and thyroid autoantibody-negative (TAb−) groups, expressed as the mean and SEM at each time point of the study. The mean and SEM of the nonpregnant control group were 2.1 ± .11. The statistical test performed was a repeated measure-mean. (Courtesy of Stagnaro-Green A, Roman SH, Cobin RH, et al: *J Clin Endocrinol Metab* 74:645–653, 1992.)

Methods.—Screening for the presence of thyroid autoantibodies was done in 552 women in the first trimester of pregnancy. Thirty-three thyroid autoantibody-positive women and 28 thyroid autoantibody-negative women were followed up prospectively 6 months into the postpartum period. Analyses of lymphocyte subsets, thyroid function, and thyroid autoantibodies were done periodically. All the women were HLA serotyped.

Findings.—Normal pregnancy was characterized mainly by reduced CD4+ T cells and increasing CD8+ T cells. This caused a significant reduction in the CD4+/CD8+ ratio in late pregnancy and post partum. Women with PPTD had a higher CD4+/CD8+ ratio, activation of T cells post partum, and significantly greater thyroid autoantibody titers. The overall incidence of PPTD was 8.8%. A significant decrease in the T-cell helper/suppressor ratio in normal pregnant women was associated with distinct T-cell subset changes. This T-cell regulation reflected an overall suppression of immune function (Figs 4–1 and 4–2).

Conclusion.—Development of PPTD was associated with a triad of immune markers: a decrease in normal immune suppression of pregnancy, enhanced postpartum T-cell activation, and increased thyroid autoantibodies. The reduction in the degree of immune suppression was a major factor in the development of PPTD.

▶ This is a fine demonstration of immunosuppression during pregnancy using modern investigative techniques. By choosing to assess the response to thyroid epitopes, suppression gives us important information about PPTD as well. Postpartum thyroid dysfunction is defined as abnormally high (hypothyroid) or low (hyperthyroid) values of hypersensitive thyroid-stimulating hormone measured at 3 and 6 months post partum. The T-cell phenotypes were identified using a monoclonal antibody technique coupled with immunofluorescence. Humeral changes were followed by enzyme-linked immunosorbent assay determination of thyroid antiglobulin and antiperoxidase assays. The incidence of antithyroid antibody was approximately 18%, and of these 102 women, a 33-member sample showed a risk of 1 in 3 having PPTD develop. Normal pregnancy was associated with a progressive suppression of overall immune activity and a decreased CD4+/CD8+ ratio in late pregnancy. Those patients destined to have PPTD showed higher levels of T-cell activation, lesser humeral and cellular immunosuppression, and both higher CD4+/CD8+ ratios and higher titers of the thyroid antibody compared with either antibody-positive or antibody-negative individuals in whom PPTD failed to develop. The technical expertise manifest here helps clear up the ambiguity noted in earlier studies (see the 1990 YEAR BOOK OF OBSTETRICS AND GYNECOLOGY, pp 181–190). Note that, of the 12 women with PPTD, all exhibited hypothyroidism, half with a transient episode of earlier hyperthyroid symptoms.—T.H. Kirschbaum, M.D.

A Survey of Zidovudine Use in Pregnant Women With Human Immunodeficiency Virus Infection

Sperling RS, Stratton P, O'Sullivan MJ, Boyer P, Watts DH, Lambert JS, Hammill H, Livingston EG, Gloeb DJ, Minkoff H, Fox HE (Mount Sinai Med Ctr, New York; Natl Inst of Child Health and Human Development, Bethesda, Md; Univ of Miami; Univ of California, Los Angeles; Univ of Washington, Seattle; et al)

N Engl J Med 326:857–861, 1992 4–2

Background.—The indications for zidovudine therapy have been expanding, which makes it important to determine its safety and toxicity in pregnant women. The results of a survey of zidovudine in pregnant women with HIV infection were reviewed.

Methods.—Pediatricians and obstetricians at the AIDS Clinical Trials Units were asked to report information on such women who were continuing their pregnancies. All cases reported occurred in women who were receiving or who had received zidovudine during gestation.

Findings.—Seventeen institutions sent reports on 43 women. The doses of zidovudine ranged from 300 to 1,200 mg/day. Twenty-four women took the drug for at least 2 trimesters. There were 2 instances of maternal toxicity—1 gastrointestinal and 1 hematological. There were no teratogenic abnormalities found in the 12 infants exposed to the drug in the first trimester. All the infants, including 2 sets of twins, were live-born. The 38 singletons born at term for whom birth weights were recorded had a mean birth weight of 3,287 g. There were 2 cases of intrauterine growth retardation among the infants delivered at term. Hemoglobin values, which were available for 31 infants, ranged from 7 to 12.4 mmol/L. Three of the 7 infants with hemoglobin values of less than 8.4 mmol/L were born prematurely.

Conclusion.—Pregnant women with HIV infection tolerated zidovudine treatment well. This drug apparently was not associated with malformations in the newborns, premature birth, or fetal distress. The newborns showed no pattern of hematological toxicity. However, the anemia and growth retardation occurring in a minority of the infants may have been partly a result of zidovudine treatment during gestation.

► With quite conclusive evidence for the usefulness of zidovudine, which usually is known as AZT, in prolonging the latent period in HIV-1 antibody–positive individuals (1), the agent has gained wide usage. It inevitably will be given to pregnant women. Fetuses certainly are subject to AZT through placenta transfer (2, 3), where its tendency to produce anemia, reduction of circulating granulocytes, and gastrointestinal ulceration and bleeding in adults are causes for concern.

In this study, the data on 45 infants resulting from 43 HIV-positive gravidas that were treated with this agent are insufficient to exclude a deleterious fetal effect, but they do make fetal side effects unlikely as a common event. Even in the 39 cases with known patterns of drug administration, fetal exposure varies. In only 9 pregnancies was drug therapy begun before pregnancy and continued throughout. In 13 cases, treatment was begun in the second trimester of pregnancy, and in 15 cases it was begun in the third trimester. Twelve women exposed their fetuses to AZT in the first trimester of pregnancy; none showed anomalous development. Anemia was noted in 6 of 45 newborns, but it was difficult to exclude prematurity or maternal nutritional problems as etiologic. Although the obstetric outcomes were diverse, they were not strikingly different from those in nondrug users; however, the power to discriminate increases in obstetric pathophysiology is very small. All in all, with the absence of compelling evidence of fetal pathology in light of the clear advantages to the infected gravida, the chances of reducing maternal-to-fetal transmission seem to justify the continued use of this agent during pregnancy, at least until more experience is amassed.—T.H. Kirschbaum, M.D.

References

1. Volberding PA, et al: *N Engl J Med* 322:941, 1990.
2. 1992 Year Book of Obstetrics and Gynecology, p 92.
3. Watts DH, et al: *J Infect Dis* 163:226, 1991.

Evaluation of Screened Blood Donations for Human Immunodeficiency Virus Type 1 Infection by Culture and DNA Amplification of Pooled Cells

Busch MP, Eble BE, Khayam-Bashi H, Heilbron D, Murphy EL, Kwok S, Sninsky J, Perkins HA, Vyas GN (Univ of California, San Francisco; Irwin Mem Blood Ctrs, San Francisco; Cetus Corp, Emeryville, Calif)

N Engl J Med 325:1–5, 1991 4–3

Background.—Voluntary exclusion from blood donation and routine antibody screening have reduced the risk of transmitting HIV-1 through nonautologous transfusion. Nevertheless, current transfusions still carry some risk. The extent to which HIV-1-infected donations may be missed by current screening procedures was determined.

Methods.—Peripheral blood mononuclear cells from fully screened donors were tested by both a highly specific viral culture technique and a highly sensitive PCR (polymerase chain reaction) proviral amplification method. Pools of cells from 50 donors were analyzed by both these methods. A total of 1,530 pools of cells were prepared from 76,500 blood donations made during a 2-year period in San Francisco.

Findings.—Among these 1,530 pools of mononuclear cells, 1,436 were successfully cultured and 873 were analyzed by the PCR technique. Only 1 pool was confirmed as being HIV-1 infected by both methods. After adjusting for sample-based estimates of sensitivity, the estimated likelihood of a screened donor being positive for HIV-1 was 1 in 61,171, with a 95% upper confidence limit of 1 in 10,695.

Implications.—The current risk of transmitting HIV-1 via blood transfusion is low—even in high-risk areas such as San Francisco. The current risk estimate is within the confidence limits of recent projections based on epidemiological models.

► The principle aim of this study, to provide reassurance regarding the safety of current blood screening methods in preventing inadvertent transmission of HIV-1 infection, is important; however, there is another message here. The study's 95% confidence range of the risk of infectivity (1/10,695 to 1/357,000) compares reasonably well with earlier estimates of maximum and minimal risks. The other concern regards the possibility that donor blood might contain HIV-1 DNA discernible only by PCR and might be infectious without evidence of host antibody formation to the virus. Such findings previously have been noted during the long period of dormancy after the retrovirus has apparently been incorporated into the host genome. In this study, the incidence of PCR-DNA–positive blood was equally infrequent to that found by culture among HIV-1-antibody–negative individuals and was essentially the same as the estimates based on antibody conversion data. Therefore, the risk of occurrence of PCR-positive blood among antibody-negative individuals can be said to be very small in this study of 76,500 donated units. The pooling of mononuclear cells necessary for economy and efficiency precludes making a precise quantitative estimate of the risk. The conclusion is, however, very reassuring.—T.H. Kirschbaum, M.D.

HIV in Pregnant Women and Their Offspring: Evidence for Late Transmission

Ehrnst A, Lindgren S, Dictor M, Johansson B, Sönnerborg A, Czajkowski J, Sundin, G, Bohlin A-B (Central Microbiological Lab of the Stockholm County Council, Stockholm; Huddinge Univ Hosp, Stockholm; Lund Univ Hosp, Lund, Sweden)

Lancet 338:203–207, 1991 4–4

Introduction.—Previous studies have estimated the relative risk of maternal vertical transmission of HIV to their offspring to range between 15% and 40%. However, it is not known how often and at which stage of the pregnancy HIV is transmitted in utero and how often it is transmitted at birth as a consequence of exposure to maternal blood and body fluids.

Patients.—HIV viremia and antigenemia during pregnancy were investigated during 47 pregnancies in 44 HIV-infected women with a mean age of 26 years. Most women were asymptomatic. Thirty pregnancies were continued, and 17 were aborted. A group of HIV studies were also performed in 12 aborted fetuses and in 27 neonates.

Results.—At some time during pregnancy, HIV was detected from plasma in 59% of women and from either peripheral blood mononuclear cells or plasma in 83%. It was not confirmed in any of the placentas or fetal tissues obtained from the aborted fetuses. None of 27 neonates had HIV viremia within the first few days of life. However, HIV was recovered from 5 of 19 children (26%) who were tested after the neonatal period but within 6 months. Thus, the mothers had a significantly higher frequency of viremia during pregnancy (83%) than their children had by 6 months of age (26%). Among the 15 children who have now reached age 18 months, 4 (27%) are known to be infected.

Conclusion.—The early detection of HIV infection in children and the absence of HIV in aborted fetuses and neonates suggest that HIV does not spread across the placenta during maternal viremia, but that vertical transmission of HIV occurs late during the pregnancy or at delivery.

▶ Although it was relatively easy to isolate the HIV virus from this group of 44 Swedish gravidas, only 1 of which had frank AIDS, it was difficult to find the virus either by direct or indirect means in the 12 abortuses and 27 newborns. Nonetheless, the anticipated 26% maternal-to-fetal transmission rate was noted (based on viral cultures at 6 months of age). This hint that newborn infection may be largely limited either to delivery or by horizontal transmission after birth is important and merits further study. If verified, it means that preterm abdominal birth and separation of the infant from the mother may decrease the risk of maternal-to-fetal transmission. Use of polymerase chain reaction to amplify viral DNA is an important adjunct to this sort of study.—T.H. Kirschbaum, M.D.

Pancreatitis Related to Severe Acute Hypertriglyceridemia During Pregnancy: Treatment With Lipoprotein Apheresis

Achard JM, Westeel PF, Moriniere Ph, Lalau JD, de Cagny B, Fournier A (CHRU, Amiens, France)

Intensive Care Med 17:236–237, 1991 4–5

Background.—During pregnancy, acute pancreatitis may develop in patients with familial hyperlipidemia as a result of increased levels of triglyceride (TG). Hypertriglyceridemia-induced pancreatitis during pregnancy is a serious complication for both the mother and the fetus. The case of a patient successfully treated with lipoprotein apheresis was reported.

Case Report.—Woman, 30, who was pregnant had high serum TG levels before and during her pregnancy; she also had a family history of the condition. She was admitted to the hospital with nausea, vomiting, fever, epigastric pain, and marked dehydration. The results of initial laboratory examinations led to a diagnosis of acute pancreatitis. Because fluid therapy and fasting did not improve her condition, a double-filtration lipoproteinapheresis was performed twice during the first 36 hours. Two lipaphereses succeeded in reducing her TG level by more than 75%. Within 48 hours, the patient's abdominal symptoms subsided and her biologic parameters returned to normal. She was placed on a low-fat diet for the remainder of her pregnancy and gave birth to a healthy infant 2 months later.

Conclusion.—Plasmapheresis has been safely performed for many other conditions in pregnant patients for a number of years. The lipaphereses in the study patient was well tolerated and appeared to lead to the patient's clinical improvement. It is important for other conditions (e.g., gallstones) to be ruled out before proceeding with this form of therapy.

▶ This interesting case report brings us a step closer to understanding the relationship between familial hypertriglyceridemia and acute pancreatitis. After somewhat more than 24 hours without benefit, selective plasmapheresis and removal of lipoprotein fractions with serum albumin replacement led to prompt subsidence of pancreatic injury (normal serum amylase and lipase, relief from abdominal pain, and return of insulin production and release). It's hard to avoid the conclusion that the high triglyceride content results in pancreatic cell injury and the release of toxic chylomicron contents that become a further toxin. Note also that management of the acute process was followed by prolonged remission from pancreatitis. It is worth remembering in an infrequent but dangerous complication of pregnancy.—T.H. Kirschbaum, M.D.

Respiratory Function in Severe Gestational Proteinuric Hypertension: The Effects of Rapid Volume Expansion and Subsequent Vasodilatation With Verapamil

Belfort MA, Anthony J, Kirshon B (Baylor Coll of Medicine, Houston; Univ of Cape Town, South Africa)

Br J Obstet Gynaecol 98:964–972, 1991 4–6

Introduction.—Severe gestational proteinuric hypertension is characterized by contracted plasma volume, low cardiac output, and high systemic vascular resistance. As a consequence, oxygen delivery may be inadequate to support normal tissue function. Increasing cardiac output with controlled volume expansion may improve tissue perfusion and respiratory function at a cellular level. The baseline respiratory function in untreated severe gestational proteinuric hypertension was defined, and the effects of volume expansion and vasodilatation on these baseline levels were assessed.

Patients.—Six women with a mean age of 26 years and a mean gestational age of 35 weeks were studied. All 6 had severe gestational proteinuric hypertension and were undergoing stabilization and delivery. Three of the women were primigravidas. None of the women had been treated before entry into the study. After assessment of baseline hemodynamic and respiratory function by invasive monitoring, the patients underwent volume expansion with a mean of 400 mL of dextran-70 to achieve a pulmonary capillary wedge pressure of 16 mm Hg; this was followed by vasodilatation with verapamil.

Results.—The baseline oxygen delivery and consumption indices were consistent with severe tissue ischemia. Volume expansion with dextran-70 normalized these variables. Subsequent vasodilatation with verapamil did not reduce these indices below the normal limits for pregnancy. Fetal outcome was favorable in all 6 cases, and the umbilical artery blood gases were all within normal limits. All 6 infants had normal neurologic and adaptive capacity scores at postpartum examination.

Conclusion.—Untreated severe gestational proteinuric hypertension is associated with prolonged tissue ischemia. Treatment with a combination of volume expansion and verapamil vasodilatation reduces the elevated blood pressure without compromising maternal respiratory function.

▶ The relationship between volume expansion, peripheral vascular resistance, and cardiac output in hypertensive pregnancy is a relatively old story (see the 1990 Year Book of Obstetrics and Gynecology, pp 73–74). Severe, untreated pregnancy-induced hypertension (PIH) is marked by low cardiac index, decreased plasma volume, and high peripheral vascular resistance. Treatment of almost any kind changes these variables in directions that are hard to predict, and past studies of such therapy have produced all of the contradictory results in the evaluation of cardiovascular function in acute PIH that are part of our literature. When volume expansion is carried out, peripheral vascular resistance decreases and cardiac output increases. Thereafter, vasodilatation produces similar but less intense changes, plus reduction of blood pressure. Vasodilators without volume expansion, in some cases, result in fetal findings suggestive of hypoperfusion. What is new here is evidence of decreased maternal oxygen consumption, calculated from maternal cardiac output and the arterial venous oxygen content difference. It appears to be reduced in severe PIH, despite reasonably normal oxygen delivery to the fetus. This means the maternal tissue oxygen extraction was impaired in these women and improved with volume expansion. This is further confirmation that severe hypertensive disease is a disturbance of end organs mediated by small vessel disease, and that central cardiovascular changes are secondary in importance. Although most patients with severe PIH appear to improve with volume expansion, a few patients with normal-to-high pulmonary wedge pressures appear to deteriorate. Be that as it may, this study provides strong suggestive evidence for the value of volume expansion, regardless of what happens to maternal blood pressure.—T.H. Kirschbaum, M.D.

Immune Thrombocytopenic Purpura in Pregnancy: A Reappraisal of Management

Cook RL, Miller RC, Katz VL, Cefalo RC (Univ of North Carolina, Chapel Hill)

Obstet Gynecol 78:578–583, 1991 4–7

Background.—Immune thrombocytopenic purpura (ITP) during pregnancy can result in serious complications to the fetus. Because low platelet counts in the fetus can lead to intracranial hemorrhage, some physicians have recommended cesarean delivery. A review of 31 pregnancies in 25 women with ITP determined the effect of mode of delivery on neonatal outcome.

Methods.—The study group was obtained from a review of records during a 10-year period. Included were pregnant women with a previous diagnosis of ITP or those with platelet counts less than 100×10^9/L on more than 1 occasion. In 27 of the 31 deliveries, obstetric indications determined the delivery method.

Results.—Of the 32 infants, 18 were delivered by cesarean and 14 were delivered vaginally. Mothers of infants delivered by cesarean had a significantly higher mean maternal platelet count at delivery than those whose babies were delivered vaginally. Six cesarean deliveries had serious delivery-related complications. Six infants were either severely thrombocytopenic at birth or became severely affected in the neonatal period—4 in the vaginal delivery group and 2 in the cesarean group. No maternal characteristic was predictive of neonatal platelet count. Maternal steroid treatment did not protect the infant from severe thrombocytopenia.

Conclusion.—It is difficult to predict which infants whose mothers receive a diagnosis of ITP will have thrombocytopenia. A 20-year literature search using MEDLINE found that the proportion of infants with intracranial hemorrhage increased as the birth platelet counts decreased. However, the data do not support the view that mode of delivery has an effect on neonatal outcome. At least for the present, patients with ITP should be managed according to obstetric indications.

▶ Although review of the 32 pregnancies complicated by ITP during this 10-year span is interesting, it's the 20-year literature review that is the most compelling part of the argument. Note that the modern definition of thrombocytopenia (platelet count, 100,00 per mm^3) was used and that exclusion criteria were chosen carefully. Predictions of fetal bleeding from maternal platelet counts would be possible only if there were good relationships between maternal and fetal counts and between fetal platelet count and neonatal bleeding. Neither proposition is true. Given newborn thrombocytopenia, the risk of clinical evidence of bleeding (approximately 30%) or intracranial hemorrhage (approximately 4%) is independent of delivery via the vaginal or abdominal route. Part of the reason that vaginal delivery is not a frequent precursor to neonatal bleeding is that the greatest risk of neonatal hemorrhage from thrombocytopenia occurs 2–4 days after birth. Because the risk of neonatal intracranial hemorrhage was roughly the same in infants with severe or moderate thrombocytopenia in this review study, the fetal scalp blood platelet counts can't be expected to be of much predictive assistance. Finally, maternal antiplatelet antibody concentrations seem to relate to neither maternal nor fetal platelet count. In light of all this, the authors' conclusions seem sound.—T.H. Kirschbaum, M.D.

Group B Streptococcus (GBS) and Neonatal Infections: The Case for Intrapartum Chemoprophylaxis

Garland SM, Fliegner JR (Royal Women's Hosp, Melbourne)

Aust N Z J Obstet Gynaecol 31:119–122, 1991 4–8

Background.—In 1979, Yow and co-workers reported that intravenous administration of ampicillin during labor prevented intrapartum transmission of group B β-hemolytic streptococcus (GBS) from mother to infant. Royal Women's Hospital in Melbourne adopted a comprehensive policy of intrapartum chemoprophylaxis for all patients identified as carriers of GBS in 1981. The results of this policy were assessed after 8 years.

Methods.—From January 1981 through December 1988, all 30,197 public patients had low vaginal swabs taken at 32 weeks' gestation for isolation of GBS. Also during that time, 26,915 private patients were admitted but were not screened or treated unless there was evidence of maternal infection. The only significant differences between the 2 groups were maternal age, with a higher percentage of public patients being younger than 20 years of age, and cesarean rate, which was lower among public patients.

Results.—There were no early onset neonatal GBS infections in any of the infants of treated asymptomatic carrier mothers in the public group; however, in the unscreened private group, there were 27 infections overall, with 8 deaths.

Conclusion.—In the absence of an effective vaccine or serological screen, GBS screening should be done antenatally at 28 weeks. Intrapartum chemoprophylaxis should be offered at least to those carriers with obstetric risk factors.

▶ Since Boyer et al. pointed to the feasibility of preventing the uncommon but devastating occurrence of neonatal GBS infection by maternal therapy (see the 1988 YEAR BOOK OF OBSTETRICS AND GYNECOLOGY, pp 231–232), there has been increasing interest in defining candidates for GBS screening who make maternal chemoprophylaxis cost-effective. Cost-effectiveness is the principle barrier to universal screening (see the 1989 YEAR BOOK OF OBSTETRICS AND GYNECOLOGY, pp 39–42 and the 1991 YEAR BOOK OF OBSTETRICS AND GYNECOLOGY, pp 30–31).

In this study, screening results at 32 weeks were used to determine penicillin/erythromycin therapy in labor; they appeared to prevent 14 cases of neonatal infection, assuming the same rate of occurrence that appeared in the control group. All 8 failures in the screened group represent either patients who failed to follow the prophylaxis protocol or cases of maternal sepsis. No cases of neonatal infection appeared in women given prophylactic antibiotic as planned. Regrettably, it's not possible to discern the rate of positive screens at 32 weeks, an important item in determining cost effectiveness. An additional problem is that approximately two thirds of all cases of newborn infection and half of all neonatal deaths came from pregnancies at or less than 32 weeks' gestation and were, therefore, unscreened. The 32-week cutoff data, chosen to reduce the number of screening cultures by a factor of two- to threefold (depending on how many earlier cultures were done) resulted in a loss of some effectiveness. The authors' recommendation that screening be done at 28 weeks on selected cases is not (strictly speaking) supported by their data, and it appears to stem from this concern. All that aside, the Melbourne group finds GBS screening effective based on its 8 years of experience.—T.H. Kirschbaum, M.D.

Haemorrhagic Problems in Obstetrics and Gynaecology in Patients With Congenital Coagulopathies

Greer IA, Lowe GDO, Walker JJ, Forbes CD (Centre for Reproductive Biology, Edinburgh; Royal Infirmary, Glasgow, Scotland; Ninewells Hosp and Med School, Dundee, Scotland)

Br J Obstet Gynaecol 98:909–918, 1991 4–9

Background.—There have been few reports of obstetric and gynecological problems arising in women who are affected by von Willebrand's disease or who carry hemophilia A and Christmas disease. The problems associated with these congenital coagulopathies were studied retrospectively.

Patients and Methods.—Through a review of 30 years of hemophilia unit records, 8 women with von Willebrand's disease, 18 obligate carriers of hemophilia A, and 5 obligate carriers of Christmas disease were identified. These subjects were identified, detailed obstetric and gynecologic histories were obtained, and case histories were reviewed. Laboratory assessments also were done. The subjects had a total of 59 pregnancies, not including first trimester losses and ectopic pregnancies.

Findings.—Seven of the patients with von Willebrand's disease had a total of 14 pregnancies. In this group, there were 4 primary and 4 secondary postpartum hemorrhages and 1 case of a large perineal hematoma that complicated episiotomy. The pregnancy-associated endogenous increase in factor VIIIc did not prevent these problems. Menorrhagia occurred in all patients with von Willebrand's disease; treatment included danazol, tranexemic acid, and oral contraceptives. Severe hemorrhage resulted from diagnostic curettage in 1 patient. Spontaneous hematomas of the broad ligament occurred in 2 patients who complained of pelvic pain and dyspareunia. Of the remaining 43 pregnancies in carriers of hemophilia A and Christmas disease, 5 were complicated by postpartum hemorrhage and 1 was complicated by a large perineal hematoma.

Conclusion.—Special obstetric and gynecological problems may arise in women with von Willebrand's disease and in obligate carriers of the hemophilias. Physicians should manage these patients in close cooperation with the local hemophilia center. Those with von Willebrand's disease need not only factor VIIIc correction, but also measurement of platelet function.

▶ Even in the time since this subject was last reviewed here (See the 1988 YEAR BOOK OF OBSTETRICS AND GYNECOLOGY, pp 106–170), a good deal has been learned about this complex set of abnormalities. As originally described, von Willebrand's disease (VW) differed from hemophilia A by resulting in soft tissue bleeding rather than joint hemorrhages, showing prolonged bleeding time with normal platelet count, and inheriting as an autosomal dominant (chromosome 12) rather than as an X-linked recessive (X chromosome). Since then, the two have proven to be interrelated in a more complex way. The plasma defect in VW originally was described as a decrease in antihemophilia globulin ([AHG-factor VIII] procoagulant [VIIIc]). Decreases in AHG antigen in plasma (type 1) and platelets (type 2) have subsequently been identified. Factor VIIIc consists of a collection of roughly 15 million molecular weight monomers, somewhat between 30 and 60 of which form the enormous multimer produced by the platelets in megakaryocytes. The multimer contains the numerous platelet sites that apparently are needed for platelet aggregation and activation at sites of endothelial damage. Both these functions are inadequate in VW.

The classification of VW reflects the presence or absence of VW antigen and factor VIIIc and their relative concentrations. Type 1 represents the heterozygous state with autosomal-dominant inheritance and all coagulation factors present but in reduced amount. Types 2A, B, and C represent discordant reductions in VW antigen and factor VIIIc (usually dominant inheritance) and, in particular, absence of large multimers of VW antigen in type 2A. Type 3 represents the homozygous state with low-to-absent VW antigen and factor VIIIc. Types 2A and 3 cause serious and cataclysmic bleeding, respectively. One variant (2C) shows sex-linked recessive inheritance reflecting the interrelationship between hemophilia A and VW. Both hemophilia and Christmas disease (absent or nonfunctional factor IX) are sex-linked recessive traits that rarely appear as homozygous states in women; heterozygous states as shown here seldom cause trouble to obstetricians. The inordinate instance of abnormal menses in women known to have these defects makes it important to look for congenital coagulopathies in young women with profuse and prolonged menses.—T.H. Kirschbaum, M.D.

Vertical Transmission of Human Immunodeficiency Virus From Seronegative or Indeterminate Mothers

Johnson JP, Vink PE, Hines SE, Robinson B, Davis JC Jr, Nair P (Univ of Maryland, Baltimore)

Am J Dis Child 145:1239–1241, 1991 4–10

Introduction.—Most HIV infections in children are vertically transmitted, and most of the children have mild or no apparent disease. Screening does not appear to identify all infected women because of the low sensitivity of the enzyme-linked immunosorbent assay used. There have been no previous reports of HIV transmission from seronegative or indeterminate individuals. The identification of infected infants born to women who were seronegative or indeterminate during pregnancy was reviewed.

Patients.—The HIV infection was identified retrospectively in 3 pregnant women. Testing for HIV was indeterminate in 2 cases and seronegative in the third. All 3 women were intravenous drug users or had had intercourse with men who were. Two of the women transmitted the infection to their children. One woman tested positive after signs of infection developed in her child, but the other woman could not be located for testing after signs developed in her infant.

Discussion.—At-risk pregnant women with seronegative or indeterminate HIV status may vertically transmit the virus to their children. Clinicians should be aware of maternal risk factors as well as serological status. Testing should be repeated several times with several assays during pregnancy, and children born to these women should be considered at risk. The lack of confirmed seropositivity in these cases may result from the window period before seroconversion, seroreversion, false negative results, or human error.

▶ This series of case reports effectively argues that, in individuals with risk factors to the infection, negative antibody testing including uncertain membrane reactivity of protein antigens transferred from polyacrylamide gel electrophoresis (Western blotting) should be treated as suspect for HIV infection. Three seronegative gravidas subsequently tested antibody positive or apparently transmitted the infection to their infants. The possibilities are seroreversion (HIV positive to HIV negative, likely in patient 1), sampling after infection but before the development of antibody, or a false negative test error. The second likelihood is particularly strong in a disease in which as many as 36 months may go by before the antibody appears after infection. What's appropriate in such women is repeated testing of both mother and infant and precautions regarding contact with patient blood despite the negative antibody status.—T.H. Kirschbaum, M.D.

Central Hemodynamic Observations in Untreated Preeclamptic Patients

Visser W, Wallenburg HCS (Erasmus Univ, Rotterdam, the Netherlands)
Hypertension 17:1072–1077, 1991 4–11

Background.—Studies of central hemodynamics in preeclampsia using a Swan-Ganz pulmonary artery thermodilution catheter have given varying results, suggesting that the hemodynamic effects of the disease are variable. These variations might, however, have resulted in part from drug treatment the women received. Central hemodynamic measurements in treated and untreated women with preeclampsia were compared.

Methods.—The study sample comprised 87 women with preeclampsia who had received no treatment and 47 who had been treated with various drug therapies and intravenous fluids. Of the untreated women, 74 were nulliparous and 13 were parous; of the treated women, 32 were nulliparous and 15 were parous. Ten pregnant women without hypertension also were studied. All were studied between 25 and 34 weeks' gestation, and all became normotensive and nonproteinuric after delivery. The women were catheterized for no longer than 72 hours, after which all patients either were treated or had delivered their babies.

Hemodynamic Profile in Untreated and Treated Preeclamptic Patients and Normotensive Pregnant Women

	Preeclamptics, untreated (n=87)	p^*	Normotensive controls (n=10)	$p^\dagger$	Preeclamptics, treated (n=47)
Systemic circulation					
Heart rate (beats·min^{-1})	74 (51–110)	<0.05	82 (68–93)	NS	85 (62–135)‡
Mean intra-arterial pressure (mm Hg)	125 (92–156)	<0.001	83 (81–29)	<0.001	120 (80–154)‡
Cardiac index (l·min^{-1}·m^{-2})	3.3 (2.0–5.3)	<0.001	4.2 (3.5–4.6)	NS	4.3 (2.4–7.6)‡
Stroke volume index (ml·beat^{-1}·m^{-2})	46 (25–75)	NS	51 (38–61)	NS	52 (32–82)‡
Systemic vascular resistance index (dyne·sec·cm^{-5}·m^{2})	3,003 (1,771–5,225)	<0.001	1,560 (1,430–2,019)	<0.005	2,212 (1,057–3,688)‡
Left ventricular stroke work index (J·beat^{-1}·m^{-2})	0.70 (0.40–1.16)	<0.005	0.54 (0.43–0.64)	<0.001	0.79 (0.48–1.27)

(continued)

Table *(continued)*

Pulmonary circulation					
Mean pulmonary arterial pressure (mm Hg)	12 (3–26)	<0.05	9 (7–13)	<0.01	13 (0.5–30)
Pulmonary capillary wedge pressure (mm Hg)	7 (−1–20)	NS	5 (1–8)	<0.05	7 (0–25)
Right atrial pressure (mm Hg)	2 (−4–10)	NS	1 (0–2)	NS	1 (−3–12)
Pulmonary vascular resistance index (dyne·sec·cm^{-5}·m^{2})	131 (47–379)	<0.005	91 (63–128)	NS	101 (8–317)‡
Right ventricular stroke work index (J·beat^{-1}·m^{-2})	0.06 (0.01–0.20)	NS	0.05 (0.04–0.08)	<0.05	0.08 (0.01–0.22)‡

The values given are median (range).
* The differences between untreated preeclamptic patients and normotensive controls.
† The differences between pharmacologically treated preeclamptic patients and normotensive controls.
‡ $P < .05$ vs. untreated nulliparous patients.
(Courtesy of Visser W, Wallenburg HCS: Hypertension 17:10722-1077, 1991.)

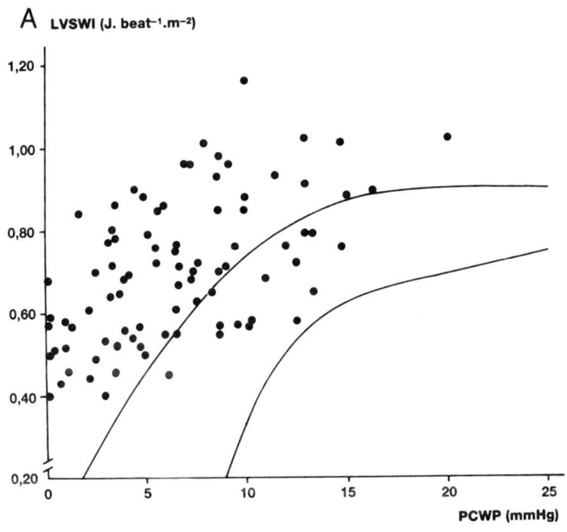

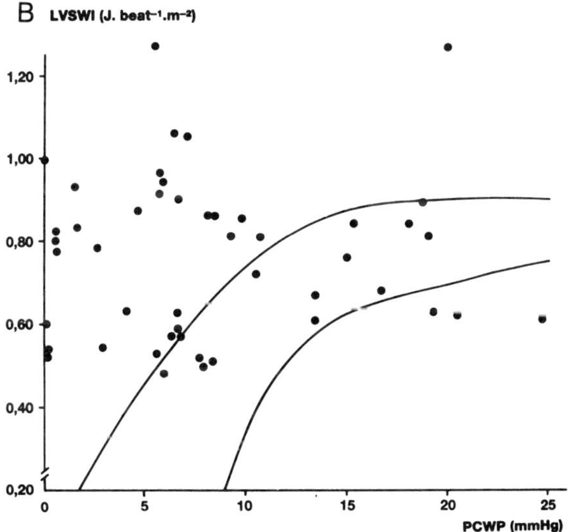

Fig 4–3.—Scatterplots showing the left ventricular stroke work index *(LVSWI)* in 87 untreated (**A**) and 47 treated (**B**) preeclamptic patients plotted against pulmonary capillary wedge pressure *(PCWP)*. The boundaries of normal, nonpregnant left ventricular function are modified from Ross and Braunwald. (Courtesy of Visser W, Wallenburg HCS: *Hypertension* 17:1072–1077, 1991.)

Results.—The cardiac index was significantly lower in the untreated patients than in the treated patients or the normotensive group: 3.3 vs. 4.3 and 4.2 $L \cdot min^{-1} \cdot m^{-2}$, respectively. The systemic vascular resistance index was significantly higher (in the untreated group) than in the other 2 groups (table). There was no significant difference in pulmonary capillary wedge pressure between the 2 preeclamptic groups. Most untreated patients had hyperdynamic left ventricular function (Fig 4–3). Untreated patients had much lower variability of all variables than the treated patients.

Conclusion.—In untreated preeclampsia, there appears to be a somewhat uniform pattern of low cardiac index, high systemic vascular resistance, and normal filling pressures. The wide variation in treated patients probably represents treatment artifacts. Parity appears to have no effect on hemodynamic findings.

▶ This study puts into more easily accessible form the previously reported experience of a careful investigative group (see the 1991 YEAR BOOK OF OBSTETRICS AND GYNECOLOGY, pp 39–41). The degree of individual variability noted in Swan-Ganz measurements in hypertensive pregnancy has been so large as to lead some to decry ever making sense of the data. This group attacks that variability by excluding prior treatment, patients with preexisting cardiovascular renal disease, labor, twins, and evidence of pulmonary edema. In doing so, a fairly homogeneous pattern emerges in untreated preeclamptic patients compared with normotensive gravidas. Systemic vascular resistance and blood pressure are increased, but cardiac index (cardiac output per unit of body-surface area) is reduced, not increased as Sibai and his co-workers have reported. The left ventricular stroke work index is increased, but to a lesser degree than after treatment for pregnancy-induced hypertension using antihypertensives and volume expansion. This is true by virtue of the greater tendency to reduce the heart rate and stroke volume noted in preeclamptic patients compared with normotensive patients with those measures. Although mean pulmonary artery pressure and pulmonary vascular resistance are increased a bit, neither right ventricular filling pressure nor stroke work index is increased.

The role of therapy with magnesium sulfate, antihypertensives, and intravenous fluids in raising the cardiac index and increasing variability is clear. It's an important new observation that the same central hemodynamic changes are seen in nulliparous women as in parous women. What this means is that, although the pathogenesis may well differ between the primigravid and multigravid woman with pregnancy-induced hypertension, the ultimate effect of pathophysiology on the vasculature is indistinguishable based on these measurements.—T.H. Kirschbaum, M.D.

Nitroprusside in Preeclampsia: Circulatory Distress and Paradoxical Bradycardia

Wasserstrum N (Baylor College of Med, Houston)

Hypertension 18:79–84, 1991 4–12

Background.—Prolonged episodes of hypotension may complicate the short-term peripartum management of hypertension with hydralazine in patients with severe preeclampsia, thereby leading to fetal distress. With

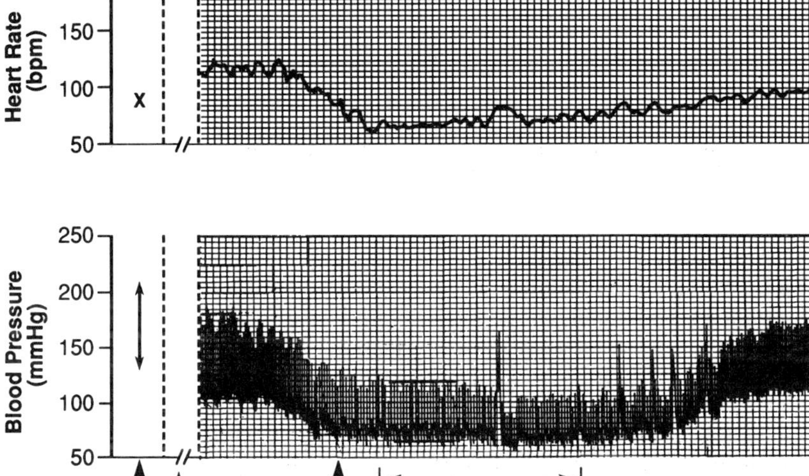

Fig 4–4.—Representative recordings illustrate time courses of decreases in systemic arterial blood pressure and heart rate in a subject from group A who was receiving nitroprusside at .50 μg/kg/min. As noted, drug infusion was discontinued after the onset of a marked reduction in blood pressure. In the interval preceding abrupt depressor response, heart rate was higher than its control, preinfusion value. (Courtesy of Wasserstrum N: *Hypertension* 18:79–84, 1991.)

its rapid onset and brief antihypertensive action, nitroprusside might reduce blood pressure in a more controlled fashion in these patients. This hypothesis was tested in 10 women with severe preeclampsia.

Methods.—The mean age of the women was 22.7 years, and their mean gestational age was 32.9 weeks. Seven were nulliparous. All had severe preeclampsia, with a mean arterial pressure (MAP) greater than 130 mm Hg and proteinuria greater than 1+. The women underwent Swan-Ganz catheterization for monitoring, after which nitroprusside infusion was begun. Infusion was begun at .02 μg/kg/min and was increased incrementally until a 10% to 20% reduction in MAP was achieved. If there was any abrupt drop in pressure, the infusion was stopped immediately.

Results.—Eight patients (group A) responded to nitroprusside with a decrease in heart rate, and 2 (group B) responded with an increase in heart rate. In group B, the sinoaortic baroreceptor reflex increased heart rate by more than 17 beats/min in response to a moderate decrease of 32 mm Hg in MAP. Their nitroprusside dose was a moderate 1.03 μg/kg/min. In group A, there was a 75-mm Hg decrease in MAP at doses of 0.35 μg/kg/min, along with a decrease in heart rate of 21 beats/min (Fig 4–4). These apparently paradoxical responses indicated severe circulatory compromise and corresponded to the cardiac and vasomotor depression characteristic of severe hemorrhage and other types of acute or severe hypovolemic hypotension.

Conclusion.—Preeclamptic patients compensate poorly for hypovolemic stimuli such as venodilators or perioperative hemorrhage. Nitroprusside may be used in severe preeclampsia only with caution and after considering the patient's blood volume. The paradoxical hemodynamic pattern described represents a cardiopulmonary baroreceptor reflex that apparently is related to the Bezold-Jarisch reflex. This response probably results from the imposition of nitroprusside's venous dilator action on the reduced blood volume of preeclampsia.

▶ Although it rests on a small number of clinical observations, this is an important warning to those who use sodium nitroprusside as an antihypertensive in acute episodes of pregnancy hypertension. The agent is a very potent, rapidly acting arterial and venous dilator. This combination, coupled with a relative hypovolemia of preeclampsia, can well lead to the abrupt decrease in cardiac output and impairment in venous filling of the heart seen in 8 of 10 of the patients studied here. Bradycardia serves as an easily recognized consequence of reduced ventricular filling. Nitroprusside is a drug to be used with great caution in pregnancy-induced hypertension.—T.H. Kirschbaum, M.D.

Early Blood Pressure Control Improves Pregnancy Outcome in Primigravid Women With Mild Hypertension

Phippard AF, Fischer WE, Horvath JS, Child AG, Korda AR, Henderson-Smart D, Duggin GG, Tiller DJ (Royal Prince Alfred Hosp; King George V Hosp, Camperdown, Australia)

Med J Aust 154:378–382, 1991 4–13

Background.—There is disagreement as to whether antihypertensive drug treatment is appropriate for pregnant women with mild-to-moderate hypertension. A double-blind, placebo-controlled study was conducted to evaluate whether strict blood-pressure control improves the outcome of pregnancy.

Methods.—The analysis included 52 primigravid women in the third trimester of pregnancy with mild-to-moderate hypertension, i.e., less than 170/110 mm Hg. Twenty-seven women were randomized to receive placebo treatment and 25 to receive action hypertensive treatment with clonidine and hydralazine. The patients remained in the hospital from entry into the trial until their infants were born. The women in the placebo group were treated if severe hypertension developed.

Results.—Nine women were withdrawn from the trial as a result of deterioration in their condition—8 in the placebo group and 1 in the treatment group (Fig 4–5). Three of the controls had proteinuria develop, but none of the treatment group subjects did. The results of in-

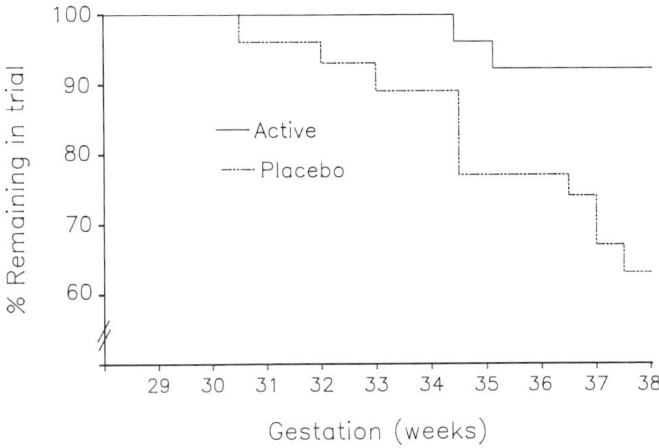

Fig 4–5.—Survival curves by treatment group for patients remaining in trial without reaching fetal or maternal end points. (Courtesy of Phippard AF, Fischer WE, Horvath JS, et al: *Med J Aust* 154:378–382, 1991.)

tention-to-treat analysis revealed that the placebo group had a significant increase in premature delivery for complications, despite treatment in the women who were withdrawn because of severe hypertension. In the placebo group, 4 infants had neonatal respiratory distress requiring intensive care, compared with none in the treatment group. None of the infants died or showed any adverse effects of treatment.

Conclusion.—Mild hypertension in pregnant women should be controlled early to prevent progression to emergency premature delivery. These results underscore the need for practical markers of preeclampsia.

▶ This prospective, blinded study attacks a common problem that is notoriously hard to research. It is important that only primigravidas are studied, because that reduces the number of women with underlying cardiovascular renal disease as the cause of their hypertension. All patients enrolled were kept hospitalized until delivery, except for occasional patients kept overnight. Because withdrawal from the study as a result of worsening hypertension, hepatic dysfunction, or intrauterine growth retardation was an important outcome measure, the extent to which decisions were blinded with respect to therapy becomes important. Those receiving antihypertensive therapy were subjected to an incremental dose scaled to obtain blood pressure control, whereas those receiving placebo were not, thereby implicitly informing physicians as to the presence or absence of drug therapy. Note that these women in their early-to-middle twenties entered with blood pressure averaging 129/84 and 126/82, with a lack of albuminuria, and with an average blood pressure of 100/60 in early pregnancy. Hypertension was, in general, diagnosable, but it certainly was mild. Regrettably, only 52 patients were studied. The results show that administration of hydralazine and clonidine in doses sufficient to decrease blood pressure resulted in fewer decisions to interrupt the study patients (2 of 25) than the placebo group (10 of 27). The risk of delivery before 38 weeks was reduced, as was the incidence of admission to the neonatal intensive care unit. This provides some justification for the treatment of women with mild preeclampsia contrasting with the lack of evidence of benefit from such therapy in gravidas with other forms of hypertension (see the 1991 YEAR BOOK OF OBSTETRICS AND GYNECOLOGY, pp 74–75).—T.H. Kirschbaum, M.D.

The Prevalence of Autoantibodies During Third-Trimester Pregnancy Complicated by Hypertension or Idiopathic Fetal Growth Retardation

Milliez J, Lelong F, Bayani N, Jannet D, El Medjadji M, Latrous H, Hammami M, Paniel BJ (Centre Hosp Intercommunal, Creteil, France)

Am J Obstet Gynecol 165:51–56, 1991 4–14

Purpose.—The prevalence of antiphospholipid and other specific autoantibodies in a general obstetric population was compared with their prevalence in pregnancies complicated by hypertension or idiopathic fetal growth retardation.

Methods.—Lupus anticoagulant, anticardiolipin, antinuclear, anti-DNA, antithyroglobulin, and antithyroid microsomal antibodies were assayed during the third trimester of pregnancy in 100 normal pregnancies and 100 pregnancies with complications. Fifty patients with pregnancy complications had fetal growth retardation, and 50 had hypertension. The hypertension included preeclampsia and gestational or chronic hypertension.

Findings.—The activated partial thromboplastin time was normal in all cases, but the lupus anticoagulant was also assayed by standard coagulation tests, tissue thromboplastin inhibition time, platelet neutralization procedure, and cephalin neutralization time. In the general obstetric population, the prevalence of the lupus anticoagulant was .27% compared with .3% in a series of 1,000 women with a history of fetal death or thromboembolic disease who did not have systemic lupus erythematosus. The prevalence of anticardiolipin antibodies in a low-risk obstetric population was 2.2%.

Conclusion.—In pregnancies complicated by hypertension, the prevalence of autoantibodies was significantly higher than in pregnancies with idiopathic fetal growth retardation or normal pregnancies. Antiphospholipid antibodies were not related to an aggravation of hypertension, an impairment of fetal growth, or a poor fetal outcome. However, patients with autoantibodies had a significantly more frequent history of fetal growth retardation during a previous pregnancy than did patients with no autoantibody.

▶ The question posed in this study is inevitable and worthy of a screening study. If lupus anticoagulant is found in .3% of gravidas without a prior history of fetal death and in approximately 2% of the normal obstetrical population, do the incidence figures for occurrence in women with hypertension and intrauterine growth retardation (IUGR) suggest a previously undetected role in those disorders? The answers are suggestive—but only for hypertensive disease. Some experimental design features have to be noted. All the patients studied had normal activated partial thromboplastin and kaolin times, the tests normally used to detect lupus anticoagulant. Only with tissue thromboplastin inhibition, platelet neutralization, and phospholipid-activated partial thromboplastin time was the diagnosis made. Antibodies to DNA, thyroglobulin, and thyroid microsomal fractions were also assayed and were found equally often in normal and hypertensive patients.

The lack of a relationship (in theory) to vascular disease makes the antithyroid findings less interesting, and grouping those results with lupus and anticardiolipin antibody holders complicates the evaluation. Exempting thyroid antibody, there is a suggestion that lupus and anticardiolipin antibodies appear more often in patients with hypertension than in normal patients, but not in those with idiopathic IUGR. An increased incidence in hypertension and IUGR is cited, but data from such patients are not given. Because the severity of hypertension was not related to the presence of antibody, the authors suggest that no special handling is indicated for these patients; however, the aggregation of patients with thyroid antibodies and the division of 8 patients into 6 categories makes the number of cases per category too small for evaluation. What all this means is that there may be an undetected autoimmune component to pregnancy hypertension involving the activation of phospholipid epitopes of clotting factors. This work enforces that hypothesis, but much more work must be done to verify it.—T.H. Kirschbaum, M.D.

Pregnancy in Patients With a History of Juvenile Rheumatoid Arthritis

Østensen M (Univ of Oslo, Norway)

Arthritis Rheum 34:881–887, 1991 4–15

Introduction.—Juvenile rheumatoid arthritis (JRA) is a rheumatic disease that starts before the age of 16 years, affects 1 or more joints or extra-articular sites, and affects slightly more females than males. Spontaneous remission of the disease occurs in approximately 70% of patients. However, the relationship between JRA and pregnancy with regard to possible reactivation of the disease, complications at delivery, and postpartum complications has not been studied in detail. Data on 76 pregnancies in 56 patients with JRA were examined retrospectively.

Findings.—In the 76 pregnancies, improvement was noted during 35, there was no change in disease activity in 34, and signs and symptoms worsened in 7 pregnancies. Inactive disease did not flare during gestation, but a small number of patients experienced a short episode of active arthritis during the first trimester. Patients with minor symptoms at conception and the majority of those with active inflammation experienced improvement or total remission in the second half of gestation. The 4 patients with JRA who had active anterior uveitis had active eye disease during pregnancy. Seventy-four of 76 pregnancies produced healthy infants of normal birth weight. One infant had low birth weight, and 1 infant was stillborn. Fifteen of 20 cesarean deliveries were related to the sequelae of JRA. A flare at 3–6 months post partum occurred in 45 pregnancies. In patients whose disease had been quiescent before or during pregnancy, this postpartum flare did not cause permanent reactivation of the disease.

Conclusion.—When 51 patients with JRA were compared with 45 age-matched female patients without children, the limiting factors in the decision for or against having children were disease severity and functional impairment. Pregnancy does not aggravate or reactivate the disease, and the disease does not harm the fetus, although multiple pregnancy carries the risk of more permanent reactivation of JRA. There is a risk for postpartum flare, even in patients with inactive disease.

► It is uncommon that enough patients with this disease can be collected to form the basis for useful generalizations in regard to its relationship with pregnancy. This report makes use of both the centralization of medical care and the relatively high incidence of rheumatoid disease in Scandinavia. The patterns are reasonably familiar. Most women experience diminution in symptoms and signs during pregnancy, except for the tendency for some to notice a mild increase in symptoms, transitionally, in the first trimester. The criteria for exacerbation of disease are relatively subtle, thereby increasing the sensitivity of the study. A postpartum flare in symptoms was seen in 45 of 50 patients available for study, and it is in this area that the reported experience is most useful. When the disease is both stable and inactive before pregnancy, the postpartum exacerbation is nearly always mild, self-contained, and unrelated to a long-term decrease in function. Only in those women with repeated pregnancies does the tendency for distinct progression appear. The data are soft in this area, but this is a fine article upon which to base the counseling of a woman with JRA who is contemplating pregnancy.—T.H. Kirschbaum, M.D.

The Influence of Pregnancy on Relapses in Multiple Sclerosis: A Cohort Study

Bernardi S, Grasso MG, Bertollini R, Orzi F, Fieschi C (Univ of Rome; Lazio Region, Rome)

Acta Neurol Scand 84:403–406, 1991 4–16

Objective.—Since the 1950s, studies have shown an overall reduction of relapses of multiple sclerosis (MS) during pregnancy but an increase in the postpartum period. To investigate further, the course of MS was analyzed during pregnancy and puerperium.

Patients.—Fifty-two women with MS were studied during pregnancy and 6 months immediately post partum. The number of relapses per person per year was determined during 66 pregnancy-years.

Findings.—Thirty-one relapses occurred, 5 during pregnancy and 26 during the puerperium. The relapse rate was significantly lower during the pregnancy-year (.38 per year) compared with the nonpregnancy-years in the same group of women. During the pregnancy-year, a heterogeneous pattern was observed, with a sharp decrease of 84% in events during pregnancy and a slight but nonsignificant increase of 22% in the puerperium. There was a total decrease of 51% in relapses during the pregnancy-year, even after considering age at onset and duration of disease.

Conclusion.—Pregnancy does not appear to be a risk factor for exacerbations of MS. On the contrary, pregnancy appears to act, on the whole, as a protective event. These data allow physicians to provide reassuring counseling to women.

▶ It's commonly believed that pregnancy reduces the incidence of relapse (worsening of old signs and symptoms or appearance of new findings lasting more than 24 hours but less than 2 years), but that the puerperium shows an increased relapse rate. This study of 66 pregnancies in 52 women who were followed for at least 1 year after delivery finds the risk of puerperal relapse heterogeneous but low, i.e., approximately 22%. Some relapses occur so soon after delivery as to make an etiological relationship to pregnancy seem likely purely on the basis of timing. The failure to demonstrate risk ratios with 95% confidence limits greater than 1 means that the risk of puerperal relapse cannot be demonstrated to be greater than that which occurs in nonpregnancy, and that the clinical impression to the contrary simply may reflect a loss of pregnancy-conferred amelioration. It is suggested that pregnancy may be an unalloyed benefit for women with MS, and that MS should not be seen as a deterrent for women with this disease who seek to become pregnant.—T.H. Kirschbaum, M.D.

Pregnancy Outcome and Ebstein's Anomaly

Donnelly JE, Brown JM, Radford DJ (Mater Misericordiae Public Hosps, South Brisbane; Prince Charles Hosp, Chermside, Queensland, Australia)

Br Heart J 66:368–371, 1991 4–17

Background.—There have been few reports of pregnancy in women with Ebstein's anomaly, an uncommon congenital cardiac abnormality. A significant proportion of these patients do reach childbearing age, and they require pregnancy advice and management.

Patients.—Twelve women with Ebstein's anomaly had 42 pregnancies, resulting in 36 live births. Ebstein's anomaly was undiagnosed until pregnancy in 6 of the patients. Associated cyanosis was present in 2 patients, and Wolff-Parkinson-White syndrome was seen in 2. Five miscarriages occurred, 4 of them in 1 patient. Dyspnea was reported in the third trimester by most patients, but only 2 received digoxin treatment. Only 1 needed treatment for palpitations. Two patients, 1 with Wolff-Parkinson-White syndrome and 1 with cyanosis, had considerable problems during pregnancy. Of the 36 live-born infants, 5 were premature and 4 more were small for gestational age. Of the 3 infants born to women with cyanosis, 2 were premature and 1 was small for gestational age. One infant died in the neonatal period.

Conclusion.—Pregnancy is usually well tolerated, with good fetal outcome, in women with Ebstein's anomaly. These women can be counseled to this effect. The risk is higher in women with arrhythmia or cyanosis, and they should be observed more closely.

▶ The abnormally low placement of the tricuspid valve in this anomaly severely restricts the stroke volume of the right ventricle. In the absence of other anomalies, this reduces blood flow to the left ventricle and, therefore, reduces cardiac output. The only adaptation to pregnancy that is possible is to increase the pulse rate. The high likelihood of tricuspid valve insufficiency in pregnancy adds to the risk by further diverting the right ventricle output from the pulmonary artery to the right atrium. That is why this report is so surprising.

The 2 deaths reported in this retrospective study were in women aged 48 and 73 years at the time of cardiologic diagnosis. The latter woman had 10 pregnancies and 6 live births. The key is that these women survived to and past the reproductive age, which is a testament to the lack of complicating co-existing cardiologic lesions and their ability to adapt, probably by increasing the right ventricular stroke volume. Arrhythmias were the only management problem in 20% of these 12 women. This is a study to remember when the rare patient with this abnormality is seen for obstetrical care.—T.H. Kirschbaum, M.D.

The Effect of Maternal Hemodynamics on Fetal Growth in Hypertensive Pregnancies

Easterling TR, Benedetti TJ, Carlson KC, Brateng DA, Wilson J, Schmucker BS (Univ of Washington, Seattle)

Am J Obstet Gynecol 165:902–906, 1991 4–18

Introduction.—Maternal hypertension can impair fetal growth, although some infants born to mothers with severe hypertension show no evidence of abnormal development. It has been hypothesized that the individual character of maternal dynamics accounts for these differences in outcome. The effects of maternal hemodynamics were reviewed in a study of 76 pregnancies.

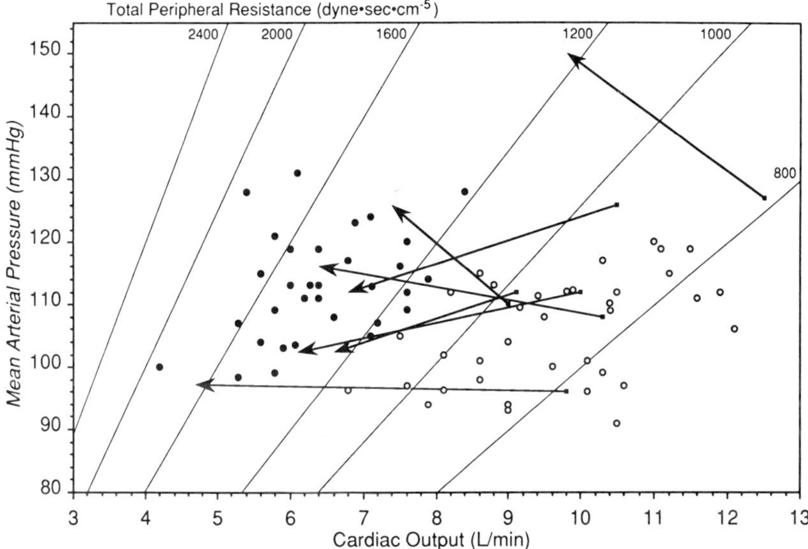

Fig 4–6.—Maternal hemodynamics. The mean arterial pressure of each subject is plotted against cardiac output. Isometric lines of vascular resistance are included so all 3 parameters can be displayed on a single figure. *Filled circles,* high-resistance subjects; *open circles,* low-resistance subjects; *square,* subject whose hemodynamics crossed over. Associated vector graphically displays the change in hemodynamics associated with crossover. (Courtesy of Easterling TR, Benedetti TJ, Carlson KC, et al: *Am J Obstet Gynecol* 165:902–906, 1991.)

Methods.—Hypertension, which was diagnosed at or before 28 weeks' gestation, was defined as a diastolic pressure of 90 mm Hg on 2 occasions that were 6 hours apart. Cardiac output was measured by the Doppler technique and blood pressure was measured by the automated cuff. All patients underwent hemodynamic measurements until the end of pregnancy. The pregnancies were characterized as high resistance hypertension (32 cases) or low-resistance hypertension (36 cases). Eight pregnancies were placed in a crossover group when subsequent measurements showed that the hemodynamic pattern changed from low- to high resistance hypertension.

Results.—The 3 groups had similar rates of nulliparity, chronic hypertension, and proteinuria. Women with low-resistance hypertension were 19 kg heavier than those with high-resistance hypertension. The mean arterial pressures were higher in both the high-resistance and crossover groups; the mean heart rates were higher in the low-resistance and crossover groups (Fig 4–6). Infants in the crossover groups had low percentile weights for gestational age and a high rate of intrauterine fetal death. High-resistance hypertension was associated with an earlier delivery (by 4 weeks) and a lower birth weight (mean, 1,058 g less) than in the low-resistance group.

Conclusion.—There are clear correlations between fetal outcome and maternal hemodynamics in hypertensive patients. Vasoconstricted maternal circulation carries a strong risk of early delivery and impaired fetal growth. The outcomes are particularly poor when there is a crossing over to high-resistance hypertension in the third trimester.

▶ Categorizing subsets of patients with pregnancy-induced hypertension using elements of the Poissette-Hagen diagram is a potentially valuable approach (see the 1990 YEAR BOOK OF OBSTETRICS AND GYNECOLOGY, pp 74–76), but there are systematic differences between the results obtained by Doppler analysis of cardiac output and the thermodilution values obtained by pulmonary artery catheter (see the 1988 YEAR BOOK OF OBSTETRICS AND GYNECOLOGY, pp 54–57). Doppler values are 10% to 20% larger than thermodilution values, and this research group declines to calculate cardiac indices, i.e., cardiac output per unit surface area. For these reasons, they report that cardiac output increased in pregnancy-induced hypertension, which is in contrast to other investigators who find the cardiac index reduced. For this reason, their upper limit of peripheral vascular resistance (1,150 dyne/sec/cm^{-5}) is much smaller than the more conventional 1,400 to 1,500 dyne/sec/cm^{-5}. Ignoring these differences, this study demonstrates that increased systemic vascular resistance during hypertensive pregnancy leads to compromise of fetal growth and survival. Although this is not an entirely surprising conclusion, it benefits by confirmation from the Seattle investigators.—T.H. Kirschbaum, M.D.

Effectiveness of Percutaneous Balloon Mitral Valvotomy During Pregnancy

Esteves CA, Ramos AIO, Braga SLN, Harrison JK, Sousa JEMR (Dante Pazzanese Inst of Cardiology, São Paulo, Brazil; Duke Univ, Durham, NC)
Am J Cardiol 68:930–934, 1991 4–19

Introduction.—Controversy exists regarding the optimal management of pregnant women with severe mitral stenosis who have medically refractory congestive heart failure. There is a significant risk of fetal death after closed or open surgical commissurotomy. The hemodynamic results and clinical outcome of balloon mitral valvotomy were examined in such patients.

Methods.—A consecutive series of 13 pregnant women underwent percutaneous balloon mitral valvotomy for the treatment of rheumatic mitral stenosis. The mean patient age was 26 years, and the mean gestational age at the time of valvotomy was 25 weeks. One woman was carrying twins. All had functional class III or IV congestive heart failure. A lead apron was used to limit fetal exposure to radiation during the catheterization procedure.

Results.—Balloon mitral valvotomy was successful in all patients. Decreases were seen immediately in mitral valve gradient, left atrial pressure, and pulmonary artery systolic pressure. The symptoms of congestive heart disease improved in all women. All 12 who had delivered by the end of the study were in functional class I. The 1 patient who had not yet given birth remained free of cardiac symptoms. Healthy infants were delivered in the singlet pregnancies, but the twins were born early (32 weeks) and died of respiratory failure at 48 hours.

Conclusion.—Excellent hemodynamic results were obtained in these young pregnant women. Their valves are unlikely to be heavily calcified or have severe subvalvular thickening, and they are thus amenable to balloon mitral valvotomy. Surgical commissurotomy of the mitral valve poses no great risk to pregnant women, but it is associated with a 15% to 33% incidence of fetal death. When performed at centers with experience in the procedure, balloon mitral valvotomy offers an effective alternative to surgery.

▶ This is a large experience, collected in just 1 year, of excellent operative results. The transseptal technique is used, entering the heart through the right atrium and puncturing the interatrial septum to gain access to the mitral valve. During balloon inflation, the atrioventricular valve is occluded, decreasing cardiac output and uterine blood flow to near zero for a few hectic moments. The good results can be attributed to several factors. More than half the cases had New York Heart Association functional class III disease, and 2 (cases 6 and 8) had relatively large mitral orifices, 1 with a nearly normal mitral pressure gradient. The less severe the lesion, the better the results. Also, the patients were young (average age, 26 years), and the lesions were of relatively short duration with no atrial fibrillation. Although one may argue with the indications for operative intervention in midpregnancy, the authors make their point. During pregnancy in properly selected cases, the procedure can safely be carried out, both from the maternal and the infant viewpoint.—T.H. Kirschbaum, M.D.

Maternal Hemodynamics in Pregnancies Complicated by Hyperthyroidism

Easterling TR, Schmucker BC, Carlson KL, Millard SP, Benedetti TJ (Univ of Washington, Seattle)

Obstet Gynecol 78:348–352, 1991 4–20

Introduction.—Hyperthyroidism in pregnancy is associated with an increased risk of stillbirth, premature delivery, and preeclampsia. Hyperthyroidism and pregnancy both increase the basal metabolic rate, and the combined impact of these 2 conditions may be expected to create a hyperdynamic state. However, the maternal hemodynamics in pregnancy complicated by hyperthyroidism have only been studied in women with severe thyrotoxicosis. The effect of drug therapy on the hemodynamics in pregnant women with less severe hyperthyroidism was studied.

Patients.—Six pregnant hyperthyroid women attending an endocrinology clinic made up the study group. The goals of therapy were to reduce the free thyroxine (T4) index to within the high-normal range and to reduce the medication dosage to the minimum required to maintain control throughout the pregnancy. The cardiac output was measured by Doppler technique. Blood pressure (BP) was measured by an automated cuff. The hemodynamic measurements obtained in the hyperthyroid women were compared at points of maximum and minimum free T4 index with those previously obtained in euthyroid pregnant women who did not have preeclampsia or gestational hypertension develop during their pregnancy.

Results.—At the maximum free T4 index, BP, cardiac output, heart rate, and stroke volume in the hyperthyroid women were significantly elevated, whereas the total systemic peripheral vascular resistance was significantly reduced compared with those values in euthyroid women. Despite normal thyroid tests at minimum free T4 index after drug therapy, the cardiac output and stroke volume remained markedly increased, and the total peripheral resistance remained reduced. There were no stillbirths, but 1 fetus died of extreme prematurity. Two other women delivered prematurely. None of the women had preeclampsia develop, but 1 woman had gestational hypertension.

Conclusion.—Although the hemodynamics in pregnant thyrotoxic women normalize with therapy, they remain significantly hyperdynamic throughout the pregnancy. The elevation in BP suggests that the increase in cardiac output is primary, and that the reduction in vascular resistance is a compensatory mechanism that reduces the BP but is unable to return it to baseline values.

▶ These 6 women were studied using Doppler-based estimates of aortic blood flow and conventional blood pressure measurements. In their validation study of Doppler measurements in hypertensive women (see the 1988 YEAR BOOK OF OBSTETRICS AND GYNECOLOGY, pp 54–57) the correspondence with thermodilution measures of cardiac output was fair, with Doppler values 10% to 20% lower than those achieved by the more conventional method. Although the cardiac index values (cardiac output per unit surface area) would have made the results more easily comparable to the work of others, the increased cardiac output, heart rate, and stroke volume are not surprising. Evidence for elevated blood pressure is equivocal here, and the authors' interpretation is somewhat clouded by the failure to differentiate preeclampsia from thyrotoxic hypertension. Increased cardiac output must result in either decreased vascular resistance or increased blood pressure. Because the pressure increment seems marginal, the decreasing peripheral vascular resistance is an unavoidable consequence of the relationship among these 3 variables. Clearly, nothing regarding the pathophysiology of preeclampsia should be inferred.

The authors refer to the work of Davis et al. (1), who reported on the results of pulmonary artery catheterization done in 4 of 7 thyrotoxic patients in heart failure. Six of these patients had no prenatal care, and their pregnancies were complicated by preeclampsia, anemia, and infection. In those patients, cardiac output was, of course, reduced, and systemic vascular resistance increased compared with normal pregnancy as a consequence of the decreased ventricular function in failure. Comparisons with the hemodynamics of the thyrotoxic patients who were not in failure seem not entirely appropriate.—T.H. Kirschbaum, M.D.

Reference

1. Davis LE, et al: *Am J Obstet Gynecol* 160:63, 1989.

HIV-I Infection in Perinatally Exposed Siblings and Twins

de Martino M, Tovo P-A, Galli L, Caselli D, Gabiano C, Mazzoni PL, Giacomelli A, Duse M, Fundarò C, Italian Register for HIV Infection in Children (Univ of Florence, Italy)

Arch Dis Child 66:1235–1238, 1991 4–21

Background.—Most cases of HIV type I (HIV-I) infection in children result from maternal transmission, mainly in utero. Only small or anecdotal reports have addressed the risk of vertical transmission in twins or second pregnancies. Data from the Italian Register for HIV Infection in Children were used to evaluate this issue.

Patients.—The study included 1,493 children born at 75 centers to HIV-I-infected mothers. A total of 823 of the children were followed prospectively from birth. There were 22 twin pairs and 56 sibships. The frequency of twin pregnancies was 1.5%, and 3.9% of women had more than 1 at-risk pregnancy. Eighteen twin pairs had a known infection status; of these, 9 were infected. Only 1 pair of dizygous twins had discordant infection status; the relative risk of infection when the other twin was infected was 23.1. There was no association between infection and gestational age, method of delivery, or birth weight.

Infection status was known in 41 sibships, including a total of 84 children. The second-born child was infected 42.3% of the time when the first-born child was infected, but only 12.5% of the time when the first-born child was uninfected. Of the children prospectively followed from birth, 22.2% of first-born and 23.8% of second-born children acquired HIV-I infection.

Conclusion.—The risk of mother-to-child HIV-I transmission does not appear to be increased in twin or second pregnancies. Perinatal infection appears to be influenced by noncausal factors in the mother, child, or both. Neither vaginal delivery nor prematurity increase the risk of infection.

▶ This study of infants whose disease status was evaluated at the age of 16.3–38 months tends to indicate a minor role for postdelivery horizontal infection between mother and infants via nursing or contact with blood or body fluids. Although the overall risks of infection, given an infected mother, were not larger for twins or siblings from the same mother, infection of 1 infant was an overwhelming determinant in either a mono- or dizygous twin. In sibs born successively after an infected neonate, no striking increase in risk compared with the risk for first singlet postinfected pregnancies was seen. Had environmental factors been important, such siblings would have shown an increased risk of infection. In fact, in 41 such sibships, roughly one third consisted of first-born infected infants followed by a second-born uninfected sibling. The findings suggest that placental access of the fetus to its mother is needed to generate the approximately 19% risk of infection now reported by this group. Although the chances of an increased risk of infection through nursing were apparent in this study in contrast to an earlier report (see the 1990 YEAR BOOK OF OBSTETRICS AND GYNECOLOGY, pp 190–199), neither preterm birth nor vaginal delivery appeared to affect outcome.—T.H. Kirschbaum, M.D.

Placental Bed Spiral Arteries in the Hypertensive Disorders of Pregnancy

Pijnenborg R, Anthony J, Davey DA, Rees A, Tiltman A, Vercruysse L, Van Assche A (Univ of Cape Town, South Africa; Univ of Leuven, Belgium)

Br J Obstet Gynaecol 98:648–655, 1991 4–22

Background.—Hypertensive disorders are a major complication of pregnancy. Lesions of the spiral arteries have a major role in the pathophysiology of these disorders, but the exact relationship between the histopathologic changes in the placental bed and the different hypertensive

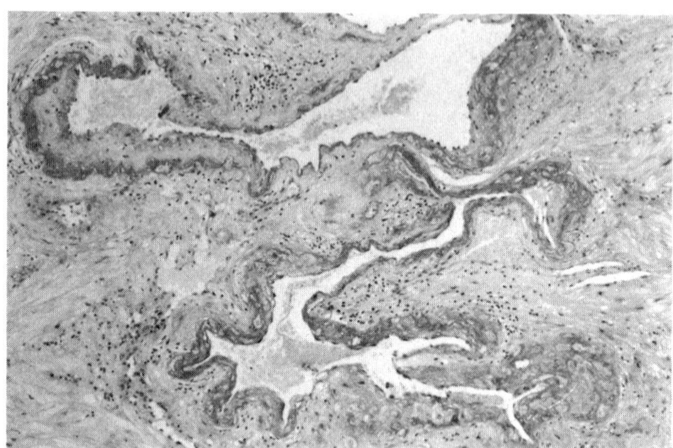

Fig 4–7.—Myometrial spiral artery of normotensive woman showing normal physiological changes of pregnancy. The vessel wall is replaced by trophoblastic cells buried in periodic acid-Schiff-positive fibrinoid material; periodic acid-Schiff × 25. (Courtesy of Pijnenborg R, Anthony J, Davey DA, et al: *Br J Obstet Gynaecol* 98:648–655, 1991.)

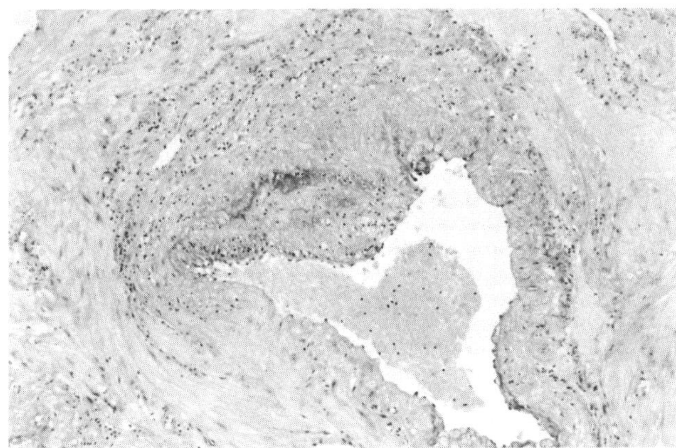

Fig 4–8.—Myometrial spiral artery of patient with gestational proteinuric hypertension showing a marked reduction of physiological changes. Only a few trophoblastic cells within some fibrinoid material are revealed by using periodic acid-Schiff staining; PAS × 25. (Courtesy of Pijnenborg R, Anthony J, Davey DA, et al: *Br J Obstet Gynaecol* 98:648–655, 1991.)

disorders classified by Davey and MacGillivray has yet to be determined. The histology of the spiral arteries of the placental bed was studied in normal pregnancies and in pregnancies complicated by hypertension.

Methods.—The observational study included 17 normal pregnant women and 43 with gestational hypertension. The latter group included 39 women with proteinuria, 17 with chronic hypertension (6 of whom had proteinuria), and 5 with unclassified hypertension. Placental bed biopsy specimens were obtained during cesarean section. The sections were stained with hematoxylin-eosin, PAS, and Lendrum's MSB.

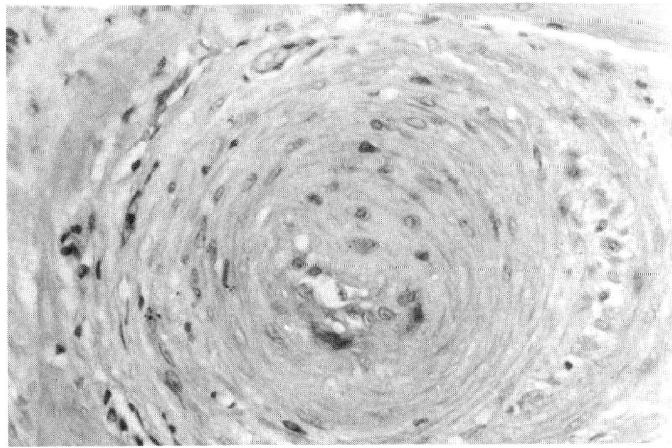

Fig 4–9.—Myometrial spiral artery of patient with gestational proteinuric hypertension showing complete absence of physiological changes and hyperplasia of the media; hematoxylin-eosin × 100. (Courtesy of Pijnenborg R, Anthony J, Davey DA, et al: *Br J Obstet Gynaecol* 98:648–655, 1991.)

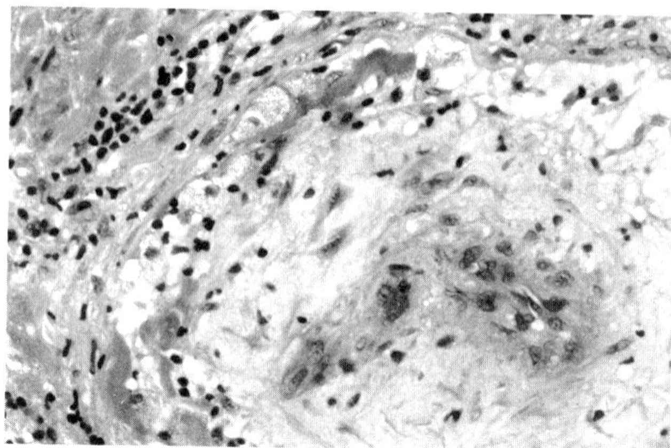

Fig 4–10.—Acute atherosis in myometrial spiral artery of patient with chronic hypertension and superimposed preeclampsia; hematoxylin-eosin; × 100. (Courtesy of Pijnenborg R, Anthony J, Davey DA, et al: *Br J Obstet Gynaecol* 98:648–655, 1991.)

Results.—Six normotensive and 44 hypertensive women had biopsy specimens that contained spiral arteries. Trophoblastic invasion was seen in 5 of 6 normotensive biopsy specimens, but not in most of those from patients with hypertension. Subintimal proliferation occurred in all normotensive biopsy specimens, but in only 8 of 28 from those with gestational hypertension and proteinuria. The other characteristics of the hypertensive biopsy specimens were medial hyperplasia, fibrin deposits, acute atherosis, endothelial vacuolation, and thrombosis (Figs 4–7 through 4–10).

Conclusion.—The absence of physiological changes may not be peculiar to preeclampsia. It may be associated with—or even be—a result of various forms of hypertension in pregnancy.

▶ This is an attempt to match the spiral arterial pathology in hypertension in pregnancy (first noted by Brosens et al. [1]) to the clinical classification of hypertensive disorders of pregnancy proposed by Davey and MacGillivray (2). The classification, which consists of 17 categories, deals with onset in relation to pregnancy and its duration (whether marked by hypertension, proteinuria, or both), presence of prepregnancy hypertension, and seizures; however, it does not deal with onset in relation to CNS system or cardiovascular changes. The biopsy technique is improved using open wedge biopsy through the incision for elective repeat cesarean section. Those who prize simplicity will be glad to know there is no regular relationship of biopsy findings to the Davey and MacGillivray classification. On the other hand, there is abundant vascular pathology in what most would call preeclampsia (28 of 39 cases) and in chronic hypertensives with (5 of 6) and without (7 of 11) incremental blood pressure increases during gestation. What is eminently clear is that disturbed uteroplacental vascular findings are common in acute hypertensive disease in pregnancy.—T.H. Kirschbaum, M.D.

References

1. Brosens I, et al: *J Path Bact* 93:569, 1967.
2. Davey DA, MacGillivray I: *Am J Obstet Gynecol* 158:892, 1988.

Fetal Cardiac Function in Intrauterine Growth Retardation
Rizzo G, Arduini D (Università Cattolica S Cuore, Rome)
Am J Obstet Gynecol 165:876–882, 1991 4–23

Background.—Fetuses with intrauterine growth retardation (IUGR) resulting from placental insufficiency have altered blood-flow velocity waveforms in several peripheral vascular beds. The concomitant changes in cardiac function were studied.

Methods.—Color and pulsed Doppler echocardiographic recordings were performed in 124 fetuses with IUGR. These fetuses had no structural or chromosomal anomalies, and they also had increased umbilical artery resistance and decreased middle cerebral artery resistance. Twenty-four fetuses were also examined weekly until the onset of antepartum late heart rate decelerations. Blood-flow velocity waveforms were obtained from the aortic and pulmonary valves, and several parameters were measured.

Results.—When compared with previously established norms, both aortic and pulmonary peak systolic velocities and the pulmonary time to peak velocity were decreased in fetuses with IUGR. Aortic time to peak velocity was increased. Left-sided cardiac output and the product of the aortic time-velocity integral multiplied by the heart rate increased, and right-sided cardiac output and the product of the pulmonary time velocity integral multiplied by the heart rate decreased, which resulted in decreased right-left ratios. Time to peak velocities and the right-left flow ratios remained stable in the 24 fetuses studied longitudinally, but the aortic and pulmonary peak velocities and cardiac output decreased significantly compared with an expected increase with advancing gestation. The reduction in cardiac output, aortic and pulmonary peak velocities, and umbilical artery pH at birth were directly related.

Conclusion.—Cardiac function abnormalities are present in fetuses with IUGR caused by placental insufficiency. These abnormalities differ between the right and left ventricles. Longitudinally studied fetuses showed a further reduction in cardiac output and pulmonary and aortic peak velocities.

▶ The errors in this study are subtle, and they can be found in the Materials and Methods section. No control observations were included, and abnormal Doppler velocity ratios were a requirement for entry as well as for the diagnosis of IUGR. This makes it relatively certain that abnormal Doppler values will prove to be part of IUGR, because they both are requirements for entry into the study. To estimate the blood-flow rate using this technology, one must multiply an integrated velocity value by the area of the conduit by a scalar representing time. However, quoting the authors, "Because valve area calculations have a relatively high coefficient of variation, cardiac flow was also expressed as the product of time, velocity integral multipled by heart rate, etc." That is to say, vessel size was ignored; therefore, what appears as changes in right ventricular and left ventricular outputs are not blood flow volumes and could represent simply pulmonary artery dilatation or aortic narrowing. Quite regularly, the pulmonary artery diameter is found to be larger than the aortic diameter. This alone could explain why there is a greater left ventricular than right ventricular flow velocity. Finally, combined ventricular outputs were not indexed to fetal weight, which means that what was recorded as decreases from norms simply could represent failure of the fetus to gain weight in utero, independent of cardiovascular events. This study does not help at all in deciding whether cardiac changes regularly exist in IUGR, or whether they are a cause or an effect.—T.H. Kirschbaum, M.D.

The Use of Prophylactic Desmopressin (DDAVP) in Labor to Prevent Hemorrhage in a Patient With Ehlers-Danlos Syndrome

Rochelson B, Caruso R, Davenport D, Kaelber A (State Univ of New York at Stony Brook)

N Y State J Med 91:268–269, 1991 4–24

Introduction.—Antepartum or postpartum hemorrhage is a major risk for some patients with the Ehlers-Danlos syndrome (EDS), a genetic disorder characterized by increased joint mobility and connective tissue compromise. Types I and IV are particularly at risk for hemorrhage. One pregnant patient with EDS type III was successfully treated with desmopressin (DDAVP) and had a vaginal delivery at term.

Case Report.—Woman, 28, with EDS type III and a long history of excessive bleeding, was seen during her second pregnancy. Except for worsening migraines, her pregnancy progressed well. At 42 weeks' gestation, with the cervix in good position, labor was induced to avoid a precipitous delivery. At 4–5 cm of dilatation, oxytocin was discontinued and 20 mg of DDAVP was given 30 minutes later. Uterine contractions increased slightly, but the fetal heart rate remained stable. Bleeding time was significantly decreased by DDAVP. The patient had a normal vaginal delivery over a median episiotomy with normal blood loss. Postpartum bleeding times worsened, necessitating daily doses of DDAVP. Although postpartum bleeding was more than average, the hematocrit remained stable at above 30%.

Conclusion.—Vaginal delivery is possible in selected patients with EDS. The use of prophylactic DDAVP in labor may prevent hemorrhage in these patients.

▶ Here is an example of a symptom complex (hyperextensible skin and joints, tendency to bruise, and impaired wound healing) with variable expression that has become understandable through molecular genetic analysis. The underlying defect is in collagen formation and may stem from deficiencies of specific collagen types, components of collagen types, chemical cross-linkages for collagen fibers, or procollagen cleavage enzymes. Because specific gene defects for those abnormalities lie on different chromosomes, inheritance may be by autosomal dominant, autosomal recessive, or sex-linked recessive mechanisms. Defective coagulation factor VIII procoagulant is linked to 1 or more of these defects and results in a von Willebrand type coagulopathy in EDS types I and IV. This accounts for the hemorrhagic tendencies seen in those variants.

This uncommon disease is particularly interesting for 2 reasons. The first is the high incidence of preterm rupture of membranes in such women and the roughly 80% chance that those patients with EDS were themselves products of pregnancies marked by preterm rupture of membranes. Because rupture of membranes is not usually associated with cervical incompetence, this points to the role of fetal collagen synthesis in this common complication of pregnancy. The second interest comes from the usefulness of this synthetic analog of arginine vasopressin in increasing endothelial factor VIII release in EDS types I and IV, as well as type I von Willebrand's disease and type A hemophilia. The risk of hypertension, potentiation of other vasopressors, antidiuresis, and uterine hypercontractility with this agent needs to be kept in mind.—T.H. Kirschbaum, M.D.

Amniotic Fluid White Blood Cell Count: A Rapid and Simple Test to Diagnose Microbial Invasion of the Amniotic Cavity and Predict Preterm Delivery

Romero R, Quintero R, Nores J, Avila C, Mazor M, Hanaoka S, Hagay Z, Merchant L, Hobbins JC (Yale Univ, New Haven, Conn)

Am J Obstet Gynecol 165:821–830, 1991 4–25

Introduction.—Microbial invasion of the amniotic cavity in women with preterm labor is associated with risks for preterm delivery and both maternal and neonatal morbidity.

Methods.—The value of amniotic fluid white blood cell count in the diagnosis of microbial invasion of the amniotic cavity was assessed in 195 consecutive patients with singleton gestation, preterm labor, and intact membranes. All patients underwent amniocentesis to retrieve fluid for culture and a white blood cell count.

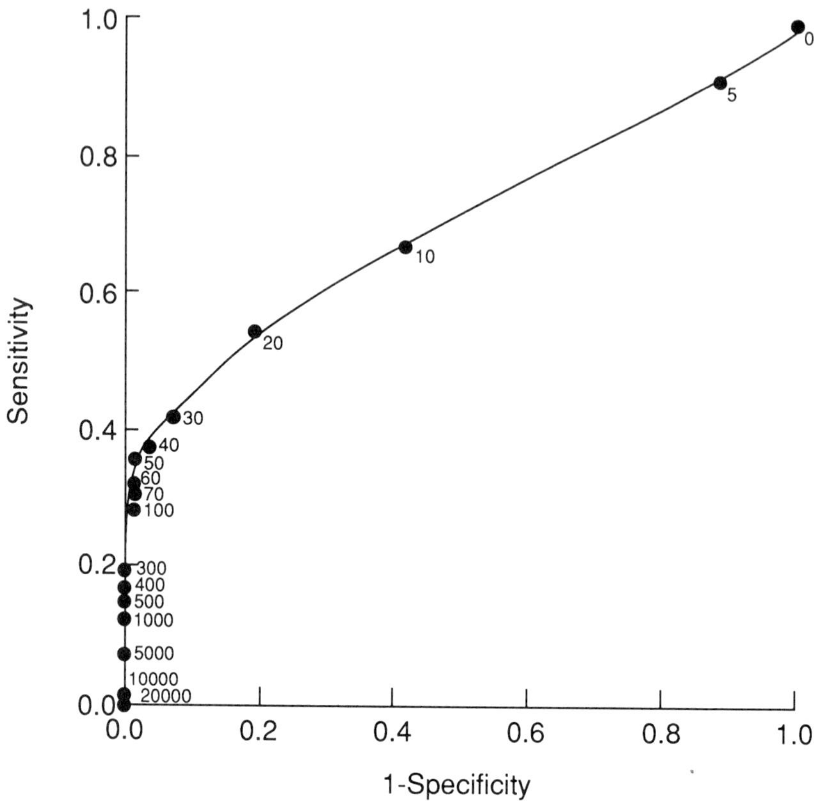

Fig 4–11.—Receiver-operator characteristic curve analysis of amniotic fluid white blood cell count in identification of a patient who will have delivery of a preterm neonate. Only patients with negative Gram stain of amniotic fluid who received tocolysis were included in this analysis. *Numbers* next to *solid dots* represent amniotic fluid white blood cell counts (cell per cubic millimeter) (area under curve, .625; SE, .044; $z = 2.810$; $P < .01$). (Courtesy of Romero R, Quintero R, Nores J, et al: *Am J Obstet Gynecol* 165:821–830, 1991.)

Results.—The prevalence of a positive amniotic fluid culture was 12.8%. Compared with patients with a negative culture, those with positive findings had a significantly younger gestational age, a more advanced cervical dilatation, and a significantly higher median amniotic fluid white blood cell count. An amniotic fluid white blood cell count of 50 cells/mm^3 or greater had a sensitivity of 80%, a specificity of 87.64%, a positive predictive value of 48.78%, and a negative predictive value of 96.75% in the detection of a positive amniotic fluid culture for microorganisms. Of 17 patients with an amniotic fluid white blood cell count of 50 cells/mm^3 or greater and a negative amniotic fluid culture, 15 had a spontaneous preterm delivery. In a subgroup of 156 patients who underwent a trial of tocolysis, all patients with an amniotic fluid white blood cell count of 500 cells/mm^3 or greater delivered a preterm neonate (Fig 4–11).

Conclusion.—The amniotic fluid white blood cell count is strongly related to microbial invasion of the amniotic cavity. A count of 50 cells/mm^3 or greater had a higher sensitivity, but a lower specificity, than the Gram stain of amniotic fluid. An increased count identifies patients at risk for failure to respond to tocolysis and deliver prematurely.

▶ The appearance of leukocytes in the amniotic fluid may be stimulated by cytokines released as a result of infection or aseptic inflammation. Examples of the latter include voided meconium, fetal-placental ischemia, or uterine trauma. This very-well-done practical study was designed to explore the predictability of the concentration of the white blood cells in the amniotic fluid in making the diagnosis of infection in the roughly 15% of cases of preterm labor in which amniotic fluid cultures proved to be positive. As always, the question is whether increased sensitivity of a predictor (the true positive rate) can be obtained without increasing the false positive rate, a question which is best handled by exploring the receiver-operator function of the assay. The authors persuasively argue that a white blood cell concentration greater than 50 cells/mm^3 yields a sharp increase in specificity compared with amniotic fluid Gram stain (false positive rate, 8.7% [17/195]; false negative rate, 2% [4/195]; positive predictive value, approximately 50%). The white blood cell count appears to be a fairly good predictor of positive amniotic fluid culture.

However, there are some other values in this study that are worthy of mention. Nearly 90% of the 17 women with white blood cell counts >50 cells/mm^3 failed tocolysis, regardless of culture results. If Gram stain of amniotic fluid was also positive, there was a 100% incidence of positive culture in the 11 women who qualified. This is the rationale for the author's recommendation that women demonstrating a positive Gram stain and more than 50 white cells/mm^3 of amniotic fluid not receive tocolysis independent of the duration of gestation. All 10 women with white blood cell counts of more than 500 cells/mm^3 delivered prematurely. The statistical inferences from data such as this are seldom so well handled.—T.H. Kirschbaum, M.D.

Severe Preeclampsia in the Second Trimester: Recurrence Risk and Long-Term Prognosis

Sibai BM, Mercer B, Sarinoglu C (Univ of Tennessee, Memphis)

Am J Obstet Gynecol 165:1408–1412, 1991 4–26

Background.—Women with severe preeclampsia-eclampsia in their first pregnancy have been reported to be at increased risk for preeclampsia in later pregnancies. They also appear to be at increased risk for chronic hypertension later in life. However, few patients included in that research had severe preeclampsia in their second trimester. The subsequent outcome of pregnancy and the remote maternal prognosis in women with severe preeclampsia in the second trimester were studied.

Patients.—A total of 125 women were followed up for a mean of 5.4 years. Seventeen had no further pregnancies, whereas 108 had 169 subsequent pregnancies.

Findings.—Thirty-five percent of those with later pregnancies were normotensive, and 65% had preeclampsia again. Among the 110 in the latter group, preeclampsia occurred in 32% in the second trimester, in 32% at 28–36 weeks, and in 36% at 37–40 weeks. Overall, 21% of the subsequent pregnancies were complicated by second trimester severe preeclampsia. A total of 35% of women had chronic hypertension with the highest incidence in those with recurrent second trimester severe preeclampsia, and the lowest incidence in those with only normotensive later pregnancies. There were 2 maternal deaths, and 2 other women had end stage renal disease that required dialysis.

Conclusion.—Women with severe preeclampsia that occurs in the second trimester are at increased risk for repeat preeclampsia, particularly in the second trimester. These women are also at increased risk for chronic hypertension and maternal morbidity and mortality.

▶ This study ignores the view of preeclampsia that has stemmed from the epidemiological work of Chesley and co-workers and has been bolstered by the endocrine experience of investigators such as Tillman (2), as well as by the renal biopsy specimen data obtained by McCartney et al. (3). This coherent body of earlier work has led to the conclusion that preeclampsia is largely confined to primigravid women, and that multigravid pregnancy-induced hypertension generally comprises some form of chronic cardiovascular renal lesion co-existing with or exacerbated by pregnancy. If one applies this series of concepts to the authors' data, correcting the authors' decision to count infants rather than pregnancies, one finds that the data do conform to those earlier basic concepts.

Of the 125 women who were followed after initial development of second trimester pregnancy-induced hypertension, 24 were multiparas and were likely to have chronic hypertension, which left 101 nulliparas for follow-up. After subtracting 17 women with no further pregnancies after the index pregnancy, 84 preeclamptics remained to be followed in subsequent pregnancies. The authors' incidence rates stem from 169 pregnancies in 109 gravidas, meaning that each pregnant woman had an average of 1½ subsequent children. Assuming that mean parity was subsequently the same in both normotensive and hypertensive pregnancies, 39 women subsequently were normotensive (169 babies × 35% normotensive × .67 to correct for multiparity). This leaves 45 women (by subtracting from 84) who had recurring PIH and were likely victims of chronic cardiovascular disease coincident with pregnancy. The incidence of chronic hypertension in these 125 women with subsequent pregnancies was 36%. This figure nicely compares with earlier work. Clearly, the more children each hypertensive woman had, the greater the rate of total hypertensive pregnancy, nevertheless, it is the risk of hypertension in women that is of interest. In clinical research, as in other pursuits, those who ignore the lessons of history are often doomed to repeat its errors.—T.H. Kirschbaum, M.D.

References

1. Chesley LC: Hypertension Disorders in Pregnancy. New York, Appleton-Century-Crofts, 1978.
2. Tillman AJB: *Am J Obstet Gynecol* 70:589, 1955.
3. McCartney CP: *Circulation* 30(suppl II):37, 1964.

Use of Acyclovir for Varicella Pneumonia During Pregnancy

Smego RA Jr, Asperilla MO (West Virginia Univ, Morgantown; Albany Med College)

Obstet Gynecol 78:1112–1116, 1991 4–27

Background.—When varicella pneumonia occurs in pregnancy, the untreated mortality may be 40% or more. Acyclovir, an antiviral agent that inhibits herpesvirus DNA synthesis, is recommended for pregnant women with this life-threatening pulmonary infection. However, data are limited on this use of acyclovir. Twenty-one cases of varicella pneumonia in pregnancy were reviewed retrospectively to evaluate the benefits and risks of intravenous acyclovir.

Patients.—Five cases were new, and 16 were found in the literature. All women became ill in their second or third trimester. The mean gestational age at the onset of pneumonia was 27 weeks; at delivery, it was 36 weeks.

Outcomes.—Twelve women needed mechanical ventilation. The mean duration of treatment was 7 days. No adverse drug effects were associated with the use of acyclovir. Three women (14%) died of uncontrolled infection or complications. Two infants whose mothers died also died: 1 was stillborn at 34 weeks and the other died of prematurity just after birth at 26 weeks. None of the infants were born with features of congenital varicella syndrome. In addition, none had active perinatal varicella infection. The onset of pneumonia in the third trimester was a risk factor for fatal maternal outcomes.

Conclusion.—Intravenous acyclovir may decrease maternal mortality and morbidity associated with varicella pneumonia in pregnancy. This treatment appears to be safe for the developing fetus when given in the second and third trimesters.

▶ Although nothing conclusive may be derived from this anecdotal account of 16 case treatments, the authors have performed a service by pointing out the hazards of this complication of pregnancy. Note the 25% mortality rate (18.7% corrected for indirect causes of death). The hazard stems from the relatively high likelihood of pneumonia when it is acquired after the second decade of life (a rate as high as 50%). The high intrinsic mortality of the disease, the tendency for lethality to be especially high in the third trimester, and the lesser in vitro activity for acyclovir against varicella compared with acyclovir against herpes simplex add to the gravity of the problem. This is a serious enough complication of pregnancy to require treatment using everything of likely merit; certainly, this includes acyclovir. The recent demonstration of the usefulness of this agent in treating varicella in normal children (1) adds to the recommendation that it be used to treat varicella pneumonia in pregnancy.—T.H. Kirschbaum, M.D.

Reference

1. Dunkle LM, et al: N *Engl J Med* 225:1545, 1991.

Perinatal Outcome in Renal Allograft Recipients: Prognostic Significance of Hypertension and Renal Function Before and During Pregnancy

Sturgiss SN, Davison JM (Univ of Newcastle-upon-Tyne, England)
Obstet Gynecol 78:573–577, 1991 4–28

Background.—In recent years, more women who have received renal allografts have subsequently become pregnant. Therefore, it is vital to clarify the prepregnancy assessment criteria for these patients and to describe other variables that may affect perinatal outcome. Gestational renal response and acute or chronic hypertension were studied and correlated to the perinatal outcome in pregnant recipients of allograft.

Patients.—The subjects were 17 women (mean age, 27 years) who received renal allografts during a 20-year period. These patients had 22 pregnancies with a duration of at least 28 weeks. All women had a prepregnancy plasma creatinine level of 1.62 mg/dL or less and a 24-hour creatinine clearance of at least 39 mL/min. Four patients who were receiving antihypertensive treatment had 6 pregnancies. The women were regularly assessed for mean arterial pressure (MAP), antihypertensive therapy, plasma creatinine, and 24-hour creatinine clearance.

Findings.—There were 10 adverse perinatal outcomes—5 stillbirths, 4 growth-retarded infants, and 1 neonatal death—and 12 satisfactory outcomes. The 2 groups had identical early-pregnancy increments and late-pregnancy decrements in renal function. Those patients with adverse outcomes had significantly higher MAP from 16–28 weeks' gestation. Hypertension, which was defined as a MAP of more than 107 mm Hg, developed in 16 cases. This occurred before 28 weeks in 7 cases and was always followed by an adverse outcome. Hypertension developed after 28 weeks in 9 cases, only 2 of which had an adverse outcome. All but 1 of 6 women receiving antihypertensive therapy had an adverse outcome.

Conclusion.—In pregnant women who have had renal allografts, there are no differences in renal function between those who have adverse or favorable perinatal outcomes. Hypertension occurring either before or early in pregnancy seems to be associated with an adverse outcome, even if the condition is controlled satisfactorily. This may result from covert cardiovascular changes, and it might be helped by more aggressive antihypertensive therapy.

▶ When experience with pregnant renal transplant patients was infrequent, all that could be said was that the results were generally favorable. Now, with larger numbers of such patient experiences, a more mixed pattern of outcomes has emerged and, furthermore, our inabilities to predict the outcome of pregnancy from conventional indices of renal function have become clear. In this study, adverse pregnancy outcome was defined for practical purposes as stillbirth or intrauterine growth retardation. What's most striking is the total lack of discriminatory capacity of either plasma creatinine concentration or creatinine clearance. In part, the same conclusion was independently reached by Drs. James Lowe and T. Terry Hyashi, who analyzed the usefulness of creatinine clearance in pregnancy before the era of renal transplantation. Even an increase of creatinine clearance in allograft recipients fails to presage a good outcome. It's tempting—but probably inappropriate—to apply these findings to patients with chronic renal disease without transplantation.—T.H. Kirschbaum, M.D.

5 Fetal Diagnosis

Medical Research Council European Trial of Chorion Villus Sampling

Grant A, for the MRC Working Party on the Evaluation of Chorion Villus Sampling) (Radcliffe Infirmary, Oxford, England)

Lancet 337:1491–1499, 1991 5–1

Background.—Compared with second-trimester amniocentesis, first-trimester chorion villus sampling can provide earlier prenatal diagnosis of genetic and cytogenetic fetal disorders, thus allowing earlier termination of affected pregnancies. However, questions remain about the comparative safety and diagnostic accuracy of these 2 techniques. A multicenter, randomized trial was performed to address these questions.

Methods.—Thirty-one centers in 7 countries participated in the trial. During a 4-year period, 3,248 women seeking prenatal diagnosis, mainly because of their age, were entered into the trial. The women were randomized into 2 diagnostic groups: 1,629 to the chorion villus sampling group and 1,619 to the amniocentesis group. Testing was not done in 5% of the chorion villus sampling group and 8% of the amniocentesis group, mainly because of spontaneous miscarriage. Thus, 1,609 women who underwent chorion villus sampling and 1,592 who underwent amniocentesis were available for analysis.

Results.—A total of 86% of the chorion villus sampling group and 91% of the amniocentesis group had a liveborn infant. After weighting for the contributions of the center, the typical difference between the groups was 4.6%. The chorion villus sampling group had significantly more spontaneous fetal deaths before 28 weeks' gestation, for a typical rate difference of 2.9%; more terminations of pregnancies for chromosomal abnormalities (1%); and more neonatal deaths (.3%). The latter resulted from a preponderance of very immature liveborn infants in the chorion villus sampling group, which also explained the longer hospital stay for that group. An abnormal diagnosis followed chorion villus analysis in 5.6% of the cases compared with 3.9% for amniotic fluid analysis, mainly because of diagnoses of trisomy 18 and placental abnormalities. There were 3 false positive terminated pregnancies, 1 in the chorion villus sampling group and 2 in the amniocentesis group. Two mosaic cases in the chorion villus group may have been false positive, and there was 1 false negative in the chorion villus group.

Conclusion.—Chorion villus sampling may allow earlier exclusive or diagnosis of some fetal disorders compared with amniocentesis. However, this advantage must be weighed against poorer safety performance, diagnostic accuracy, and the need for further testing. Despite these risks, many women will continue to seek first-trimester sampling.

▶ This is a comparative, prospective, randomized study of 2 alternative, frequently used approaches to fetal diagnosis. This study parallels a comparable Canadian effort (published in 1989) that consisted of fewer cases (2,019). Its results, although similar, showed fewer differences than in the European study. An unavoidable design problem is the difference in time between expected delivery and the time of performance of chorionic villi biopsy (CVB) vs. amniocentesis, because the former is used earlier in pregnancy. The time difference alone could be predicted to result in more pregnancy terminations and more fetal deaths before 28 weeks' gestation, with fewer fetal deaths unsampled in the CVB group; those results are indeed seen.

The price that is paid for earlier diagnosis with CVB is abundantly clear in this study of 320 women, the vast majority of whom were seen at an age older than 35 years. Chorionic villi biopsy suffers in terms of safety, accuracy, and the need for repeat procedures beyond the impact of the earlier time of the procedure in the CVB group. A total of 17% of all CVBs were described as difficult, with 31% requiring repeat insertions. The comparable figures for second trimester amniocentesis are 5% and 6%, respectively. In CVB, accuracy is compromised by the need to confirm trisomies and some other euploidies by fetal blood and amniotic fluid studies that were designed to rule out placental mosaicism (see the 1989 YEAR BOOK OF OBSTETRICS AND GYNECOLOGY, pp 176–7). The surplus of CVB pregnancy losses is caused by both the performance of therapeutic abortion in that group and the more spontaneous fetal deaths before 28 weeks' gestation. In a rigorous sense, beyond the broad qualitative considerations that the authors indicate, the results of the 2 approaches aimed at different goals in time are not wholly comparable.—T.H. Kirschbaum, M.D.

6 Fetal Complications of Pregnancy

The Outcome of Congenital Cytomegalovirus Infection in Relation to Maternal Antibody Status

Fowler KB, Stagno S, Pass RF, Britt WJ, Boll TJ, Alford CA (Univ of Alabama, Birmingham)

N Engl J Med 326:663–667, 1992 6–1

Objective.—Congenital cytomegalovirus (CMV) infection, the most common intrauterine infection, results in more frequent and severe sequelae when it is symptomatic. Transmission of the virus is not prevented by maternal antibody, but serious injury is prevented to an unknown degree. The outcomes were compared in 2 groups of CMV-infected children: those whose mothers acquired primary CMV infection during pregnancy and those whose mothers were immune to CMV infection.

Methods.—A total of 197 children with congenital CMV infection were studied. Serum samples collected before pregnancy (usually cord serum from previous deliveries) and samples collected before delivery were used to define maternal infection. Women with seroconversion or

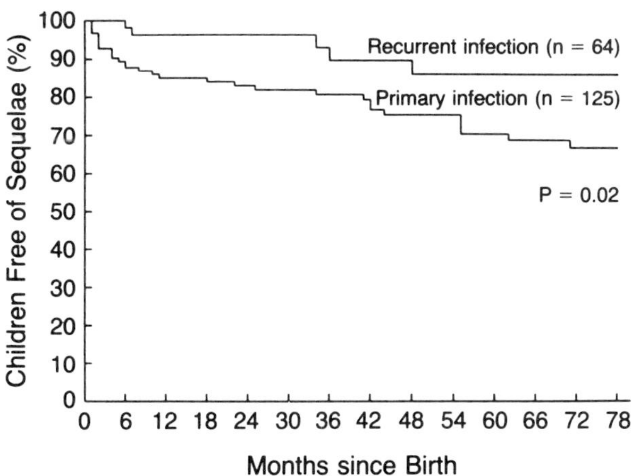

Fig 6–1.—Percentage of children with congenital CMV infection who remained free of sequelae, according to type of maternal infection. The *P* value was obtained by log-rank test. (Courtesy of Fowler KB, Stagno S, Pass RF, et al: *N Engl J Med* 326:663–667, 1992.)

CMV-specific IgM antibodies were classified as having primary CMV infection. Those with IgG antibodies in stored serum were classified as having recurrent infection. The virus was isolated during the newborn period in all children. The children's medical records for the first month of life were reviewed, and most children were routinely followed up for sequelae of CMV infection at a special clinic. The mean follow-up was 4.7 years.

Results.—There were 125 infants in the primary-infection group and 64 in the recurrent-infection group. Symptomatic CMV infection was present at birth in 18% of the primary-infection group vs. none in the recurrent-infection group. The incidence of sensorineural hearing loss was 15% vs. 5%, respectively. Thirteen percent of the primary-infection group had an intelligence quotient of 70 or less vs. no mental impairment in the recurrent-infection group. The incidence of chorioretinitis was 6% vs. 2%. Microcephaly was the only neurological sequela in the recurrent-infection group. The overall incidence of sequelae was 25% in the primary-infection group vs. 8% in the recurrent-infection group (Fig 6–1), with none of the latter children having more than 1 sequela.

Conclusion.—The presence of maternal antibody to CMV appears to protect the fetus and reduce the severity of sequelae of CMV infection. Vaccination of seronegative women may prevent many damaging CMV infections. The variable persistence of IgM antibody may have caused some of the recent primary infections to be classified as recurrent.

▶ Although this group has previously provided us with similar conclusions in qualitative form (1), this study sharpens that earlier work by providing more cases and better estimates of rates of newborn sequelae. The large volume of maternal and cord blood serum samples maintained in archival fashion from pregnancy (occurring as long as 20 years ago) enables the distinctions between primary and recurrent maternal infection to be made with unique certainty. In this study, primary infection means either conversion from negative to positive status for IgG to CMV or the demonstration of IgM during pregnancy in IgG-negative women. Recurrent CMV is denoted by the presence of both IgG and IgM antibody in the maternal blood. Fetal infection was proven by urine viral culture. The results show that primary infection carries a greater risk of symptomatic newborn disease, hearing loss, intelligence quotient impairment, chorioretinitis, and multiple sequelae. Those infants from recurrently infected gravidas failed to show bilateral hearing loss, intelligent quotient less than 70, and neurological sequelae exempting microcephaly. This study sets the stage for the development of a program of active immunization of seronegative women of childbearing age; such a program may sharply reduce the number of infants damaged by this very common fetal infection.—T.H. Kirschbaum, M.D.

Reference

1. Stagno S, et al: N *Engl J Med* 306:945, 1982.

Management of Fetal Hemolytic Disease by Cordocentesis: II. Outcome of Treatment

Weiner CP, Williamson RA, Wenstrom KD, Sipes SL, Widness JA, Grant SS, Estle L (Univ of Iowa, Iowa City)

Am J Obstet Gynecol 165:1302–1307, 1991 6–2

Introduction.—Since 1985, fetal intravascular transfusion has been the method of choice for the treatment of fetal hemolytic disease at the University of Iowa. Of the 128 pregnancies complicated by maternal red blood cell alloimmunization, 48 with fetuses that had severe anemia were identified with cordocentesis and were treated by fetal intravascular transfusions. Thirteen (27%) fetuses had hydrops when therapy was begun.

Treatment.—A total of 142 simple intrauterine intravenous transfusions were initiated when the fetal hematocrit was less than 30%. Each fetus received pancuronium and furosemide. Transfused blood was negative for cytomegalovirus, hepatitis B, and HIV; compatible with mother and fetus; buffy coat poor; washed in saline solution; irradiated; and resuspended in saline solution. The mean gestational age at the first transfusion was 28 weeks (range, 18–36).

Outcome.—The overall survival rate was 96%, and 77% of the survivors received 2 or more transfusions before delivery. The survival rate for fetuses with hydrops was 85%. With intravascular transfusion, the fetal red blood cells were replaced with adult red blood cells and fetal erythropoiesis was suppressed. The percentage of circulating fetal red blood cells was less than 1% by the completion of the second transfusion, and the mean reticulocyte count was less than 1% within 3 weeks of the second transfusion. Excluding the first transfusion, the rate at which fetal hematocrit decreased after a transfusion correlated inversely with gestational age, allowing a 4–5-week interval between transfusions after 32 weeks' gestation. Of the survivors, 78% were delivered at term. Compared with neonates who were transfused only once antenally, those transfused more than once required less phototherapy and, when delivered at term, required fewer hospital days. All transfusion attempts were successful. Transfusion was well tolerated. There were only 2 complications: amnionitis and fetal bradycardia (8%). Bleeding from the uterine and umbilical cord puncture sites was not clinically significant. The only 2 deaths were in fetuses with severe hydrops.

Conclusion.—Treatment of fetal anemia by simple intrauterine intravascular transfusion is associated with high perinatal survival and allows term delivery with low perinatal morbidity.

▶ This 5-year experience in the management of erythroblastosis fetalis—almost solely by percutaneous umbilical transfusion—is remarkable in several respects. Umbilical vein sampling could be used for an average of 3 times per pregnancy. This makes estimates of transfused volume less demanding and also provides fertile material for investigation, because repeated sampling can then be used to judge the effect of the expansion of the fetal red cell mass on measures of fetal well-being. Four of 48 cases experienced fetal bradycardia, 2 of which resulted in fetal death and a third that required emergency cesarean section. The fetal deaths occurred in hydropic infants and led to safeguards against volume overload and the metabolic consequences of transfusion of blood rendered acidotic by anticoagulant and the erythrocyte storage lesion. An 85% survival rate for hydropic infants constitutes a fine result, as does the 100% survival of nonhydropic infants. Both rates are a function of the bold decision to allow alloimmunized pregnancies to go to term—provided the umbilical vein hematocrit is in the range of 45% to 50%. This experienced group has established a mark of excellence against which the rest of us must weigh our efforts.—T.H. Kirschbaum, M.D.

Maternal Left Ventricular Dimension in Pregnancies Complicated by Fetal Growth Retardation

Veille J-C, Morton MJ, Paul MS (Case Western Reserve Univ, Cleveland; Oregon Health Sciences Univ, Portland)

Obstet Gynecol 78:265–269, 1991 6–3

Background.—Small heart volume is a risk factor for premature birth and fetal growth retardation, but studies of this relationship have not addressed the fact that small women have smaller hearts, less blood volume, and smaller infants than women of average size. M-mode echocardiography was used to evaluate cardiac size and function in normal pregnant women and those with suspected fetal growth retardation.

Methods.—The subjects were 79 healthy volunteers in the third trimester of pregnancy and 42 women with suspected fetal growth retardation. In the latter group, women with grossly abnormal and symmetrically small fetuses were excluded. All fetuses were followed to delivery, and those weighing at least 2 standard deviations (SDs) below the mean were considered to be small for gestational age (SGA). All subjects underwent M-mode echocardiography to obtain a left ventricular study at the level of the chordae tendineae.

Results.—In the suspected fetal growth retardation group, 23 of the fetuses were within 2 SDs of SGA, and 19 were lower than 2 SDs. None in this group had chromosomal abnormalities or congenital infection. The 3 groups showed no difference in time from echocardiography to delivery. Neither were there any significant differences in hemodynamic characteristics.

Conclusion.—There appears to be no difference in left ventricular size and function in women whose fetuses are affected by idiopathic asymmetrical fetal growth retardation. There may still be some associated cardiovascular maladaptation, but the current results fail to implicate the heart in the pathogenesis of growth retardation.

► Earlier Scandinavian publications in 1959 and 1962 (1, 2) estimated maternal heart volume from frontal and lateral x-rays of the heart and calculated total heart volume from 3 cardiac diameters, assuming the shape of an ellipsoid. The volume changes in the cardiac cycle were ignored as irrelevant, and a single constant was used for all x-ray tube-to-object distances to convert for parallax error in the films. Most of the comparisons were made with premature births, although a few cases who had what would now be called intrauterine growth retardation (IUGR) were included. The calculations, which were based on M-mode echocardiography of the left ventricle and differences in the volume in systole and diastole calculated from an empiric formula, failed to show any relationship between heart volume and IUGR. That is not particularly surprising.

The original explanation for the purported relationship rested with the development of the intervillous space as being both essential to the low total vascular resistance of pregnancy and a stimulant to the increase in blood volume. With imperfect placentation and, therefore, defective intervillous space, the plasma volume would not expand and the diastolic ventricular volume would not increase. One would expect such placental maldevelopment to result occasionally in abortion or premature birth. Nevertheless, this study helps exclude cardiogenic causes as being common in IUGR.—T.H. Kirschbaum, M.D.

References

1. Raiha CE: *Biol Neonate* 1:113, 1959.
2. Hedberg E, Radberg C: *Acta Obstet Gynecol Scand* 41:48, 1962.

Global and Depth Resolved Phosphorus Magnetic Resonance Spectroscopy to Predict Outcome After Birth Asphyxia

Moorcraft J, Bolas NM, Ives NK, Ouwerkerk R, Smyth J, Rajagopalan B, Hope PL, Radda GK (John Radcliffe Hosp, Oxford, England)

Arch Dis Child 66:1119–1123, 1991 6–4

Introduction.—Phase modulated rotating frame imaging (PMFRI), a modification of MR spectroscopy, provides depth-resolved biochemical information. A correlation between PMRFI results and the severity of encephalopathy after birth asphyxia was previously reported.

Methods.—To determine whether spatially localized PMRFI data improved the accuracy of global MR spectroscopy in predicting death or morbidity in a larger group of asphyxiated infants, global and depth-resolved phosphorus MR spectroscopy were used to study 12 normal and 32 asphyxiated neonates.

Results.—Of the asphyxiated infants, 8 died or survived with major neurodevelopmental abnormalities. A global phosphocreatinine-to-inorganic phosphate ratio below the range obtained from normal infants predicted these adverse outcomes with a sensitivity of 88%, a specificity of 83%, and a positive predictive value of 64%. Global inorganic orthophosphate-to-adenosine triphosphate ratios had a predictive value of 88%, a sensitivity of 96%, and a specificity of 88%. Spatially localized MR spectroscopy data obtained during PMFRI showed that cerebral energy metabolism was more abnormal in deep regions than in superficial regions after birth asphyxia. None of the regional metabolite concentrations were better than the global data for predicting outcomes.

Conclusion.—In this study, the prognostic sensitivity of the global metabolite ratios was high, and it was not improved by the regional data obtained by PMRFI. Conventional ^{31}P MR spectroscopy is, therefore, a useful prognostic technique for infants asphyxiated at birth.

▶ For a relatively concise discussion of magnetic resonance spectroscopy with ^{31}P, see the 1990 YEAR BOOK OF OBSTETRICS AND GYNECOLOGY, pp 206–207. In brief, hypoxemia of the brain, as it affects the analysis of organic phosphates, is reflected in a decrease in phosphocreatinine (PC), an energy store that is the source for adenosine triphosphate (ATP). Adenosine triphosphate is a source of the high energy phosphate bonds that are essential in providing the energetics of intracell processing. In releasing its available energy quantum, ATP becomes ADP + inorganic phosphate (Pi).

Hypoxemia first reduces PC and increases Pi as the capacity to generate PC is impaired and existing energy stores are consumed in cell operations. With continued hypoxemia, ATP is reduced in concentration, but this change reflects a high likelihood of cell injury and death. For these reasons, the increased ratio of Pi/ATP is a most sensitive index of permanent adverse outcome, reflecting the gravity of reduced ATP and its relationship to the abolition of cellular work. The resulting sensitivity, specificity, and predictive value of positive indices in these 44 cases reflect the excellent predictability of the findings, given an increase in this ratio. When this method is applied to the measurement of differential results through the bulk of the brain, it fails to confirm the subcortical strata as being the most metabolically active. The biphasic changes in intracellular organophosphates noted with serial measurements (see the 1990 YEAR BOOK mentioned above) were not noted in this study consisting of single measurements of 1- to 5-day-old infants. This approach remains the best method of detecting hypoxic brain injury that is currently available to investigators.—T.H. Kirschbaum, M.D.

Prenatal Diagnosis of Fetal Cytomegalovirus Infection

Lynch L, Daffos F, Emanuel D, Giovangrandi Y, Meisel R, Forestier F, Cathomas G, Berkowitz RL (Mount Sinai Med Ctr, New York; Institut de Puericulture de Paris; Mem Sloan-Kettering Cancer Inst, New York)

Am J Obstet Gynecol 165:714–718, 1991 6–5

Introduction.—Intrauterine cytomegalovirus (CMV) infection affects an estimated 1% of all live births in the United States, and approximately 10% of infants congenitally infected with CMV are symptomatic at birth.

The recent development of effective antiviral agents against human CMV could enable the treatment of infected fetuses in utero. However, before this approach can be considered, it is necessary to accurately diagnose fetal CMV infection. Experience with the prenatal diagnosis of CMV infection was described.

Patients.—Twelve fetuses were evaluated by ultrasonography, amniocentesis, and blood sampling for possible CMV infection. Seven fetuses were studied because the mother had a documented primary maternal CMV infection, and 5 fetuses were studied because abnormal ultrasonography findings suggested fetal CMV infection.

Results.—Only 1 of the 7 fetuses exposed to primary maternal CMV infection was infected in utero. All 7 fetuses had normal ultrasonography findings. A correct diagnosis was possible by combining viral cultures of amniotic fluid and assessment of CMV-specific immunoglobulin M (IgM), total IgM, platelet count, and γ-glutamyl transpeptidase in the fetal blood samples. The pregnancy with the infected fetus was terminated. The 6 remaining fetuses of infected mothers were delivered at term, and 5 of them were appropriately grown. None had clinical manifestations of CMV infection at birth. Specific IgM and viral cultures were negative in all neonates. None of the 5 fetuses with abnormal ultrasonography findings survived. Three pregnancies were terminated, and the 2 live-born infants died within a few days. Cytomegalovirus infection was confirmed by isolation of the virus from fetal tissues after pregnancy termination and in the urine of the live-born infants during the first week after birth.

Conclusions.—Prenatal diagnosis of fetal CMV infection is possible with a combination of amniocentesis and fetal blood sampling. Once the diagnosis of CMV infection has been made, abnormal ultrasonography findings herald a very poor prognosis for intact fetal survival.

▶ Because of the 1% frequency of intrauterine CMV infection and the devastating effects it can have, albeit on a minority of such infants, this is an important topic that is infrequently represented in our literature. Although maternal infection before pregnancy, marked by the presence of IgM or IgC to CMV, does not prevent fetal infection, it sharply decreases the likelihood of devastating fetal consequences. The incidence of severely damaged fetuses appears disproportionately high in women from upper socioeconomic strata, in which the incidence of seroconversion to CMV tends to occur later in life than for other women. The most serious problems occur in primary maternal infection in early pregnancy (less than 27 weeks). Demonstration of maternal CMV IgM is a necessary, but not sufficient, criterion for the diagnosis of primary infection. Fetal blood analysis for total IgM and CMV IgM suffices to make the diagnosis of intrauterine infection and fetal CMV infection, respectively.

Where this report charts new grounds is in the abilities of amniotic fluid studies, fibroblast culture techniques, and PCR amplification of DNA to allow hybridization techniques to make a specific diagnosis. In 2 to 3 cases, those approaches were far more successful than in cases reported by others. More experience is needed to evaluate the possibility that amniocentesis may prove equal to PUB in the diagnosis of fetal infection, an obviously desirable occurrence. The results of ultrasound were nonspecific; however, one should bear in mind that oligohydramnios, intrauterine growth retardation, cerebroventricular dilatation, microcephaly, and brain calcification, all of which are common features of litigation for obstetrical professional liability, result far more often from fetal CMV than is recognized.—T.H. Kirschbaum, M.D.

Prophylactic Amnioinfusion as a Treatment for Oligohydramnios in Laboring Patients: A Prospective, Randomized Trial

Schrimmer DB, Macri CJ, Paul RH (Univ of Southern California, Los Angeles)
Am J Obstet Gynecol 165:972–975, 1991 6–6

Background.—There are several current indications for amnioinfusion. The effect of prophylactic amnioinfusion on the incidence of operative intervention for fetal distress, fetal outcome, and the incidence of intrapartum and postpartum infection was investigated.

Methods.—A randomized sample of 305 women with oligohydramnios who were in labor was studied. Of these women, 175 had amnioinfusion, and the remainder served as controls. In the treatment group, amniotic fluid was titrated to an amniotic fluid index of more than 10 cm.

Outcomes.—Women who had amnioinfusion had significantly less operative intervention for fetal distress and fewer cesarean sections. They also had increased umbilical artery pH at the time of delivery. The rates of amnionitis and endometritis did not differ significantly between the groups, although the length of hospitalization was significantly lessened in the treatment group.

Conclusion.—Prophylactic amnioinfusion is a safe, simple method that may be used to treat oligohydramnios in women in labor. Prophylactic amnioinfusion reduces the rate of operative intervention for fetal distress, the rates of cesarean section, and the length of stay. It apparently has no adverse effects on the fetus or mother, and it does not increase the rates of maternal infection.

▶ Note that, in this report, those patients with moderate or severe variable decelerations were excluded from entry. This deprives the study of demonstrating more than that the procedure is safe as used, grants a reasonable duration of labor, and reduces the risk of operative delivery. The frequency with which variable decelerations are abolished with amnioinfusion is potent evidence for cord occlusion to be their etiology, especially with oligohydramnios. This abolition, in turn, reduces the chances of emergency cesarean section for the diagnosis of fetal distress based on progressively severe variable decelerations. Amnioinfusion may not have been begun in cases with suspect fetal distress, and this is likely to be the reason for the favorable results in this study. Note that there is no purported virtue of amnioinfusion given to fetuses exhibiting late fetal decelerations.—T.H. Kirschbaum, M.D.

Shoulder Dystocia: Should the Fetus Weighing ≥ 4000 Grams Be Delivered by Cesarean Section?

Langer O, Berkus MD, Huff RW, Samueloff A (Univ of Texas Health Sciences Ctr at San Antonio)

Am J Obstet Gynecol 165:831–837, 1991 6–7

Introduction.—The optimum method of delivery of the fetus weighing 4,000 g or more remains controversial. A total of 75,979 women who had vaginal delivery from 1970 to 1985 were evaluated.

Methods.—The patients were classified into diabetic and nondiabetic groups, and they were further subdivided into birth weight categories at intervals of 250 g. The effects and relative contribution of the risk factors for diabetic and nondiabetic subjects were evaluated using logistic regression analysis.

Findings.—The overall incidence of macrosomia (≥ 4,000 g) was 7.6% among the 74,390 nondiabetic subjects and 20.6% among the 1,589 diabetic subjects. Dystocia occurred in .5% of the nondiabetic subjects compared with 3.1% in diabetic women. Compared with nondiabetic women, the relative risk of dystocia in diabetic women was 2.6-fold higher when birth weight was less than 4,000 g and 3.6-fold when birth weight was 4,000 g or more. Approximately 40% of shoulder dystocia in the nondiabetic group occurred in infants weighing less than 4,000 g.

In the diabetic group, the cumulative incidence of shoulder dystocia was 76% when fetal weight was 4,250 g or more. If all these infants were delivered by cesarean section, the overall cesarean section would increase by only .26% and would eliminate 76% of the cases of shoulder dystocia. In contrast, no definitive weight category in the nondiabetic group was identified as the optimal threshold for cesarean section delivery to reduce cases of shoulder dystocia. Using the current recommended weight of 4,500 g or more for elective delivery by cesarean section in nondiabetic patients, only 19.5% of the cases of shoulder dystocia would be prevented, with an overall increase of 1.2% in the cesarean section rate. Even at 4,000 g, approximately half the cases of shoulder dystocia would be missed, with an alarming increase of 7.5% in the overall cesarean section rate. Birth weight, diabetes, and labor abnormalities were the principal risk factors contributing to shoulder dystocia.

Conclusion.—For diabetic women, elective cesarean section is strongly recommended when estimated fetal weight is 4,250 g or more. This approach will eliminate 80% of cases, with a minimal increase in cesarean section rate; however, in nondiabetic women, prevention of shoulder dystocia by elective cesarean section will leave the majority of cases undetected. A trial of vaginal delivery for fetuses weighing 4,000 or more is recommended for nondiabetic patients, being watchful of labor abnormalities with macrosomic fetuses.

▶ The uncertainty as to whether a birth weight of 4,000 or 4,500 g constitutes an appropriate definition of macrosomia that would be useful in preventing birth trauma rests with the multiple variables that impact on the incidence of such trauma (prolonged labor, forceps delivery, postdatism, anesthesia). The authors provide a fair amount of clarification simply by controlling for an important determinant-maternal diabetes. The comparison benefits by the much lower incidence of shoulder dystocia seen in infants weighing less than 4,000 g in diabetic pregnancies than in nondiabetic pregnancies. What evolves when controlling for diabetes only is that the appropriate definition for macrosomic infants is equal to or greater than 4,500 g in nondiabetic pregnancies and is greater than 4,250 g in diabetic pregnancy. Looking carefully at Table 5 in the original article, using 4,500 g as an indication for cesarean section in diabetes appears to halve the incidence of cesarean section at the cost of increasing shoulder dystocia from 24% of 4,000 g in those weighing 4,250 g to 36% in those weighing 4,500 g at birth. When the day comes when we can diagnose fetal weight greater than 4,000 g with enough precision to discriminate this 250-g difference preoperatively, it will become important in therapy. In general, this paper argues for the 4,500-g definition of macrosomia, all things being equal.—T.H. Kirschbaum, M.D.

Herpes Simplex Virus Infection of the Placenta: The Role of Molecular Pathology in the Diagnosis of Viral Infection of Placental-Associated Tissues

Schwartz DA, Caldwell E (Emory Univ, Atlanta)

Arch Pathol Lab Med 115:1141–1144, 1991 6–8

Introduction.—A herpes simplex infection of the placenta is a rare occurrence; therefore, its symptoms and pathologic characteristics may not be easily recognizable. A patient with a herpes simplex viral infection of the placenta's decidualized tissue, characterized by lack of inflammation and by the absence of viral inclusions on conventional laboratory staining methods, was evaluated. The use of molecular biological testing methods, such as in situ DNA hybridization, aided the diagnosis of herpes simplex virus infection.

Case Report.—A pregnant woman, 18, who was gravida 3 and para 2002, required medical care because of uterine contractions and a possible herpes infection of the genitals. She had had confirmed genital herpes 11 months earlier. After a cesarean delivery of a male infant without signs of congenital herpes, the patient had postpartum endometritis that responded to antibiotics. The patient's laboratory results appeared negative for herpes simplex.

Methods.—The molecular biological methods of immunohistochemical antibody to herpes simplex type 2 and in situ DNA hybridization for herpes simplex virus analyzed the placenta for herpes simplex virus infection.

Results.—The placenta and fetal membranes appeared normal on physical examination. Microscopic examination of the placental tissue found no abnormalities related to viral infection. The maternal erythrocytes in the intervillous space demonstrated sickling-type changes, and rare plasma cells appeared in the patient's decidualized tissues. The in situ DNA hybridization samples showed cell groups with well-stained nuclei in the subchorionic maternal tissue from the decidua capsularis, indicating the presence of herpes simplex virus. The immunohistochemistry studies also demonstrated clearly marked areas of intranuclear staining, also within the decidua capsularis. These latter cells were the same ones stained by the in situ DNA hybridization method.

Conclusion.—These results suggest that the herpes simplex virus may infect the placenta and related tissues more often than was previously suspected. The testing of placental tissues using molecular biology methods in women with clinical signs of herpes simplex infection can aid in understanding the incidence of this disease.

▶ It's a mistake to make too much of a single case report, but this one is of uncommon interest. In a woman with recurrent vulvar herpes in term labor, maternal cervical culture, physical examination of the newborn, and standard gross and microscopic examination of the placenta failed to demonstrate evidence of herpesvirus infection. The use of chromogen-complexed DNA probes hybridized in vitro and immunohistochemistry using a rabbit monochromal antibody to herpes simplex virus types 1 and 2 antigen led to easy recognition of viral antigen in decidual tissue. There was no evidence of inflammatory reaction in the tissue containing viral antigen. The presence of what appears to be a latent or subclinical endometrial infection is an observation worth confirming in larger numbers. If verified, it means that herpes simplex virus is capable of long-term residence within the endometrium without evoking an inflammatory reaction, and also serves as a possible focus for periodic infection of the genitalia.

At least 1 other investigator (1) has found similar evidence of herpes simplex virus antigen in pregnant and nonpregnant human endometria, placentas, umbilical cords, and neonatal tissues; frequency ranged from approximately 25% to nearly 65%, depending on the selection factors for study tissues. This observation points to an unexpectedly high incidence of latent herpes simplex virus infection in endometria, and to a remarkable combination of viral biology and/or host defenses that maintain it apparently innocuous for periods of time.—T.H. Kirschbaum, M.D.

Reference

1. Robb JA, et al: *Hum Pathol* 17:1210, 1986.

Numeric Analysis of Heart Rate Variation in Intrauterine Growth-Retarded Fetuses: A Longitudinal Study

Snijders RJM, Ribbert LSM, Visser GHA, Mulder EJH (Univ Hosp Groningen, The Netherlands)

Am J Obstet Gynecol 166:22–27, 1992 6–9

Introduction.—Previous research has demonstrated that fetuses affected by intrauterine growth retardation (IUGR) may have a heart rate (PHR) that falls within normal limits. These cross-sectional studies did not determine the actual sequence of changes in FHR patterns with increasing deterioration. The FHR and its variation were measured longitudinally in fetuses with IUGR to determine changes that occur with time and progressive deterioration.

Methods.—Thirteen pregnant women were selected retrospectively because they had had 1 hour of FHR recordings, had undergone cesarean delivery because of late fetal heart decelerations, and had an infant with a birth weight below the 10th percentile (as corrected for sex and parity) and no congenital malformations. Most of the 13 patients delivered their infant before the 35th week of gestation. Each woman had noted fetal movements on a record sheet.

Results.—A small but significant increase in basal FHR occurred on each deceleration. Over time, the FHR decreased, with the median value falling below the normal value (30 ms) at approximately the time each deceleration appeared. Subjective responses were higher for fetuses with symmetric IUGR. The interfetal differences in FHR appeared high, although birth weights were similar for this fetal population. In most patients, the pulsatility index for the umbilical artery increased slowly over time before the occurrence of decelerations.

Conclusion.—Progressive deterioration of the fetus with IUGR occurs over time and before the initial decelerations. These events are accompanied by a gradual decrease in the variation of FHR. A study of the reductions in FHR variation allows identification of those fetuses with IUGR that may benefit from further development in utero. Using each fetus as its own control for late deceleration measurements has been suggested.

▶ This further exploration of the numerical analysis of the beat-to-beat variability of fetal heart rate (see the 1989 Year Book of Obstetrics and Gynecology, pp 117–118 and the article by Dawes et al. in Abstract 7–3 of this Year Book) succeeds in clouding the issues. An important design fault is arranging the data assays around the occurrence of late decelerations in heart rate, which may or not have a predictable relationship to fetal hypoxemia or acidosis from case to case. In this study, the trends in heart rate variability, which were measured by the mean range of minutes in milliseconds, are reported despite the fact that the large variability among fetuses deprives the data of any significance. Although both Dawes (cited above) and Smith et al. (1) failed to demonstrate a relationship between heart rate variability and fetal hypoxemia and/or acidosis, a relationship is posited here without benefit of pH measurement. Because longitudinal measurements are reported only for 2 fetuses and the data sets show marked differences, there appears to be no support for the authors' conclusions.—T.H. Kirschbaum, M.D.

Reference

1. Smith JH, et al: *Br J Obstet Gynaecol* 95:980, 1988.

Management of Fetal Hemolytic Disease by Cordocentesis: I. Prediction of Fetal Anemia

Weiner CP, Williamson RA, Wenstrom KD, Sipes SL, Grant SS, Widness JA (Univ of Iowa, Iowa City)

Am J Obstet Gynecol 165:546–553, 1991 6–10

Background.—The premise that assessment of fetal blood rather than amniotic fluid would predict more accurately the severity of fetal disease and the need for transfusion was first examined in 1985. A management scheme for red blood cell alloimmunization based on fetal blood testing was planned. It was speculated that such direct testing would minimize the number of invasive procedures and prevent unnecessary preterm delivery.

Methods.—A total of 128 women with pregnancies complicated by maternal red blood cell alloimmunization were referred between 1985 and 1990. Two hundred seventy-two diagnostic cordocenteses were done, with the timing of repeat procedures being based on retrospectively developed criteria. These criteria included fetal hematocrit values, reticulocyte counts, and direct Coombs' test results, and they were derived from the first 84 pregnancies and confirmed on the next 44.

Findings.—Four hematological patterns were identified in the 98 antigen-positive fetuses on the basis of the first blood sample. In pattern 1, with an incidence of 11%, the fetuses were at low risk for significant antenatal anemia. These fetuses had normal hematocrit values and reticulocyte counts and negative or trace-positive direct Coombs' results. None of these fetuses had significant antenatal anemia. In pattern 2, which was found in 31%, the fetuses had an intermediate risk of anemia. These fetuses had a normal hematocrit value, a direct Coombs' titer of 1 or 2+, and a normal or low reticulocyte count. Twenty-one percent of the fetuses in this group had significant antenatal anemia. Those fetuses with patterns 3 and 4 had the greatest risk of severe anemia. Pattern 3 fetuses had normal hematocrit values associated with either reticulocyte counts higher than the 97.5 percentile for gestation or a direct Coombs' test of at least 3+. Pattern 4 fetuses had these features or a mild anemia. Pattern 3 occurred in 50% of patients and pattern 4 occurred in 10%. Eighty percent of the pattern 3 fetuses and 90% of pattern 4 fetuses had a hematocrit value of less than 30%.

Conclusion.—Cordocentesis appears to be an acceptable alternative to optical density measurements of 450 nm. Assessing fetal hemolytic disease with a fetal blood specimen allows identification of fetuses at high risk of antenatal anemia.

▶ For almost 30 years, the predictive capacity of optical absorption of amniotic fluid at 450 nm has been the cornerstone of clinical management in estimating fetal anemia caused by erythroblastosis fetalis. Now its role is being questioned from 2 points of view. The first is by advocates of real-time ultrasound evaluation of the fetal cardiac consequences of anemia hypoxia, as manifest by cardiac dilatation, pericardial, and pleural fluid. The second is by the direct determination of fetal anemia through fetal blood obtained by cordocentesis.

This analysis of 272 percutaneous umbilical blood samplings (PUBs) done in 127 alloimmunized pregnancies doesn't lead to an unequivocal answer regarding its relative value compared with other approaches; however, it nicely portrays the issues. The advantages of PUB include a direct, rather than inferential, diagnosis of fetal anemia; a probable reduction in the number of invasive procedures needed for diagnosis; and access to the umbilical circulation for direct transfusion. The authors also propose evidence that the cord blood reticulocyte count, normalized to gestational age, and the semiquantitative magnitude of the fetal direct Coombs' reaction are predictive of the severity of alloimmunization. The principle hazard comes from the risk of cord spasm on puncture (2.8% for the umbilical vein; 15% for an umbilical artery), and the apparently enhanced likelihood of fetal-to-maternal antigen transfer as measured by the maternal serum α-fetoprotein concentration.

This study group finds PUB to be an acceptable alternative, although emergency cesarean section for bradycardia resulted from a PUB done at 28 weeks. A decision to replace amniocentesis with PUB in the management of this problem rests primarily with the technical expertise of the obstetrician and the experience with fetal bradycardia from umbilical vessel spasm.—T.H. Kirschbaum, M.D.

Prenatal Diagnosis in Multiple Gestation: 20 Years' Experience With Amniocentesis

Anderson RL, Goldberg JD, Golbus MS (Univ of California, San Francisco)
Prenat Diagn 11:263–270, 1991 6–11

Introduction.—It has generally been thought that prenatal diagnosis by amniocentesis should not be performed in cases of multiple gestation because of an increased risk of fetal loss. Accurate risk data on this question were sought in a review of 339 cases of amniocentesis in multiple gestation.

Methods.—The patients were seen at the study institution between 1969 and 1990. The incidence of multiple gestation in pregnant women undergoing amniocentesis was 1 in 65. Because ultrasound was not routinely used early in the study period, 23 cases of multiple gestation were unrecognized before amniocentesis was performed. The multiple pregnancies were compared with singleton pregnancies for the incidence of fetal loss and perinatal death.

Results.—The 339 multiple gestations included 330 sets of twins and 9 sets of triplets. Seven abnormal fetuses were selectively terminated. Three couples chose to terminate both fetuses when only 1 had a karotypic abnormality. There were 12 spontaneous abortions of both fetuses before 28 weeks. This rate of loss (3.57%) was higher than that in the singleton pregnancies (.60%). Perinatal mortality was similar for the multiple gestation (12.6/1,000) and singleton (12.1/1,000) groups. No perinatal loss occurred in the 9 triplet pregnancies. The average gestation time was 35 weeks for triplets, 37 weeks for twins, and 39 weeks for singletons.

Conclusion.—Although there was an increase in the risk of pregnancy loss after amniocentesis in cases of multiple gestation, this increase does not appear to exceed the normal biologic loss rate in twins. Parents should be counseled about the potential risks of the procedure and about the increased chance of having a karotypically abnormal offspring in a multiple gestation.

▶ The question posed as the basis for this study ("Is amniocentesis more hazardous in twin than in singlet pregnancy?") proves difficult to answer. The rate of abortion after first trimester amniocentesis is the sum of the spontaneous abortion rate during the time interval and the rate of abortion induced solely by the procedure. In this study, the total risk of abortion for twins subject to amniocentesis before 28 weeks is 6 times larger than the risk for singlets during the same time period. Regrettably, the spontaneous abortion rate for twins to 28 weeks is not known, but it probably is larger than for singlets. Rather than reflecting the biology of multiple gestation, the relatively low perinatal mortality rate for multiple pregnancies (12.6 per 1,000 live birth) more likely reflects the presence of a small obstetrics service with a large number of mature women who are relatively socioeconomically favored. Women bearing twins deserve to know that amniocentesis is probably more hazardous to them than to those women bearing singlets. To what extent it is more hazardous is still uncertain.—T.H. Kirschbaum, M.D.

Double Jeopardy: Twin Infant Mortality in the United States, 1983 and 1984

Fowler MG, Kleinman JC, Kiely JL, Kessel SS (Natl Ctr for Health Statistics, Hyattsville, Md)

Am J Obstet Gynecol 165:15–22, 1991 6–12

Introduction.—The United States Linked Birth/Infant Death Data Sets: 1983 and 1984 Birth Cohorts from the National Center for Health

Statistics were used to identify the maternal and infant characteristics related to twin infant mortality.

Data Analysis.—The analyses used were on twin-pair characteristics rather than on individual twins. Of 135,051 twins on the 1983 and 1984 birth files, 41,544 white and 10,062 black twin pregnancies with both members born alive were successfully paired with respect to county and state of birth and residence, maternal race, age, prior live births, month prenatal care began, education, marital status, and father's race, age, and education. Monozygotic twins could not be identified from among the like-gender twin pairs; their increased risk for complications could account for the increased risk of mortality for like-gender twins. Twin infant mortality was analyzed in relation to summary levels of low, moderate, or high maternal demographic risk developed for singletons. The low-risk group included married primiparous women 20–29 years of age and low-parity multiparous women who were older than 20 years of age and had 13 or more years of education. The high-risk group included unmarried teenagers, primiparous women older than 30 years of age, and high-parity multiparous women with fewer than 12 years of education. Approximately half the white twin births and two thirds of the black twin births had low birth weights. Nine percent of white and 16% of black twin births were in the very-low-birth-weight (VLBW) category. There were 3,911 (47.1 per 1,000) white and 1,595 (79.3 per 1,000) black twin deaths. Three fourths of the deaths in both races occurred in the VLBW category.

Conclusion.—The overall infant mortality rates were approximately 5 times the rates for singletons. Three fourths of the deaths were infants in the VLBW category. Twins who were born to high-risk women were twice as likely to die as were twins born to low-risk women. Strategies to decrease twin infant mortality must address both maternal and infant risk factors.

▶ Although it benefits by the very large numbers of cases derived from the 1983 and 1984 Birth Infant Death Data Sets, this analysis from the National Center for Health Statistics suffers from the limited data of sometimes uncertain fidelity that appear on birth and death certificates. These faults particularly preclude an attempt to deal with cause-specific causes of death beyond the fact that 53% of deaths stem from causes related to low birth weight. Another way of looking at this is that the 9% of white and 16% of black twin births with birth weights less than 1,500 g accounted for 75% of all deaths. The increased hazard to like-sex compared with unlike-sex twins, white or black, probably stems from the vascular anastomoses of the monochorionic placenta which increase twin morbidity. Others have shown that black twin mortality rates are lower than white rates at birth weights less than 1,500 g, but are greater at birth weights greater than 1,500 g. It should also be noted this study shows that, in 25% of cases, twin B is of greater weight than twin A. In general, not many clues to improving twin survival are revealed from this massive data collection.—T.H. Kirschbaum, M.D.

Indomethacin for Preterm Labor: Fetal Toxicity in a Dizygotic Twin Gestation

Hallak M, Reiter AA, Ayres NA, Moise KJ Jr (Baylor College of Medicine, Houston)

Obstet Gynecol 78:911–913, 1991 6–13

Background.—Indomethacin is an effective treatment for preterm labor and symptomatic polyhydramnios, but there has been concern about its possible constrictive effect on the fetal ductus arteriosus and reduction in fetal urine output. Fetal toxicity from maternal indomethacin use in a twin gestation was studied.

Case Report.—A woman with confirmed twin gestation was treated with 2.5 mg of terbutaline every 4 hours and 200 mg of indomethacin per day for preterm labor at 34 weeks' and 5 days' gestation. Initial ultrasound studies showed normal growth, development, and amniotic fluid volume in both fetuses. After 7 days of treatment, repeat sonography showed severe oligohydramnios in both amniotic sacs and cardiomegaly in the female fetus. In the female fetus, echocardiography showed closure of the ductus arteriosus, tricuspid regurgitation, right ventricular dysfunction, and pericardial effusion. All abnormalities resolved within 7 days of discontinuation of medications. The infants were delivered vaginally at 37 weeks' gestation, and both are alive and well at age 2 months.

Conclusion.—The use of high doses of indomethacin for prolonged periods late in pregnancy may cause deleterious side effects in the fetus. All fetuses of mothers treated with indomethacin, especially those with multiple gestations, should be closely monitored for early evidence of decreased amniotic fluid volume and constriction of the ductus arteriosus. Fetal toxicity with indomethacin is reversible once the medication is discontinued.

▶ This case report provides a nice counterpoint to the report of Besinger (1) concerning the effect of chronic use of indomethacin on fetal right ventricular function. The use of 200 mg of indomethacin every day for 7 days appeared to be a responsible response to oligohydramnios in both twins and to ductus arteriosus constriction in the female twin. With pulmonary vascular constriction maintained during fetal life by the normally low pulmonary artery Po_2, ductus constriction caused by the inhibition of prostaglandin production in its endothelium and the musculature needed to maintain its patency produced a problem. Ductus constriction in fetal life sharply increases resistance to right ventricular outflow. The only compensations possible to the fetus are right chamber dilatation, increased right atrial pressure, and increased right-to-left shunting to the left atrium. Without these, the fetal heart would fail. Note that, at 35 weeks, the cardiac findings reverted to normal within 5 days of interdiction of indomethacin.—T.H. Kirschbaum, M.D.

Reference

1. Besinger RE: *Am J Obstet Gynecol* 164:981, 1991.

The Prevalence, Aetiology and Clinical Significance of Pseudo-Sinusoidal Fetal Heart Rate Patterns in Labour

Murphy KW, Russell V, Collins A, Johnson P (John Radcliffe Hosp, Oxford, England)

Br J Obstet Gynaecol 98:1093–1101, 1991 6–14

Introduction.—The fetal heart rate (FHR) usually fluctuates during labor and delivery. The sinusoidal pattern (as seen in the FHR recording) may indicate a serious loss of the beat-to-beat variability. Fetal heart rate patterns were assessed to determine the prevalence of sinusoidal and pseudosinusoidal patterns in women monitored during labor.

Methods.—The study population included all women who underwent fetal monitoring during labor in a 6-month period. A total of 1,520 patients were identified. In some patients, intrapartum ultrasound was used to determine whether fetal sucking or mouth movements occurred during a pseudosinusoidal pattern recording. Every tenth woman who was monitored and did not have a sinusoidal or pseudosinusoidal FHR pattern served as a control.

Results.—Among a total of 1,520 cardiotocographs (CTGs) reviewed during the study period, there was not 1 case of an FHR sinusoidal pattern. A total of 230 pseudosinusoidal FHR patterns were recorded, however, for a prevalence of 15%. Among the 230 pseudosinusoidal FHR patterns, 219 were rated as minor occurrences, but 11 were judged as intermediate (Fig 6–2). The mean time for the pattern was 21 minutes.

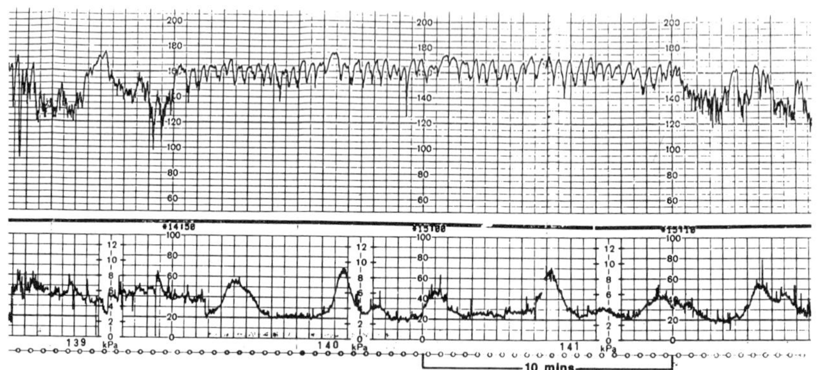

Fig 6–2.—Intermediate pseudosinusoidal FHR pattern showing oscillations with amplitude of 15–20 beats/min and frequency of 2–3 cycles/min. The baseline pattern was caused by non-nutritive, fetal sucking. Fetal outcome was normal. FHR: internal electrocardiographic recording; tocograph: external recording; paper speed: 1 cm/min. (Courtesy of Murphy KW, Russell V, Collins A, et al: *Br J Obstet Gynaecol* 98:1093–1101, 1991.)

Most of the pseudosinusoidal FHR patterns occurred during the first stage of labor. Women with pseudosinusoidal FHR patterns and controls differed significantly in the percentage who received 100 mg of intramuscularly administered pethidine (60% compared with 36%, respectively), in the percentage who received an epidural analgesic (57% compared with 39%), in the percentage who received oxytocin (65% compared with 51%), and the duration of labor, with the pseudosinusoidal FRH-patterned population having a longer labor. The intermediate pseudosinusoidal FRH pattern occurred during fetal sucking in utero.

Conclusion.—It appears that pseudosinusoidal FHR patterns may arise to compensate for the hypoxia experienced by the cardiac center in the medulla. Most fetuses will have a normal outcome, even after having a recorded pseudosinusoidal FHR pattern; however, careful fetal assessment is mandatory.

▶ True sinusoidal FHR patterns occur with a frequency of 2–4 per minute in a fixed long-term pattern, alternating with smooth flat baseline intervals exhibiting a profound loss of beat-to-beat variability. They are very rare, and their association with fetal anemia and/or hypovolemia is well known. The more one deviates from these rigid criteria, the more often sinusoidal patterns are seen with variously perserved beat-to-beat variability. Called pseudosinusoidal FHR patterns here, this becomes relatively common—seen in 15% of the cases reported in this study. Pseudosinusoidal patterns generally are benign and do not warrant operative intervention in the course of labor. The associations with pseudosinusoidal patterns are nicely outlined here. Epidural anesthesia, Demerol, Nisentil, and sleep/state changes are the most often identified coincidental events. No one has succeeded in indicting fetal hypoxemia as their cause. The lesson here is clear. If one decides to act on the presence of sinusoidal FHR patterns in labor, he must be certain that his diagnostic criteria match the rigorous classical criteria used to define them, as described in this paper.—T.H. Kirschbaum, M.D.

Follow-Up and Prognancy Outcome After a Diagnosis of Mosaicism in CVS

Breed ASPM, Mantingh A, Vosters R, Beekhuis JR, Van Lith JMM, Anders GJPA (State Univ of Groningen; Univ Hosp, Groningen, The Netherlands; Rijnstate Hosp, Arnhem, The Netherlands)

Prenat Diagn 11:577–580, 1991 6–15

Background.—The chromosomal mosaic patterns encountered in chorionic villus sampling (CVS) are usually restricted to extraembryonic tissues. When normal cell lines are involved, an aberrant cell line generally is not confirmed in the amniotic fluid or fetal tissues. A series of pregnancies with this finding was followed up to assess the significance of the abnormal cells.

Findings.—Between November 1984 and January 1, 1990, a total of 2,103 consecutive CVS specimens were prepared by direct or long-term culture, or both. Twenty-six samples had a mosaic pattern involving a cell line with a normal cytogenetic complement, for a rate of 1.2%. Two pregnancies were terminated; 1 of them involved a 46,XY/47,XY,+9 pattern in the amniotic fluid and umbilical cord blood. Among the remaining 24 pregnancies, there were 4 spontaneous abortions, for a rate of 16.7%. There also were 2 immature newborns who survived and 3 small-for-dates children.

Conclusion.—Placental mosaicism appears to be associated with fetal loss; the presence of these abnormal cells appears to compromise the viability of chromosomally normal fetuses. Counseling for patients in whom CVS discloses mosaicism includes a possible higher risk of complications and further invasive procedures.

▶ This experience supports the conclusion of Schwinger et al. (see the 1991 YEAR BOOK OF OBSTETRICS AND GYNECOLOGY, pp 201–202), which was based on 14 personal cases and 185 cases gleaned from the literature. In 24 cases proven by CVS and normal amniocentesis, there was 1 early fetal loss and 3 spontaneous abortions, a high rate of pregnancy loss given pregnancies with sufficient maturity to undergo CVS. The outcome of such pregnancies with respect to the development of intrauterine growth retardation is not discussed. There is growing reason for concern that placental mosaicism affords a disadvantage to the euploid fetus to which it is connected.—T.H. Kirschbaum, M.D.

Second Trimester Amniotic Fluid Oestriol, Dehydroepiandrosterone Sulphate, and Human Chorionic Gonadotrophin Levels in Down's Syndrome

Cuckle HS, Wald NJ, Densem JW, Canick J, Abell KB (St Bartholomew's Med College, London; Womens and Infants Hosp, Providence, RI)
Br J Obstet Gynaecol 98:1160–1162, 1991 6–16

Introduction.—Decreased maternal serum levels of alpha-fetoprotein (AFP) and unconjugated estriol (uE_3) and increased levels of human chorionic gonadotropin (hCG) suggest the presence of fetal Down's syndrome. To determine why these levels vary from normal in women carrying a Down's syndrome fetus, stored amniotic fluid samples from normal and affected pregnancies were compared.

Methods.—The amniotic fluid samples from all subjects who had an amniotic fluid AFP test between 1975 and 1983 were analyzed for levels of uE_3, total estriol (tE_3), dehydroepiandrosterone sulfate (DHEAS), and hCG. During this time period, 48 Down's syndrome pregnancies had occurred, and sample material from 45 cases was provided. Most of the hormones and metabolites were measured by radioimmunoassay, and the concentrations were expressed as multiples of the median (MoM).

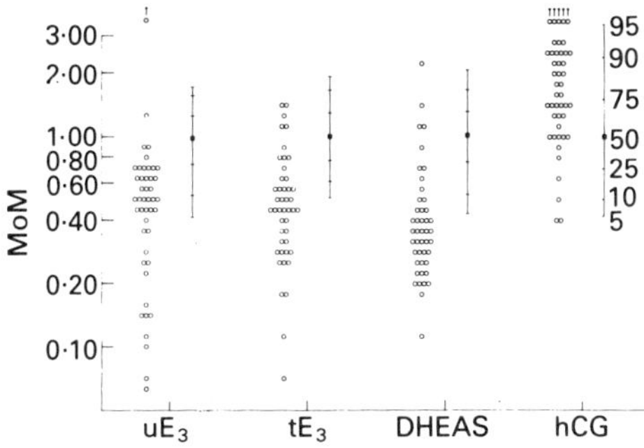

Fig 6–3.—Individual amniotic fluid values in 45 Down's syndrome pregnancies and selected centiles in 224 controls (*vertical lines*). (Courtesy of Cuckle HS, Wald NJ, Densem JW, et al: *Br J Obstet Gynaecol* 98:1160–1162, 1991.)

Results.—Figure 6–3 presents the MoM outcomes for the Down's syndrome pregnancies in relation to some controls. The differences in hormone levels between the Down's syndrome cases and the subjects with normal pregnancies were significant. The median levels of uE_3 and tE_3, and the DHEAS levels all appeared significantly lower than in normal pregnancies. For the Down's syndrome pregnancies, both the amniotic fluid and the maternal serum demonstrated low concentrations of uE_3.

Conclusion.—Maternal serum concentrations of tE_3 may serve as a marker for fetal Down's syndrome, although it does not possess the specificity of uE_3. It appears that the lower levels of uE_3 in the serum of women carrying a Down's syndrome fetus result chiefly from problems with the fetal adrenal gland's synthesis of DHEAS, and that the higher levels of hCG in the maternal serum result from overproduction of this hormone by the placenta.

▶ This study deals with a subject of continuing interest, because the majority of infants with Down's syndrome continue to result from pregnant women younger than 35 years of age, despite the low rate of incidence of Down's syndrome in that age group. The problem is to make the infrequent diagnosis accurately and precisely in women of younger age, but to do so at low cost—despite the large number of negative results anticipated. The problem is unsolved to date, but this paper represents a genuine step in understanding the endocrinological findings in gravidas with infants with Down's syndrome. Serum uE_3 values are better predictors than total estriol concentrations, because the latter better reflect maternal, rather than fetal, estrogen production.

The reduced concentration of amniotic fluid and maternal serum uE_3 in Down's syndrome suggests reduced production of estriol rather than impaired placental secretion into the maternal blood. This conclusion is confirmed by the low concentrations of DHEA sulfate, the major fetal contribution to the enhanced production of estrogen in pregnancy, in amniotic fluid. The reverse seems to be true of placental hCG production, with the placenta serving as nearly the entire source of that protein hormone. Because increased hCG is equally increased in the amniotic fluid and maternal serum, it's likely that trophoblastic production of hCG is augmented in this syndrome. The relationship between impaired fetal adrenal steroid precursors and increased placental HCG production may contain a clue to facilitating the diagnosis of Down's syndrome in fetuses of young gravidas.—T.H. Kirschbaum, M.D.

7 Fetal Surveillance

The Acute Response of the Umbilical Artery Pulsatility Index to Changes in Blood Volume in Fetal Sheep

van Huisseling H, Muijsers GJJM, de Haan J, Hasaart THM (Univ Hosp Maastricht, The Netherlands)

Eur J Obstet Gynecol Reprod Biol 43:149–155, 1992 7–1

Introduction.—Absent or reversed end-diastolic flow in Doppler umbilical artery waveforms is associated with fetal and neonatal morbidity and mortality. The flow velocity waveform is the result of several interacting factors, and changes in one of these might influence the flow velocity waveform indices. However, to what extent the changes in any of these factors influence the umbilical artery waveform in vivo is unknown. The effects of acute changes in fetal circulating blood volume on the umbilical artery pulsatility index (PI) were investigated.

Methods.—Six sheep between 117 and 125 days' gestation were provided with an electromagnetic flowmeter for measurement of the umbilical venous blood flow, catheters for the determination of arterial blood pressure and umbilical venous pressure, and a 5-MHz Doppler trans-

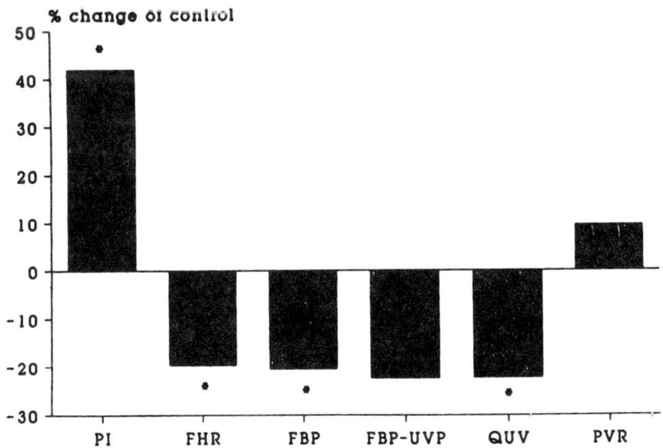

Fig 7–1.—The percent changes from control in umbilical artery PI, fetal heart rate, fetal blood pressures, umbilical blood flow, and placental vascular resistance after withdrawal of 50 mL of fetal blood. *$P < .05$ (Wilcoxon's matched pairs signed ranks test). (Courtesy of van Huisseling H, Muijsers GJJM, de Haan J, et al: *Eur J Obstet Gynecol Reprod Biol* 43:149–155, 1992.)

ducer placed around 1 umbilical artery for umbilical artery flow velocity analysis. A few days after instrumentation, fetal hypervolemia was induced by infusing 50 mL of maternal blood, and hypovolemia was induced by withdrawing 50 mL of fetal blood.

Results.—Hypervolemia resulted in an increase in arterial pressure and umbilical venous pressure, whereas the PI, the umbilical blood flow, and the calculated placental vascular resistance remained unchanged (Fig 7-1). Hypovolemia resulted in a decrease in fetal heart rate, arterial pressure, umbilical venous pressure, and umbilical blood flow. The PI increased by 42%, and the placental vascular resistance was unchanged. Thus, a 10% to 15% increase in fetal circulating blood volume did not affect the umbilical artery PI or the placental vascular resistance, whereas an acute reduction in fetal blood volume with the same amount was associated with an increase in the umbilical artery PI without a change in placental vascular resistance.

Conclusion.—Increased umbilical artery blood velocity indices are not necessarily related to pathologic changes in placental vessels, but they may be a sign of fetal hypotension.

▶ This is another in a series of animal experiments demonstrating the failure of Doppler indications of the changes in vascular resistance to correspond to resistance measured classically by the ratio of blood pressure/blood flow rate (see the 1992 YEAR BOOK OF OBSTETRICS AND GYNECOLOGY, pp 145–46). Because the observations are based solely on the physics of blood flow, there seem to be few hazards in projecting work done of necessity in animal fetuses to the human. The change in circulatory dynamics was transient (less than 30 minutes), because only blood volume changes of the magnitude of 10% to 15% of the estimated blood volume were imposed. Pulsatility index in the umbilical arteries increased primarily because of the reduction in both heart rate and end diastolic flow velocity, the latter reaching nearly 0 in one case. Despite this average increase of 45% in PI, umbilical vascular resistance did not increase significantly (approximately 8%). The authors inferred, but did not directly measure, a decrease in cardiac output from the reduction in blood volume. If this is correct, 0 or negative end diastolic flow velocity may represent either bradycardia, reduced fetal blood pressure, or both, instead of a change in placental resistance.—T.H. Kirschbaum, M.D.

Extremely High Maternal Serum Alpha-Fetoprotein Levels at Second-Trimester Screening

Killam WP, Miller RC, Seeds JW (Univ of North Carolina, Chapel Hill, NC)

Obstet Gynecol 78:257–261, 1991 7–2

Background.—Maternal serum α-fetoprotein (MSAFP) screening is primarily used to identify pregnancies at increased risk of an open neural tube defect (NTD). However, recent studies have shown that MSAFP increases to 5 or more multiples of the median (MoM) are associated with a range of fetal anomalies and adverse pregnancy outcomes. The pregnancy outcomes were examined in a cohort of women with mid-pregnancy MSAFP levels of greater than 8 MoM.

Methods.—During a 5½-year study period, 40,676 pregnancies were screened for MSAFP and 44 (.1%) had MSAFP levels of greater than 8 MoM. Maternal blood was drawn between 15 and 19 weeks' estimated gestational age. The medians were calculated from regional data. The 44 women ranged in age from 15 to 37 years, and the mean age at MSAFP sampling was 25 years. The outcomes for all 44 pregnancies (42 singleton and 2 twin sets) were determined and classified into 5 primary diagnostic categories.

Results.—Of the 44 pregnancies with MSAFP levels of greater than 8 MoM, 20 (45%) had a major fetal anomaly, 11 (25%) had a spontaneous fetal death before 20 weeks' gestation, 7 had placental anomalies, 4 had obstetric complications, and 2 had inappropriately low estimated gestational age by the last menstrual period. Of the 20 pregnancies with a major fetal anomaly, 10 had an NTD, 9 had ventral wall defects, and 1 had renal agenesis. The overall positive predictive value of an MSAFP level of 8 or more MoM for NTDs was 22.7%. There were only 16 live births among the 46 fetuses. Among the 16 live-born infants, 31% had a major anomaly, 19% had intrauterine growth retardation and an anomaly, 12.5% had intrauterine growth retardation without an anomaly, and 25% were preterm.

Conclusion.—Pregnancies with MSAFP values of 8 or more MoM are associated with a high incidence of adverse outcomes. Diagnostic ultrasound plays a definitive role in the management of these patients.

▶ With reasonably clear interpretations of what is meant by moderately increased and low MSAFP established, this study of 44 pregnancies, representing .1% of all screened patients at Chapel Hill, deals with what's left. The values of MSAFP of 8 or more MoM correspond to pregnancies in which neural tube defects and ventral wall abnormalities are either very large or are associated with each other, with or without gross placental anomaly. No single simple class of abnormalities is defined by such MSAFP values, but the magnitude of the change bespeaks a terrible prospect for survival. To this point, note the fetal death rate of 65%, which is falsely high by virtue of the inclusion of therapeutic abortion for anomaly and the perinatal mortality figure of 63/1000 live births. In this series, antenatal ultrasound appeared to detect all in utero problems (except for minor anomalies concealed by major ones) and slightly more than half the placental abnormalities. The real difficulty comes from the rare occasion when no antenatal abnormality is seen on ultrasound in women with very high concentrations of MSAFP. In fairness, that couple must be warned of a possible poor outcome and the fallibility of antenatal diagnosis.—T.H. Kirschbaum, M.D.

Computerized Analysis of Episodic Changes in Fetal Heart Rate Variation in Early Labor

Dawes GS, Rosevear SK, Pello LC, Moulden M, Redman CWG (John Radcliffe Hosp, Oxford, England)

Am J Obstet Gynecol 165:618–624, 1991 7–3

Background.—Loss of baseline fetal heart rate (FHR) variation has been shown to be a reliable sign of impending death before birth. Reduced FHR variation appears to be the single most reliable sign of hypoxemia, developing acidemia, and imminent intrauterine death before onset of labor. A computerized analysis of the episodic changes in FHR variation in early labor was reported.

Methods.—A total of 136 women at 37–42 weeks' gestation were enrolled in a study. Variation of FHR in early labor was measured using computerized analysis in cyclic episodes of low or high variation.

Results.—The amplitude in episodes of low variation was 20.6 ms. In high variation, it was 57.3 ms. The duration of low episodes was less than that of high episodes, but it sometimes was more than 1 hour. In

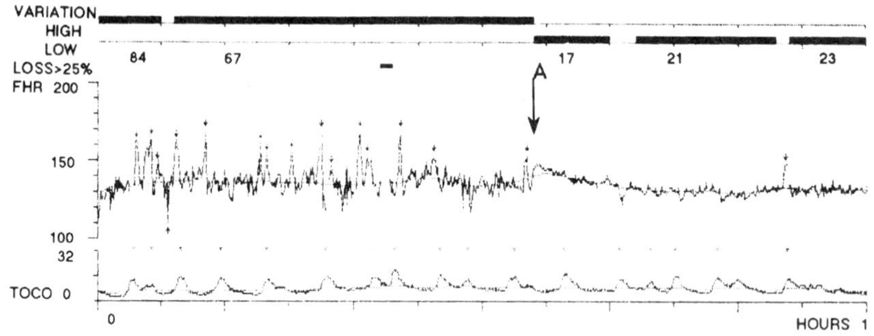

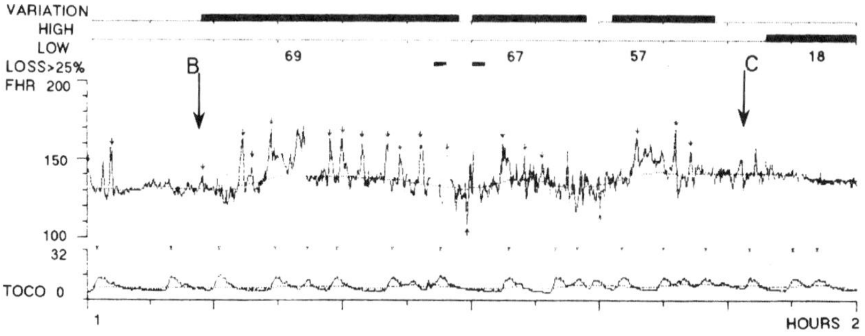

Fig 7–2.—Computer analysis of 2 hours in the early first stage of labor at 40 weeks' gestation shows successive episodes of low (*A–B*) and high (*B–C*) FHR variation. The mean range of long-term variation was 50 ms, although episodes of low variation averaged 20.7 ms and high variation averaged 66 ms. No analgesia was given; at delivery, umbilical arterial pH was 7.26 and base deficit was 7 mmol/L. (Courtesy of Dawes GS, Rosevear SK, Pello LC, et al: *Am J Obstet Gynecol* 165:618–624, 1991.)

episodes of low variation, the amplitude was less than 5 beats per minute in the long term for 11% of the fetuses and less than 2.5 ms in the short term in 8%. If persistent before birth, these measures would predict intrauterine death (Fig 7–2).

Conclusion.—The use of reduced FHR variation as a diagnostic sign of acute fetal hypoxemia in labor is incorrect. Changes of this size occur randomly as a result of fetal sleep states. Fetal heart rate variation during the last hour of labor was not significantly correlated with umbilical arterial base deficit on delivery.

▶ Ordinarily, FHR variability, both in the long and short term, is visually assayed by noting the variations of the integrated FHR inscribed on a strip recorder. This approach, originating at Oxford (see the 1989 YEAR BOOK OF OBSTETRICS AND GYNECOLOGY, pp 117–118), relies on statistically analyzing the digitized records of the interval between fetal heart excursions (sampled 10 times per second each 3.7 seconds), calculating a baseline FHR interval, and measuring the deviation from baseline as the deviation from that mean. The variability of these deviations is taken as a measure of FHR variability. Filtering is used to exclude sharp accelerations and decelerations that would distort the averaging in techniques. What results are observations that cannot be made by visual inspection and that threaten the validity of years of similar prior interpretations.

In this study, reduced beat-to-beat variability means hypoxemia, hypoxia, and fetal acidosis. Note that the results are different for infants with intrauterine growth retardation, and hypoxemia, in whom reduced beat-to-beat variability seems to be related to the degree of acidemia. In particular, Smith et al. (1) found very little FHR variability in such infants (short-term variability averaged less than 2.5 ms) to be diagnostic of impending death. As Professor Dawes adds to his illustrious career as a premier fetal physiologist with these studies, his results are important to all of us.—T.H. Kirschbaum, M.D.

Reference

1. Smith JH, et al: *Br J Obstet Gynaecol* 95:980, 1988.

Sinusoidal Fetal Heart Rate Pattern During Labor

Egley CC, Bowes WA Jr, Wagner D (St Francis Med Ctr, Peoria, Ill; Univ of North Carolina, Chapel Hill)

Am J Perinatol 8:197–202, 1991 7–4

Background.—Sinusoidal heart rate (SHR) pattern is an ominous sign in antepartum monitoring of the rhesus immunized pregnancy, but its significance in nonimmunized pregnancies is unclear. The incidence and factors associated with the SHR pattern during labor were examined.

Methods.—All fetal heart rate tracings obtained by means of a scalp electrode during a 6-month period were reviewed. Only cases of typical

SHR, defined as a frequency of 2–5 per minute, amplitude of 5–10 bpm, and short-term viability of less than 2 bpm, were sought. Fifty-four such cases were found, for an incidence of 4.2%. This group of patients was compared with those who did not exhibit the SHR pattern.

Results.—In the SHR group, the pattern was present for more than 90 minutes in 7 cases, 6 of them during oxytocin administration. There was no difference between the 2 groups in Apgar score, incidence of other fetal heart rate abnormalities, or passage of meconium. Of 3 fetuses with SHR in whom scalp pH was measured, all had a pH greater than 7.3. Administration of alphaprodine during labor was associated with the SHR pattern, but administration of other narcotics was not.

Conclusion.—In antenatal fetal monitoring, the development of an SHR pattern in a nonsensitized pregnancy does not appear to be an ominous sign. Such infants should be assessed for signs of congestive heart failure, but the typical SHR pattern does not appear to be a sign of fetal hypoxia. Scalp pH sampling should be done if an atypical pattern (sine waves of amplitude greater than 15 bpm) is noted.

► This manuscript makes an important point that is seldom recognized. When rigorously defined as in this study, an SHR pattern is seldom a sign of fetal compromise—with some important exceptions. The exceptions are fetal blood isosensitization, vasa previa, and other less common causes of fetal anemia. Provided the absence of vaginal bleeding and the ability to exclude potential causes of fetal anemia, careful definition of SHR patterns finds them neither uncommon (4.2% of laboring women in this case) nor particularly ominous.—T.H. Kirschbaum, M.D.

Relation of Fetal Blood Gases and Data From Computer-Assisted Analysis of Fetal Heart Rate Patterns in Small for Gestation Fetuses

Ribbert LSM, Snijders RJM, Nicolaides KH, Visser GHA (King's College Hosp, London; Univ Hosp Groningen, The Netherlands)

Br J Obstet Gynaecol 98:820–823, 1991 7–5

Background.—Computerized analysis of fetal heart rate (FHR) may help overcome the variable interpretation of various patterns. A relationship between FHR variation and umbilical cord blood PO_2 obtained at elective cesarean section has been reported, but this may have been affected by delays between FHR analysis and blood sampling, among other factors. Cordocentesis enabled this relationship to be assessed in utero.

Methods.—Monitoring of FHR was done immediately before cordocentesis in 25 pregnancies (mean gestation, 31.5 weeks) for assessment of suspected severe intrauterine growth retardation. Amniotic fluid volume, as evaluated by ultrasonography, was reduced in 18 cases, 9 of

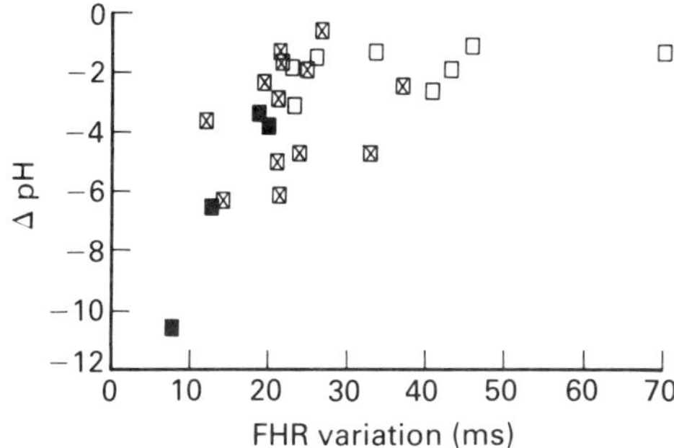

Fig 7–3.—Relation of FHR variation and umbilical vein blood Δ pH in 25 small-for-gestational-age fetuses. *Open squares,* decelerations absent plus accelerations present; *squares with an x,* decelerations plus accelerations present; *filled squares,* decelerations present accelerations absent. (Courtesy of Ribbert LSM, Snijders RJM, Nicolaides KH, et al: *Br J Obstet Gynaecol* 98:820–823, 1991.)

which were oligohydramniotic. All infants were beneath the 5th percentile in birth weight.

Results.—The mean Po_2 was 2 standard deviations (SD) below normal, and the mean pH was 3.4 SD below normal. Significant associations were found between FHR variation and both umbilical vein blood Po_2 and pH (Fig 7–3). Those infants with no acceleration in their FHR tracings had significantly lower Po_2 and pH: −1.69 and −2.85 SD, respectively. However, fetal blood gas values could not be predicted accurately by FHR patterns because of the wide scatter of values around regression lines. However, in all infants with FHR variation less than 20 ms, there was severe fetal hypoxemia and acidemia.

Conclusion.—In severely growth-retarded fetuses, reduced FHR variations, decelerations, or absence of accelerations appear to be associated with hypoxemia and acidemia. Further investigations, such as serial FHR, other noninvasive tests, or cordocentesis, are needed to determine the significance of FHR variation less than 20 ms.

▶ This study contains 2 important contributions. Ordinarily, data of this sort compare characteristics of fetal heart traces with cord blood analyses at the time of delivery, which necessitates impossible inferences about fetal blood values several minutes or hours before delivery. Cordocentesis allowed more proximate evaluation of the relationship between cord blood values and antenatal testing in these infants with severe IUGR, defined as a birth weight less than the fifth percentile for sex and gestational age at delivery. The results show a high likelihood of acidosis and hypoxemia of the umbilical vein blood in such infants. This does not necessarily mean that tissue hypoxia occurred, because increased umbilical artery extraction of oxygen and changes in umbilical vein blood flow rates are capable of compensating for the concentration change noted.

A nice relationship of FHR variation to acidosis was seen, but the methods of FHR analysis introduced by Dawes and colleagues need to be understood (see the 1989 YEAR BOOK OF OBSTETRICS AND GYNECOLOGY, pp 117–118). In this study, variation in beat-to-beat FHR is calculated as an average over 1 hour, but the pulse interval, which is reciprocal of the heart rate, and is measured in milliseconds around the calculated baseline with accelerations and decelerations, is eliminated. It's precisely the need to use such well-defined quantitative expressions of FHR variability that allows this sort of careful search for relationships between cardiovascular-respiratory function and heart rate of the fetus to be done. Note, however, that Dawes and co-workers (Abstract 7–3) failed to find such relationships using the same analytic techniques, although they used measurements of acid-based status at the time of delivery as dependent variables.—T.H. Kirschbaum, M.D.

Umbilical Artery Resistance Index as a Screening Test for Fetal Well-Being: I. Prospective Revealed Evaluation

Pattinson R, Dawes G, Jennings J, Redman C (John Radcliffe Hosp, Oxford, England)

Obstet Gynecol 78:353–358, 1991 7–6

Introduction.—Examination of the antenatal fetal heart rate (FHR) is used to assess fetal well-being. However, this nonstress test (NST) is time consuming and difficult to interpret. It has been reported that an increased umbilical artery resistance index (UARI) derived from flow velocity patterns measured by Doppler ultrasound techniques precedes an abnormal FHR pattern. The usefulness of the UARI as a first screening test of fetal well-being was studied prospectively.

Patients.—During a 10-month period, 369 pregnant women underwent 1,354 assessments at 26–42 weeks' gestation to monitor fetal well-being. All women were at high risk for fetal compromise. Each examination included a computerized antenatal FHR analysis and a continuous-wave Doppler ultrasound examination. However, clinical management was based strictly on the NST results.

Results.—The mean duration of each NST was 27 minutes compared with 6 minutes for the Doppler ultrasound examination. Twenty-nine of the 1,354 NSTs obtained were abnormal. The UARI was increased in 27 of the 29 fetuses with abnormal NSTs and was normal in the 2 with abnormal NSTs. The UARI also was increased in 293 fetuses with normal NSTs. When the NST was considered the gold standard, the value of the UARI in predicting an abnormal NST had a sensitivity of 93.1%, a specificity of 77.9%, a positive predictive value of 8.4%, and a negative predictive value of 99.8%. An increased UARI identified those fetuses with an abnormal NST or a clinical diagnosis of antenatal distress with a high sensitivity and a high negative predictive value. Because 40 women had abnormal UARIs without antenatal fetal distress, Doppler ultrasound umbilical artery scanning appeared to have a high false positive rate. However, this high false positive rate was reduced when fetal distress in labor was included as a third end point.

Conclusion.—Doppler ultrasound scanning of the umbilical artery may be a good screening test for the assessment of fetal well-being. Further randomized controlled trials are needed, because this study population included only pregnant women at high risk for fetal compromise.

▶ The authors' conclusions that Doppler study of the umbilical artery velocity patterns "may be a good screening test of fetal well-being" seems hard to understand. In predicting abnormal NST, increased Doppler "resistance" has a false positive rate of 91.5%; in predicting fetal distress, the false positive rate is 78% before and 83% during labor. The high negative predictive values stem almost entirely from low prevalence rates. The incidence of abnormal NST was 2.1%, and the incidence of fetal distress was about 3.5%. That means that if no testing were done but all 381 patients seen for antenatal testing simply were labeled normal, those predictions would be correct in 97.9% and 96.5%, respectively. Against that background, Doppler evaluation contributes little. That's consonant with a companion paper (1) in which preliminary screening of suspect patients with Doppler failed either to improve perinatal outcome or to save time.—T.H. Kirschbaum, M.D.

Reference

1. *Obstet Gynecol* 78:359, 1991.

Computerized Fetal Heart Rate Analysis in Labor

Pello LC, Rosevear SK, Dawes GS, Moulden M, Redman CWG (Nuffield Dept of Obstetrics and Gynecology, Oxford, England)

Obstet Gynecol 78:602–610, 1991 7–7

Background.—Several studies have shown that interobserver and intraobserver variations in interpretation of fetal heart rate (FHR) tracings are unacceptably high. It was previously shown that computerized analysis can provide an objective means to differentiate normal from abnormal tracings. A preliminary study of the relationship between simple FHR variables and outcome was assessed.

Methods.—The subjects were 394 patients at 37 or more weeks' gestation who had measurement of umbilical arterial and venous blood gas parameters. Continuous monitoring was done in most patients, most commonly because of induction of labor or epidural analgesics. All tracings were recorded on line and were analyzed for associations between pattern and outcome, as reflected by umbilical arterial base deficit or Apgar score on delivery. The influence of Syntocinon and pethidine and/or epidural analgesia was analyzed separately.

Results.—There was a great range of normality and many diverse patterns among infants delivered without acidemia (Fig 7–4). Neither Syntocinon nor pethidine had a significant effect on FHR pattern. Among women who had epidural analgesia compared with those who did not,

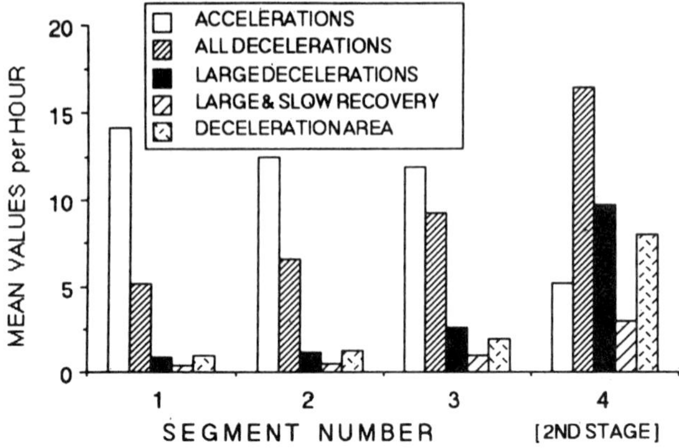

Fig 7–4.—Observations on 66 patients with neither analgesia nor metabolic acidemia on delivery. All the deceleration measures show large, statistically significant ($P < .05$) increases with the progress of labor. (Courtesy of Pello LC, Rosevear SK, Dawes GS, et al: *Obstet Gynecol* 78:602–610, 1991.)

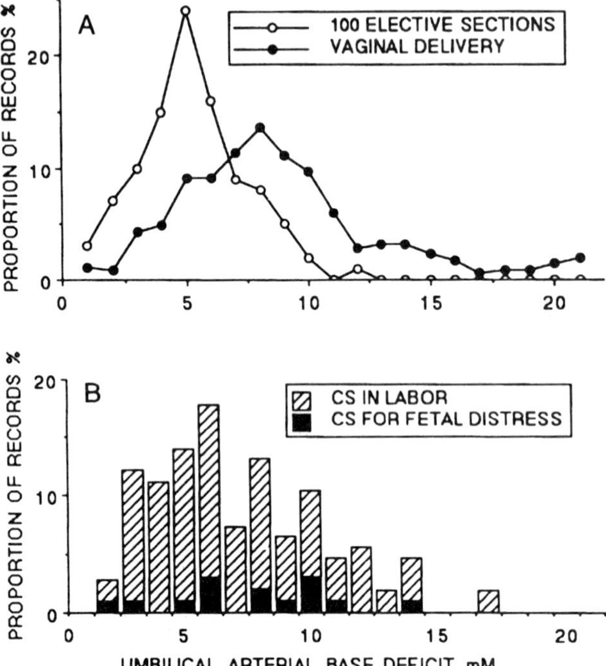

Fig 7–5.—Frequency distribution of umbilical artery blood base deficit values from cesarean (CS) in labor (**B**). The heights of the columns show the overall incidence; the *filled bars* indicate the contribution of fetal distress to the total. **A** shows the frequency distribution for 100 elective cesareans in the absence of labor or fetal distress and for 340 vaginal deliveries. The most acidemic fetuses were delivered vaginally. mM = mmol/L. (Courtesy of Pello LC, Rosevear SK, Dawes GS, et al: *Obstet Gynecol* 78:602–610, 1991.)

spontaneous vaginal delivery was less common, the first and second stages of labor were longer, cesarean delivery was 3 times as common, and operative deliveries were more common. Fetal heart rate in women who had epidural analgesia showed a significantly higher basal heart rate, less range of variation, and fewer accelerations. However, there were no differences in the condition of the fetus at delivery.

There was no association between the diagnosis of fetal distress and the finding of severe acidemia (Fig 7–5). Acidemia occurred in patients with reduced long-term FHR variation and a basal rate below 160 bpm, which may have been associated with sleep states. There was no correlation between base deficit on delivery and basal FHR or long-term FHR variation, nor between lag time and pH or base deficit. Less than one third of acidemia cases were identified by lag time. Eighteen fetuses had end stage bradycardia; acidemia was mild or moderate/severe in 13 of these. Among infants born with severe acidemia, duration of labor was longer in those with birth asphyxia.

Conclusion.—Epidural analgesia appears to be an important confounding variable. The conventional FHR attributes, including late deceleration, are insufficient to predict fetal acidemia. The high intervention rate in infants without acidemia may be explained in part by an increase in basal FHR, perhaps resulting from an increase in maternal temperature.

▶ Here is yet another example of the objectified computer-based analysis of continuous fetal heart records from the Nuffield Department in Oxford. Although such an analysis usually is conducted with a subjective approach to visual pattern recognition, this approach is rigorous to define accelerations and decelerations, to measure the area and duration of decelerations relative to computed average baseline, and to measure the mean variations from that baseline averaged over intervals of 3.75 seconds (16 times per minute) as measures of long-term variability. Analyses from 3 phases of stage 1 and 1 phase of stage 2 labor were compared with respect to a series of independent variables. It's reassuring that the expected pattern of increasingly large and prolonged decelerations with increasing accelerations emerged from the analysis of normal labor viewed this way.

The results conflict in many respects with the analysis of FHR tracings with other techniques. Neither oxytocin nor meperidine affects FHR relativity. Epidural anesthesia increases the baseline rate and decreases long-term variability. The reduced long-term FHR variability may represent hypoxemia, but it is often enough compensated and confused with fetal state changes that the findings are not reliably associated with severe acidemia. There was no correlation between delayed recovery from decelerations (late decelerations) and either cord blood pH or base deficit. Of 9 fetuses delivered with cord blood pH less than 7, conventional fetal heart rate analysis failed to predict that outcome. This is not to say that there may not be gifted clinicians who can make clinically useful interpretations from visual FHR inspection on the basis of the long years of experience. The approach the authors submit may prove to be more advantageous to those who lack that degree of skill.—T.H. Kirschbaum, M.D.

Multicenter Randomized Clinical Trial of Home Uterine Activity Monitoring for Detection of Preterm Labor

Mou SM, Sunderji SG, Gall S, How H, Patel V, Gray M, Kayne HL, Corwin M (Univ of Missouri—Kansas City; State Univ of New York, Syracuse; Univ of Illinois, Chicago; Boston Univ; Boston City, Hosp)

Am J Obstet Gynecol 165:858–866, 1991 7–8

Background.—Preterm labor is often detected too late for effective tocolysis. Many studies have attempted to evaluate the effectiveness of home uterine activity monitoring in detecting preterm labor, but most have included intensive perinatal nursing support. Home uterine activity monitoring was evaluated as the sole addition to current high-risk obstetric care.

Methods.—The study included 377 women from 3 centers. All were at risk for preterm labor and were reviewed at their initial visit, at 22–26 weeks' gestation, and at 32 weeks' gestation. The patients were randomly assigned to receive high-risk prenatal care alone (nonmonitored) or high-risk care plus twice-daily home uterine activity monitoring without increased nursing support (monitored). Monitoring was done from 24 weeks to 37 weeks or delivery (if delivery occurred before 37 weeks).

Results.—The monitored and nonmonitored groups were similar in terms of medical condition and demographics at entry into the study and in routine and nonroutine visits and gestational age at diagnosis of preterm labor. Labor occurred before term in 41 of 198 monitored and 39 of 179 nonmonitored patients. The mean cervical dilatation was greater in the nonmonitored group than in the monitored group: 2.5 cm vs. 1.4 cm. The infants of the women in the monitored group had greater birth weight, spent fewer days in neonatal intensive care, and were less likely to need oxygen therapy and mechanical ventilation.

Conclusion.—Home uterine activity monitoring may increase the chances of diagnosing preterm labor before advanced cervical dilatation, thereby providing a better chance to initiate tocolytic therapy and thus improve neonatal outcome. The benefits are consistent for a medically and demographically diverse study population and for all outcome variables.

▶ This is an important study, because the authors claim it was the basis of the Food and Drug Administration's consideration of the use of a home monitoring device in the prevention of preterm labor. Certainly, it's a more significant piece of work than most of what has gone before. Previous studies simply tended to express the biases of those with a particular interest in the device. In this study, questions arise with respect to patient selection and comparability of the monitored and nonmonitored groups. Because 9% appears to be a reasonable estimate of preterm birth in this country, the total expected incidence of preterm labor in 2,316 screened pregnancies is 208. Therefore, this study dealt with only 40% of the anticipated fetal risk, having excluded about 125 cases in an effort to isolate a population with what proved to be a 25% chance of preterm labor. That's understandable, but it means—at best—that this is not a generally applicable conclusion, because it deals with only a fraction of the study population at risk.

Random assignment to monitored and nonmonitored cases should lead to equal numbers of comparable independent variables in each group. Therefore, it is hard to understand why 60% of the University of Illinois cases were monitored. Those patients who were not monitored consisted of larger numbers of nonwhite patients without a high school education and with a greater use of alcohol, cocaine, heroin, and tobacco. More seriously, 45% of monitored cases had proven prior preterm labor, whereas 54.8% of nonmonitored cases showed prior history of PTL. These differences proved, as they usually do, to be predictive of PTL, because 71.8% of the nonmonitored cases with PTL had a positive history. See de Haus et al. (1) for a nice review of the risk factors for preterm labor. Although the authors claim no significant differences between groups, I found a significant difference with respect to this element of history.

The results rest on a small number of cases (12 cases with birth weight less than 2.5 kg and 7 cases less than 2 kg between monitored and nonmonitored cases), which makes one wonder about the presence of 9 more women with prior preterm labor in the monitored group than in the nonmonitored group. No conclusion can be drawn from these data, because Table 1 in the original article should have been constructed around the 334 women whose preterm labor status was known, omitting the 43 patients in whom preterm labor was not possible or was unknown. Given a sample of women whose preterm labor status was ultimately known (biased in the direction apparent in the 377 enrolled), all the subsequent observations might easily be explained by that bias alone, independent of any value of home monitoring. Perhaps this study proved convincing to the Food and Drug Administration committee; however, there certainly are a large number of unanswered questions and a good deal of unconvincing data.—T.H. Kirschbaum, M.D.

Reference

1. de Haus I, et al: *Am J Obstet Gynecol* 165:1290, 1991.

Doppler Flow Velocity Waveform Analysis in High Risk Pregnancies: A Randomized Controlled Trial

Newnham JP, O'Dea MR-A, Reid KP, Diepeveen DA (King Edward Mem Hosp for Women, Perth, Western Australia)

Br J Obstet Gynaecol 98:956–963, 1991 7–9

Objective.—The effects of the introduction of Doppler waveform analysis on the neonatal morbidity and obstetric management in an ultrasound department of a tertiary level hospital were evaluated in a randomized controlled trial.

Subjects.—A group of 505 women with high-risk pregnancies who were referred for fetal investigation during the third trimester was randomly assigned to have or not to have continuous-wave Doppler studies of umbilical and uteroplacental arterial circulations. The main outcome measure was the duration of neonatal stay in the hospital. Other outcome parameters, such as the number and type of fetal heart rate monitoring studies, obstetric interventions, frequency of fetal distress, birth weight, Apgar scores, and the need for neonatal intensive care, were compared between the study and control groups. The 2 groups were comparable for maternal age, height, parity, smoking, and gestational age at enrollment.

Outcome.—The duration of neonatal stay in the hospital did not differ significantly between groups. However, small trends in obstetric management were observed in the study group, including fewer contraction stress tests, less likelihood of antepartum fetal distress, and greater likelihood of fetal distress after induction of labor leading to emergency cesarean section. Depressed Apgar scores occurred more frequently in the study group.

Discussion.—The introduction of Doppler waveform studies did not reduce neonatal morbidity in this study, although it did provide a small but not significant effect on obstetric management. Although previous studies have suggested that Doppler studies provide information useful in obstetric management and that their introduction does not increase the number of preterm births or obstetric interventions, there is still little evidence of improved outcome from the use of Doppler waveform analysis in late pregnancy.

▶ In an extraordinary approach to the evolution of new techniques in obstetrics, clinicians in Western Australia agreed not to purchase Doppler systems until they are demonstrated to be of proven value in a series of studies centered in and around the King Edward Memorial Hospital for Women in Perth. Remarkably, they have clung to the notion that the instrumentation designed to improve perinatal outcome should be capable of producing improved perinatal outcome. What an example for American obstetricians! The prospective randomized use of Doppler waveform analysis provides new information for decision-making and helps make possible the diagnosis of intrauterine growth retardation and changes in patterns of evaluation (fewer contraction stress tests–nonstress tests). It also appears to decrease the prelabor diagnosis of fetal distress and increase the number of emergency cesarean sections for fetal distress in labor. However, no differences in the frequency distribution of gestational age at birth, fetal and neonatal death rates, neonatal intensive care unit admissions, and neonatal respiratory support were seen as a result of the use of Doppler instrumentation. Inexplicably, the instances of

APGAR scores less than 7 were significantly more common in the Doppler study group than in the controls; neonatal brain injury was more common in that group as well, although the numbers were small. Once again, here's evidence failing to support the value of routine Doppler testing for fetal well-being in pregnancy.—T.H. Kirschbaum, M.D.

Doppler Investigation of Uteroplacental Blood Flow Resistance in the Second Trimester: A Screening Study for Pre-Eclampsia and Intrauterine Growth Retardation

Bewley S, Cooper D, Campbell S (King's Coll Hosp Med School, London)
Br J Obstet Gynaecol 98:871–879, 1991 7–10

Background.—Preeclampsia and intrauterine growth retardation, major causes of maternal and perinatal mortality and morbidity, are poorly defined conditions with poorly understood underlying pathologies. Several Doppler studies screening for these complications have been reported, but their results have varied widely. The screening properties of a mid-trimester uteroplacental Doppler scan were studied in a normal, unselected population.

Methods.—A group of 977 women at 16–24 weeks' gestation was enrolled in the study. An averaged resistance index (AVRI) was measured from 4 sites with continuous wave Doppler ultrasound. The main outcome measures were intrauterine death, birth weight, pregnancy-induced hypertension, and antepartum hemorrhage.

Results.—A total of 97% of the women were followed up. Those women with high AVRI values had a higher prevalence of proteinuric hypertension, placental abruption, small-for-gestational-age babies, and fetal loss. Women with AVRIs greater than the 95th percentile had an overall risk of pregnancy complications of 67% and a risk of a severe complications of 25%. However, the test's sensitivity for these complications was only 13% and 21%, respectively. For an individual with a high AVRI, the risk of a complication developing was increased by as much as 9.8 times.

Conclusion.—Doppler screening is able to detect a unifying defect that results in perinatal death, preeclampsia, growth retardation, and placental abruption. However, the predictive values do not yet justify its use as a routine test.

▶ This is another attempt to appraise the usefulness of screening uteroplacental Doppler signals in 16- to 24-week pregnancies (1). Although the authors conclude the tests detect "a unifying defect leading to prenatal death, preeclampsia, growth retardation, and placental abruption," there is no evidence for such a singular defect and not much more support for screening this signal than what evolved from the work of Hanretty et al. The crucial observation is the low prevalence rates for these abnormalities among the population of 977 gravidas. The prevalence generates the high specificity ratio but the sensitivity rates—largely in the range of 10% to 25%—demonstrate the usefulness of the procedure. The single sensitivity figure outside this range (38%) represents the successful prediction of adverse outcome in 3 of 8 abruptions. The high relative risk factors reflect a fraction in which the large number of true negatives in the numerator (reflecting the predominance of normal gravidas) is divided by the smaller number reflecting true positives, false positives, and false negatives. This study from King's College yields the same conclusion as does the Glasgow study. Doppler investigation of "utero-placental blood flow" has no role in routine screening for OB abnormalities.—T.H. Kirschbaum, M.D.

Reference

1. Hanretty KP, et al: *Br J Obstet Gynaecol* 96:1163, 1989.

Randomized Controlled Trials of Home Uterine Activity Monitoring: A Review and Critique

Grimes DA, Schulz KF (Univ of Southern California School of Medicine, Los Angeles; Ctrs for Disease Control, Atlanta)

Obstet Gynecol 79:137–142, 1992 7–11

Objective.—Home uterine activity monitoring has been suggested as a means of early recognition of incipient labor, thereby aiding in the reduction of the incidence of preterm birth. Five randomized studies have addressed the effectiveness of this technique. The results of these studies were analyzed.

Methods and Findings.—The 5 studies appeared in peer-reviewed journals from 1987 to 1991. Each report was evaluated to establish how well it met the criteria for such studies. None of the studies explicitly stated the principal outcome of interest or the size difference in rates that was sought. Two trials did not address sample size and power; only 1 described its technique of randomization, and it was inadequate and unblinded. All the studies were prone to selection bias similar to that of an observational study. Withdrawals, which ranged from 2% to 67%, were not well handled. This is important because of the likelihood that noncompliance was related to the treatment method. Although each study described its treatment regimen sufficiently, only limited details on the diagnosis and management of incipient preterm labor were given. Three studies made no attempts at blinding, and the other 2 did not report their degree of blinding. Problems relating to defining the outcome of interest, faulty statistical analysis, lack of relative risks with confidence intervals, and no mention of complications were also noted.

Discussion.—Recent controlled trials of home uterine activity monitoring do not meet the standards of scientific rigor. In addition, most suggest that the technique is not effective. One of the 5 trials evaluated showed a benefit, but this may have resulted from the greater nursing attention given to the electronic monitoring group. Home uterine activity monitoring should not be used until its efficacy has been established.

▶ This subject, reviewed before (see the 1987 YEAR BOOK OF OBSTETRICS AND GYNECOLOGY, pp 62–64; and the 1989 YEAR BOOK OF OBSTETRICS AND GYNECOLOGY, pp 113–114), is comprehensively treated in this publication in a fashion that could serve as a prototype for the evaluation of clinical research results. Historically, a lack of control of observer bias has been a repetitive part of the initial evaluation of new obstetrical treatments and, especially, instrumentations. The authors of this study concisely discuss the need to exclude the impact of measures other than home monitoring—the independent variable—on measured outcomes. The need for care in the blinded random assignment of cases, especially when the treatment cannot be blinded from evaluators, is especially critical. With regard to evaluation, the criteria for the diagnosis of failed monitoring and, because it effects some possible outcomes, the mode of treatment, become very important. The need to handle withdrawals of patients from the protocols correctly becomes important, because in some cited studies, two thirds of the patients who were enrolled did not complete the study. This analysis provides the best support to date for the position that home uterine monitoring, despite the contrary view of its enthusiasts, is of unproven benefit in the management of threatened preterm labor.—T.H. Kirschbaum, M.D.

Fetal Monitoring in Perinatal Sepsis

Day D, Ugol JH, French JI, Haverkamp A, Wall RE, McGregor JA (Univ of Colorado, Denver; Denver Gen Hosp)
Am J Perinatol 9:28–33, 1992 7–12

Background.—Perinatal infection present at birth is a common cause of neonatal mortality and morbidity. If this condition could be identified by electronic fetal heart rate monitoring (EFM) patterns, treatment that might improve perinatal outcome could be initiated before birth. The usefulness of EFM in detecting presumed intrapartum perinatal sepsis manifested soon after birth was analyzed. An assessment of the predictive value of antepartum and intrapartum complications was also performed.

Methods.—Of 9,249 patients delivered between 1984 and 1985 in 2 hospitals, 18 patients had documented neonatal sepsis acquired in utero and available intrapartum fetal monitor tracings, which were reviewed. These neonates were compared with 18 matched control newborns.

Results.—No significant differences were found between the groups, based on analysis of the fetal monitor tracings, of the overall impression of labor. Overall, 61% of the tracings from cases with sepsis were judged to have reassuring fetal heart rate patterns. No pattern characteristic of intrapartum fetal sepsis was consistently identified. Fetal tachycardia occured in 22% of the cases. Meconium together with fetal tachycardia was not correlated with neonatal sepsis. No antepartum or intrapartum complications significantly predicted neonatal sepsis. Chorioamnionitis together with neonatal sepsis was not accompanied by EFM abnormalities. No differences between frequency of vaginal examinations during labor, internal monitoring, premature rupture of membranes, prolonged labor, preterm labor, maternal fever, chorioamnionitis, or preterm delivery were seen between cases and controls. Nine of 10 newborns with sepsis caused by group B *Streptococcus* organisms had reassuring EFM tracings. Prematurity and low birth weights were associated with a markedly increased risk of mortality among newborns with sepsis.

Conclusion.—No intrapartum fetal heart rate pattern predicting presumed intrauterine perinatal sepsis was found. No antepartum or intrapartum complication was found associated with neonatal sepsis.

▶ Although this retrospective, observer-blinded, case-controlled study is somewhat restricted by the small number of cases, its study subjects are uncommon and the questions posed are very important. If sepsis were to produce a distinctive pattern of fetal heart rate abnormality, our management of fetuses infected with group B *Streptococcus* organisms, which are the cause of nearly half the cases of fetal sepsis, would be facilitated. Furthermore, the question emerges in some cases of professional liability litigation with considerable impact. In this study by the redoubtable Dr. Haverkamp et al., no significant changes in baseline heart rate, accelerations, decelerations, or beat-to-beat variability were discerned specific to the various stages of labor. This observation has the further advantage of confirming the clinical impressions of those of us who have speculated about it.—T.H. Kirschbaum, M.D.

Reproducibility of Ultrasonic Measurement of Fetal Cardiac Haemodynamics

Beeby AR, Dunlop W, Heads A, Hunter S (Princess Mary Maternity Hosp, Newcastle upon Tyne, England; Freeman Road Hosp, New Castle upon Tyne, England)

Br J Obstet Gynaecol 98:807–814, 1991 7–13

Background.—Ultrasonic techniques have been used to measure fetal cardiac hemodynamics, although the accuracy of ultrasonic measurement of cardiac blood flow in the fetal heart has not been validated. The reproducibility of ultrasonic estimates of volume flow in the human fetal heart was examined, and the method's potential for detecting abnormal flow was evaluated.

Methods.—Twenty-seven pregnant women were recruited for the study and divided into 3 equal groups according to the range of gestation: 19–21 weeks, 29–31 weeks, and 38–40 weeks. Using a combination of cross-sectional and Doppler echocardiography, 2 observers made independent estimates of volume flow across all 4 heart valves in the 27 fetuses.

Results.—One observer obtained 61% and the other obtained 78% of the 108 possible estimates of volume flow, with varied success rates in the different gestational groups. Although the mean values of each observer were similar, there were considerable differences between values obtained from individual fetuses. Considerable within-observer variability was mainly a result of errors in cross-sectional measurements. Discrepancies between observers in volume flow estimation arose from inconsistency both in cross-sectional and Doppler measurements.

Conclusion.—The measurement of volume flow in the fetal heart would be of great clinical value, but the reliability of the method examined here is not sufficiently accurate. The problem of obtaining good flow data is usually an unfavorable fetal position.

▶ This study confirms the reservations voiced here earlier (see the 1987 YEAR BOOK OF OBSTETRICS AND GYNECOLOGY, pp 42–43) regarding the hazards of estimating fetal endocardiac flow rates with this technique. Both intraobserver and interobserver differences as large as 300% are occasionally recorded in this work. The problems are the difficulty in measuring irregularly shaped valve orifices (which change in size and shape with the cardiac cycle) and the error introduced by assuming the Doppler signal measures the linear nonturbulent column of blood with uniform velocity profile amenable to electronic averaging. This technique is not adequate to such measurements.—T.H. Kirschbaum, M.D.

Fetal and Umbilical Flow Velocity Waveforms Between 10–16 Weeks' Gestation: A Preliminary Study

Wladimiroff JW, Huisman TWA, Stewart PA (Academic Hosp Rotterdam-Dijkzigt, Rotterdam, The Netherlands)

Obstet Gynecol 78:812–814, 1991 7–14

Introduction.—With the advent of transvaginal pulsed Doppler systems, fetal flow velocity waveforms can be studied as early as 10 weeks of gestation.

Methods.—Maximal flow velocity waveform recording was attempted in the umbilical artery, fetal descending aorta, and the fetal intracerebral level using a cross-sectional study design in 77 normal singleton pregnancies between 10–16 weeks of gestation. The relationships between each of the flow velocity waveform indices and the fetal heart rate were also evaluated.

Results.—Technically acceptable waveforms were obtained in the umbilical artery in 79% of women, in the fetal descending aorta in 65%, and at the intracerebral levels in 34%. At 10–12 weeks of gestation, end-diastolic flow velocity waveforms were always absent in the fetal descending aorta and the umbilical artery, but they were observed in 58% of fetal intracerebral arteries, suggesting a relatively low cerebral vascular resistance. The pulsatility index at all 3 levels decreased significantly with advancing gestational age, suggesting a reduction in fetal and umbilical placental vascular resistance during the late first and early second trimesters of normal pregnancy. There was no correlation between the different waveform indices and fetal heart rate.

Conclusion.—Transvaginal flow velocity waveform recording can be successfully performed up to 14 weeks of gestation. The documentation of normal flow velocity waveforms in the fetal intracerebral arteries, descending aorta, and umbilical artery will allow studies on peripheral dynamics in complicated pregnancies.

▶ Operating with vaginal Doppler, these investigators have generated some interesting data. Their conclusions, however, that "waveform changes were not related to fetal heart rate" seem incorrect. Their studies were performed in the range of gestational age in which the endogenous myocardial rate is slowed by the increasing functional attainment of autonomic modulation. Note they find a coefficient of linear correlation in the regression of fetal heart rate on gestational age of −.72, with $P < .001$. This means that, as noted in the 1992 YEAR BOOK, fetal heart rate slows with development between 10 and 16 weeks' gestation. This rate change could well be the cause of the reductions in waveform indices others have noted (see the 1990 YEAR BOOK OF OBSTETRICS AND GYNECOLOGY, pp 127–129, 140–146), and it could simply reflect the decrease in heart rate. The authors' contention that, at a fixed gestational age, there is no relationship between pulsativity index and fetal heart rate says nothing about the developmental changes and may simply reflect little variability in fetal heart rate or pulsatility index, or both, at stated gestational age. An additional possibility stems from an error from sampling a small sample size. The Doppler velocity indices are heavily determined by fetal heart rate.—T.H. Kirschbaum, M.D.

Maternal Angiotensin Sensitivity and Fetal Doppler Umbilical Artery Flow Waveforms

Cook CM, Trudinger BJ (Univ of Sydney, Westmead, New South Wales, Australia)

Br J Obstet Gynaecol 98:698–702, 1991 7–15

Introduction.—Abnormal umbilical flow velocity waveforms (FVWs) can be demonstrated in 66% to 75% of fetuses subsequently born small for gestational age. It is generally assumed that pregnancy-induced hypertension reduces uteroplacental perfusion, which in turn causes fetal morbidity resulting from vascular deprivation. However, abnormal umbilical FVWs are often demonstrated before clinical preeclampsia occurs. A previous study reported no response to the angiotensin infusion sensitivity test (AIST) in women with a normal pregnancy and an enhanced pressor response in preeclamptic women. The placental vascular lesion identified by abnormal umbilical FVWs was examined to determine whether it precedes preeclampsia.

Patients.—The AIST was performed in 36 normotensive women with a singleton pregnancy of 24–38 weeks' gestation and umbilical Doppler FVWs suggestive of placental vascular disease. Flow velocity waveforms were recorded at least every 2 weeks until delivery.

Results.—Eighteen women had a positive pressor response to the AIST, and 18 had a negative response. The mean gestational age at delivery was 38.5 weeks among women with a negative AIST and 35.3 weeks among those with a positive AIST response. The mean birth weight was 3,048 g for infants born to women with a negative AIST and 2,010 g for infants born to women with a positive AIST. Fetal distress in labor occurred in only 1 woman with a negative pressor response, but it occurred in 4 women in the positive pressor response group. All differences were statistically significant. The Doppler umbilical systolic-diastolic (S-D) ratio decreased with gestation among women with a negative AIST, suggesting continuing placental growth and expansion. In contrast, the S-D ratio increased in women with a positive pressor response, indicating vascular obliteration.

Conclusion.—Among normotensive pregnant women with a high umbilical artery S-D ratio, a positive pressor response to the AIST predicts those at risk of fetal morbidity associated with placental vascular pathology.

▶ The logic is relatively tangled in this study. Abnormalities in umbilical artery velocity waveforms are those derived from "uteroplacental arteries" that, regrettably, have proven relatively ineffective in predicting the ultimate presence either of intrauterine growth retardation or pregnancy-induced hypertension in the experience of others. The angiotension pressor response has some capacity to predict eventual pregnancy-induced hypertension, but it is ordinarily applied earlier in pregnancy than in the 31.3 ± 3.7 weeks' gestational age range where positive results were obtained in this study. There is a relationship between hypertensive disease of pregnancy and intrauterine growth retardation, especially for chronic hypertensives, but it is impossible to tell how many of the 22 of 36 multiparous patients in this study had chronic hypertension. Neither is it possible to tell whether AIST successfully predicted pregnancy-induced hypertension in this experience. Of the 18 women in the AIST-positive group, the elective cesarean section rate was 44%, resulting in a mean birth weight of 2,010 ± 966 g (both vastly more variable and smaller) than those in the AIST-negative patients; births occurred at an average of 35 weeks' gestation. The latter infants were born with a cesarean section rate of 16.7% at 38.5 weeks. There was no difference in the perinatal death rates between the 2 groups.

The criteria for obstetrical management are not detailed, but it appears that the independent variables (AIST and Doppler wave forms) were used as criteria for management in a fashion which led to premature delivery and determined the dependent variable (low birth weight) without evident patient benefit. In part, the results—at least for the 20 average-for-gestational-age infants and maybe some of the 16 small-for-gestational-age infants—represent self-fulfilling prophecies imposed by the study design. It is hard to know what, it anything, one should make of all this.—T.H. Kirschbaum, M.D.

8 Labor, Surgery, and Delivery

Long-Term Effects of Vacuum and Forceps Deliveries

Seidman DS, Laor A, Gale R, Stevenson DK, Mashiach S, Danon YL (Sheba Med Centre, Tel-Hashomer, Israel; Israeli Defence Forces Med Corps; Biku Cholim Hosp, Jerusalem; Stanford Univ, Calif; Tel-Aviv Univ, Israel)

Lancet 337:1583–1585, 1991 8–1

Background.—The use of forceps delivery and vacuum extraction is increasing, but there are few data on the long-term effects of these obstetric interventions. A 17-year follow-up of infants born by instrumental deliveries was reported.

Methods.—During an 8-year period, 55,993 infants were born in 4 study hospitals. At age 17 years, 52,282 (93.4%) were seen for their draft board medical examination. Some of the missing subjects were hospitalized for severe chronic or psychiatric illness, thus introducing a source of possible selection bias. The examination addressed intelligence scores as well as physical health.

Results.—Of the study sample, 47,500 were delivered spontaneously, 2,098 by cesarean section, 1,747 by vacuum, and 937 by forceps. Before adjustment for confounding factors, the vacuum- and forceps-delivery groups had higher mean intelligence scores than the other 2 groups. However, these differences disappeared after adjustment by stepwise multiple regression (table). Those subjects delivered with forceps had significant functional impairment of the feet, vision, and retina, and

Mean (SE) Intelligence Test Scores at 17 Years of Age in Subjects Born in Jerusalem Between 1964 and 1970

Obstetric intervention	Unadjusted	Adjusted*
Spontaneous delivery (n = 29 136)	105·4 (0·1)	105·7 (0·1)
Forceps delivery (n = 567)	108·2† (0·7)	104·6 (0·40
Vacuum extraction (n = 1207)	109·6† (0·5)	105·9 (0·4)
Caesarean section (n = 1335)	105·4 (0·4)	103·7† (0·1)

* Results after adjusting by multiple regression for confounding effects of sex, birth weight, ethnic origin, birth order, maternal age, paternal and maternal education, and social class.

† $P < .0001$ compared with spontaneous delivery.

(Courtesy of Seidman DS, Laor A, Gale R, et al: *Lancet* 337:1583–1585, 1991.)

those delivered with vacuum had significant impairment of the legs compared with those who were delivered spontaneously. However, these differences were small.

Conclusion.—Vacuum or forceps delivery does not appear to increase the individual's risk of cognitive or functional impairment in adulthood. Despite the possible selection bias, the view that, except in a small minority of cases of birth asphyxia, events at delivery do not significantly affect cognitive outcome was strengthened.

▶ This study benefits from competent statistical analysis and from an excellent record system making intelligence testing results available for children of both sexes subject to the compulsory draft registration in Israel. Note that large numbers of cases were studied and, after confounding variables were excluded, no differences in intelligence tests results were noted among those delivered spontaneously or by forceps or vacuum extraction. Among the confounding variables were sex, birth weight, ethnicity, birth order, mother's age, parental education, and social class. Only those born by cesarean section showed significantly lower intelligence scores; however, indications for operative birth were unknown and were certainly compelling enough to justify emergency procedures. This means that the number of normal pregnancies was certainly fewer than in the spontaneous-birth group.

This study should be compared with a less sophisticated one (1) in which analysis of 110 cases of cesarean section without elimination of confounders led to the conclusion that "a detrimental effect of increasing length of trial labor" on intelligence existed. Seidman et al. are correct in pointing out that events at delivery are not important in determining adult cognitive outcome. Indeed, development psychologists routinely find that, by 3–4 years of age, environmental determinants are strong enough to cause any noncatastrophic birth event to lose significant relationship to the intelligent quotient.—T.H. Kirschbaum, M.D.

Reference

1. Roemer FJ, et al: *Obstet Gynecol* 77:653, 1991.

Birthweight-Specific Infant Mortality Risk in Cesarean Section

Atrash HK, Hogue CJR, Becerra JW (Ctrs for Disease Control, Atlanta)

Am J Prev Med 7:227–231, 1991 8–2

Introduction.—The role of cesarean section delivery in reducing infant mortality in the United States from 26 deaths per 1,000 live births in 1960 to 12.6 deaths per 1,000 live births in 1980 has not been proved. Data on the association between the method of delivery and infant survival were studied using population-based information from birth and death records.

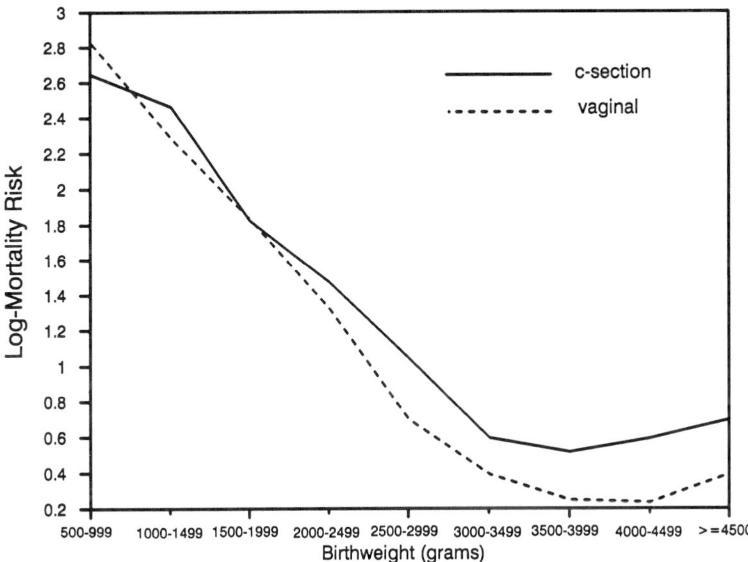

Fig 8–1.—Neonatal mortality risk by birth weight and method of delivery. Blacks, selected states, United States, 1980. (Courtesy of Atrash HK, Hogue CJR, Becerra JW: *Am J Prev Med* 7:227–231, 1991.)

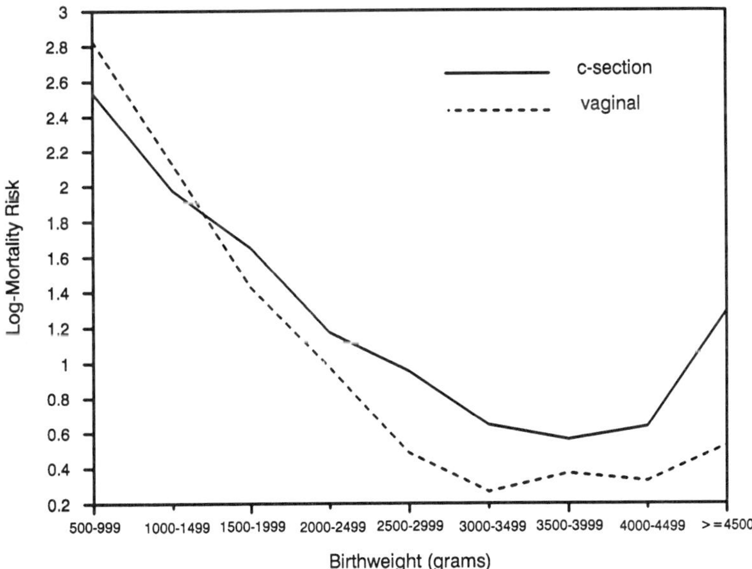

Fig 8–2.—Neonatal mortality risk by birth weight and method of delivery. Whites, selected states, United States, 1980. (Courtesy of Atrash HK, Hogue CJR, Becerra JW: *Am J Prev Med* 7:227–231, 1991.)

Methods.—Data on infant deaths, including birth weight, age at death, and delivery method, were obtained from the National Infant Mortality Surveillance (NIMS) project. This program collects information from 53 vital statistics reporting areas. Nineteen of the 50 states contribute data on delivery method. Because the NIMS data represent a birth cohort and not actual numbers, mortality risk better describes this factor than mortality rate. The relative risks resulted from factoring the death risk for 1 infant group and dividing this number by the death risk from another group.

Results.—The total infant mortality risk and neonatal mortality risk for singleton births were significantly greater for infants delivered by cesarean section than for those delivered vaginally for both blacks and whites. However, the infant and neonatal mortality risks were significantly lower for cesarean deliveries than for vaginal deliveries among infants weighing 500–1,499 g, especially for black infants (Fig 8–1). White infants weighing between 500 g and 999 g had a lower mortality risk (Fig 8–2). When the data were controlled for the delivery method, the black newborns had a significantly lower neonatal mortality risk than white infants in all birth weight categories up to 2,500 g. The mortality risk appeared significantly lower for multiple-delivery infants delivered by cesarean section than for those born vaginally.

Conclusion.—Although cesarean section delivery has actually increased infant mortality and morbidity, very-low-birth-weight infants have a better outcome when delivered by cesarean section. However, this does not hold true for other birth weight divisions. Additional studies that control for all maternal and infant conditions requiring cesarean delivery are recommended.

▶ This study of birth-death certificate data from the neonatal infant mortality surveillance project of the Centers for Disease Control updates us with information from 1980. Of course, the customary problems in interpretating this sort of information persist. The infant mortality risk of cesarean section cannot be separated from the risk to an infant's well-being caused by the obstetrical abnormality that motivates the operative birth. Infants that are delivered vaginally and weigh less than 1,500 g tend to reflect the obstetrician's judgment that survival, for 1 reason or another, is relatively unlikely. It is for this reason that, although the authors' data show an increased likelihood of survival for infants delivered abdominally and weighing less than 1,500 g, the authors believe that these problems of interpretation mitigate against recommending cesarean section in such cases. Two things are clear from this information, however. There is no impact of cesarean section on postneonatal mortality, because that apparent relationship vanishes with correction for low birth weight. Second, the black-white difference in infant mortality can't be explained by racial differences when deciding whether to use cesarean section, because the risk ratio for infant death after cesarean section is lower for blacks than for whites.—T.H. Kirschbaum, M.D.

Patient-Controlled Epidural Analgesia: Demand Dosing

Ferrante FM, Lu L, Jamison SB, Datta S (Brigham and Women's Hosp, Boston; Harvard Med School, Boston)

Anesth Analg 73:547–552, 1991 8–3

Introduction.—Analgesics can be delivered through various modes, such as intravenous demand dosing, self-administered fixed dosing, and continuous infusion plus demand dosing. Studies have shown that patient-controlled epidural analgesia (PCEA) used during labor and delivery has similar results to continuous epidural infusions (CEI). The results of using pure demand-dose PCEA were compared with the use of CEI for pain relief during labor and delivery.

Methods.—All participating patients had a singleton fetus in the vertex presentation at term and an uncomplicated pregnancy. Epidural catheterization was performed with the catheter placed at the L3-4 or L2-3 interspace. All the patients received an initial dose of bupivacaine to establish anesthesia. The 40 patients were then randomized to receive .125% bupivacaine with 2 μg of fentanyl per mL, through CEI at 12 mL/hr, or through demand-dose PCEA. Patients using PCEA could demand 3 mL every 10 minutes without restriction. The patients had an interview every 30 minutes to assess the adequacy of analgesia.

Findings.—Both study groups had a comparable duration of the first and second stages of labor, and newborns had similar Apgar scores 1 and 5 minutes after birth. The pain scores and degree of motor blockade during the first and second stages of labor were also similar for the 2 treatment groups. The total amount of bupivacaine and fentanyl used by the 2 groups was markedly different; the dosage reductions were 45% and 55%, respectively, for the PCEA patients. No significant complications occurred during this study.

Conclusion.—The use of demand-dose PCEA produces a significant dose-sparing effect compared with a conventional CEI protocol for administration of analgesia during labor and delivery. This dose-sparing effect occurred without impaired analgesic efficacy or any reduction in the amount of motor blockade.

▶ This report expands the evidence of usefulness of patient control for postoperative analgesia (see the 1991 YEAR BOOK OF OBSTETRICS AND GYNECOLOGY, pp 138–139) to include epidural anesthesia during labor and delivery. Patients were blinded to the study by inactivating the demand button in those selected for the control group. The resulting nearly 50% reduction in the amount of bupivacaine and fentanyl consumed by demand (as compared with continuous infusion) is further testament to the improvement in anesthesia and analgesia that flows from patients who believe that they have personal control of their own pain relief. It also shows once again how objectively and responsibly women behave in that regard when allowed the opportunity to exercise that control.—T.H. Kirschbaum, M.D.

The Effect of Cesarean Section on Intraventricular Hemorrhage in the Preterm Infant

Anderson GD, Bada HS, Shaver DC, Harvey CJ, Korones SB, Wong SP, Arheart KL, Magill HL (Univ of Tennessee, Memphis; Memphis State Univ, Memphis)

Am J Obstet Gynecol 166:1091–1101, 1992 8–4

Background.—The relationship of the route of delivery to the pathogenesis of periventricular-intraventricular hemorrhage in the neonate has now been well studied, and the frequency of hemorrhage is independent of the mode of delivery. The role of active-phase labor and the development of periventricular-intraventricular hemorrhage were examined in women undergoing cesarean sections.

Methods.—A total of 106 infants of 85 women were studied. Twenty-seven infants were born during active-phase labor, 33 during latent-phase labor, and 46 infants were in a no-labor group. Head ultrasonography was done at delivery; at 1, 6, 12, and 24 hours; and daily for the first 7 days of life. Infants with no hemorrhage were compared with those with periventricular-intraventricular hemorrhage.

Results.—There were no between-group differences in frequency of early hemorrhage, late hemorrhage, or overall periventricular-intraventricular hemorrhage. However, infants born during the active phase of labor had a significantly higher frequency of grade 3 or 4 hemorrhage and progression of hemorrhage than those whose mothers had no labor or latent-phase labor. Infants with early periventricular-intraventricular hemorrhage also had a higher frequency of progression of hemorrhage.

Conclusion.—Performing cesarean section before the active phase of labor does not change the overall frequency of hemorrhage in the neonate. However, it does result in a lower frequency of progression to grade 3 or 4 hemorrhage. These findings do not support a policy of performing more cesarean sections for preterm delivery to prevent progression of periventricular-intraventricular hemorrhage in preterm infants.

▶ This study is most noteworthy for its failure to show any benefit from cesarean section in this experience. This finding is particularly impressive, because the study design is biased in a direction that would be expected to exaggerate an unfavorable outcome in cases where cesarean section was done after the onset of labor. Although the indications for cesarean section during active labor are not defined, it seems likely they at least include the 8 cases of abruption, 2 cases of placenta previa, and 17 cases of fetal distress with a mean aggregate birth weight of approximately 1,100 grams. One would expect these cases would confer a relatively high risk for intraventricular hemorrhage on the sectioned subset. The authors ignore the uncertainty and arbitrariness of the diagnosis of latent-phase labor, which accounts for 30% of the group. No impact of cesarean section on either the occurrence of intraventricular hemorrhage or its timing was seen. A total of 50% of all hemorrhages occur at or beyond 48 hours of life. The authors' conclusion that those incidents of cesarean section done in active labor have a greater likelihood of progression of hemorrhage is not true for those cases in which initial ultrasound shows Papile grade 4 hemorrhage shortly after birth. Furthermore, the distinction between Papile classes 2 and 3, which is critical to this interpretation, is highly subjective. Despite the intriguing title, this report says little of value concerning the role of cesarean section in preterm delivery.—T.H. Kirschbaum, M.D.

Electrocardiographic Changes During Cesarean Section Under Regional Anesthesia

McLintic AJ, Pringle SD, Lilley S, Houston, Thorburn J (Western Infirmary; Glasgow; Western Gen Hosp, Edinburgh; Royal Hosp for Sick Children, Glasgow)

Anesth Analg 74:51–56, 1992 8–5

Introduction.—During cesarean section using regional anesthesia, there are changes in the maternal ECGs. One study reported that such changes develop in 37% of patients, and it suggested that this may be a result of myocardial oxygen supply and demand. The results of a prospective study of 25 patients who underwent elective cesarean section and were assessed for myocardial ischemia using echocardiography were reviewed.

Methods.—The 25 healthy patients scheduled for elective cesarean delivery were first assessed by ECG and then by both ECG and echocardiography for any signs of myocardial ischemia. Before administration of regional anesthesia, each patient underwent attachment to an ambulatory ECG recording device. After induction of anesthesia, the patient was also monitored by echocardiography.

Results.—Of the 25 patients fitted with these myocardial assessment devices, 16 had significant ST-segment depression at the modified V_5 lead. A large temporal relationship developed between the sinus tachycardia at delivery and the ST-segment deviation, with ST-segment depression of 1–30 minutes (mean, 7.5 minutes). Patients with this ST-segment depression had a higher mean heart rate than those without ST-segment deviation. The difference between these 2 patient groups became significant at delivery. The mean rate pressure product also reached its highest value at delivery.

Conclusion.—Many patients who undergo elective cesarean delivery using regional anesthesia experience ST-segment depression. However, the ECG changes do not result from myocardial ischemia, indicating that ST depression represents nonspecific results.

► These findings, although perhaps not useful in themselves, are important when chest pain occurring at or shortly after delivery necessitates ECG examination of the recently delivered parturient. Roughly two thirds of women showed ST-segment depression on 2 precordial leads, which was suggestive of myocardial ischemia. The average duration of such findings (7.5 minutes) was derived from instances in which the change lasted as long as 30 minutes. To the extent that ECG examination of the heart could be used to exclude dysfunction of the ventricular walls, there was no evidence of functional impairment—nor was there subsequent confirmation of myocardial infarction. It's important to remember that the ST-segment changes were nonspecific and very likely, in retrospect, represented respiratory alkalosis at the time of delivery; the changes persisted postpartum until the return to normal acid base balance occurred.—T.H. Kirschbaum, M.D.

Effect of Active Management of Labor on the Incidence of Cesarean Section for Dystocia in Nulliparas

Boylan P, Frankowski R, Rountree R, Selwyn B, Parrish K (Univ of Texas, Houston)

Am J Perinatol 8:373–379, 1991 8–6

Introduction.—Active management of labor (AML) involves a defined policy of managing labor in nulliparas that has been associated with consistently low rates of cesarean section (CS) in several countries. The approach consists of close involvement of the senior obstetric staff, a personal nurse for each patient in labor, early diagnosis of labor, early rupture of membranes, and a specified dose of oxytocin when cervical dilation is less than 1 cm/hr. The effect of AML in reducing the incidence of CS for dystocia in nulliparas was studied in a Texas hospital.

Methods.—Over 2 years (4 consecutive 6-month periods), 3,901 births to nulliparous women were studied. The criteria for AML were vertex presentation, singleton pregnancy, and no evidence of fetal distress. In the first year, the women were managed by prevailing, undefined meth-

Numbers and Percent Distributions of Delivery Type of Nulliparous Women in Control and AML Intervention Periods

Delivery	*Control Periods* *July 1984–June 1985*	*AML Intervention* *July 1985–June 1986*
Cesarean	448 (24.3%)	387 (18.8%)
Spontaneous vaginal	735 (39.9%)	1049 (51.0%)
Forceps vaginal	660 (35.8%)	621 (30.2%)
Total	1843 (100%)	2057 (100%)

(Courtesy of Boylan P, Frankowski R, Rountree R, et al: *Am J Perinatol* 8:373–379, 1991.)

ods. In the second year, all patients were managed according to the principles of AML. Rates of CS and other related outcome variables were compared for the 2 methods of management.

Results.—In the 2 control periods, the incidence of CS was 23% and 24%. The institution of AML reduced the incidence of CS by 4.4% in the initial AML period and by 5.5% during the entire 2-year period. The incidence of dystocia decreased by 10.3%, and the incidence of dystocia for CS decreased by nearly one fifth. Reporting of fetal distress as an indication for CS was stable during the control period, but it increased by 6.9% during the intervention period. With AML, the incidence of forceps delivery decreased by 5.6% (table). No significant differences were noted in indicators of fetal outcome.

Conclusion.—The principles of AML appear to significantly reduce the incidence of CS in nulliparas with no negative effects on either mother or child. A multicenter randomized trial would be needed to prove this finding scientifically. Decreasing the incidence of CS in first deliveries is the best way to decrease total incidence of CS.

▶ This approach to managing primigravid labor is, as the senior author avows, "practiced in its purest form" at the National Maternity Hospital in Dublin. In this study, a senior obstetrician from that distinguished center (Dr. Peter Boylan) demonstrates the usefulness of the method in Houston, Texas. The results are quite impressive. What evolved was an 18% reduction in the incidence of CS for dystocia, a 23% reduction in the CS rate, a 5.6% reduction in operative forceps deliveries, and a 5.5% increase in spontaneous vaginal births. The cost was a 6.9% increase in the incidence of CS done for fetal distress, which is, naturally, the heart of the study. Fetal deaths and asphyxial neonatal deaths were so infrequent as to preclude comparative analysis, although admissions to the neonatal intensive care unit were increased during the time of this study. The diagnosis of asphyxia was decreased in incidence (from 1.95% to 1.8%), as was the incidence of neonatal seizures (from .43% to .19%), although not statistically significantly so. It seems hard to deny that the principles of AML contain elements of care in labor which might well result in a reduction in operative births if applied widely in this country.—T.H. Kirschbaum, M.D.

A Controlled Trial of a Program for the Active Management of Labor

López-Zeno JA, Peaceman AM, Adashek JA, Socol ML (Northwestern Univ, Chicago)

N Engl J Med 326:450–454, 1992 8–7

Introduction.—During the past 20 years, the rate of cesarean section in the United States has increased from 5% to 25% of deliveries, primarily because of the increased frequency of dystocia. The active management of labor, which involves patient education, accurate diagnosis of labor, early amniotomy, early use of relatively high doses of oxytocin, and rigorous peer review, decreases the rate of cesarean delivery.

Methods.—To determine the safety and efficacy of active management, 351 nulliparous patients who were in spontaneous labor at term were randomly assigned to active management and were compared with 354 similar patients assigned to traditional management. Spontaneous labor was defined as regular uterine contractions occurring at least once every 5 minutes, combined with complete cervical effacement or spontaneous rupture of membranes. This definition did not include the degree of cervical dilation, but the rate of dilation was assessed during labor.

Active management involved amniotomy of the intact membranes within 1 hour of the diagnosis of labor. Based on cervical examinations performed hourly for 3 hours and every 2 hours thereafter, the rate of cervical dilation was determined. If the rate was less than 1 cm per hour during the first stage, or if the fetal head was arrested for 1 hour in the second stage, then oxytocin administration was initiated at 6 mU per minute and was increased to 36 mU per minute, or until 7 contractions occurred every 15 minutes. Traditional management was generally based on the judgment of the attending obstetrician; however, an arrest of progress was defined as 2 hours without further cervical dilation, and oxytocin administration was initiated at 1 mU per minute and increased until 8 contractions occurred every 20 minutes.

Results.—The active management group had a 10.5% rate of cesarean section compared with 14.1% in the traditional management group; this difference resulted from a decreased frequency of arrest disorders. After controlling for numerous potential confounding variables, the reduction in the rate of cesarean section was statistically significant. Active management was not associated with increased complications of labor or with increases in neonatal morbidity.

Conclusion.—Active management of labor is safe and effective in reducing dystocia and, thereby, in reducing the rate of cesarean delivery. It is possible that the unblinded nature of this study might have prodded the management of the control patients toward a more active approach. Although the results of a previous study suggested that active management of labor might be associated with an increased rate of neonatal seizures, this study was not sufficiently powerful to evaluate this.

▶ Whenever a structured clinical trial demonstrates a beneficial outcome, it is necessary to weigh the relative role of the new intervention against the possible impact of Hawthorne effect—the tendency for interest and focused activity in themselves to result in an improved outcome independent of what's done. This paper is a nice demonstration of the Hawthorne effect.

Labor management differs strikingly from the "active management of labor" as originally described by O'Driscoll (see the 1989 YEAR BOOK OF OBSTETRICS AND GYNECOLOGY, pp 139–40). Labor was defined by uterine contractions and cervical effacement or rupture of the membranes, not by reference to cervical dilatation as per O'Driscoll. Amniotomy was routine for the test group, and the management of controls differed from the test group only in regard to amniotomy and the lesser rates of oxytocin infusion used in the control cases. The resulting decreases in cesarean section rates from 22.4% before the study to 10.5% for the test group and to 14.1% for the control cases (all primigravidas) indicate the value of relatively large rates of oxytocin infusion and attainment of a rate of cervical dilatation equal to or greater than 1 cm per hour in preventing dysfunctional labor. This conclusion seems true even when confounding relationships are excluded. Emphasis on the problem of dysfunctional labor without "active management" also resulted in a considerable reduction of the cesarean section rate in the control group.

In all, this was a well-designed, randomized, prospective study, replete with power calculations and the proper treatment of withdrawn study patients. By design, blinded observations were not possible. However, it is clear that those who cared for patients in the control group had heightened concern for the development of dysfunctional labor, which likely was based on the observation of test patients. This study should be compared with that by Boylon et al. in the *American Journal of Perinatology* (see Abstract 8–6).—T.H. Kirschbaum, M.D.

Sonographic Diagnosis of the Large for Gestational Age Fetus at Term: Does It Make a Difference?

Levine AB, Lockwood CJ, Brown B, Lapinski R, Berkowitz RL (Mount Sinai School of Medicine, New York)

Obstet Gynecol 79:55–58, 1992 8–8

Background.—Accurate prediction of fetal weight is important, particularly of large-for-gestational-age (LGA) fetuses. There have been many attempts to identify the optimal way to predict LGA fetuses. A study group of 406 women was reviewed to determine the accuracy of ultrasound in identifying LGA fetuses and to determine whether this prediction influenced obstetric management.

Methods.—All women underwent ultrasound examination after 36 weeks' gestation, usually indicated by previous cesarean delivery or diabetes. The Hadlock formula was used to estimate fetal weight, and LGA was defined as fetal weight equal to or greater than the 90th percentile for gestational age. To assess the effect of sonographic prediction on management, true negatives were compared with false positives and false negatives with true positives.

Results.—Sonographic diagnosis of LGA had a sensitivity of 50%, a specificity of 90%, and a positive predictive value of 52%. Sixty-eight women received a diagnosis of having an LGA fetus. Thirty percent of them had diagnosed labor abnormalities vs. 19% of women without a diagnosed LGA fetus. Epidural anesthesia was used in 74% of women with a diagnosed LGA fetus vs. 57% without, and 53% required cesarean delivery vs. 32%, respectively. A false positive diagnosis of LGA had a significant effect on the diagnosis of labor abnormalities and the incidence of elective cesarean delivery.

Discussion.—Sonographic prediction of LGA often is inaccurate; this may be related to inaccurate assessment of gestational age, which reflects the clinical situation in which management decisions must be made. Sonographic estimation of fetal weight is related to the management of labor and delivery, although no true cause-and-effect relationship can be concluded. These estimations should be used cautiously in making management decisions.

▶ There is no reason to believe that those who work at Mount Sinai Hospital are any worse at ultrasonic evaluation of fetal weight than the rest of us. Granting that, this study casts the same doubts on the ability to estimate LGA infants based on ultrasound as is true for abdominal palpation. That is, a positive predictive value of 51.5% is little better than the random alternate assignment of the diagnosis of macrosomia. Comparison between false positives and true negatives is an ingenuous analytical concept, and it indicates that the presence of the ultrasonic diagnosis of macrosomia alone, even in average-for-gestational-age infants, is associated with at least part of the increased incidence of elective abdominal birth and the diagnosis of labor abnormality seen in those thought to be LGA. Once again, here is confirmation that the advantages of ultrasound evaluation of the fetus do not extend to precision in the diagnosis of macrosomia.—T.H. Kirschbaum, M.D.

Efficacy of the Fetal-Pelvic Index in Nulliparous Women at High Risk for Fetal-Pelvic Disproportion

Morgan MA, Thurnau GR (Univ of Oklahoma College of Medicine, Oklahoma City)

Am J Obstet Gynecol 166:810–814, 1992 8–9

Background.—Fetal-pelvic disproportion increases the rates of maternal and perinatal morbidity and mortality. Of the numerous methods of identifying fetal-pelvic disproportion, the fetal-pelvic index has been most successful. The efficacy of this index was evaluated in 137 nulliparous women at high risk for fetal-pelvic disproportion.

Methods.—Women with either an unengaged fetal presentation, clinically suspected fetal macrosomia, a small maternal pelvis, or an indication for labor induction or augmentation were included. The blinded fetal-pelvic index values and 2 other methods of identifying fetal-pelvic disproportion (ultrasonography-derived, estimated fetal weight ≥4,000 gm and Mengert's index) were related to delivery outcome. All patients had an adequate trial of labor.

Results.—Spontaneous vaginal deliveries were possible in 64 patients. The remaining women required operative intervention, either cesarean section (65) or operative vaginal (8). The mean gestational age at delivery and mean birth weight were significantly greater in the operative delivery group than in the spontaneous delivery group. Fifty-five of the patients requiring operative delivery had a positive fetal-pelvic index, yielding a sensitivity of 75% for the index. Sixty-two of the 64 women who had a spontaneous vaginal delivery had a negative fetal-pelvic index, for a specificity of 96%. The overall predictability of delivery outcome for the index was 85%. Ultrasonography alone yielded a sensitivity of 22%, a specificity of 98%, and an overall predictability of 58%. The corresponding values for Mengert's index were 30%, 95%, and 61%.

Conclusion.—Prolonged labor trials as a result of fetal-pelvic disproportion often lead to adverse outcomes. The fetal-pelvic index compares the size of the passage (maternal pelvis) with the size of the passenger (fetus) and can predict which patients would benefit from early operative intervention.

▶ This study compares 2 imprecise estimates of fetal-pelvic disproportion and, ignoring the several assumptions that stretch reality, finds their method to be superior. Calculations of circumferences of the fetal head, inlet, and midplane were done by averaging anteroposterior and lateral diameters and using the relationship between the diameter and circumference of a circle. Neither the oval of the pelvic inlet nor the fetal head are appropriately estimated with this technique. Estimating the circumference of the midplane (with its irregular shape encompassing the elastic sacrosciatic notches) and the space formed by the urogenital diaphragm (between the diverging inferior rami of the pubis) certainly is a far more crude estimate.

The Colcher-Sussman x-ray pelvic measurement technique relies on positioning the pelvis in semirecumbency to put the transfer diameter of the inlet and the interspinous measurements in the same plane, equidistant from the x-ray film and in the same plane as the reference bar. When this is done, correction for parallax error is possible. Unfortunately, the x-ray method works well only for normal gynecoid pelvises. Finally, the authors assumed that all failure of vaginal delivery is the result of fetal-pelvic disproportion in considering outcome, thereby reducing dystocia caused by uterine malfunction to an impossibility. To say that this approach constitutes a useful means of predicting cephalic-pelvic disproportion is to stretch credulity, regardless of the reported 75% sensitivity value.—T.H. Kirschbaum, M.D.

The Cesarean Birth Rate: Influence of Hospital Teaching Status

Oleske DM, Glandon GL, Giacomelli GJ, Hohmann SF (Rush-Presbyterian-St Luke's Med Center, Chicago; Southern Illinois Univ, Springfield; MMI, Inc, Bannockburn, Ill)

Health Serv Res 26:325–337, 1991 8–10

Background.—A knowledge of how cesarean birth rates vary by hospital characteristics may help modify some of the components of newborn

TABLE 1.—Cesarean Birth Rates by Selected Characteristics According to Hospital Teaching Status, Illinois, 1986

Characteristic	*Hospital Teaching Status*	
	Teaching Hospital Cesarean Birth Rate†	*Other Hospital Cesarean Birth Rate*†
Cesarean birth rate		
Total	20.4	23.1*
Primary	14.4	15.6*
Age group of mother (in years)		
<20	13.4	18.3*
20–24	18.2	21.2*
25–29	21.0	23.4*
30–34	24.1	25.6††
≥35	26.3	28.5
Expected primary payer		
Self-pay	14.6	17.4*
Medicaid	18.1	21.8*
All other payers	22.1	24.3*

* $P < .001$.
† Number of births by cesarean procedure per 100 hospital newborn deliveries.
‡ $P < .01$.
(Courtesy of Oleske DM, Glandon GL, Giacomelli GJ, et al: *Health Serv Res* 26:325–337, 1991.)

delivery services to reduce the necessity of birth by cesarean section. The effect of certain hospital characteristics on cesarean section rates were studied.

Methods.—Data on hospital newborn deliveries in Illinois for 1986 among 130,249 patients aged 10–50 years were obtained from computerized hospital discharge abstract files. Hospital characteristics were obtained from the annual American Hospital Association survey.

Findings.—Adjustment was made for mother's age at delivery; presence of pregnancy, labor, and delivery complications; the expected primary payer; and hospital size. Women who delivered in hospitals with a teaching status were less likely to have a primary cesarean birth than those delivering in hospitals without this designation. The cesarean birth rate in teaching hospitals was also significantly lower in women of all age groups, in Medicaid and non-Medicaid women, and for most categories of delivery complications (Tables 1 and 2).

Conclusion.—Researchers should now identify the programmatic, technological, and manpower functions associated with hospital teaching status that could reduce the likelihood of a primary cesarean delivery. Changes directed toward the manner of diagnosis, monitoring, and management of pregnancy and delivery complications may also decrease the cesarean birth rate.

TABLE 2.—Relative Odds of Primary Cesarean Birth in Hospital With Teaching Status by Indication

Indication	*Adjusted Odds Ratio* * *(95% Confidence Limits)*	p-*Value*
Breech	0.88 (0.72–1.07)	.19
Dystocia	0.78 (0.73–0.85)	<.001
Fetal distress	0.52 (0.46–0.58)	<.001
Other pregnancy or labor-delivery complication	0.79 (0.73–0.86)	<.001
Other nonpregnancy–nonlabor and delivery complication	0.55 (0.39–0.78)	<.001

Note: Excluded from this analysis were 12,320 women who underwent repeat cesarean delivery.
* Adjustment for all factors that entered regression model with $P < .10$. (Adjustment of the nonsignificant odds ratio included teaching status plus all other significant variables from the model.)
(Courtesy of Oleske DM, Glandon GL, Giacomelli, GJ, et al: *Health Serv Res* 26:325–337, 1991.)

▶ This survey of data collected from 130,249 births in Illinois in 1986 was done to explore a paradox reported by others; that rates for general surgical procedure are higher in teaching hospitals, but that the cesarean section rates are lower compared with nonteaching institutions. Repeat cesarean sections without trial of labor were excluded. Teaching affiliation was identified by hospital membership in the Council of Teaching Hospitals (COTH) recorded in American Hospital Association files. Membership in COTH means that a hospital sponsors or participates in at least 4 residency-training programs. The implicit questions are whether differences in patient characteristics, pregnancy, labor complications, or other hospital characteristics (number of beds, numbers of deliveries, incidence of Medicaid payment, etc.) might be confounding in the relationship between teaching status and cesarean section rate. Examination of crude primary and total cesarean section rates showed them to be lower in teaching hospitals, lowest for self-pay and Medicaid as primary payers, and higher for third-party payers. However, the important conclusions stem from logistic regression analysis where patient characteristics, pregnancy, pregnancy abnormalities, peer class, and bed size could be controlled.

The likelihood for cesarean section for all pregnancy abnormalities except breech presentation was significantly lower in COTH hospitals than in others. The difference was particularly striking for cesarean section done for fetal distress and roughly half as likely in teaching hospitals as the others. On the other hand, the diagnosis of fetal distress was made twice as often in COTH hospitals than in nonteaching hospitals, which probably explains the difference (12.9 vs. 5.9%). Note that the results were obtained despite the higher incidence of pregnancy abnormalities in teaching hospitals (79.4%) vs. nonteaching hospitals (68.4%). The authors sugggest peer review programs, a difference in accessibility of technology, or increased numbers of medical personnel may be the reason for the difference. Whatever the mechanism, nonteaching hospitals status joins private patient operator, hospital bed size fewer than 500 deliveries a year, and proprietary hospital ownership as important factors in determining cesarean section rates in this country. (See the 1992 YEAR BOOK OF OBSTETRICS AND GYNECOLOGY, pp 159 and 160.)—T.H. Kirschbaum, M.D.

A Comparative Study of X-Ray Pelvimetry and CT Pelvimetry

Raman S, Samuel D, Suresh K (Univ Hosp, Kuala Lumpur, West Malaysia)
Aust NZ J Obstet Gynaecol 31:217–220, 1991 8–11

Introduction.—Obstetricians have used radiographic pelvimetry in the management of pregnancy for more than 80 years. The results of conventional radiographic pelvimetry were compared with those of CT pelvimetry in 24 pregnant patients to assess the routine use of the latter method.

Methods.—Twenty-four prospective patients underwent cesarean section delivery because of a variety of obstetric reasons. The CT pelvimetry technique used less radiation than the conventional radiographic method. The images taken in CT pelvimetry included true conjugate (anteroposterior diameter), anteroposterior outlet diameter, and transverse diameter of the pelvic inlet. A section through the femoral head fovea

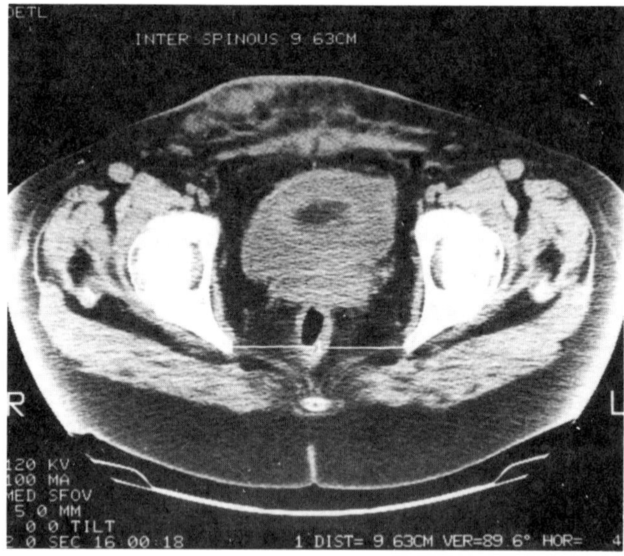

Fig 8–3.—An axial section through the fovea of the femoral heads clearly demonstrating both the ischial spines and the measurement. (Courtesy of Raman S, Samuel D, Suresh K: *Aust NZ J Obstet Gynaecol* 31:217–220, 1991.)

provided the axial measurement of the interischial spinal distance (Fig 8–3). Three independent observers read the radiographs.

Results.—The 24 patients had a mean age of 25 years. The radiographs and the CT assessments were analyzed by 3 review groups. Statistical analysis of the outcomes of the reading of these 2 sets of test demonstrated no significant differences between the 2 pelvimetry methodologies. However, 41.7% of the conventional erect lateral radiographs produced unsatisfactory results. The images from CT pelvimetry usually are of good quality with a properly operating CT scanning system.

▶ Stewart and Kneale's (1) 1970 publication of a purported relationship between x-ray pelvimetry and childhood cancer proved impossible to duplicate in other hands, and the radiation dosage from the procedures subsequently have diminished sharply during the past 30–35 years. The infrequency with which the procedure is currently performed is likely part of the ever increasing tendency in modern obstetrics to treat dystocia with abdominal delivery. Given a woman with a fetus presenting by the vertex, an arrest of cervical dilatation at 5 cm, and station minus 2, it would seem useful to know that both the pelvic inlet, which lies approximately 2 cm below the biparietal diameter of the head, and the ischial spines, which lie 5 cm or so below the biparietal diameter, were normally spaced as background to the decision of whether to stimulate labor or do cesarean section for management.

Knowledge of pelvic shape is often valuable in deciding on the appropriate maneuvers in a midforceps procedure done from a position other than OA or OP. The evidence that trial of labor is very effective in patients with prior cesarean section for cephalopelvic disproportion supports the value of postpartum pelvimetry in such cases as a guide to management of future pregnancies. By and large, publications during the past 15 years have tended to fail to demonstrate the value of x-ray pelvimetry, results which are attributable either to the lack of skill of using the method or to the technique per se. This study is noteworthy for showing that, given an experienced staff of obstetricians, radiologists, and medical officers, the results of x-ray pelvic mensuration are as good as those obtainable by the far more expensive computer-based tomography. It seems likely that pelvimetry, by whatever modality, is an underused approach in modern obstetrics.—T.H. Kirschbaum, M.D.

Reference

1. Stewart A, Kneale CW: *Lancet* 1185, 1970.

Anesthetic Modification of Hemodynamic and Neuroendocrine Stress Responses to Cesarean Delivery in Women With Severe Preeclampsia

Ramanathan J, Coleman P, Sibai B (Univ of Tennessee, Memphis)

Anesth Analg 73:772–779, 1991 8–12

Introduction.—General anesthesia (GA) administered during cesarean delivery can cause serious neuroendocrine and hemodynamic changes in healthy women. Pregnant patients with severe preeclampsia also appear to have significant hemodynamic problems under GA, but not with the use of epidural anesthesia (EA). The results of a prospective study comparing lumbar EA and GA in 21 women with severe preeclampsia undergoing a cesarean delivery were evaluated.

Methods.—The 21 participants with severe preeclampsia were scheduled for cesarean delivery. All patients underwent laboratory tests upon admission to the obstetric unit. Preoperative medication was controlled. Intravenously administered ephedrine was used to treat any decrease in the woman's systolic pressure below 100 mm Hg. The patients participated in the decision of which anesthesia they would undergo (GA or EA).

Results.—Ten of the 21 women received GA, and 11 were given the EA. The EA group demonstrated a significantly longer induction of anesthesia to delivery time. The patients given EA also received significantly more fluids than the patients given GA. Figure 8–4 gives the mean arterial pressure values for both patient groups. The patients given EA experienced a significant decrease in mean arterial pressure, both during anesthesia administration and later at delivery. At the skin incision, those patients given GA demonstrated significant increases in adrenocortico-

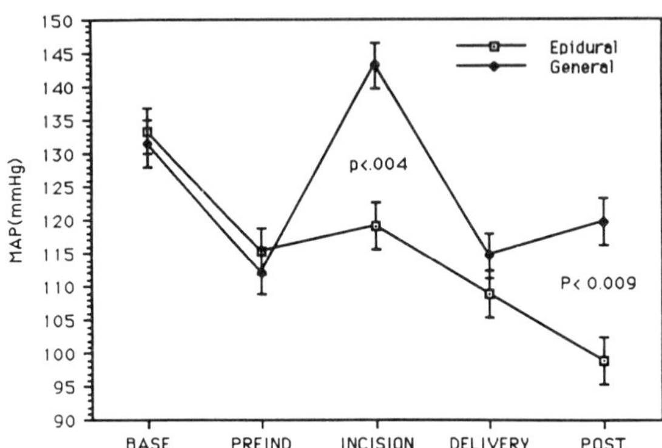

Fig 8–4.—Changes in mean arterial pressure (*MAP*) in the study groups. *Abbreviations*: *BASE*, baseline values; *PREIND*, in the general anesthesia group = MAP obtained after pretreatment with labetalol or nitroglycerin and in the epidural anesthesia group = MAP with T-4 sensory block; *INCISION*, at skin incision; *DELIVERY*, at delivery of infant; *POST*, post partum. (Courtesy of Ramanathan J, Coleman P, Sibai B: *Anesth Analg* 73:772–779, 1991.)

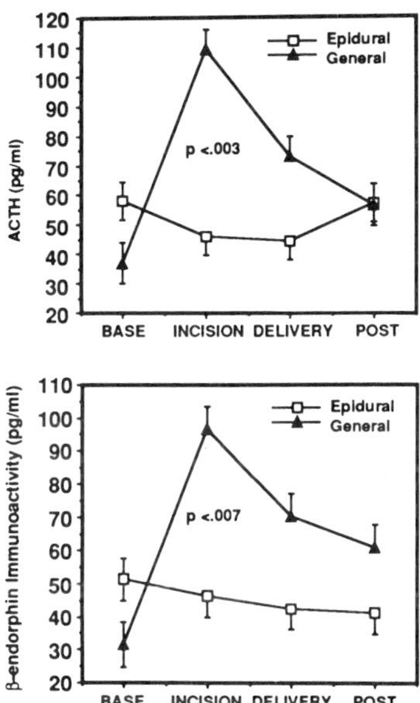

Fig 8–5.—The changes in the levels of adrenocorticotropic hormone and β-endorphin-like immunoactivity in the 2 study groups: before induction of anesthesia (BASE), at skin incision (INCISION), at delivery of infant (DELIVERY), and post partum (POST). (Courtesy of Ramanathan J, Coleman P, Sibai B: *Anesth Analg* 73:772–779, 1991.)

tropic hormone and β-endorphin levels compared with their baseline concentrations; however, the patients given EA did not (Fig 8–5). Cortisol levels also increased significantly in both groups of patients. The GA group had significantly more infants born with Apgar scores less than 7 at 1 minute, but this difference disappeared at 5 minutes after birth.

Conclusion.—The administration of EA up to the T-4 dermatome can lead to a reduction of both the neuroendocrine and hemodynamic stress responses to the cesarean method of delivery in patients with severe preeclampsia. However, this type of anesthesia did not affect the stress hormone levels in the infants at birth.

▶ Much depends on the skill with which these techniques are applied to pregnant women. Nonetheless, the differences noted in this study are impressive. Epidural anesthesia to T-4 runs the risk of hypoperfusion associated with the abrupt loss of autonomic vasomotor tone, the stimulation of the sympathetic nervous system that comes from tracheal intubation needed to reduce the risk of aspiration. Managed by volume expansion and ephedrine (thiopental), GA avoids this risk, but it introduces a different challenge. Even when that problem is negotiated (with an antihypertensive supplement to succinyl choline, in this case) surgical incision results in striking increases in catecholamine, adrenocorticotropic hormone, and β-endorphin concentrations as the CNS responds appropriately—even with consciousness obtunded. These responses are particularly strong in hypertensives. As much as anything, the trade-offs often depend on the familiarity and skill of the anesthesiologist in dealing with these problems.—T.H. Kirschbaum, M.D.

Epidural Analgesia and Cesarean Section for Dystocia: Risk Factors in Nulliparas

Thorp JA, Eckert LO, Ang MS, Johnston DA, Peaceman AM, Parisi VM (Univ of Texas, Houston)

Am J Perinatol 8:402–410, 1991 8–13

Purpose.—The use of epidural analgesia in labor has increased dramatically during recent years; however, its effect on the rate of cesarean section remains controversial. A previous study found a significant increase in the incidence of cesarean section for dystocia associated with epidural analgesia in nulliparous labor. The risk factors associated with the increased incidence of cesarean section done for dystocia were studied retrospectively.

Patients.—The records of the first 500 consecutive nulliparas who met the study's inclusion criteria were analyzed. The inclusion criteria were term nulliparous, singleton gestation, cephalic presentation, spontaneous onset of labor, and 5 cm or less of cervical dilation on admission. The patients were then grouped according to their rate of cervical dilation in early labor and the timing of epidural placement.

Results.—Of the 500 patients, 294 had epidural analgesia and 206 did not. Statistical analysis revealed that epidural analgesia had no effect on the incidence of cesarean section for fetal distress. However, the incidence of cesarean section for dystocia was 15.6% among patients who were given epidural analgesia and 2.4% among patients who did not receive it. The greatest effect was seen among nulliparas who dilated at slower rates in early labor and who had epidural analgesia placed at 5 cm or less of cervical dilation. Both the rate of cervical dilation before epidural placement and the extent of dilation at epidural placement were significantly correlated with the frequency of cesarean section for dystocia.

Conclusion.—The use of epidural analgesia in labor, especially in early labor, may increase the incidence of cesarean section for dystocia in nulliparas.

▶ This was a controversial presentation at the annual clinical meeting of the American College of Obstetricians and Gynecologists in 1989, and it is just now seeing publication. Remember that it is a nonrandomized, retrospective study in which comparability with respect to race, age, height, and weight among groups was relatively good. Some small differences in mean birth weight are probably not significant, but the observations aggregated by the rate of cervical dilatation and epidural use as a function of cervical dilatation could not be blinded. This means that observer bias regarding the role of epidural analgesia in the diagnosis of dystocia cannot be excluded. Nevertheless, it is a well-structured retrospective analysis, valid only for primigravidas in whom dystocia is most common at the spontaneous onset of labor.

Most would agree (on the basis of personal experience) that epidural given before 5 cm in the face of slow primigravid labor increases the risk of the diagnosis of dystocia, despite the increase in need to use oxytocin wherever epidural is compared with nonepidural management. The real surprise comes in comparing all cases who received an epidural for pain relief with those who did not. In this study, the incidence of cesarean section for the diagnosis of dystocia was nearly 5 times higher than in those without epidural analgesia. Note that no increases in cesarean section for fetal distress or other indications were noted, nor was there evidence of adverse effect on the newborn as a result of the epidural administration. Ultimately, the question becomes one of the adequacy of the use of oxytocin supplementation with epidural analgesia. Only if an obstetrician believes he/she does a better job than this group at the University of Texas at Houston can he/she fail to heed the warning implied in this study regarding the use of epidural analgesia in primigravid labor.—T.H. Kirschbaum, M.D.

The Effects of the Addition of Sufentanil to .125% Bupivacaine on the Quality of Analgesia During Labor and on the Incidence of Instrumental Deliveries

Vertommen JD, Vandermeulen E, Van Aken H, Vaes L, Soetens M, Van Steenberge A, Mourisse P, Willaert J, Noorduin H, Devlieger H, Van Assche AF (Katholieke Universiteit, Leuven, Belgium; St Elisabeth Hosp, Turnhout, Belgium; St Anna Hosp, Anderlecht, Belgium; St Lucas Hosp, Assebroek, Belgium; Heilig Hart Ziekenhuis, Roeselare, Belgium; et al)

Anesthesiology 74:809–814, 1991 8–14

Introduction.—Although epidural anesthesia is considered safe for labor and delivery, it may increase the incidence of instrumental deliveries. To determine whether the addition of the opioid sufentanil to epidural bupivacaine with epinephrine would reduce the total amount of local anesthetic and the incidence of instrumental delivery, 695 women were enrolled in a double-blind, randomized, prospective, multicenter study.

Results.—Addition of 30 μg of sufentanil significantly reduced the incidence of instrumental deliveries and improved the quality and duration of analgesia without affecting the neurobehavioral status of the baby. Pruritus was the only side effect; it occurred more frequently with sufentanil than without it.

Conclusion.—Epidural injection of sufentanil with bupivacaine and epinephrine improved the quality of analgesia and reduced the incidence of instrumental deliveries without increasing the risk to either mother or baby.

▶ This study from Belgium is nicely representative of a number of reports on the usefulness of fentanil or sufentanil combined with epinephrine to the local anesthetic used in epidural anesthesia. What results is more effective, longer lasting analgesia. Although the rate of onset of analgesia is faster, the differences are small. Whether the incidence of operative delivery is altered depends primarily on obstetric, rather than anesthetic, practices. In moderate doses, it is impossible to discern adverse fetal effects. The only side effect of sufentanil is the somewhat puzzling pruritus, which usually neither needs nor responds to therapy. All in all, it looks to be a useful complement to current obstetric epidural anesthetic techniques.—T.H. Kirschbaum, M.D.

9 Genetics

Physiatric Management of Two Neonates With Limb Deficiencies and Prenatal Cocaine Exposure

Sheinbaum KA, Badell A (Long Island Jewish Med Ctr, New York)

Arch Phys Med Rehabil 73:385–388, 1992 9–1

Background.—Congenital limb deficiencies related to intrauterine maldevelopment in the first 2 months of pregnancy may be inherited, of unknown etiology, or the result of a teratogen. Two patients with unilateral limb malformations had positive urine toxicology screenings for cocaine.

Case 1.—A boy was born at 36 weeks' gestation to a woman, 29, with a history of multiple drug use, including cocaine. The delivery was vaginal and spontaneous. At 4 weeks of age, the infant's Apgar scores were 8 and 9 at 1 and 5 minutes, respectively. His urine proved positive for cocaine and opiate metabolites. He had no family history of congenital limb deficiency, and he had terminal transverse complete adactylia of the right upper extremity and partial hemimelia of the right lower extremity. His left extremities were normal structurally. An occupational treatment program was prescribed for developmental stimulation, and caregiver training was begun.

Case 2.—An infant boy seen a few hours after birth, was born to a woman, 21, who denied drug use. The infant's urine toxicology screening was positive for cocaine metabolites. His Apgar scores were 9 at 1 minute and 10 at 5 minutes. There was no family history of congenital limb deficiency, and his vital signs were stable. On physical examination, the infant was sleepy with occasional spontaneous eye opening. He had terminal transverse partial aphalangia, syndactyly of the second to fifth digits, and an amniotic band remnant at the proximal interphalangeal (PIP) joints of these digits on the right hand. He had 1 distal phalanx extending from the proximal interphalangeal joints and an intact thumb. His right foot, which was smaller than the left, had a partially flexible equinovarus deformity with metatarsus adductus; the left extremities were normal. A developmental stimulation program was initiated for this patient also.

Conclusion.—Fetal exposure to cocaine may result in limb reduction deficits. Physiatrists should be alerted to a possible increase in the incidence of limb malformation related to cocaine use during pregnancy.

▶ In 1990, Hoyme, Jones, and Dixon (1) predicted that congenital limb reduction in fetuses exposed to cocaine in utero may be expected to occur as a result of the acute increase in sympathetic tone and vasoconstriction. They reasoned that this might well critically influence terminal digit development during the 35th to 45th day of gestation. Here are 2 cases that are consonant but do not prove the hypothesis. Several publications since 1988 have pointed to the increased risk of minor limb reduction noted in infants born after early chorion villus biopsy, in comparison with external controls collected years earlier. The possibility that these findings are related to illicit drug use and are only coincident with chorion villus biopsy must be borne in mind when evaluating these data.—T.H. Kirschbaum, M.D.

Reference

1. Hoyme HE, et al: *Pediatrics* 85:743, 1990.

Chorionic Villus Sampling and Limb Abnormalities

Dolk H, Bertrand F, Lechat MF (Eurocat, School of Public Health, UCL, Brussels)

Lancet 339:876–877, 1992 9–2

Background.—Associations between chorionic villus sampling (CVS) and limb abnormalities have been studied. This possible relationship was further investigated.

Methods and Findings.—Seven European Registration of Congenital Anomalies and Twins registries were contacted. These registries surveyed more than 600,000 births in geographically defined populations. A total of 336 cases of limb reductions were evaluated. Four of these, or 1.2%, involved exposure to CVS. In 11,883 cases of other congenital anomalies, 78, or .66%, involved exposure to CVS, for an odds ratio of 1.8. The increase in risk was not statistically significant. Three of the 4 cases of limb reduction involving exposure to CVS had exposure after 66 days of gestation. The 4 cases of limb reduction consisted of isolated agenesis of the second, third, and fourth left toes, with hypoplasia of nails on the remaining left toes; partial amputation of 4 fingers of the left hand; amniotic disruption sequence with total aplasia of the left leg, hypoplasia of the left pelvis, left diaphragmatic hernia, imperforate anus and vagina, pulmonary hypoplasia, kidney anomaly, persistent left superior vena cava, and drainage of the right pulmonary vein into the right atrium; and Moebius syndrome with syndactyly of right and left hands, agenesis of the second to fourth fingers of the right hand, posterior cleft palate, and micrognathism.

Conclusion.—Chorionic villus sampling exposure was not definitely known for all cases of limb reduction or hypoperfusion anomaly. Exposed populations are probably at greater risk of malformation than the unexposed. The data from the European Registration of Congenital Anomalies and Twins suggest that, if there is a risk as high as 1% for all

CVS and 1.7% for early CVS, then it must be related to specific procedures or the timing of exposure.

▶ Early last year, the Radcliffe Maternity Hospital reported 4 cases of oromandibular-limb hypogenesis and 1 case of terminal transverse limb reduction anomaly among 289 pregnancies; in-home transabdominal CVS was performed between 50 and 66 days' gestation (1). This incidence of 1.7% was larger than the .05% to .06% reported incidence of such limb anomalies reported from the British Columbia registry of anomalous births (2).

The Italian Multicenter Birth Defects Registry reports a surplus of CVS among pregnancies associated with transverse limb reduction defects; however, without a denominator, no incidence figure can be calculated (3). This report from a registry of 7 European countries and based on more than 600,000 births finds an odds ratios for CVS between limb reduction and other anomalies to lack statistical significance; it reports an incidence figure of .05%. Several other reports distribute themselves variously with respect to the presence or absence of an association with CVS. Few reports subsequent to the Radcliffe experience dealt with the oromandibular-limb anomaly but rather, they dealt solely with transverse reduction defects. About all that can be said is that the results are uncertain and contradictory, and that limb differentiation in the human is ordinarily complete at 52 days' gestation for the arms and 56 days for the feet and legs before the bulk of the 50 to 66-day interval. It seems prudent to refrain from CVS before 10 weeks' gestation until this question is fully resolved.—T.H. Kirschbaum, M.D.

References

1. Firth HV, et al: *Lancet* 337:762, 1991.
2. Canadian Collaborative CVS-Amniocentesis Clinical Trial Group: *Teratology* 39:127, 1989.
3. Mastroiacovo P, Cavalcanti DP: *Lancet* 337:1091, 1991.

Application of PCR Amplification of DNA From Paraffin Embedded Tissue Sections to Linkage Analysis in Familial Retinoblastoma

Onadim Z, Cowell JK (Inst of Child Health, London)

J Med Genet 28:312–316, 1991 9–3

Background.—In the familial form of retinoblastoma (Rb), the tumor phenotype segregates as an autosomal dominant trait. The Rb gene has been mapped to chromosome region 13q14. Analysis of the gene, RB1, has shown structural rearrangements within the genomic sequence and mRNA in approximately 30% of tumors. Because the complementary DNA does not identify polymorphic sites for restriction enzymes, a series of unique-sequence intragenic DNA probes were made for gene tracking in families and to detect unaffected Rb gene carriers.

Objective.—A family segregating for the Rb predisposition gene was analyzed using the polymerase chain reaction (PCR) technique to exclude a son as an affected gene carrier. The affected child, who would have served to establish phase in a linkage study, died of a second tumor before DNA analysis was available. The only tissue available was a paraffin-embedded, formalin-fixed specimen of the second tumor.

Results.—It proved possible to isolate DNA from the histopathologic specimen and to amplify the DNA flanking 2 polymorphic restriction enzyme sites, thereby establishing alleles that cosegregated with the Rb predisposing gene. Genomic DNA fragments containing the polymorphic *Bam*HI site and the polymorphic *Xba*I site were amplified.

Implications.—This approach makes it possible to use archival material to provide informed genetic counseling to families. If DNA is available from key deceased family members, the linkage phase can be established.

▶ The remarkable contribution of this study is not the genetic analysis, but the methodology in which enough DNA is extracted from formalin-fixed, paraffin-embedded tissue to subject it to recombinant DNA techniques and investigation. What's needed are thick sections from paraffin blocks of formalin-fixed, embedded tissue. Extensive knowledge of the composition of the gene at issue, as well as those primers suitable to allow amplification of a gene segment containing a polymorphic sequence (where the chances of specific gene identification are optimal), is also necessary. The success of this sort of undertaking opens the door to studies of tumor identity, carcinogenesis, and tumor classification from archival material, as well as to the improvements in genetic counseling to which the authors point.—T.H. Kirschbaum, M.D.

Direct Diagnosis by DNA Analysis of the Fragile X Syndrome of Mental Retardation

Rousseau F, Heitz D, Biancalana V, Blumenfeld S, Kretz C, Boué J, Tommerup N, Van Der Hagen C, DeLozier-Blanchet C, Croquette M-F, Gilgenkrantz S, Jalbert P, Voelckel M-A, Oberlé I, Mandel J-L (Institut National de la Santé et de la Recherche Médicale [INSERM] Unité 184, Strasbourg, France; INSERM Unité 73, Paris; Ulleval Hosp, Oslo) JF Kennedy Inst, Glostrup, Denmark; Institut Universitaire de Génétique Médicale, Geneva; et al)
N Engl J Med 325:1673–1681, 1991 9–4

Background.—The most common inherited cause of mental retardation is the fragile X syndrome, which results from increased size of the Xq27.3 DNA fragment of the X chromosome. The fragment is usually larger than 600 base pairs in the full mutation and as large as 500 base pairs in carriers. Of females who are obligate carriers, only 55% have a detectable fragile X site; the premutation transmutes to the full mutation only when the gene is transmitted by the mother. In women, the premutation or normal sequence is methylated only on the inactive X chromosome. Direct DNA analysis was used to identify carriers of the fragile X syndrome.

Methods.—A total of 511 subjects from 63 families with the fragile X syndrome were studied. Southern blotting with a probe adjacent to the mutation target was used to disclose mutations and abnormal methylation. Double DNA digestion using *Eco*RI and *Eag*I was able to clearly differentiate between normal genotype, premutation, and full mutation.

Findings.—In all samples, this analysis was able to establish the genetic status of the fragile X locus. Analysis of DNA was far more reliable and effective than either cytogenetic testing or segregation studies using closely linked polymorphic markers. Among subjects with premutations, the frequency of mental retardation was similar to that found in the general population. All 103 males and 31 of 59 females with the full mutation were mentally retarded. Some cells carried premutation only in approximately 15% of the subjects with the full mutation. The mothers of affected children all carried either a premutation or a full mutation.

Conclusion.—The DNA analysis described is a direct, efficient, and reliable primary test for the fragile X syndrome. It will be useful both for testing after birth and for prenatal diagnosis and counseling. Future studies must address the role of cytogenetic analysis.

▶ This paper very nicely summarizes the considerable progress that this group has made in understanding the biology of the fragile X syndrome (see the 1987 YEAR BOOK OF OBSTETRICS AND GYNECOLOGY, pp 227–228; the 1988 YEAR BOOK OF OBSTETRICS AND GYNECOLOGY, p 176; and the 1991 YEAR BOOK OF OBSTETRICS AND GYNECOLOGY, pp 155–156). The methodology replaces karyotypic cell culture analysis in the face of deficient folic acid, in which a probe hybridized to the DNA adjacent to the mutation site underlying this abnormality allows Southorn blottings of DNA fragments obtained by restriction enzyme digestion. That site is a 200 base-pair tandem (1 after another) repeat of the base sequence cytosine-guanine-guanine (CGG). Expression of the fragile X defect is affected by the size of the mutation, abnormal methylation of the base sites, sexual imprinting, and mosaicism. Mutation at the q27.3 site of the X chromosome yielding an increase in the size of this tandem repeat segment to 600 or more base-pairs results in the full expression of the syndrome, provided abnormal methylation occurred. The latter takes place only with maternal transmission of the gene mutation, and then only when the defect is housed on the inactive member of the X chromosome pair in the female carrier.

Mosaicism, which is present in 10% of females and nearly twice as often in males, may further reduce the expression of the mutation. Those mutations with less extensive replications of the CGG tandem repeat, which are in the range from 200 to 500 base-pairs, are called premutations here; they rarely result in mental retardation. These premutations, however, are often converted to the longer full-mutation pattern when the gene is passed from mother to male child, thereby evoking the changes in methylation that are described above. Presence of the full mutation will result in mental retardation in 100% of males and 50% of females, depending on whether it rests on the active X chromosome. Although that progression is common in this experience, the development of new mutations from normal premutated X chromosomes was a rare event in the pedigrees studied.

What all this means is that the diagnosis of fragile X syndrome can now be made definitively, using recombinant DNA techniques. The approximate 50% inability to diagnose the carrier state using karotypic analysis is now replaced by definitive tests for recognition and expression in females and female carriers. This is an enormous series of steps in our understanding of this common disorder and a very important body of new knowledge for those who undertake counseling in families exhibiting mental retardation.—T.H. Kirschbaum, M.D.

Sonographic, Clinical and Genetic Aspects of Prenatal Diagnosis of Cystic Kidney Disease

Reuss A, Wladimiroff JW, Niermeyer MF (Erasmus Univ, Rotterdam, The Netherlands)

Ultrasound Med Biol 17:687–694, 1991 9–5

Introduction.—The pathologic, macroscopic, and clinical picture of cystic kidney disease can vary considerably, from solitary cysts to several forms of multicystic and polycystic kidneys. An accurate diagnosis requires examination of the kidneys and liver, clinical data, family history, and a search for associated anomalies. The perinatal manifestations of cystic kidney disease that may be diagnosed with prenatal ultrasound were examined.

Renal Cystic Disease.—A common classification of cystic disease of the kidney is based on genetic considerations. Nongenetic or multifactorial types of the disease include multicystic kidney, multilocular cyst, simple cyst, pyelogenic cyst, and acquired renal cystic disease in chronic hemodialysis patients. An important genetic form is polycystic kidneys, a term applied to 2 separate inherited disorders in which evidence of dysplasia is not found: autosomal recessive polycystic kidney disease (ARPKD) and autosomal dominant polycystic kidney disease (ADPKD). Renal cystic changes can also be a sign of inherited multiple malformation syndromes.

Sonographic Diagnosis of ARPKD and ADPKD.—The severity of ARPKD can be quite varied, although it tends to be constant within a given family. Prenatal sonographic diagnosis is not always possible because of the variability in time of onset in utero and the difficulty in excluding the disease with certainty. Such diagnosis should be based on the presence of kidney enlargement in combination with the typical hyperechogenic texture of the renal parenchyma. The most common form of renal cystic disease, ADPKD, is characterized by bilateral involvement and progressive enlargement of renal cysts. Cysts of the liver occur in as many as 50% of patients. Diagnosis is usually made after 30 years of age; it is rarely discovered in the infant or fetus. Chorionic villus sampling before DNA studies offers the only reliable prenatal diagnosis in a fetus at risk.

Conclusion.—It may be quite difficult to distinguish between ARPKD and ADPKD. Imaging studies, morphologic studies, clinical data, family history, and examination of both liver and kidneys are recommended. A final diagnosis is important for its impact on prognosis, as well as for determination of the inheritance pattern.

▶ Here is an example of advances in genetics that have the effect of complicating (though correcting) previous naive, simple concepts. Polycystic renal disease expressing autosomal recessive inheritance usually appears in infancy—but not always. Similarly, although autosomal dominant inheritance usually is diagnosed in the fourth decade of life, it may appear in infancy. The recessive form is associated with hepatic fibrosis, the dominant form with hepatic cysts. The dominant inherited form is more common, and the only reliable prenatal genetic diagnosis for this type is based on the restriction fragment polymorphism studies on chromosome 16; it is neither highly specific, nor is chromosome 16 always apparently involved. In brief, as information emerges about this cluster of disorders, it has become increasingly difficult to make a precise diagnosis from fetal ultrasound. This means that genealogical, clinical, and morphological studies are needed to establish the diagnosis with precision. It also decreases somewhat the possibility of establishing a diagnosis that is firm enough to allow fetal therapy in many of these cases.—T.H. Kirschbaum, M.D.

Maternal Plasma Corticotrophin-Releasing Hormone Elevated in Preterm Labour but Unaffected by Indomethacin or Nylidrin

Kurki T, Laatikainen T, Salminen-Lappalainen K, Ylikorkala O (Univ Central Hosp of Helsinki)

Br J Obstet Gynaecol 98:685–691, 1991 9–6

Background.—Corticotropin-releasing hormone (CRH) may be a factor in initiating labor through an effect on the pituitary-adrenal axis or other means of promoting fetal maturity. The role of CRH in preterm labor was studied in women randomly assigned to receive treatment with indomethacin or with nylidrin.

Methods.—The women were between 26 and 33 weeks' gestation. Eleven were given indomethacin, and 12 were given nylidrin, a β-sympathomimetic agent.

Findings.—When compared with 23 control pregnancies matched for gestational age but without uterine contractions, the maternal plasma level of CRH was higher in the preterm group before treatment. After 3 and 24 hours of treatment, the levels of CRH were reduced by 10% in

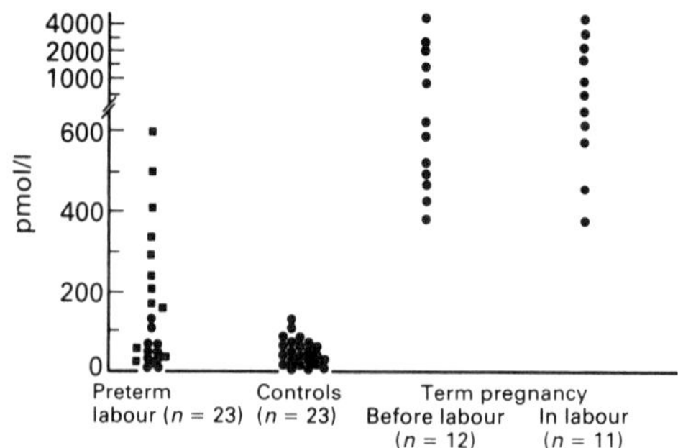

Fig 9–1.—Levels of CRH in 4 groups of pregnancies: 23 in preterm labor, 23 controls matched for gestational age, 12 before labor at term, and 11 in labor at term. In group 1, 12 were delivered preterm (*filled squares*) and 11 were delivered at term (*filled circles*). The levels of CRH were significantly higher in the preterm labor group than in the control group. (Courtesy of Kurki T, Laatikainen T, Salminen-Lappalainen K, et al: *Br J Obstet Gynaecol* 98:685–691, 1991.)

the indomethacin group and by 10% to 20% in the nylidrin group. These changes were not statistically significant. After uterine contractions stopped during tocolysis, 12 women gave birth preterm. Their pretreatment levels of CRH were higher than those of women whose pregnancies proceeded to term. In another group, full-term labor was not associated with any changes in maternal levels of CRH. Umbilical plasma levels of CRH were 1.1% to 9.8% of the paired maternal levels, and they did not increase as gestational age advanced. In addition, the type of delivery had no effect on fetal levels of CRH, and levels of CRH were unrelated to levels of cortisol in mother and fetus (Fig 9–1).

Conclusion.—The maternal level of CRH is increased in preterm labor, and the maternal level of CRH is little affected by treatment with indomethacin or nylidrin. The fetal level of CRH appears to be of no significance in the initiation of preterm or term labor.

▶ This study provides some most interesting data on the relationship of CRH to labor. The increase in maternal concentration during pregnancy with parallel but decreased concentration increase in umbilical blood, together with abundant CRH in amniotic fluid, make it likely the placenta is the source of the peptide. Because umbilical artery and vein concentrations are roughly the same, the fetus appears to be a passive recipient of this placental product. The levels of CRH are increased in preterm labor, and the size of the increase appears to have some predictive strength in ruling out false labor. Because tocolytics fail to decrease elevated maternal CRH concentration, it seems unlikely that either prostaglandins or catecholamines, which have been shown to increase CRH secretion in placental cell culture, are the cause of the change in maternal blood. Oxytocin—the only other agent that is active in vitro in increasing CRH concentration—has not been excluded as causative here. Although the maternal blood concentration of CRH is high at term, it does not appear to be increased after labor and, therefore, is not likely produced by uterine contractions. The CRH and maternal cortisol concentrations are not interrelated; therefore, CRH changes do not appear to be stress related. The role of binding proteins that inactivate CRH needs to be clarified, because it may influence the results. This series of facts is awaiting a hypothesis that fits them. This may be the beginning of an experimental framework with real promise in the elucidation of the onset of preterm labor.—T.H. Kirschbaum, M.D.

Prevention of Neural Tube Defects: Results of the Medical Research Council Vitamin Study

MRC Vitamin Study Research Group
Lancet 338:131–137, 1991 9–7

Background.—For many years, it has been suspected that diet has an etiological role in neural tube defects. Previous studies have suggested that folic acid or other vitamins may reduce the recurrence rate of these defects. A multicenter, randomized, double-blind trial with a factorial design was done to determine whether supplementation with folic acid or other vitamins could prevent neural tube defects.

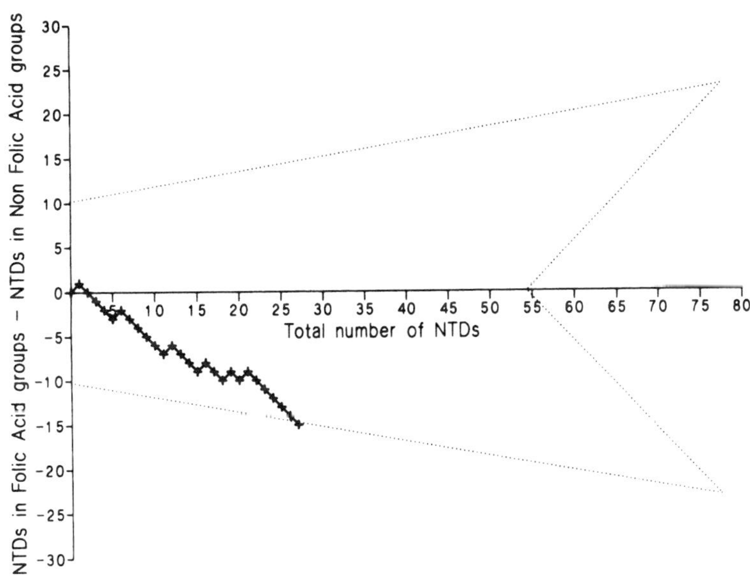

Fig 9–2.—Sequential analysis showing the cumulative difference between the number of neural tube defects (NTDs) in folic acid and non-folic-acid groups plotted against the total number of NTDs. Boundaries of diagram define stopping points of study. The upper and lower boundaries of figure were constructed by use of approximation that the number of events in the folic acid groups minus the number in the groups without folic acid follows gaussian distribution with mean N(1−r)/1+r) and variance N, where r is relative risk and N is total number of NTDs in study. By taking the parameters of this gaussian distribution, equations given by Armitage can be used to specify the upper and lower boundaries of figure. (Courtesy of MRC Vitamin Study Research Group: *Lancet* 338:131–137, 1991.)

Methods.—The study was performed at 33 centers in 7 countries. The subjects were 1,817 women who were at high risk of having a pregnancy with a neural tube defect because of a previous affected pregnancy. The women were randomized to 1 of 4 supplementation groups: folic acid; a mixture of vitamins A, D, B_1, B_2, B_6, C, and nicotinamide; both folic acid and the other vitamins; or neither. Supplementation began near the time of conception, and the patients were evaluated every 3 months until the twelfth week of pregnancy. Each woman remained in the trial until she had a pregnancy in which it could be determined whether a neural tube defect was present—an "informative" pregnancy—or until the end of the trial. The trial was halted after approximately 8 years, when sufficiently conclusive results emerged.

Results.—There was a total of 1,195 informative pregnancies. Of these, 27 were found to have a neural tube defect, 6 in the groups receiving folic acid and 21 in the other 2 groups (Fig 9–2). The prevalence of neural tube defects was 1% in women who received folic acid compared with 3.5% in those who did not. Folic acid had a 72% protective effect, and the other vitamins had no significant protective effect. Exclusion of women who reported they had stopped taking their capsules before their last scheduled visit yielded similar prevalence results. Folic acid supplementation appeared to cause no demonstrable harm, although the study had limited ability to detect rare or slight adverse effects.

Conclusion.—Neural tube defects can be prevented by folic acid supplementation. Supplementation with folic acid, beginning before pregnancy, is recommended for all women who have had a pregnancy with a neural tube defect. Public health measures should be taken to ensure adequate amounts of folic acid in the diets of all women of childbearing age.

▶ This is a great rarity in the literature on the nutritional impacts on pregnancy: a prospective, randomized, blinded study that yields a solid conclusion. The result is not surprising in view of the well-known relationship between neural tube defects (NTD) and antifolate medication during pregnancy. Of the 23 cases of NTD, 3 should be excluded, because these women entered the study less than 2 weeks before their last menstrual period and were already pregnant when they began medication. Their exclusion appropriately results in a small relative risk ratio for NTD, comparing those who received folate with those who didn't. Comparing groups A and C (neither of which received prenatal vitamins, but A received folate) yields a significant risk ratio in favor of folate use. The same comparison between B and D, the former receiving folate and both receiving vitamins, failed to show such an effect; however, the study was not designed to test the effect of vitamin supplementation overall. As has become conventional in such studies, the ethics of blinded exclusion of an agent of possible preventive value was handled with sequential analysis, stopping the study when sufficient cases to detect halving of the relative risk at the probability level equal to .05 with 75% power was reached.—T.H. Kirschbaum, M.D.

A Newly Defined X Linked Mental Retardation Syndrome Associated With α Thalassaemia

Gibbons RJ, Wilkie AOM, Weatherall DJ, Higgs DR (John Radcliffe Hosp, Oxford, England)

J Med Genet 28:729–733, 1991 9–8

Introduction.—Severe α thalassaemia usually occurs in individuals with a Mediterranean or Oriental background. In 1981, 3 northern European families were found to have this condition in 1981, which manifested as severe mental retardation and hemoglobin H (Hb H) disease. The Hb H disease produces a more than 50% reduction in α globin chain synthesis in the adult. By 1990, the α thalassaemia and mental retardation (ATR) syndrome had occurred in 13 reported cases, with 2 additional pedigrees published as an X-linked ATR syndrome (ATR-X). The studies of the total 16 cases of ATR to date were evaluated.

Methods.—An analysis of the clinical features of the ATR-X syndrome demonstrated a severe total retardation from infancy, although the pregnancy and birth appeared normal. Other characteristics of the syndrome from the published studies sometimes included dysmorphic facies, geni-

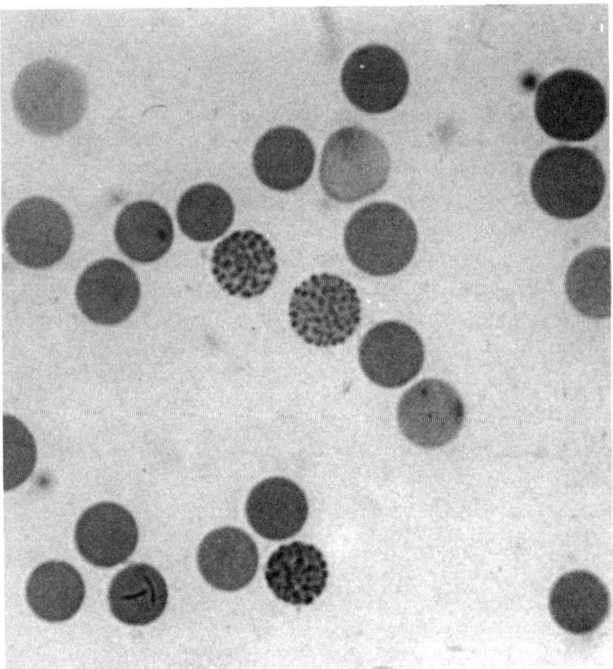

Fig 9–3.—Photomicrograph of the peripheral blood of a patient with X-linked α thalassaemia and mental retardation syndrome showing some cells containing hemoglobin H inclusions. (Courtesy of Gibbons RJ, Wilkie AOM, Weatherall DJ, et al: *J Med Genet* 28:729–733, 1991.)

tal anomalies, skeletal abnormalities, and food regurgitation. Those with the ATR-X syndrome had very mild Hb H disease.

Results.—The cases determined by the dysmorphic facies and related clinically diagnosed abnormalities indicated some of the patients to have normal or only slightly abnormal hematological parameters. The Hb H inclusion appeared after incubation of the red blood cells with 1% brilliant cresyl blue (Fig 9–3) showing a 0% to 6.7% Hb H level of electrophoresis testing. All 9 of the affected subjects with ATR-X syndrome were male. One of these families had a recorded history of frequent miscarriages and deaths of male fetuses in utero.

Conclusion.—A normal hemoglobin level and red blood cell count do not indicate that the patient does not have the condition. The X-linked α thalassaemia and mental retardation syndrome outlines a distinct hematological condition with identifiable dysmorphism. Boys with severe undiagnosed mental retardation accompanied with other ATR-X symptoms should undergo a blood test for the presence of Hb H inclusions in blood cells.

▶ Infants with hypotonia, feeding disturbances, delayed motor development and cortical atrophy combined with mental retardation not infrequently form the basis for claims against obstetricians' professional liability. For this reason, this syndrome, which was newly defined only 10 years after first being reported, should be borne in mind. The important association is with the presence of Hb H in newborn infant blood. In Hb H, the globin moeity is composed of 4 β chains instead of the normal composition of hemoglobin A ($\alpha_2\beta_2$) or hemoglobin F (garma 4). When resulting from deletion of the gene for α globin chains on the short (petit) arm of chromosome 16, the defect results in severe problems in oxyhemoglobin transfer (see the 1991 YEAR BOOK OF OBSTETRICS AND GYNECOLOGY, pp 91–93). In the newly defined syndrome, the defect appears to lie on the X chromosome, inheritance is by the sex-linked recessive mechanism, and expression of the defect is confined to males. Hematological and acid/base values are usually normal, perhaps because the occurrence of Hb H-containing red blood cells, seen with brilliant cresyl blue staining, is relatively infrequent. Dysmorphic facial features are seen, but they are variable in occurrence and extent. Stain for Hb H should be added to the evaluation of infants who exhibit brain maldevelopment and mental retardation in the early neonatal period.—T.H. Kirschbaum, M.D.

Correlation Between Omphalocele Contents and Karyotypic Abnormalities: Sonographic Study in 37 Cases

Getachew MM, Goldstein RB, Edge V, Goldberg JD, Filly RA (Univ of California, San Francisco)

AJR 158:133–136, 1992 9–9

Background.—Fetuses with omphaloceles often have a variety of concomitant visceral malformations and chromosomal abnormalities, both of which adversely influence outcome. However, when the omphalocele is seen as an isolated defect, it usually can be repaired surgically after birth with excellent results. Recent studies have found that the absence of liver in the omphalocele is strongly correlated with the presence of fetal karyotypic abnormalities and perinatal mortality. This study further examined the relationship between the contents of an omphalocele and chromosomal abnormalities.

Methods.—Between 1984 and 1990, omphaloceles were detected in 37 fetuses with gestational ages ranging from 15 to 34 menstrual weeks. The omphalocele was detected at or before 24 weeks' gestation in 24 of the 37 fetuses. Sonographic examinations were performed with real-time sonography. The sonograms were studied retrospectively for the contents and transverse diameter of the omphalocele, associated abnormalities, and the volume of amniotic fluid. Fetal echocardiography was performed only when the pregnancy was not terminated electively.

Results.—Nine fetuses had concomitant morphological abnormalities that were characteristic of the amniotic band syndrome on the sonograms. All these pregnancies were terminated electively. Confirmatory pathologic data were available for 5 of the 9 aborted fetuses. Four of the 9 aborted fetuses had normal karyotypes. The 28 remaining fetuses had omphaloceles confirmed at autopsy or postnatal follow-up. Karyotypic correlation was available for 22 fetuses, and the karyotype was abnormal in 5 of these (23%). Twenty-two omphaloceles contained liver, and 6 omphaloceles contained bowel only. Sixteen fetuses with omphaloceles containing liver were tested for karyotype, and the karyotype was abnormal in only 1 of these. In contrast, 4 of 6 fetuses with omphaloceles containing only bowel had abnormal karyotypes. All 4 fetuses had additional morphological abnormalities. The 2 fetuses with normal karyotypes and omphaloceles containing bowel only were well after surgical repair. Excluding the 9 fetuses with amniotic band syndrome, sonograms showed concomitant anomalies in 15 fetuses with liver-containing omphaloceles and the karyotype was abnormal in only 1 of these.

Conclusion.—Karyotypic abnormalities are more common in association with omphaloceles that contain only bowel compared with those that contain only liver.

▶ Increasingly common use of maternal serum α-fetoprotein testing and fetal ultrasound has led to the increasingly frequent diagnosis of fetal ventral wall defects. The distinction between gastroschisis and omphalocele is important, because infants with gastroschisis usually lack other forms of anomalous development, whereas those with omphalocele occasionally (10 of 26 or approximately 40% here) bear karyotypic abnormality. The most severe of these (trisomies 13 and 18) are incompatible with normal life, and the ability to predict these abnormalities from fetal ultrasound is what makes this paper important. The authors confirm and provide additional cases to the experience reported by Benacarraf et al. (1), which points to omphaloceles (containing only bowel loops and, therefore, representing a defect in recovery of intestinal loops from their normal position inside the cord in the 10th week of development) as being suggestive of aneuploidy. When the other features of those trisomies are difficult to deduce, this may be an important finding in diagnosis and counseling.—T.H. Kirschbaum, M.D.

Reference

1. Benacarraf BR, et al: *Obstet Gynecol* 75:317, 1990.

Fetal and Neonatal Effects of Treatment With Angiotensin Converting Enzyme Inhibitors in Pregnancy

Hanssens M, Keirse MJNC, Vankelecom F, Van Assche FA (Univ of Leuven, Belgium; Leiden Univ, The Netherlands)

Obstet Gynecol 78:128–135, 1991 9–10

Introduction.—Since the introduction of captopril in 1977, the class of angiotensin-converting enzyme inhibitors for the treatment of hypertensive disorders has grown to more than 15 agents. Both captopril and enalapril appear to cross the placenta in humans with potential harmful effects. All available reports on the use of angiotensin-converting enzyme inhibitors in human pregnancy were reviewed.

Data Analysis.—A total of 25 publications reported 85 pregnancies in 81 women in which angiotensin-converting enzyme inhibitor had been used. Fourteen of 25 publications were primary publications, and the remainder were abstracts or letters. In 47 pregnancies, women had received treatment in the first trimester of pregnancy. These cases had a spontaneous loss of 9% and total loss of 13%. Oligohydramnios was documented in 11 pregnancies and was associated with IUGR in 5 cases. There were 3 cases of lung hypoplasia and a high frequency (23%) of very preterm delivery. Available data on the birth weight of 64 infants showed 36% with a weight below the tenth percentile and 17% below the fifth percentile. Of 11 deaths that occurred in 82 fetuses, 6 were stillbirths and 4 occurred in the neonatal period. The perinatal mortality rate was 85, or 97 per 1,000.

Conclusion.—There was no evidence that use of angiotensin-converting enzyme inhibitors during pregnancy increased the likelihood of low birth weight for gestational age, respiratory distress syndrome, or persistent ductus arteriosus. The agents can cause severe disturbance of fetal and neonatal renal function, such as oligohydramnios, pulmonary hypoplasia, and long-lasting neonatal anuria. The renal dysfunction may result from inhibition of the autoregulatory mechanism of the efferent arteriole and appeared to be more common with enalapril than with captopril. Extreme caution should be used in prescribing angiotensin-converting enzyme inhibitors during pregnancy.

▶ This class of agents has been clearly identified as useful in the treatment of congestive heart failure and of possible use in chronic hypertension. For these reasons, it is likely to appear among the array of drugs to which pregnant or potentially pregnant women are exposed. This review article makes clear the risk from this agent to which the human fetus is exposed. Among those risks are oligohydramnios, intrauterine growth retardation, pulmonary hypoplasia, preterm labor, and fetal and neonatal death. The early immediate cause identified to date is interference of the role of angiotensin in regulating glomerular filtration through modulation of vascular resistance in the efferent glomerular arteriole of the fetal kidney. Although there is reason to be concerned about the risk of anomaly, the 47 cases exposed to the drug in the first trimester of pregnancy are insufficient to establish that an increased risk of teratogenicity exists. This is an agent to be avoided in pregnancy.—T.H. Kirschbaum, M.D.

Prenatal Diagnosis With Fetal Cells Isolated From Maternal Blood by Multiparameter Flow Cytometry

Price JO, Elias S, Wachtel SS, Klinger K, Dockter M, Tharapel A, Shulman LP, Phillips OP, Meyers CM, Shook D, Simpson JL (Univ of Tennessee, Memphis; Integrated Genetics, Framingham, Mass)

Am J Obstet Gynecol 165:1731–1737, 1991 9–11

Introduction.—Medical geneticists have long attempted to create prenatal testing techniques that did not cause harm to the fetus. Both amniocentesis and chorionic villus biopsy are considered invasive methods with accompanying risks to the pregnancy. Several noninvasive methods assaying fetal cells from the maternal circulation appear promising. A procedure to sort fetal nucleated erythrocytes from maternal blood using flow cytometry, followed by DNA characterization with polymerase chain reaction technology, was studied.

Methods.—Volunteers provided venous blood specimens just before chorionic villus biopsy. Part of the blood sample underwent flow cytometry measurement, whereas separated fetal cells were exposed to polymerase chain reaction methodology. Positive selection of cells under flow cytometry required the sample cells to have the 4 characteristics of cell size, cell granularity, glycophorin-A cell surface molecule, and transferrin receptor. The umbilical cord blood samples served as controls. The background signal level of the Y-specific probe was measured by in situ DNA hybridization.

Case Report.—Woman, 42, underwent prenatal testing at 10.8 weeks' gestation because of her age. Flow-sorted cells tested by in situ hybridization with various probes (Fig 9–4) resulted in an 8.7% single hybridization signal to the Y probe and a 90.3% no signal to the X probe, with an overall profile indicating a male fetus with trisomy 18. The patient elected to terminate the pregnancy, which led to the confirmation of the fetal diagnosis of 47,XY,+18.

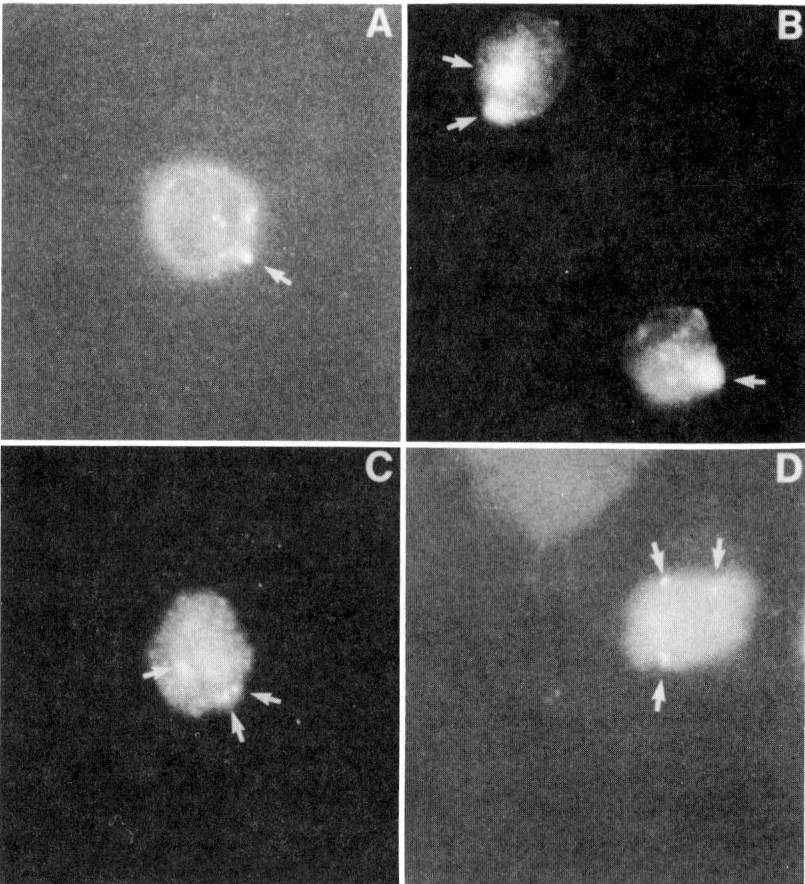

Fig 9–4.—Flow-sorted cells hybridized to various chromosome-specific probes. The probes were labeled with biotin and visualized with fluorescein isothiocyanate—streptavidin. All cells were from a single blood sample and were analyzed in coded fashion. **A,** male cell of fetal origin. Fluorescent signal (*arrow*) in a cell hybridized to pDP97 probe, which identifies a repetitive sequence in the heterochromatic region on the long arm of the Y chromosome. **B,** female cell of maternal origin (*upper left*) showing 2 signals (2 *arrows*) and male cell of fetal origin (*lower right*) showing single signal (*arrow*). The cells are hybridized to the X-chromosome-specific cosmid probe, which identifies pericentromeric repeat sequence on X chromosome. **C** and **D,** trisomy 18 fetal cells sorted from maternal blood. Fluorescent signals (3 *arrows*) in cells hybridized to chromosome 18—specific cosmid contig probe, which identifies single-copy sequence on distal long arm of chromosome 18. (Courtesy of Price JO, Elias S, Wachtel SS, et al: *Am J Obstet Gynecol* 165:1731–1737, 1991.)

Results.—The results of the flow cytometry in the umbilical cord samples demonstrated a cell positive value of 21%, whereas first trimester cells had a positive value of .4% and a second trimester value of 2.2%. Approximately 10% of the fetal cells could be extracted from the woman's blood sample. The polymerase chain reaction method correctly identified male fetuses 12 of 12 times and female fetuses 5 of 6 times among the 18 patients tested. The background signal level of the Y-specific probe occurred in 5% of the sorted female cord blood samples that led to a correct fetal sex identification in 68% of the cases.

Conclusion.—Analysis of fetal cells extracted from the pregnant woman's circulation may permit a noninvasive means of fetal diagnosis.

▶ Here is another significant step in the exciting prospects for genetic analysis of fetal cells obtained from cell sorting of maternal blood (see the 1990 YEAR BOOK OF OBSTETRICS AND GYNECOLOGY, pp 178–80). In this instance, the efficacy of cell sorting has been improved to the point of demonstrating 1 fetal nucleated red blood cell among 10^7 to 10^8 maternal cells. Polymerase chain reaction applied to primers flanking segments of the Y chromosome allowed prediction of male gender based on positive recognition in all 12 cases, and 5 of 6 females identified by negative recognition, for an overall 94% success rate. More importantly, it was possible to demonstrate hybridization of complimentary probes to the X and Y chromosomes and chromosomes 21 and 18. This led to the correct diagnosis of a male who was trisomic for chromosome 18 and another who was trisomic for chromosome 21. As efficiency continues to increase in this procedure, we come ever closer to the prospect of fetal diagnosis in the first trimester of pregnancy without invading the amniotic sac.—T.H. Kirschbaum, M.D.

Endoluminal Catheter-Assisted Transcervical US of the Human Embryo: Work in Progress

Ragavendra N, McMahon JT, Perrella RR, Tessler FN, Hansen GC, Kimme-Smith C, Grant EG, Crandall BF (UCLA School of Medicine, Los Angeles; Eve Surgical Ctrs, Los Angeles; UCLA–Olive View Med Ctr, Sylmar, Calif)
Radiology 181:779–783, 1991 9–12

Introduction.—Although transvaginal ultrasonography (US) enables the evaluation of cardiac activity in very small embryos and early prenatal diagnosis of some congenital anomalies, its ability to depict anatomical details in early embryos is less than satisfactory. To enhance visualization of anatomical structures in the human embryo, a new technique called endoluminal catheter-assisted transcervical (ELCAT) sonography was used.

Technique.—The ELCAT US is performed with a commercially available US catheter originally intended for intravascular use. The catheter consists of an outer polyethylene sheath housing a metal drive shaft containing the transducer at its tip. A motor in the imaging device rotates the metal drive shaft. The catheter-based high-frequency US transducer is introduced via the cervix into the endometrial cavity of the uterus.

Patients.—Seven women who were about to undergo voluntary termination of a first-trimester pregnancy agreed to participate in the study. The object of the examination was to confirm the intrauterine location of the pregnancy, with particular attention to visualizing the anatomical parts of the embryo. The study was recorded on videotape.

Results.—The imaging catheter could be passed without difficulty in all 7 cases, and there were no complications. The embryos ranged from 5.2 to 10 weeks' menstrual age. Cardiac pulsations were observed in 6 of the 7 embryos, with 1 fetal death. The US catheter did not rupture any of the fluid-filled chorionic/amniotic cavities. In 2 cases, the measurements of the embryonic disk could be obtained without difficulty, but there were problems in obtaining the crown-rump lengths. The most prominent anatomical structures visualized were the heart and neural tube.

Conclusion.—The preliminary findings of this investigation show that ELCAT US can successfully image structures of the developing human embryo.

▶ This report of a work in progress documents a further refinement of the ability to scan the human embryo without disruption of the chorion. A scanning unit housed in a 3-mL-diameter catheter represents application of a technique in use to investigate intravascular and, especially, atherosclerotic lesions to reproduction science. Clear definition is limited to 1-cm distance from the sensor, and images are interpretable to a distance of 2 cm. The importance of techniques to scan embryos with respect to diagnosis and research in defective development has received comment earlier in this book. This approach increases the ability to explore embryonic structure, normal or abnormal, by an order of magnitude.—T.H. Kirschbaum, M.D.

10 The Puerperium

Drug Screening of Newborns by Meconium Analysis: A Large-Scale, Prospective, Epidemiologic Study

Ostrea EM Jr, Brady M, Gause S, Raymundo AL, Stevens M (Wayne State Univ, Detroit)

Pediatrics 89:107–113, 1992 10–1

Introduction.—Identification of neonates that have been exposed to illicit drugs is difficult. A method was recently developed to identify drugs and their metabolites in the meconium of neonates; this method is easy, specific, and sensitive. It was used in a large-scale, prospective screening of newborns to determine the prevalence and epidemiological characteristics of drug use in a high-risk, urban population.

Methods.—The meconium of 3,010 neonates was analyzed for the presence of metabolites of cocaine, morphine, and cannabinoids. The infants were delivered at a tertiary perinatal center in Detroit from 1988 to 1989. Demographic, clinical, and laboratory data on the mothers and newborns were compiled and analyzed.

Results.—Of the newborns, 44% were positive for cocaine, morphine, or cannabinoids; 31% were positive for cocaine, 21% for morphine, and 12% for cannabinoid. Only 11% of mothers gave self-reports of illicit drug use during pregnancy. Maternal drug users were significantly more likely to be service patients, single, multigravid (more than 3) with little or no prenatal care, and to have had meconium-stained amniotic fluid. Cocaine users had a significantly shorter duration of labor than other women. The presence of more than 1 drug was demonstrated in 32% of all positive test results. Among neonates, positive results were associated with a significantly higher incidence of prematurity, low birth weight, smaller length and head circumference, and an Apgar score of less than 6 at 1 minute. Meconium test results were positive in 88% of newborns whose mothers admitted drug use during pregnancy compared with 52% with positive urine test results.

Conclusion.—This technique detected the presence of drug metabolites in 44% of specimens of neonatal meconium, which was 4 times more than the 11% rate of drug usage obtained from maternal self-report. This discrepancy may be partly based on the use of self-report during the routine maternal history taken by the physician, although other methods can provide more accurate information on maternal drug use. Because many newborns exposed to drugs in utero may appear normal at birth and may have mothers who deny drug use, drug screening and a high index of suspicion may be necessary to detect newborns at risk.

▶ During the past 4 years, this group has been at the forefront in developing a meconium assay using radioimmunoassay for cocaine, opioid, and cannabinoid derivatives. The advantages of this approach are many. The illicit drug is transferred from the mother to the fetus, where hepatic metabolism takes place and bilinary excretion of fetal metabolites ensues. The telltale metabolites languish in the bowel content for weeks and become obtainable with the first voided stool in the immediate neonatal period. Whereas the search for metabolites of these agents is carried out in the maternal blood and urine, rapid clearance through the urinary tract and rapid transients of concentration in both sources decrease the likelihood of finding them present in contrast to the meconium assay, which reflects a longer period of possible exposure.

Comparisons between maternal hair analysis and meconium assays are reasonably concordant, and positive findings (44% with a 32% incidence of multiple agents) reveal more frequent drug usage in pregnancy than usually is reported. Certainly, the 11.1% of women who admitted to drug use are relying on the probability that their remote use will not be detected by medical attendants. Among those 11% who were acknowledged drug users, 88% showed meconium-positive findings, whereas only 52% showed detectable urinary metabolites. As an interesting aside, 12% of infants born of mothers with a positive history of drug use were meconium negative, suggesting significant false positive errors as judged by patient accounts of drug use. The authors provide an important diagnostic approach to critical medical and social problems, which will sharpen our diagnostic capabilities in the puerperal diagnosis of illicit drug use.—T.H. Kirschbaum, M.D.

Gastric Emptying in the Postpartum Period

Gin T, Cho AMW, Lew JKL, Lau GSN, Yuen PM, Critchley JAJH, Oh TE (Chinese Univ of Hong King, Shatin)

Anaesth Intensive Care 19:521–524, 1991 10–2

Background.—Pregnant women at term are at increased risk of acid aspiration caused by multiple factors. Many of these risk factors are believed to persist in the postpartum period, but no specific guidelines suggest when these factors revert to normal and precautions against acid aspiration before general anesthesia are no longer necessary. To help establish appropriate fasting guidelines for elective surgery during the postpartum period, the gastric emptying was measured at 1 and 3 days post partum.

Methods.—Eight women were studied on the first and third day post partum using the technique of paracetamol absorption. Six women also had gastric emptying assessed at 6 weeks post partum.

Results.—The women had a median age of 30 years, a median weight of 65 kg, and a median gestation of 39 weeks. All patients at all testing dates had similarly shaped paracetamol concentration-time curves. Pharmacokinetic analyses showed that gastric emptying was rapid even at 1 day post partum, although the metabolism of paracetamol seemed to be faster than at 6 weeks post partum.

Conclusion.—Gastric emptying seems to be rapid in patients 1 day post partum. No special fluid fasting guidelines may be necessary for these patients in preparation for elective surgery.

▶ Acetaminophen (paracetamol) is not absorbed in the stomach but is rapidly absorbed in the jejunum. The interval between oral administration and maximum plasma concentration therefore can be used as an indirect measurement of the duration before gastric emptying in pregnancy. These results indicate that delays of gastric emptying during pregnancy apparently are abolished within 12–30 hours after delivery. This somewhat surprising finding would have been bolstered by measurements in pregnancy, which would have provided internal controls rather than necessitating comparisons with the work of others. The direct application of this information is to assure obstetricians and anesthesiologists that the hazards of gastric aspiration are quickly diminished post partum—an important item in the conduct of postpartum sterilization. Additionally, because hormonal regressive changes are not striking so soon after delivery, these data raise questions regarding the nonhormonal effects of pregnancy on gastric emptying.—T.H. Kirschbaum, M.D.

Duplex Ultrasound of the Common Femoral Vein in Pregnancy and Puerperium

Duddy MJ, McHugo JM (Birmingham Maternity Hosp, Queen Elizabeth Medical Centre, Birmingham, England)

Br J Radiol 64:785–791, 1991 10–3

Background.—Fatal pulmonary embolus in pregnancy is comparable to hypertensive disease of pregnancy as the most common cause of maternal death in the United Kingdom. Earlier detection of thrombus in the veins of the pelvis and legs has been proposed. One report states that reduced flow in the femoral vein detected by noninvasive methods is an indication for anticoagulant treatment. The effects of the enlarged uterus in late pregnancy and early puerperium on the Doppler characteristics of the common femoral vein (CFV) and on the Doppler and caliber response of the CFV to the Valsalva maneuver were studied.

Methods.—Sixty-eight CFVs in 34 women were assessed by ultrasound. Ten were at 8 to 9 weeks' gestation; 19 were at 28 to 40 weeks' gestation; and 5 were between 2 and 10 days' post partum. All were healthy volunteers with no signs of deep vein thrombosis (DVT). The cross-sectional areas of the veins were measured while the women were

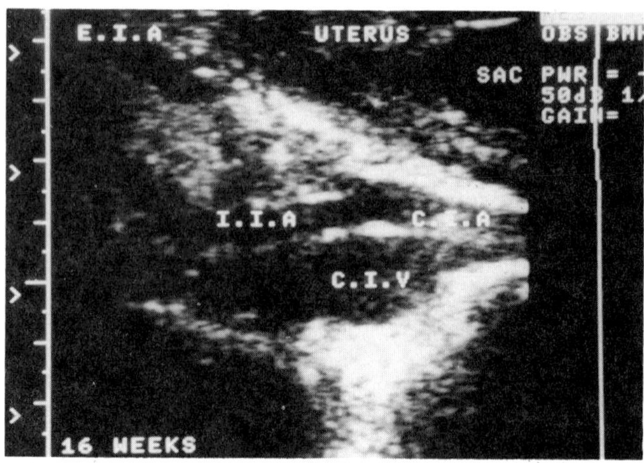

Fig 10–1.—Sonogram of the iliac vessels through a 16-week-gestation gravid uterus as an acoustic window. *Abbreviations: CIV*, comon iliac vein; *CIA*, common iliac artery; *IIA*, internal iliac artery; *EIA*, external iliac artery. (Courtesy of Duddy MJ, McHugo JM: *Br J Radiol* 64:785–791, 1991.)

at rest in the supine position and also during a Valsalva maneuver. Pulsed Doppler ultrasound also was used to assess the veins.

Findings.—During the Valsalva maneuver in the supine position, the caliber response of the CFV was unreliable in women late in pregnancy and early puerperium. Examination with the patient in the decubitis position may be more likely to exclude iliac vein occlusion. Doppler assessment was better than caliber change measurement in excluding iliac thrombosis (Fig 10–1).

Conclusion.—Doppler examination is superior to caliber response assessment during the Valsalva maneuver for excluding an isolated iliac occlusion late in pregnancy and early in puerperium. If Doppler findings are abnormal or equivocal, the patients should be examined in the decubitus position. Pulsatile flow in the CFV may be present in pregnancy in the absence of cardiac disease. In late pregnancy, retrograde flow during a Valsalva maneuver may be present in the absence of diseased venous valves.

▶ Because pulmonary embolus is now the leading cause of maternal death in this country, the detection of pelvic phlebothrombosis has taken on new urgency. This paper summarizes 2 sets of ultrasound approaches to the diagnosis of iliofemoral thrombosis, the most common site of intrapartum and postpartum thrombosis. It's possible to image the bifurcation of the common iliac arteries and, adjacent to them, the iliac veins. Organized thrombi yield an intraluminal echo, but this is so unreliable as to be of little use. The Valsalva maneuver causes the iliac vein to distend, but the authors' contention is that criteria for normal distensibility are uncertain. Their argument is that pulsed Doppler evaluation of the veins can be used to demonstrate zero flow with Valsalva, accelerated flow after its release, and transmission of respiratory blood flow cycles conducted through the inferior vena cava and enhanced flow on lower leg compression. All these can be used as evidence for patency of iliofemoral veins and can at least decrease the number of patients who require venography for the diagnosis of iliofemoral thrombosis. It's worth keeping in mind in relation to this most common of potentially lethal postpartum complication.—T.H. Kirschbaum, M.D.

Diagnostic Imaging in Puerperal Febrile Morbidity

Lev-Toaff AS, Baka JJ, Toaff ME, Friedman AC, Radecki PD, Caroline DF (Temple Univ Hosp; Hahnemann Univ Hosp, Philadelphia)

Obstet Gynecol 78:50–55, 1991 10–4

Background.—Imaging studies have not been widely used in the management of postpartum febrile morbidity. The value of ultrasound, CT, and MRI in the diagnosis and management of such patients was performed.

Patients.—The medical records and imaging studies of 31 patients referred with puerperal febrile morbidity that did not respond to antibiotic treatment were reviewed; they accounted for .4% of deliveries during the study period. Thirty of the patients were black, and 11 were adolescents. A total of 42% of the women delivered prematurely, and 74% delivered by cesarean section. Forty-five percent had bleeding requiring blood transfusions.

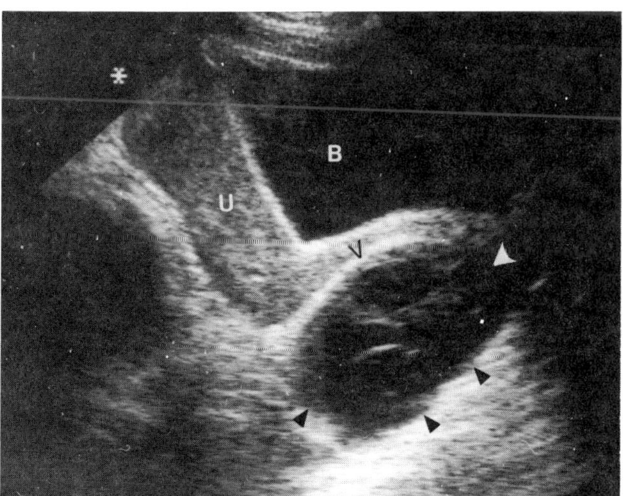

Fig 10–2.—Rectovaginal septum hematoma. Midsagittal sonogram showing a complex mass (*arrowheads*) posterior to the vagina (*v*). This hematoma was followed by sonography to resolution. *U* = uterus; *B* = bladder. (Courtesy of Lev-Toaff AS, Baka JJ, Toaff ME, et al: *Obstet Gynecol* 78:50–55, 1991.)

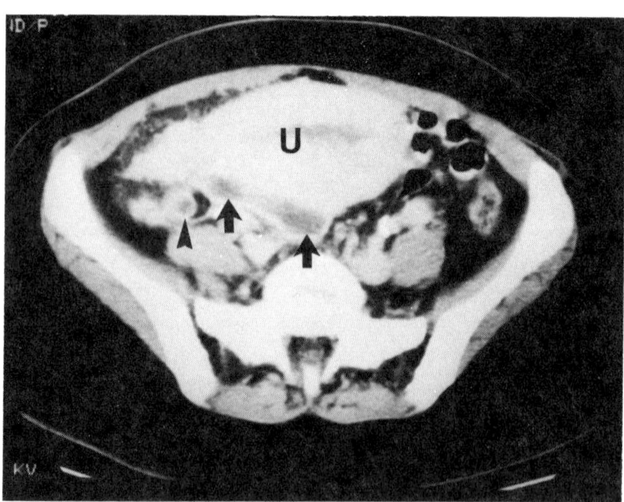

Fig 10–3.—Right ovarian venous thrombosis and septic pelvic thrombophlebitis. A CT scan through the pelvis shows thrombosed pelvic (*arrows*) and right ovarian vein (*arrowhead*). Sonography confirmed a tortuous thrombosed ovarian vein without Doppler signal. *U* = uterus. (Courtesy of Lev-Toaff AS, Baka JJ, Toaff ME, et al: *Obstet Gynecol* 78:50–55, 1991.)

Findings.—Eleven patients were found to have hematomas, 6 of whom were delivered by cesarean, 2 by cesarean hysterectomy, and 3 vaginally. Rectovaginal septum hematoma disclosed by ultrasound in 1 case was managed conservatively and followed by ultrasound (Fig 10–2). There were 7 abscesses, 2 cases of ovarian venous thrombosis (Fig 10–3), and 1 case each of small-bowel obstruction, vesicouterine fistula, and subcutaneous seroma. Endomyometritis was found in 21 patients, 13 of whom had other extrauterine abnormalities, including 6 cases of abscess, 4 of hematoma, and 1 each of ovarian venous thrombosis, vesicouterine fistula, and small bowel obstruction. Two patients were found to have retained placental tissue. Imaging studies were negative in only 2 patients, and in most it led to a specific diagnosis and allowed definitive therapy.

Conclusion.—Imaging studies can be useful in the evaluation of women with puerperal fever. Ultrasound is the first imaging study for most patients. Either CT or MRI may be required for obese patients or if skilled personnel are unavailable. Ultrasound readily helps in diagnosing bladder-flap hematoma.

▶ This is a look into a new epoch in the management of febrile postpartum morbidity. It is uncommon for a postpartum temperature increase to last longer than 72 hours with antibiotics, but when it does, the usual pattern in the absence of localizing signs is to treat for endomyometritis, with heparin therapy used for phlebothrombosis. In this admittedly small group of patients, approximately half had no localizing signs and symptoms, and the other half usually complained of abdominal and/or pelvic pain. The finding of unsuspected hematomas in 35%, abscesses including perinephric and subphrenic collections in 20%, and 2 cases of ovarian-vein thrombosis make it clear how much imaging has to offer over hopeful expectation. Then too, guidance in needle aspiration of abscesses and in transvaginal drainage of pelvic hematomas are potential secondary gains. It is a good idea to begin scouting with ultrasound after 48 hours of postpartum fever—if you are *not* certain you are merely treating endometritis or urinary-tract infection. Finding extrapelvic causes for fever is certain to become more common with this approach. Only half the cases of endomyometritis were capable of confirmation through imaging. That is not surprising for a problem where the pathology is dominantly microscopic, but it makes for an uncomfortable number of false negative results in the clinical management of such patients.—T.H. Kirschbaum, M.D.

Maternal Employment Effects on Family and Preterm Infants at Three Months

Youngblut JM, Loveland-Cherry CJ, Horan M (Case Western Reserve Univ, Cleveland; Univ of Michigan, Ann Arbor; Grand Valley State Univ, Allendale, Mich)

Nurs Res 40:272–275, 1991 10–5

Introduction.—More than half of all mothers with children younger than 3 years are employed, some because of necessity. Past studies of the effect of maternal employment on healthy children have yielded conflicting results. The effects of the mother's degree of choice and satisfaction with her work on her child and family were investigated.

Methods.—The mothers of 110 families with a premature infant (younger than 37 weeks of gestation) rated their degree of choice about work and their satisfaction with that choice. Family cohesion, adaptability, and relationships were assessed. Child outcome was measured using the Bayley instrument.

Results.—Neither family functioning nor child development correlated with whether the mother was employed, unemployed, or on leave of absence from work. The infant's motor development correlated positively with the number of hours the mother worked per week, and also with her degree of choice when employed. When the mother was unemployed, motor development correlated negatively with choice.

Conclusion.—Maternal work does not adversely affect the development of preterm infants at age 3 months. Working may in fact be beneficial, particularly if the mother has a choice in the matter. Longer term studies are needed for nurses to appropriately advise parents.

▶ For most young mothers who must, or choose to, work after delivery, the effect of employment and of time away from infant care is a frequent source of anxiety and guilt. Because care needs are greater for premature than for mature neonates, the authors' decision to study the development of premature infants makes sense. On the other hand, if care in the neonatal intensive care unit is necessary for most of the 3-month follow-up period, in this study, the maternal contribution to total care needs is diminished; however, it probably is still important. What is reassuring is that a mother's employment shows no deleterious effect on mental or motor development. Indeed, the mean scores for both dimensions of developmental gain are larger for infants of working than for nonworking mothers, although not statistically significantly so. This is an important basis for reassurance to working puerperas.—T.H. Kirschbaum, M.D.

11 The Newborn

Perinatal Hepatitis B Virus Infection Caused by Antihepatitis Be Positive Maternal Mononuclear Cells

Shimizu H, Mitsuda T, Fujita S, Yokota S (Yokohama City Univ; Yokohama City Maternity Hosp, Japan)

Arch Dis Child 66:718–721, 1991 11–1

Introduction.—The Japanese national project for prevention of mother-to-infant transmission of hepatitis B virus (HBV) with vaccination has protected 90% to 95% of the offspring of hepatitis Be antigen (HBeAg)-positive HBV-carrier mothers. In contrast, although HBeAg-negative mothers comprise three quarters of pregnant hepatitis B carriers, no prophylaxis is recommended for their infants. Regardless of HBeAg status, the quantity of circulating HBV-DNA is directly related to HBV infectivity. The infectivity of HBV from mothers to infants was investigated.

Methods.—The HBV-DNA in plasma and peripheral mononuclear cells from 28 antihepatitis Be–positive, hepatitis B surface antigen-positive carrier mothers was examined by a highly sensitive polymerase chain reaction/Southern hybridization technique.

Findings.—There was HBV-specific DNA detected in 3 maternal mononuclear cell samples, but not in plasma. Of 4 infants born to 3 mothers who carried the HBV-DNA positive mononuclear cells, 2 had acute or fulminant hepatitis developed within 3 months of birth. In the 25 infants of mothers who were HBV-DNA negative in both plasma and mononuclear cells, there were no HBV markers or increased activity of transaminases during follow-up of as long as 3.5 years. There was a specific association between the HBV-DNA expression in maternal peripheral mononuclear cells and the HBV infection of their infants.

Conclusion.—Even asymptomatic, anti-HBe–positive pregnant women may carry HBV-DNA positive mononuclear cells in the peripheral blood that can transmit infectious HBV to their offspring. It may be prudent to treat infants of HBV-DNA mononuclear-cell–positive mothers with both HBIg and HBV vaccine.

▶ It has been a piece of conventional wisdom that efforts to prevent the 95% chronic infant HBV carrier state and risk of hepatic carcinoma in infants should focus on those cases in which the mother is both HBsAg and HBeAg positive (see the 1990 YEAR BOOK OF OBSTETRICS AND GYNECOLOGY, pp 95–96, 199–200; and the 1991 YEAR BOOK OF OBSTETRICS AND GYNECOLOGY, pp 177–179). In such cases, the risk of maternal-to-fetal transmission is now recognized to be in the range of 75% in the absence of maternal antibody to the E antigen (anti-HBe), which confers partial protection against fetal infection. This study follows up a Japanese report indicating that 10% of infants born to women who are HBsAg positive but HBeAg negative have acute or fulminant hepatitis develop (1). Such infants should therefore also receive hepatitis B immunoglobulin (HBIg) at birth, followed by HBV vaccine.

This study's exploration of pathogenesis finds, using polymerase chain reaction, evidence that HBV-DNA can be found in maternal monocytes independent of maternal HBe antigen or antibody, and that the amount of such viral DNA is proportional to evidence of fetal infectivity. This work suffices to broaden the need for infant prophylaxis to all cases where maternal blood is HBsAg positive. It also offers an improved, albeit expensive, test for evaluating maternal-fetal infectivity.—T.H. Kirschbaum, M.D.

Reference

1. Shiraki K, et al: *Acta Paediatr Jpn* 28:338, 1986.

Cerebral Palsy: MR Findings in 40 Patients

Truwit CL, Barkovich AJ, Koch TK, Ferriero DM (United States Army Med Dept, Academy of Health Sciences, Houston; Univ of California, San Francisco)

AJNR 13:67–78, 1992 11–2

Background.—Numerous clinical, neuropathologic, and neuroradiological studies have been done on cerebral palsy. However, neuroradiological studies have been limited in their usefulness, mostly because of the limited abilities of neuroimaging before CT and MRI were introduced. The MR findings in patients with CP were studied.

Methods.—Forty patients, aged 1 month to 41 years, were scanned with MR. The findings were correlated with clinical histories for each patient.

Findings.—Eleven patients who had been born prematurely had periventricular white matter damage, indicating hypoxic-ischemic brain injury. The chronology of this was difficult to determine. Three major patterns were seen among the 29 patients who had been born at term. The first consisted of gyral anomalies suggesting polymicrogyria, which was consistent with mid-second–trimester injury. The second pattern consisted of isolated periventricular leukomalacia, reflecting late second- or early third-trimester injury. In the third pattern, watershed cortical or deep gray nuclear damage was seen, consistent with late third-trimester, perinatal, or postnatal injury. Fifty-five percent of those who had been born at term had MR findings of intrauterine brain damage. In more than half these patients, MR showed developmental anomalies, which is almost twice the rate previously reported in CT studies.

Conclusion.—These findings support the growing consensus that cerebral palsy in infants born at term often results from prenatal factors and, less commonly, from perinatal factors. The consideration of prenatal and, occasionally, postnatal causes may be useful in determining the time of brain injury in patients with cerebral palsy.

▶ Although this is a retrospective study based on referrals to the faculty of pediatric neurology and neuroradiology at University of California, San Francisco, the findings are important in providing structural confirmation of the growing body of information regarding the etiology of cerebral palsy. Findings in preterm births (11 cases) were stingingly different from those in term births (29 cases). All but 2 of the preterm births were at or before 32 weeks. Here, 9 of 11 cases (82%) showed evidence of periventricular leukomalacia reflecting in utero pathophysiology, which may have been associated with the cause of preterm birth or handicap in the newborn in his or her postnatal adjustment.

Of the infants born at term, 16 of 29 cases (55%) showed evidence that was compatible with in utero pathology and, in 10 cases, of developmental anomaly. Six cases showed periventricular leukomalacia, again reflecting in utero pathology before delivery. In 2 of these 16 cases, there was evidence of additional postnatal injury stemming from apnea secondary to sudden infant death syndrome. In only 7 cases (24%) was there evidence of postnatal injury (deep focal gray matter lesions, cortical thinning, cystic encephalomalacia, etc.). One of these cases had co-existing developmental abnormality (polymicrogyria). In only 5 of these 7 cases (12% of the total) was there both history and magnetic resonance evidence of perinatal asphyxia associated with cerebral palsy. This finding is very similar to the 3% to 13% figure from Nelson (1) and the 4.9% to 8.2% figure from the Western Australia Cerebral Palsy registry study (2).—T.H. Kirschbaum, M.D.

References

1. Nelson KB: *J Pediatr* 112:572, 1988.
2. Blair E, Stanley FJ: *J Pediatr* 112:515, 1988.

HIV Replication During the First Weeks of Life

Krivine A, Firtion G, Cao L, Francoual C, Henrion R, Lebon P (Hôpital Saint-Vincent-de-Paul, Paris; Clinique Universitaire Port-Royal, Paris)

Lancet 339:1187–1189, 1992 11–3

Background.—Human immunodeficiency virus infection can be diagnosed in children born to HIV-positive mothers during the first 12 months. However, few studies have examined HIV status during the first weeks of life.

Methods.—Fifty infants born to HIV-1 seropositive women were enrolled in a prospective, longitudinal study. Blood samples were taken at birth and at 4–9 weeks and 5–9 months of age. Testing for HIV-1 consisted of polymerase chain reaction (PCR), viral culture, and p24 antigen measurements.

Findings.—Sixteen children had HIV infection by 4–9 weeks of age, according to PCR and culture. Infection could be detected in only 5 children at birth. No change in HIV status occurred between 4–9 weeks and 5–9 months of age in the 44 infants available for retesting.

Conclusion.—Using PCR or viral culture, perinatal HIV-1 infection can be diagnosed in the first 2 months of life. In nearly 70% of the infants subsequently found to be infected, HIV-1 infection could not be detected at birth, thereby suggesting an active replication of HIV in the first weeks of life. The findings may favor the hypothesis that HIV-1 transmission occurs at the end of pregnancy or at delivery.

▶ This experience, together with the search for IgA to HIV-1 (see Abstract 11–14), helps to allow separation of passive and active newborn antibody formation in infants born of HIV-1–positive gravidas. The value of this approach is that it avoids the 15- to 16-month wait otherwise recommended to differentiate passive and active newborn antibody. Use of polymerase chain reaction (PCR) applied to DNA from circulating infant mononuclear cells using primers specific to HIV-RNA, complemented by viral culture, provided the basis for the early diagnosis. None of the 45 infants who were tested at a mean of 5.7 days of life and were found to be PCR negative had positive cultures or antibody to the p24 viral antigen. When retested at 4 to 9 weeks of age (37.2 days), 16 of 44 infants were now PCR positive, and all were either culture positive then or at reexamination in the interval from 5–9 months of life. There are 2 alternatives that explain this course of events. Infection could have occurred in late pregnancy or at delivery, resulting in latency of infection in early neonatal life. It also could have occurred through horizontal transmission resulting from neonatal contacts with the mother or other environmental agencies. Regrettably, there is no way to choose between these 2 alternatives. Either way, these data suggest prevention of infant transmission must focus on delivery and the early neonatal period.—T.H. Kirschbaum, M.D.

Survival and Cerebral Palsy in Low Birthweight Infants: Implications for Perinatal Care

Stanley FJ (Univ of Western Australia, Perth)
Paediatr Perinat Epidemiol 6:298–310, 1992 11–4

Introduction.—The decrease in neonatal mortality in several countries appears to be linked to an increase in the occurrence of cerebral palsy. One hypothesis suggests that as more infants with lower birth weights survive, they sustain postnatal brain damage from complications of extreme immaturity. The other hypothesis is that cerebral palsy and preterm birth have their origins in pregnancy, and that more of these chil-

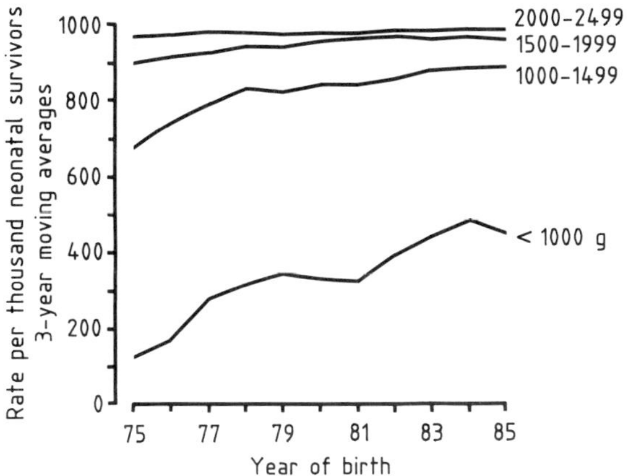

Fig 11–1.—Low-birth-weight neonatal survivor rates per 1,000 live births in Western Australia, 1975–1985 (3-year moving averages). (Courtesy of Stanley FJ: *Paediatr Perinat Epidemiol* 6:298–310, 1992.)

Low-Birth-Weight Cerebral Palsy Rates per 1,000 Neonatal Survivors, 1975–1985 (Grouped Years)

	Birthweight (g)				
	<1000	1000–1499	1500–1999	2000–2499	Total <2500
1975–1978 (4 years)					
Neonatal survivors	56	261	741	2839	3879
Cerebral palsy					
No.	2	7	25	19	53
Rate	35.7	26.8	33.7	6.7	13.6
1979–1982 (4 years)					
Neonatal survivors	93	363	857	3062	4375
Cerebral palsy					
No.	7	13	17	19	56
Rate	75.3	35.8	19.8	6.2	12.8
1983–1985 (3 years)					
Neonatal survivors	113	358	761	2545	3777
Cerebral palsy					
No.	11	27	11	17	66
Rate	97.4	75.4	14.5	6.7	17.5

(Courtesy of Stanley FJ: *Paediatr Perinat Epidemiol* 6:298–310, 1992.)

dren who were compromised before birth now are surviving. Determining whether the increase in cerebral palsy has antenatal or postnatal causes could have a direct influence on neonatal care practices. Regional data on increased survival, cerebral palsy, and timing of brain damage were assessed.

Method.—Data from the Western Australian Cerebral Palsy Register and from the Maternal and Child Health Research Data Base for stillbirths, neonatal deaths, and survivors were examined. Only data on infants born between 1975–1985 in Western Australia were renewed. The 10-year span was divided into epochs of 4 years each.

Results.—Both antenatal and postnatal complications are important in the increase in cerebral palsy in low-birth-weight infants. For infants who weighed between 1,500 and 1,999 g, cerebral palsy rates decreased along with neonatal mortality. For infants who weighed more than 2,000 g there has been some improvement in mortality, but there was no change in the cerebral palsy rates (Fig 11–1; table). The proportion of all cerebral palsy occurring in very-low-birth-weight (less than 1,500 g) infants increased from 5.6% in 1975–1978 to 26% in 1983–1985.

Conclusion.—Analysis of data on infants in Western Australia suggests that both antenatal and postnatal complications are important in the increases in cerebral palsy in low-birth-weight infants. Although better prenatal care may prevent a certain proportion of postnatally damaged low-birth-weight survivors, other infants may be damaged before birth with remote possibilities for prevention. Future studies of low-birth-weight infants with cerebral palsy should include antenatal factors, the etiological pathways to preterm birth, randomized controlled trials of neonatal intervention, and identification of better neonatal predictors of brain damage.

► In both the United States and Western Australia, perinatal survival rates are improving, resulting in large part from the improved rate of survival in infants born weighing less than 1,500 g, which provides the disproportionate part of the increase. This report demonstrates the simultaneous increase in incidence of cerebral palsy occurring predominantly in the very-low-birth-weight range. In that respect, similar conclusions have been generated by 3 European countries as well (1–3). These data are quite convincing and consist of the diagnosis of cerebral palsy established on 5-year follow-up.

In our 3 grouped intervals from 1975 to 1985, the stillbirth rate decreased in Western Australia, and perinatal survival increased only in those infants weighing 2,000 g or less at birth. During the same interval, survival at less than 1,000 g of birth weight has increased from 20% to 50%, and for birth weights from 1,000 to 1,500 g, from 75% to 89%. At birth weights above 1,500 g, little improved survival is reported. In the birth weight range less than 1,500 g, the rate of cerebral palsy per 1,000 surviving infants increased sharply as well. The lesser rates of increase of aggregate cerebral palsy per 1,000 live births suggests, but does not prove, that postnatal and perinatal events are more likely than antenatal factors to matter in causation.

Because the total cerebral palsy incidence figures for all birth weights are not given, it's not possible to tell whether the .2% incidence of cerebral palsy for all live births, which was stable for nearly 30 years in Western Australia, has increased as a result (see the 1989 YEAR BOOK OF OBSTETRICS AND GYNECOLOGY, pp 172–174). These trends are a source of concern and raise important issues in ethics and patient management of very-low-birth-weight infants.—T.H. Kirschbaum, M.D.

References

1. Hagberg B, et al: *Acta Paediatr Scand* 78:283, 1989.
2. Pharoah POD, et al: *Arch Dis Child* 65:602, 1990.
3. Dowding V, Barry C: *Irish Med J* 81:25, 1988.

Risk Factors for Mother-to-Child Transmission of HIV-1

Peckham CS, for the European Collaborative Study (Inst of Child Health, London)

Lancet 339:1007–1012, 1992 11–5

Introduction.—The rates of transmission of HIV type 1 (HIV-1) from mother to child range from 7% to 39%. The stage of maternal infection

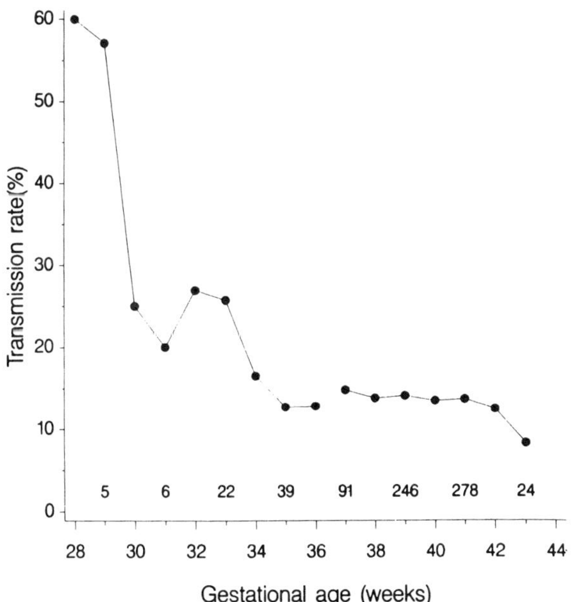

Fig 11–2.—Transmission rate by gestational age. The figure has been smoothed by plotting 3-point averages; e.g., value at 36 weeks is the observed transmission rate for 35–37 weeks. Numbers born by gestational age are shown in 2-week intervals. (Courtesy of Peckham CS, for the European Collaborative Study: *Lancet* 339:1007–1012, 1992.)

or breast-feeding may pose a risk of increased transmission. The risk factors for mother-to-child transmission of HIV-1 were investigated.

Method.—From 1984 to 1991, 1,005 children from 19 centers were enrolled in the study. The HIV status was determined in 721 children of 701 mothers. Associations between clinical and immunological status of the mother during pregnancy, maternal characteristics of age, parity, and race; length of gestation; mode of delivery; and breast-feeding with HIV-1 transmission were analyzed.

Results.—The rate of vertical transmission of HIV-1 was 14.4%. Vertical transmission was not significantly associated with parity, race, maternal age at delivery, or intravenous drug use. The risk of infection was greatest for infants born to 13 women with AIDS. The odds ratios for transmission were 2 in 25 in breast-fed children compared with never-breast-fed children, 3 in 80 in children born before 34 weeks of gestation, and 0 in 56 in children delivered by cesarean section. The duration of breast-feeding did not affect risk. The mechanism for the higher risk of infection found in children born before 34 weeks was unclear (Fig 11–2). Transmission was associated with maternal p24-antigenemia and a CD4 count of less than 700 μL. Transmission was also higher in children born of vaginal deliveries in which episiotomy, scalp electrodes, or instruments were used, but only in centers where these procedures were not routine.

Conclusion.—Women infected with HIV with p24-antigenemia or a low CD4 count have an increased risk of vertical transmission of HIV-1. The higher rate of infection found in children born before 34 weeks of gestation corresponds with a decrease in transmission with gestational age. In utero HIV infection may affect fetal development and lead to premature delivery. Alternatively, women with AIDS or antigenemia may be more likely to deliver before 34 weeks of gestation, or concurrent infections may increase both the risk of premature delivery and the risk of transmission of HIV infection. The significance of the twofold increase in risk of infection in breast-fed children has not been defined.

▶ This is an update of data from the European Collaborative Study, which has now expanded to include 19 participating countries (see the 1990 YEAR BOOK OF OBSTETRICS AND GYNECOLOGY, pp 196-198). With more case material, the reported rate of maternal-to-fetal transmission is now less than the earlier estimate of 24%. The tendency for a higher rate of fetal transmission at less than 24 weeks of gestation may relate to the impact of more advanced maternal infection in very long labor, diminished fetal capacity for immune protection, or the relationship between intravenous drug abuse and a predisposition for preterm labor. Presence of CD4 lymphocyte counts below 700 per μL, and antigenemia of p24, a major viral core protein for HIV, increased the likelihood of fetal infection. The hazard of fetal infection via breast milk is again confirmed by multivariate analysis, but the protective effect of cesarean section presumed by some fails the test of statistical significance. The data are suggestive of benefit from reducing contact with the birth canal in infected women. This report is of considerable value in the difficult manner of counseling HIV-1–positive gravidas.—T.H. Kirschbaum, M.D.

Respiratory Disease in Very-Low-Birthweight Infants After Prenatal Thyrotropin-Releasing Hormone and Glucocorticoid

Ballard RA, Ballard PL, Creasy RK, Padbury J, Polk DH, Bracken M, Moya FR, Gross I, and the TRH Study Group (Mount Zion Hosp and Med Ctr, San Francisco; Yale Univ, New Haven, Conn; Univ of Texas Health Science Ctr, Houston; Harbor Med Ctr, Torrance, Calif)

Lancet 339:510–515, 1992 11–6

Background.—Despite prenatal glucocorticoid therapy, respiratory distress syndrome (RDS) and chronic lung disease (CLD) may develop in very-low-birth-weight infants. In a multicenter, blinded, randomized trial, the effect of additional prenatal treatment with thyrotropin-releasing hormone (TRH) was investigated.

Methods.—Eligible study participants were women with threatened preterm delivery at less than 32 weeks' gestation. Of the 404 women enrolled, 198 received betamethasone plus TRH (4 doses of 400 μg every 8 hours), and 206 were given betamethasone plus placebo. Complete data were available for 114 infants delivered to 99 women in the treatment group and for 117 infants of 105 women in the control group.

Results.—The 2 groups (TRH + betamethasone and betamethasone alone) had no significant differences in birth weight, gestational age, mortality, gender, or racial distribution. In neonates of less than 1,500 g birth weight, TRH treatment did not affect the total incidence of RDS (47% vs. 58% in controls) or of severe RDS (13% vs. 25% in controls); however, CLD developed in significantly fewer TRH-treated infants (18%) than in controls (44%). The TRH + betamethasone group had significantly fewer adverse outcomes, defined as death or continuing oxygen requirement, than the betamethasone only group, both at 28 days' and at 36 weeks' postconceptional age. Other complications of prematurity occurred at similar rates in the 2 groups. Women in the TRH + betamethasone group experienced more side effects (nausea, vomiting, and flushing) than those in the betamethasone only group.

Conclusion.—Prenatal treatment with TRH plus glucocorticoid substantially reduces the occurrence of CLD in very-low-birth-weight infants. There were no fetal deaths associated with TRH therapy and only minor maternal side effects.

▶ In vitro and animal experimental data have shown a role for T-3, T-4, thyroid-stimulating hormone, prolactin, insulin, and a few other substances in supporting fetal lung maturation. How important these agents may be in preventing respiratory distress syndrome (RDS) when compared with glucocorticoids has been a lingering question. This collaborative, prospective, double-blinded study goes a long way toward answering those questions. Thyroid stimulating hormone given to gravidas crosses the placenta and, in the 9 cases where cord plasma was assayed 2–6 hours after the last dose of maternal TRH, all showed significant increases in concentration of the measured variables, excepting only prolactin. The addition of TRH had no effect on the incidence or severity of respiratory distress syndrome, intracranial hemorrhage, patent ductus arteriosus, retinopathy, or necrotizing enterocolitis. In infants with birth weights of less than 1,500 g, TRH appeared to reduce the duration and need for both oxygen administration and ventilatory assistance. Because both of these are important determinants of chronic lung disease in infants, this study and a few others seem to make the case for supplementing glucocorticoids with 4 doses of 400 μg of TRH administered intravenously every 8 hours when the estimated fetal weight is less than 1,500 g. No significant difference in effectiveness by infant sex or race were noted.—T.H. Kirschbaum, M.D.

Improvement of Outcome for Infants of Birth Weight Under 1000 g

Kitchen WH, for the Victorian Infant Collaborative Study Group (Univ of Melbourne, Australia)

Arch Dis Child 66:765–769, 1991 11–7

Background.—Perinatal care in the Australian state of Victoria has improved since 1979/1980, when the survival rate of extremely-low-birth-weight (ELBW) infants was 25.4%, and only 49.4% of survivors were free of neurological disabilities at 2 years. Those born at level III centers did better than those born elsewhere. A comparable cohort born from 1985 to 1987 was studied to compare survival rates and rates of neurological impairment and disability.

Methods.—Of 182,719 infants born in the state during a 3-year period, 560 were ELBW, for an incidence of .306%. Extremely low birth weight was defined as birth weight ranging from 500 to 999 g. Data were gathered from many sources, as in the previous study, and they were cross-checked with the state's level III centers, in which all but 1 of the survivors spent some time. At 2 years of age, the children were assessed for psychological, developmental, and neurological outcome.

Results.—By 1985 to 1987, 2-year survival increased from 25.4% to 37.9%. The proportion of those who survived to 2 years with no neurological disabilities increased from 12.5% to 26.2%. Survival increased in association with greater birth weight. As in the earlier study, the later study showed higher survival among infants born in level III centers, and this advantage remained after adjusting for birth weight. In the later study, fewer infants were born outside of level III centers. For those born elsewhere, the rate of severe neurological disabilities was no longer significant. The rates of sensorineural impairment decreased slightly, but the difference was not significant.

Conclusion.—In Victoria, the survival of ELBW infants has improved as neurological morbidity has decreased. Immediate care for infants born outside of level III centers has probably improved. In the later study, ventilator support was sometimes withdrawn if cranial ultrasound showed a major intracranial hemorrhage. The absolute number of patients surviving with severe disabilities has not increased, but the number of survivors free of disabilities has more than doubled.

▶ This study is superior to many similar studies in that the authors collected sufficient cases to allow analysis in 100-g birth-weight intervals, and there apparently are excellent patient descriptive data. Note there has been no survival below 600-g birth weight. The report displays the improved outcome in level III compared with level I and II birth centers, the increasing incidence of level III referral, and the attainment of the same improved survival of referred ELBW infants as that obtained by those inborn in tertiary-care centers. The rates of neurosensory impairment were lower in the 1985 to 1987 group than in the 1979 and 1980 group, but they do not differ significantly. Because the total number of ELBW infants was increased in the more recent material, the number of intact survivors (rate of intact survival multiplied by the number of cases) was significantly increased. It is important that the 2 groups were found not to differ in rates of twins, male births, malformations, socioeconomic stratum, maternal age, non-English speaking origin, and educational and occupational level. What is most encouraging, beyond the evidence of effective transfers to tertiary-care centers, was evidence of improved survival in primary and secondary units resulting from improved pediatric training, available cranial ultrasound and CT, and improvements in respiratory assistance. As the authors emphasize, those changes, together with educational efforts that are directed at pediatricians and underlie improved use of tertiary referral, "do not come cheaply."—T.H. Kirschbaum, M.D.

Postnatal Transmission of Human Immunodeficiency Virus Type 1 From Mother to Infant: A Prospective Cohort Study in Kigali, Rwanda

Van de Perre P, Simonon A, Msellati P, Hitimana D G, Vaira D, Bazubagira A, Van Goethem C, Stevens A-M, Karita E, Sondag-Thull D, Dabis F, Lepage P (Natl AIDS Control Program, Kigali, Rwanda; Centre Hospitalier, Kigali; Univ of Bordeaux II, France; Univ of Liege, Belgium)

N Engl J Med 325:593–598, 1991 11–8

Background.—The transmission of HIV type 1 (HIV-1) from mother to infant during pregnancy and delivery is well documented. However, little is known about the possible transmission of HIV-1 during the postnatal period.

Methods.—A total of 212 HIV-1-seronegative mother-infant pairs were enrolled in the prospective cohort study. All infants were breastfed. The pairs were followed up at 3-month intervals with Western blot

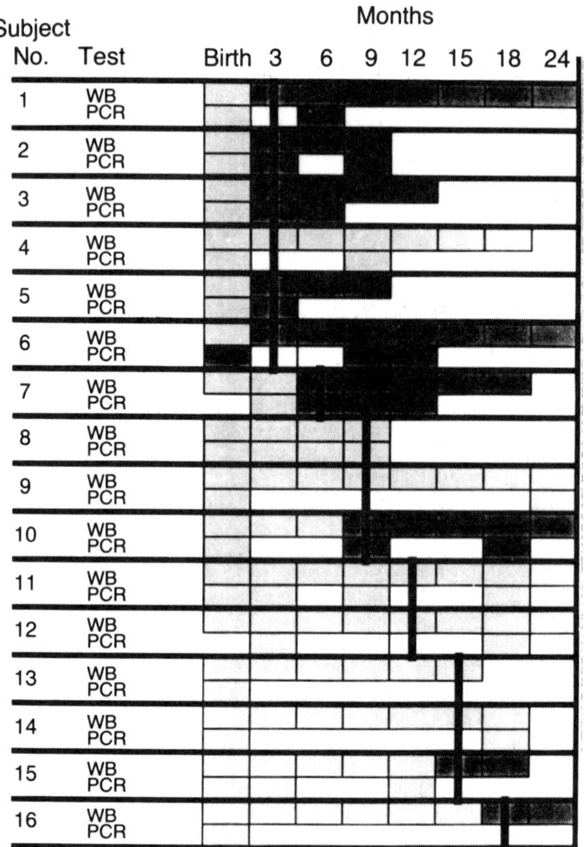

Fig 11–3.—Sequential results of HIV serologic tests and PCR in 16 infants born to mothers who seroconverted. Lightly shaded boxes indicate a negative test, and heavily shaded boxes, positive test. For all infants, PCR was performed at birth or at age 3 months, before the mother's seroconversion. In addition, sequential mononuclear cell samples were available for analysis by PCR for some infants. Subjects were numbered according to the time of the mother's seroconversion, as indicated by *wide vertical bars*. *Abbreviation:* WB, Western blot assay. (Courtesy of Van de Perre P, Simonon A, Msellati P, et al: *N Engl J Med* 325:593–598, 1991.)

assays for antibodies to HIV-1 and testing of mononuclear cells by a double polymerase chain reaction (PCR) involving 3 sets of primers. Each mother who seroconverted was matched with 3 seronegative control women.

Results.—At a mean follow-up of 16.6 months, 16 mothers became seropositive for HIV-1. Nine of their infants became seropositive. One of these infants was excluded from further analysis because of a positive test on the blood sample taken at birth. Postnatal seroconversion occurred in 4 of the 5 infants born to mothers who seroconverted in the first 3 months after delivery and in 4 infants of 10 mothers who seroconverted between 4 and 21 months (Fig 11–3). Infants seroconverted in the same 3-month period as the mothers in all cases. Being single was the main risk factor for maternal seroconversion.

Conclusion.—Mothers may transmit HIV-1 infection to their infants during the postnatal period. Colostrum and breast milk many be efficient routes of transmission from recently infected mothers to their infants.

▶ This prospective study, conducted in Central Africa with the support of the AIDS Task Force of the European Economic Community, provides important information that tends to cast postpartum horizontal transmission of HIV as a greater concern than was previously thought (see the 1991 YEAR BOOK OF OBSTETRICS AND GYNECOLOGY, pp 199–200). Additionally, it suggests that polymerase chain reaction (PCR) in newborn blood may be a less important approach to the study of the epidemiology of this disease than was earlier envisioned (see the 1990 YEAR BOOK OF OBSTETRICS AND GYNECOLOGY, pp 66–67). The cases of special interest include the 16 women who converted from negative to positive HIV-antibody status after delivery and 9 of their 16 infants who seroconverted after birth. In only 1 of those 9 cases was PCR useful in demonstrating viral infection not demonstrated by Western blot. That finding was useful in establishing case number 6 as a situation in which antepartum vertical infection occurred in an infected woman without HIV-antibody response during pregnancy. In 4 of 9 cases of postpartum infant infection, that is 44% of the total, based on seroconversion at or after 6 months of life; there is strong suggestive evidence for external environmental infection. The probable—but not certain—source was virus borne in the cellular components of breast milk. However important they may be, the findings rest with very few cases.

It is comforting to realize that all that's known of AIDS epidemiology need not be redone using PCR to augment the viral DNA present in the blood of subjects to the point of discernment by other techniques. This study will lend imperativeness to the need to interdict nursing by women who are AIDS antibody positive, and to expand the number of studied cases of newborn seroconversion beyond those reported here.—T.H. Kirschbaum, M.D.

Incidence of Intrauterine Cocaine Exposure in a Suburban Setting

Schutzman DL, Frankenfield-Chernicoff M, Clatterbaugh HE, Singer J (Mercy Catholic Med Ctr, Darby, Pa)

Pediatrics 88:825–827, 1991 11–9

Introduction.—The incidence of cocaine use in pregnant women is increasing. The incidence of intrauterine cocaine exposure in a socioeconomically mixed suburban setting was determined, and the effectiveness of an anonymous questionnaire in eliciting information on maternal use of illicit drugs during pregnancy was evaluated.

Methods.—Between February and May 1990, meconium was collected from 500 consecutively born infants and analyzed for the presence of benzoylecgonine, the primary metabolite of cocaine. An anonymous 2-page questionnaire was distributed to all postpartum mothers.

Results.—Of the infants, 59 (11.8%) tested positive for cocaine, including 23 (6.3%) whose mothers had private insurance and 36 (26.9%) whose mothers had no insurance or were covered by Medicaid. The questionnaires were returned by 316 (75.4%) of 419 mothers, including 73.4% with private insurance and 26.4% who had no insurance or were covered by Medicaid. None of the mothers with private insurance and only 5 of the mothers with no insurance or who were covered by Medicaid admitted using cocaine. If the questionnaires had been answered truthfully, 15 mothers with private insurance and 23 mothers with Medicaid or no insurance would have admitted to using cocaine.

Conclusion.—Intrauterine cocaine exposure may be a much more serious problem than was previously thought, not only in the inner city but also in the suburbs. Anonymous maternal self-reporting through a questionnaire is not effective in identifying infants who are at risk for illicit exposure to drugs.

▶ This study documents both the high incidence of cocaine use in pregnancy (even in nonmetropolitan areas) and its vast underreporting (even when anonymity is offered). Newborn drug screening from voided meconium has the advantage of offering access to long-term screening for drug use, because it may reflect drug exposure many weeks before birth (see Abstract 10–1). There is a good likelihood that some of the underreporting here may have come from women who, because they had not used cocaine in the 24 hours before testing, may have believed that earlier drug use could not be detected. The failure of reporting by all 23 cocaine users with private insurance, by 86% of the 36 cocaine users without insurance, plus the roughly 12% overall incidence of cocaine use makes a strong argument for routine newborn drug testing for narcotic exposure in contemporary America.—T.H. Kirschbaum, M.D.

Tentorial Subdural Hemorrhage in Term Newborns: Ultrasonographic Diagnosis and Clinical Correlates

Huang C-C, Shen E-Y (Natl Cheng Kung Univ Hosp, Tainan, Taiwan; Mackay Mem Hosp, Tainan, Taiwan)

Pediatr Neurol 7:171–177, 1991 11–10

Background.—Tentorial tearing is a common cause of subdural hemorrhage in the newborn period. Such tearing, which causes the underlying sinus or bridging veins to rupture, may result from abnormal pressure exerted by vacuum, forceps, or breech presentation on the molded skull during delivery.

Patients and Outcomes.—In 9 term newborns, cranial ultrasonography and CT were used to diagnose tentorial subdural hemorrhage with its supratentorial and infratentorial extensions. In 6 cases, vacuum extraction or forceps were used for delivery. In 8 patients, abnormal neurological manifestations appeared after a period of normality. The most common presentation was increased intracranial pressure. All patients had bleeding at the falcotentorial junction near the incisura. Five also had bleeding around the tentorial leaflet. Posterior fossa retrocerebellar subdural hemorrhage occurred in 5 patients. Posterior interhemispheric subdural hemorrhage developed in 4. All 6 patients treated conservatively had normal neurodevelopmental outcomes. The other 3 underwent suboccipital craniotomies, and only 1 of the 3 had a normal outcome. Although ultrasonography localized the tentorial subdural hemorrhage at the incisura area or tentorial leaflet, it did not identify all patients with retrocerebellar or posterior interhemispheric subdural hemorrhage.

Conclusion.—Ultrasonography and CT are complementary in the diagnosis of tentorial subdural hemorrhage in term newborns. Surgical decompression of the posterior fossa subdural hematoma is needed only when acute hydrocephalus or signs of brain stem compression are present.

▶ There are several surprises here, especially for those who believe that rupture of the great Galen vein is a priori evidence of birth trauma. In 3 of 9 cases, the injury followed spontaneous vaginal delivery of infants weighing from 2,600 to 3,000 g, and in 1 case, vacuum extraction of an infant weighing 3,600 g at 42 weeks. Such findings suggest that subdural hemorrhage may be considerably underdiagnosed. Apgar scores were normal, with only 1 case with an Apgar score less than 7 at 1 minute and no cases with an Apgar less than 8 at 5 minutes. Six of 9 infants were neurodevelopmentally normal on follow-up. Both ultrasound and CT appear necessary for evaluation, although CT is preferable for detection. Ultrasound, despite its high false negative rates, is useful for localization. Because their results with conservative, nonsurgical management were so good, the authors believe surgical evacuation is warranted only for acute hydrocephalus and brain stem herniation.—T.H. Kirschbaum, M.D.

Lack of Evidence of Vertical Transmission of Human Immunodeficiency Virus Type 2 in a Sample of the General Population in Bissau

Poulsen A-G, Kvinesdal BB, Aaby P, Lisse IM, Gottschau A, Mølbak K, Dias F, Lauritzen E (Univ of Copenhagen; Hvidovre Hosp, Copenhagen; Laboratório Nacional de Saúde Publica, Bissau, Guinnea-Bissau)

J Acquir Immune Defic Syndr 5:25–30, 1992 11–11

Background.—Human immunodeficiency virus type 2 (HIV-2), found primarily in West Africa, is assumed to be transmitted like HIV-1, by sexual contact, blood contact, and from mother to child during pregnancy or delivery. A previous study (begun in 1987) of the epidemiology of HIV in Guinea-Bissau was unable to document vertical transmission of HIV-2, despite a high prevalence among the adult population and positive findings for heterosexual transmission and transmission by blood transfusion. Vertical transmission of HIV-2 was investigated further.

Methods.—Twenty-nine HIV-2 seropositive women in Bissau were each matched for age and marital status with 2 HIV-2 seronegative women. The clinical and pregnancy histories of the 2 groups were compared. Western blot and enzyme-linked immunosorbent assays for HIV-1 and HIV-2 antibodies were performed on serum samples. Lymphocytes were assessed for the presence of CD4 and CD8 by immunocytochemical labeling.

Results.—Seropositive women had a mean age of 39.7 years; seronegative women had a mean age of 40.2 years. The 2 groups were similar as to the total number of pregnancies, live children, dead children, and abortions. Both groups had the same risk of having had at least 1 abortion or 1 dead child. Children from HIV-2 seropositive and seronegative mothers had no significant differences in mortality. Significantly more HIV-2 seropositive women had lower T-helper cell number and H/S ratios than HIV-2 seronegative women, but none was severely immunodeficient. Seven children born to seropositive women were not born with detectable HIV-2 infection. Based in part on retrospectively identified children of HIV-2 infected mothers, a rough estimate of the rate of vertical transmission was 0% to 4%.

Conclusion.—Among these Guinean women, little evidence of vertical transmission of HIV-2 was found. This may be because of the specific biological properties of HIV-2 or the absence of disease and immunodeficiency in this population.

▶ The demonstration of a second HIV type (HIV-2) has raised the spector of a double-barreled attack by this extraordinarily dangerous class of infectious agent. There are many structural similarities between HIV-1 and HIV-2, as marked by the roughly 50% nucleotide sequence homology and cross-reactivity with viral envelope and, particularly, core antigens. This paper, however, is representative of the emerging evidence for sharp epidemiological differences between HIV types 1 and 2. In nearly 50 cases of HIV-2 seropositive women, no instances of viral transmission to the fetus occurred, and passive maternal antibody transfer appears to be uncommon, with more rapid disappearance of passively transferred antibody than is the case with HIV-1. This good news appears to stem from the lesser degree of immune inhibition that occurs with HIV-2 compared with the earlier recognized HIV-1. Should this viral strain appear in this country in considerable numbers, it will apparently be easier to deal with than HIV-1.—T.H. Kirschbaum, M.D.

Cocaine/Polydrug Use in Pregnancy: Two-Year Follow-Up

Chasnoff IJ, Griffith DR, Freier C, Murray J (Northwestern Univ, Chicago;

Natl Association for Perinatal Addiction Research and Education, Chicago)
Pediatrics 89:284–289, 1992 11–12

Background.—It is generally agreed that cocaine use in pregnancy increases the risk of maternal and fetal/neonatal complications. The data on the long-term outcome of affected neonates are conflicting, however, as to whether there are permanent effects on growth. The growth and developmental outcome of infants exposed to cocaine in utero was assessed after 2 years of follow-up.

Methods.—A total of 106 infants born to women who used cocaine, and usually also marijuana, alcohol, or tobacco, were compared with 45 infants born to mothers who used marijuana and/or alcohol but no cocaine, and to 81 infants born to mothers who did not use illicit drugs or alcohol. All mothers had similar racial and demographic characteristics and received prenatal care as part of a therapeutic drug treatment program. Neonates were examined blindly for weight, length, head circumference, and on the Bayley Scales of Infant Development at 3, 6, 12, 18, and 24 months of age.

Results.—At birth, the cocaine-exposed infants had reductions in weight, length, and head circumference; however, after birth, cocaine-exposed infants recovered growth. At 3 months of age, the mean length of cocaine-exposed infants was similar to that of the other groups. At 1 year of age, the cocaine-exposed infants had also caught up to the other infants in weight. Head circumference in both drug-exposed groups remained less than in the control group at 2 years after birth. No significant differences were found on the Bayley Scales of Infant Development among the groups through 2 years of age. In infants between 12 and 24 months of age, head size was significantly correlated with Bayley developmental scores. During the first 12 months of life, cocaine exposure was the best predictor of reduced head circumference.

Conclusion.—Intrauterine exposure to cocaine appears to reduce head growth at least through 2 years of age, and head growth seems correlated with developmental outcome. Although no significant effect of cocaine use was seen in infants' development using the Bayley scales, they may not provide an accurate assessment of the problems of cocaine-exposed infants.

▶ This is a very clear demonstration of the role of intrauterine drug exposure on some objective elements of the infant function. It's important to point out that multiple drug exposure was the selection factor in this study (alcohol, tobacco, marijuana), that the newborn results with or without cocaine against that background are not much different, and that the differences rest between drug-free pregnancy and that associated with multiple drug use. The principle defects are reduced head circumference manifest from the 24th week of pregnancy and retardation in mental and psychomotor development that reaches statistical significance at 6 months of age. Thereafter, catch-up growth and development follows as environmental variables begin to correct the defects of intrauterine life. This is about as far as one can go with developmental studies of pregnancy influences. Any more lasting effects that exist are likely to be swamped by the enormous diversity of environmental determinants of subsequent growth and development in the infant past the age of 2–3 years.—T.H. Kirschbaum, M.D.

Incidence and Neurodevelopmental Outcome of Periventricular Hemorrhage and Hydrocephalus in a Regional Population of Very Low Birth Weight Infants

Hanigan WC, Morgan AM, Anderson RJ, Bradle P, Cohen HS, Cusack TJ, Thomas-McCauley T, Miller TC (Univ of Illinois College of Medicine at Peoria; Univ of Illinois College of Medicine, Chicago; Univ of Cincinnati Med Ctr)
Neurosurgery 29:701–706, 1991 11–13

Introduction.—Beginning in January 1984, very-low-birth-weight (VLBW) infants admitted to a state-designated Level III Neonatal Intensive Care Unit underwent cerebral sonographic evaluation. The incidence of periventricular hemorrhage (PVH) and hydrocephalus in infants admitted in 1984–1987 was assessed, and their neurodevelopmental outcomes were reviewed.

Methods.—Cerebral sonography was performed in a standardized sequence and graded with the Papile scale. The term VLBW included infants who weighed 1,500 g or less at the time of admission to the neonatal intensive care unit. All VLBW infants discharged from the unit were scheduled for multidisciplinary follow-up evaluation at approximately 6 months, 12 months and, when possible, at 3 years corrected age.

Results.—Of 2,525 infants admitted to the neonatal intensive care unit, 459 were VLBW. The finding of PVH in these infants decreased from a peak of 26.6% in 1985 to 16.4% in 1987. The mortality rate in VLBW infants with PVH decreased from a peak of 11 (47.8%) in 1984 to 4 (19%) in 1987. The primary cause of death for all VLBW infants was respiratory insufficiency and/or sepsis, not PVH. Follow-up data were obtained for 66 of the 69 VLBW infants with PVH who survived initial hospitalization. Only 1 of 16 VLBW infants with high-grade PVH had normal motor and cognitive development. All grades of PVH were associated with an increased risk of abnormal neurodevelopmental outcome.

Conclusion.—The decrease in the incidence and mortality of VLBW infants with PVH was associated with an increase in the incidence of inborn VLBW infants. Hydrocephalus developed in 15.8% of the VLBW infants with PVH who survived initial hospitalization. The developmental prognosis for these infants was poor, despite measures to control intracranial pressure.

► This 4-year experience in infants weighing less than 1,500 g portrays a worst-case picture of the consequences of intraventricular hemorrhage (IVH). Even within this weight range, the relationship of low birth weight to impaired function is apparent. In this population of 459 infants, 97 showed ultrasonic evidence of IVH, 28 of whom expired. With only minor hemorrhage (Papile grade I–II) only 25% showed distinct developmental abnormality after 3 years' follow-up. Its a major strength of this study that such an extended follow-up was possible in 95.7% of the children. With high grade (Papile III) IVH, the picture is catastrophic. Only 1 of 16 children was developmentally normal, and 75% were frankly abnormal at 3 years of age. The overall incidence of hydrocephalus was 15.8%. Approximately one fourth of all IVHs in surviving VLBW infants were of the high grade type. Although this unit and many others report improving statistics in recent years, the hazards of being born VLBW are very clear in this study.—T.H. Kirschbaum, M.D.

Early Diagnosis of Perinatal HIV Infection by Detection of Viral-Specific IgA Antibodies

Quinn TC, Kline RL, Halsey N, Hutton N, Ruff A, Butz A, Boulos R, Medlin JF (Natl Inst of Allergy and Infectious Diseases, Bethesda, Md; Johns Hopkins Univ, Baltimore, Md; et al)

JAMA 266:3439–3442, 1991 11–14

Introduction.—More than 3 million women of reproductive age are infected with HIV, and many live in developing countries. A major problem in the diagnosis of the children born to them is the lack of a dependable IgG antibody assay for HIV. The results were examined of a clinical study of the use of HIV-IgA serological assay in the diagnosis of HIV among infants delivered of women who were HIV positive from the United States and Haiti.

Methods.—The serum from 116 children born to HIV-positive women at the Johns Hopkins Hospital in the United States and from 62 similar

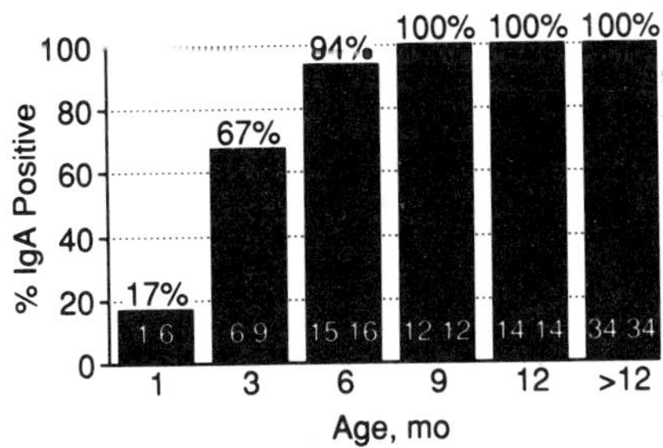

Fig 11–4.—The percentage of HIV-infected children who were positive for IgA antibodies to HIV-specific proteins by age of serum sample collection in 47 children with perinatally acquired HIV infection. *The numbers within each bar* represent the number of children who were IgA-HIV positive compared with the number of HIV-infected children tested during that time period. (Courtesy of Quinn TC, Kline RL, Halsey N, et al: *JAMA* 266:3439–3442, 1991.)

children born in Port-au-Prince, Haiti, underwent HIV testing with a human IgA antibody test. Serum samples from 42 Haitian infants born to women who were HIV seronegative also were studied. The results of this HIV-IgA blood test were then compared with the outcome of the standard IgG Western blot analysis and the clinical diagnosis of the Centers for Disease Control.

Results.—Results of the HIV-IgA assay showed 71 of 116 children as HIV seronegative and clinically HIV negative and 34 as HIV seropositive. Of the 152 samples from children who were HIV seropositive, 145 samples were IgA positive. All 119 samples from the patients who were HIV seronegative resulted in a negative IgA test. Of the 7 children who were HIV-positive with a negative IgA outcome, all had had samples taken before 6 months of age. Of the 162 infants born to HIV-positive women in Port-au-Prince, Haiti, 130 were serologically and clinically HIV negative. Four of the children from Haiti had at least 1 sample that was IgA discordant with the clinical diagnosis. The sensitivity and specificity for the IgA assay for the combined results from American and Haitian children were 97.6% and 99.7%, respectively. Only 1 sample that was IgA HIV positive was taken within the first month of life (Fig 11–4).

Conclusion.—The HIV IgA assay has a high sensitivity, specificity, and prognostic value for those children sampled after the first few months of life. Because the early diagnosis of the HIV infection in children remains exceedingly important in avoiding opportunistic infections, this rapid, less costly, and simple assay can aid in the care of these children at risk.

▶ This study offers considerable help in the matter of differentiating passive from active newborn IgG to HIV-1 in infants born of HIV-1 antibody-positive mothers. Previous studies have shown that newborn IgG passively transferred to the fetus takes 15–24 months to disappear from newborn blood (see the 1990 Year Book of Obstetrics and Gynecology, p 196, 207; and the 1991 Year Book of Obstetrics and Gynecology, p 96). The variability in duration depends on the degree of certainty of the absence of type I error that is posited in the analysis. However, IgA-HIV exists in large dimeric or trimeric aggregates that preclude placental transfer and passive fetal immunization. This class of antibody, which is involved in membrane immunoreactivity and antibody secretion, apparently is not important in the biology of HIV infection. However, when it appears past 3 months of age, it serves as a useful indicator of active infant immunoreactivity and, therefore, presumably infection. For infants at risk, this means shortening the interval of uncertainty by nearly a year through the demonstration of IgA to HIV in infant blood. This constitutes a major contribution to the medical and social implications of the dreadful problem of judging, as quickly as possible, the presence of newborn infection from this virus.—T.H. Kirschbaum, M.D.

Comparison of Maternal and Newborn Serologic Tests for Syphilis

Rawstron SA, Bromberg K (Children's Med Ctr of Brooklyn, NY; State Univ of

New York, Brooklyn)
Am J Dis Child 145:1383–1388, 1991 11–15

Introduction.—New York State has recently experienced a significant increase in congenital syphilis, which prompted the state health agency to require cord blood syphilis testing for all infants. Because only anecdotal evidence and a few studies have been reported on the correlation between maternal syphilis and cord blood disease, the results of using cord blood, newborn serum, and maternal serum for the diagnosis of congenital syphilis were compared.

Methods.—A rapid plasma reagin (RPR) test was used on neonate cord blood and maternal serum to determine the presence of syphilis. If the patient or newborn had a positive RPR, a fluorescent treponemal antibody absorption test was performed. The records of all patients with RPR-positive results were reviewed for the present study. Congenital syphilis was defined by using presumptive categories.

Results.—Of the 9,421 births during a 22-month period, 429 (5%) of the mother-infant pairs had a positive RPR test result for either one of the pair. A total of 348 pairs were analyzed. The results were RPR positive for both cord and maternal serum in 226 (65%) pairs, but only 95 of 171 newborn serum samples tested positive when the maternal serum had a positive RPR outcome also. Eighty-seven of 171 samples of both newborn cord blood and newborn serum were RPR positive, whereas 115 infants' cord blood did not react in the RPR test when the maternal serum tested positive. However, 7 infants had RPR-positive cord blood when the mother had RPR nonreactive results. Among the 348 maternal-newborn pairs with available cord and maternal samples, 33 newborns had congenital syphilis (4 confirmed and 29 presumptive). Twenty-nine infants had RPR-positive cord blood results, and 4 had RPR-nonresponsive cord blood at birth. Among the mother-infant pairs that tested positive, 7 infants had cord serum syphilis titers 4 times greater than the maternal sample at delivery; however, only 4 of these newborns had congenital syphilis.

Conclusion.—Maternal serum provides a better material than newborn serum for the identification of infants at risk for congenital syphilis. Screening of the women and their infants at birth for syphilis to identify all those at risk for this disease is advocated.

▶ The increasing incidence of congenital syphilis has stimulated increasing concern for the means by which the diagnosis can be made as early after birth as possible. The easy availability of cord blood makes it a popular testing substrate but, as this study shows, it's often misleading. In this 22 months' experience, the incidence of RPR-positive samples in either, or both, mother and fetus was 4.5%. Of the 81% of such cases with adequate records, discordant RPR and fluorescent titer antibody absorption occurred in 3.7%. Of those, one third of the infants born of mothers who were RPR positive were RPR negative. In 7 cases (2%), RPR-positive infants had mothers who were RPR negative. However, three fourths of these latter 7 PRP-positive infants proved to be RPR negative on retesting. There were 4 confirmed congenital leutic children (based on identification of *Treponema pallidum*) and 29 presumptive diagnoses. Four of these 23 infants had RPR-negative cord serum. Compared with newborn serum, cord serum had a false positive RPR rate of 10% and a false negative rate of 5%. These results make it clear that the diagnosis of congenital syphilis is best based on maternal and neonatal serum, together with physical and other laboratory examination of the newborn. Cord blood results made be confirmatory, but they are a tenuous basis on which to make this important diagnosis.—T.H. Kirschbaum, M.D.

Outcome of Confirmed Symptomatic Congenital Cytomegalovirus Infection

Ramsay MEB, Miller E, Peckham CS (PHLS Communicable Disease Surveillance Ctr; Inst of Child Health, London)

Arch Dis Child 66:1068–1069, 1991 11–16

Introduction.—The outcome of symptomatic congenital cytomegalovirus infection was prospectively determined in 65 children and correlated with specific neonatal signs and symptoms.

Methods.—Only those infants in whom cytomegalovirus was isolated or specific IgM was detected before age 21 days and with signs consistent with congenital cytomegalovirus infection in the first 4 weeks of life were studied. The median patient age at follow-up was 3.5 years (range, 1–6.4 years).

Results.—In 29 (45%) children, there was definite neurological impairment, including 22 (34%) with gross motor or psychomotor problems and 7 (11%) with sensorineural deafness. Definite handicap was present in 16 (73%) of 22 infants with abnormal neurological signs in the neonatal period, 13 (37%) of 35 infants with hepatomegaly, splenomegaly, or purpura but no neurological signs in the neonatal period, and none of the 8 infants with microcephaly and/or respiratory problems and without neurological signs in the neonatal period.

Conclusion.—The prognosis of infants with symptomatic congenital cytomegalovirus infection is better than previously reported. The prognosis is worse for infants with neurological signs in the neonatal period, but is relatively good among infants with respiratory problems or microcephaly.

▶ This follow-up of neonates with evidence of cytomegalovirus (CMV) infection within the first 21 days of life should be compared with an earlier study from the CMV Study Group at Birmingham, Alabama (1). The current cases were drawn from reports of the Communicable Disease Surveillance Centre for England and Wales from 1983 to 1987. Of 125 such cases, there was

54% follow-up for 3–4 years. The American series stemmed from referrals and primary case findings in a very large comprehensive research program in Alabama. Because only symptomatic infants were reported in the 1980 American study, the 8 asymptomatic group 3 infants must be omitted from the comparison.

Whereas the death rate in the Alabama experience is 29%, it is not possible to discern the infant death rate in cases reported from London. The American data indicate that only 10% of symptomatic neonates were without handicap, whereas the English report 50% without abnormality. The difference rests with the evaluation of isolated microcephaly, which Ramsay et al. did not include as a definite handicap. If the 16 cases were listed as significant abnormalities, the total figure for significantly damaged infants became 78% for the London series, which was not much less than the 90% American figure. In either cases, symptomatic CMV infection at birth presages a small chance for intact survival as measured at 4 years of age.—T.H. Kirschbaum, M.D.

Reference

1. Pass RF, et al: *Pediatrics* 66:758, 1980.

12 Fetal Therapy

In-Utero Transplantation of Fetal Liver Stem Cells Into Human Fetuses

Touraine J-L (Hôpital Edouard Herriot, Lyon, France)
Hum Reprod 7:44–48, 1992 12–1

Introduction.—The postnatal transplantation of fetal liver cells, alone or combined with syngeneic fetal thymic cells, can fully restore immunological function to patients with severe combined immunodeficiency disease, and it can improve other patients with various congenital or hematological disorders. The procedure is especially useful when a compatible donor is unavailable to provide a marrow transplant.

Patients.—Three fetuses, 2 with severe immunodeficiency disease and 1 with thalassemia major, received transplants of human fetal liver stem cells in utero. Both fetuses with immunodeficiency disease were diagnosed in midgestation, and the fetus with thalassemia was treated at 12 fertilization weeks.

Results.—All transplant procedures were followed by engraftment, and there were no adverse effects. One of the infants with immunodeficiency disease had cell-mediated immunity restored and is living normally at home. The other infant and the infant with thalassemia, treated more recently, have not yet exhibited a complete effect. The latter infant has received a single transfusion and has a total level of hemoglobin slightly below normal.

Implication.—These cases demonstrate the feasibility of in utero fetal liver transplantation and provide hope for significant improvement in patients with a wide range of inherited disorders.

▶ This extraordinary paper points the way to a new chapter in fetal therapy and underlines the urgent need for research in the biology of fetal tissue transplantation, which has been precluded by misguided actions of this country's federal executive. Fetal transplantation of fetal liver and thymic stromal cells have the advantage of eluding rejection reactions, which are primitive if operative at all in fetuses of the second trimester. Furthermore, the slow growth of ingrafted cells takes place in several weeks in utero, a residence that is far superior to the best plastic bubble ever devised.

These 3 exploratory cases represent attempts of intact survival in which the only other management options were abortion or neonatal death. The diagnosis of severe congenital immunodeficiency disease was made in 2 cases when cordocentesis demonstrated fetal lymphocytes with major histocompatibility complexes lacking—in one case, both HLA class I and II antigens (absent T- and B-cell activity, respectively)—and absent T-cell immunoreactivity. In the first case, a single in utero transplant appears to have produced a fine response, albeit 16 months of isolation were needed after delivery until sufficient IgM and IgG production took place. In the second case, engraftment took place, but adequate cellular immunity had not developed at the time of the report. In the third case, sufficient production of hemoglobin A resulted from transplantation at 14 weeks' menstrual gestational age to result in an infant with β-thalassemia major who is normal to 1 year of age.

These preliminary findings point to the possibility that a wide range of inherited disorders of metabolism and hematological development may be cured or vastly improved by the application of in utero grafting of fetal stem cells in the second trimester of pregnancy.—T.H. Kirschbaum, M.D.

Fetal Surgery for Cleft Lip: A Plea for Caution

Longaker MT, Whitby DJ, Adzick NS, Kaban LB, Harrison MR (Univ of California, San Francisco)

Plast Reconstr Surg 88:1087–1092, 1991 12–2

Background.—Members of the Fetal Treatment Program at the University of California, San Francisco, have performed fetal surgery in only 27 of more than 300 potential candidates since 1981. Although there is considerable interest in correcting congenital defects in utero, the benefits of fetal surgery remain unproven. Findings from previous fetal surgery experience were applied to fetal surgery for cleft lip and palate repair.

Patients and History.—The 27 fetuses operated on ranged from 18–28 weeks' gestation. All had life-threatening anatomical malformations, including severe bilateral obstructive uropathy (9), congenital diaphragmatic hernia (15), congenital cystic adenomatoid malformation of the lung (2), and sacrococcygeal teratoma (1). Attempts at fetal surgery were preceded by more than 1,000 operations on pregnant sheep and monkeys. After more than a decade of experimental studies, guidelines were established that weighed the potential benefits of surgery against maternal and fetal risks.

Risks of Fetal Surgery.—The principal risk in open fetal surgery is to the mother. Although there has been no maternal mortality or significant long-term morbidity in this study, preterm labor has been a persistent problem with all cases. Another concern is the effect of surgery on the mother's fertility and ability to carry further pregnancies.

Fetal Surgery for Cleft Lip and Palate.—Because facial clefts may be associated with severe abnormalities incompatible with life, the natural history of fetuses with clefting diagnosed in utero may differ from that of infants with clefting diagnosed at birth. Thus, it is important for other severe abnormalities to be ruled out before proceeding with fetal surgery. Animal models do not prove that in utero surgery allows complete correction of cleft lip and palate.

Conclusion.—Based on the fact that fetal surgery for cleft lip and palate repair carries the same risks as surgery for lethal conditions, the procedure is not recommended at the present time. The benefit of scarless healing appears insufficient when weighed against the potential risks.

▶ Fetal wounds differ from those of the adult in the pattern of collagenous deposition and the repair that follows. In the fetus, collagen is formed in a reticular pattern that leaves, at most, only an epithelial depression and, in hair-bearing areas, an absence of follicles as a residuum of wound healing. In the adult, the densely packed complex bundles of newly formed collagen leave the possibility of scar formation and distortion of the adjoining tissue through retraction. The appeal of fetal surgery for the repair of fusion defects of the lips and palate is obvious, because it would avoid the scarring that often compromises surgery carried out on the infant.

The author who had led the active Fetal Treatment Program as senior surgeon raises some appropriate questions from his extensive experience and lists the 5 criteria his group uses in considering fetal surgery. His concerns are with justifying the maternal risks (including preterm labor) for a nonlethal fetal condition, the difficulty in excluding related anomalies that may be severe, and the lack of development of a satisfactory animal model on which the surgical details and experience may be based. This study is an important set of concepts and a fine review of the state of the art by one of its premier performers.—T.H. Kirschbaum, M.D.

Fetal Supraventricular Tachycardia and Hydrops Fetalis: Combined Intensive, Direct, and Transplacental Therapy

Hallak M, Neerhof MG, Perry R, Nazir M, Huhta JC (Pennsylvania Hosp, Philadelphia)

Obstet Gynecol 78:523–525, 1991 12–3

Background.—The mortality rate in nonimmune hydrops fetalis is high, but one of the more treatable causes of the condition is tachydysrhythmia. Depending on the gestational age at diagnosis, intrauterine treatment seems warranted. The case of an infant survived after treatment with digoxin and procainamide was reviewed.

Case Report.—Woman, 30, was referred at 25 weeks' gestation because of fetal tachycardia and hydrops fetalis. Ultrasound revealed no anatomical abnormalities in the fetus. Echocardiography showed supraventricular tachycardia of 270 beats per minute with 1:1 atrioventricular conduction and a mildly dilated right atrium. The fetal heart rate remained high after digoxin was administered intravenously to the mother at .5 mg every 6 hours for 24 hours. A decision thus was made to start fetal therapy. The fetus received, by intramuscular injection, a total of 20 μg of digoxin in 3 divided doses at 8-hour intervals for the next 24 hours. Improvement was seen within 1 hour, and oral therapy to the mother then was continued. Procainamide was added to the regimen 2 weeks later when severe hydrops fetalis persisted. It took 7 weeks for the hydrops to resolve completely. Labor was induced at 36 weeks' gestation, and a male infant was delivered. Although there was no evidence of hydrops at birth, the infant later had recurrent supraventricular tachycardia. At 6 months, he still required digoxin for control of the condition.

Conclusion.—Direct fetal therapy is of value in some cases of fetal tachycardia and hydrops fetalis. Maternal treatment also is required, and the infant may need further digoxin therapy after delivery.

▶ Information is continuing to evolve in this area of placental-mediated treatment of fetal supraventricular tachycardia with digoxin, ever since the uncertain effectiveness of this approach was first noted here (see the 1987 YEAR BOOK OF OBSTETRICS AND GYNECOLOGY, pp 150–151). Few, if any, have reported the good results attained by Kleinman and associates (see the 1988 YEAR BOOK OF OBSTETRICS AND GYNECOLOGY, p 215). Several reports like this one have, through percutaneous umbilical blood (PUB) sampling, reported evidence of variable and, at times, poor placental transfer of digoxin from mother to fetus in the human. Because many of these cases involved instances of hydrops fetalis, providing the rationale for PUB, fetal cardiovascular failure, and/or placental cotyledonary edema may be the problem. These authors point to fetal intramuscular digoxin as a way out in this remarkable case in which recovery from severe hydrops took place over 7 weeks. Only when it becomes possible to measure placental permeability in the human in vivo (flux per unit concentration gradient, placental surface area, and membrane thickness) will it become possible to show that the diffusion coefficient is decreased with placental hydrops and will we fully understand this transfer problem.—T.H. Kirschbaum, M.D.

Clinical Outcome of Fetal Uropathy. I: Predictive Value of Prenatal Echography Positive for Obstructive Uropathy

Paduano L, Giglio L, Bembi B, Peratoner L, D'Ottavio G, Benussi G (Istituto per l'Infanzia "Burlo Garofolo", Trieste, Italy)

J Urol 146:1094–1096, 1991 12–4

Objective.—The diagnostic accuracy of prenatal echography positive for obstructive uropathy was evaluated in 73 neonates.

Methods.—Postnatal echography usually was performed on day 3 or 4 of life. Neonates with positive findings were investigated further with excretory urography and voiding cystourethrography, and those with negative findings underwent a second echography after 2 months.

Outcome.—Forty-two neonates had prenatal suspicion of unilateral hydronephrosis, but postnatal studies showed obstructive uropathy in 15 and multicystic dysplastic kidneys in 2. Ten patients had prenatal suspicion of bilateral hydronephrosis; however, only 1 had true bilateral obstruction, and 2 had unilateral obstruction on postnatal studies. In addition, 1 had multicystic dysplastic kidney, 1 had bilateral cystic dysplasia, and 2 had massive bilateral vesicoureteral reflux. Of the 8 patients with prenatal suspicion of cystic disease, postnatal evaluation showed obstructive uropathy in 2, multicystic dysplastic kidney in 2, and simple renal cyst in 4. Thirteen patients had prenatal suspicion of anatomical and obstructive abnormalities, but a definitive abnormality can be established in only 8 patients. Overall, of the 52 fetuses with a prenatal suspicion of obstructive uropathy, obstructive uropathy was confirmed postnatally in only 18 patients.

Implications.—The predictive value of prenatal echography positive for obstructive uropathy is 34.6%. As a diagnostic tool for obstructive uropathy, echography has several limitations, such as its ability to detect mostly anatomical defects but not functional abnormalities, and its difficulty in differentiating between multicystic dysplastic kidney and hydronephrotic dilatation.

▶ The message here is fairly clear. Ultrasonic evaluation of the fetal urinary tract is very reliable for the diagnosis of simple or multiple cystic dysplasia and other structural abnormalities. Where it often fails is in the diagnosis of abnormal function and, in particular, urinary tract obstruction. In only 35% of cases of unilateral and 10% of bilateral fetal hydronephrosis could obstruction be confirmed after delivery. Almost 40% had normal findings or showed minor variants of normal on delivery. In only 23.3% of the infants who were of concern during fetal life was early surgical therapy ultimately required. Again, it is a rare case in which obstructive uropathy can be established in fetal life with sufficient assurance to warrant fetal intervention and therapy.—T.H. Kirschbaum, M.D.

Intrauterine Transfusion Treatment of Nonimmune Hydrops Fetalis Secondary to Human Parvovirus B19 Infection

Sahakian V, Weiner CP, Naides SJ, Williamson RA, Scharosch LL (Univ of Iowa, Iowa City)

Am J Obstet Gynecol 164:1090–1091, 1991 12–5

Introduction.—Human parvovirus B19, first identified in 1975, is the cause of a number of diseases including nonimmune hydrops fetalis. Congenital human parvovirus B19 infection resulting from aplastic anemia at 20 weeks' gestation was successfully treated with intrauterine transfusion.

Case Report.—Woman, 23, with her first pregnancy, underwent routine ultrasonography at 20 weeks. The examination revealed anhydramnios and frank anasarca characterized by subcutaneous edema, fetal ascites, and cardiomegaly with a pericardial effusion. Cordocentesis results were consistent with a viral infection. The umbilical venous pressure was elevated and indicated congestive heart failure. Intravascular transfusion therapy normalized the umbilical venous pressure and stabilized the fetal hematocrit. Two weeks later, there was clear improvement in the results of liver function studies and a decrease in the total level of IgM from 46 to 15 mg/dL. A healthy male infant was delivered at term.

Conclusion.—Recovery in a hydropic fetus after transfusion suggests that a good outcome is possible if the fetus survives the acute infectious episode. This appears to be the third fully documented case of antenatal diagnosis, treatment by intrauterine transfusion, complete resolution of hydrops, and a normal infant.

▶ This is one of several reports of successful treatment of this severe early fetal abnormality. YEAR BOOK readers have seen the rapid growth of information regarding this problem over the past 2 years (see the 1990 YEAR BOOK OF OBSTETRICS AND GYNECOLOGY, pp 59–60, 122–123; and the 1991 YEAR BOOK OF OBSTETRICS AND GYNECOLOGY, pp 88–90). Although the B19 strain has a predilection for endothelium and erythroid marrow elements, suppression of platelet and leukocyte production has increasingly been reported from fetal umbilical blood sampling of hydropic infants. The majority of such cases have been noted at 20 to 24 weeks' gestation. As in this case, fetal serum bilirubin is not elevated, nor are reticulocytes increased, denoting inhibition of erythropoesis rather than hemolysis. Although the myocardium and liver may be infected by the virus, so far there is little convincing evidence that anything other than marrow and endothelial cell damage is important as primary pathology. Fortunately, fetuses who survive the congestive heart failure apparently caused by anemic hypoxia show no apparent side effects up to 1 year of age.

Intrauterine transfusion has become the treatment of choice for fetal hydrops resulting from this agent. If transfusion takes place in the absence of extensive damage to other organs and, perhaps, at the point where, as in this case, IgM production marks the appearance of competent fetal immunological responsiveness, it may well lead to a subsequently normal infant. The risk of maternal to fetal transmission of virus to the point of clear clinical findings appears to be approximately 10% to 15%.—T.H. Kirschbaum, M.D.

In Vivo Transfer of the Human Cystic Fibrosis Transmembrane Conductance Regulator Gene to the Airway Epithelium

Rosenfeld MA, Yoshimura K, Trapnell BC, Yoneyama K, Rosenthal ER, Dalemans W, Fukayama M, Bargon J, Stier LE, Stratford-Perricaudet L, Perricaudet M, Guggino WB, Pavirani A, Lecocq J-P, Crystal RG (Natl Heart, Blood, and Lung Inst, Bethesda, Md; Transgene SA, Strasbourg, Institut Gustave Roussy, Villejuif Cedex, France; Johns Hopkins School of Med, Baltimore)
Cell 68:143–155, 1992 12–6

Background.—Cystic fibrosis (CF) is a common, lethal, recessive hereditary disorder. Its manifestations predominantly are abnormalities of the airway epithelial surface. The gene responsible for CF is the CF transmembrane conductance regulator (CFTR) gene, which is localized on chromosome 7 at q31. Direct transfer of the normal CFTR gene to airway epithelium was studied.

Methods and Results.—A replication-deficient recombinant adenovirus (Ad) vector containing normal human CFTR cDNA (Ad-CFTR) was used to assess direct transfer. In vitro Ad-CFTR–infected CFPAC-1 CF epithelial cells expressed human CFTR mRNA and protein. Correction of defective cyclic adenosine monophosphate–mediated $C1^-$ permeability was demonstrated. Two days after in vivo intratracheal introduction of Ad-CFTR in cotton rats, human CFTR gene expression was demonstrated in lung epithelium on in situ analysis. Polymerase chain reaction amplification of reverse transcribed lung RNA showed human CFTR transcripts derived from Ad-CFTR. Northern analysis of lung RNA showed human CFTR transcripts for up to 6 weeks. With antihuman CFTR antibody, human CFTR protein was detected in epithelial cells 11–14 days after infection.

Conclusion.—In vivo CFTR gene transfer appears to be a feasible treatment for the pulmonary manifestations of CF. The safety and efficacy of this treatment have yet to be determined.

▶ This exciting study points the way to possible gene replacement therapy in human fetuses homozygous for the mutated gene causing cystic fibrosis (CFTR). In an extraordinary accomplishment, that gene has been identified on the long arm of chromosome number 7 and has been characterized (1). The normal gene regulates membrane conductants and probably represents a chloride channel activated by cyclic adenosine monophosphate. Failure of its normal expression changes the capacity of ciliated pulmonary epithelial cells to secrete a normal product. The resultant thick tenacious product, dense and adherent because of its high DNA content, results in the often lethal pulmonary problems that ensue in childhood and early adult life.

Three bits of serendipity have added to the chances of success in gene therapy for this disease. First, transfer of the normal gene product has been shown to have the capacity to override the defective chloride secretion capacity in vitro of pulmonary epithelial cells from individuals with cystic fibrosis—an uncommon event. Second, each pulmonary epithelial cell appears to contain a small number of chloride channels per cell (approximately 2), increasing the likelihood of benefit from transfection. Finally, it has been possible to complex the normal gene to an adenovirus (normally infective of pulmonary epithelium) modified to prevent its replication and production of disease. This step makes widespread dissemination of the gene-virus complex likely with bronchial installation in a fetus. Instilling the vector into the trachea of rats results in evidence of gene expression in a respiratory epithelium as judged by radioautography, in vitro hybridization to complementary probes applied to respiratory epithelium, PCR and application of human anti-CFTR antibody.

What remains is to explore the consequences of excessive gene expression in transfected cells and to develop techniques for generalized deposition of the cloned normal gene. Then, cautiously, some human trials might be done. The prospects for fetal diagnosis and gene replacement in homozygotes preventing human CF in otherwise doomed infants appears, so far, to be a possibility.—T.H. Kirschbaum, M.D.

Reference

1. Rommens JM, et al: Science 245:1059, 1989.

GYNECOLOGY

13 Operative Gynecology

Prevalence of Simple Adnexal Cysts in Postmenopausal Women

Wolf SI, Gosink BB, Feldesman MR, Lin MC, Stuenkel CA, Braly PS, Pretorius DH (Univ of California Med Ctr, San Diego; Portland State Univ, Portland, Ore)

Radiology 180:65–71, 1991 13–1

Background.—The presence of an ovarian cystic lesion in a postmenopausal woman raises suspicion of a neoplasm. However, there is as yet no systematic study defining the prevalence of simple cysts in asymptomatic postmenopausal women.

Study Design.—In a prospective study, transabdominal and transvaginal ultrasound were performed on 149 unselected, asymptomatic women 50 years and older to assess the prevalence of unilocular, nonseptated adnexal cysts ("simple cysts") in postmenopausal women. Patients were classified according to hormone replacement regimens (no hormones, unopposed estrogen, continuous daily estrogen and progesterone, and sequential estrogen and progesterone) and length of menopause (less than 5 years, 5 to 10 years, or longer than 10 years).

Results.—Twenty-two women had simple adnexal cysts, for a relative frequency of 14.8% and prevalence of 14,800 patients with cysts per

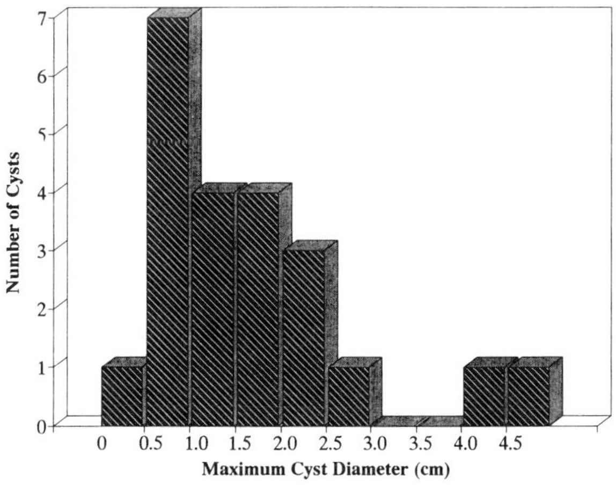

Fig 13–1.—Histogram of unilocular cyst diameters. (Courtesy of Wolf SI, Gosink BB, Feldesman MR, et al: *Radiology* 180:65–71, 1991.)

100,000 patients. Unilocular cysts varied in size from .4 to 4.7 cm (Fig 13–1). Combining both transabdominal and transvaginal ultrasound identified 68% of the ovaries, but neither transabdominal nor transvaginal ultrasound alone was optimal for identifying cysts. The occurrence of cysts was independent of the hormone replacement regimen and length of menopause.

Conclusion.—Ovarian cysts are remarkably common in postmenopausal women, regardless of age, hormone replacement status, and duration of menopause. Whether they possess the potential to be malignant is unknown. Both transabdominal and transvaginal ultrasound are required to visualize these cysts.

▶ This study is a good beginning to answering a very important question, i.e., the prevalence of ultrasonically definable simple cysts in postmenopausal women. The authors report a relative frequency of 15%, which did not seem to vary with age or hormone replacement status. This prevalence is higher than in previous reports, but the authors attribute this in part to combining abdominal and vaginal ultrasound. None of the patients had bilateral cysts; 21 of 22 patients with cysts had a single cyst. All but 2 of the cysts were less than or equal to 3 cm in size. The patient with a 4-cm cyst underwent surgery and was found to have a papillary serous cystadenoma. The patient with the 4.7-cm cyst refused surgery. Her cyst decreased to 2.3 cm at 3 months' follow-up. Four patients had other adnexal abnormalities; 2 of the 4 underwent surgery (hydrosalpinx; 1.8-cm dermoid) and 2 did not (ovarian asymmetry). Simple cysts less than 3 cm in diameter in postmenopausal women rarely represent ovarian neoplasias.—C.P. Morrow, M.D.

Laparoscopic Management of Ovarian Cysts: An Endocrinologist View

Thornton KL, DeCherney AH (Yale Univ, New Haven, Conn)

Yale J Biol Med 64:599–606, 1991 13–2

Background.—The traditional surgical approach to ovarian cysts often has been quite radical. Over time, this approach has become more conservative, in great part because of improvements in the laparoscopic surgical technique, which requires improved ability to predict the benign nature of the cysts. The differential diagnosis of ovarian cysts in women of child-bearing age, the ability of ultrasound to predict their benign vs. malignant nature, and their laparoscopic management were reviewed.

Differential Diagnosis.—The differential diagnosis includes follicular cyst, corpus luteum cyst, hemorrhagic ovarian cyst, benign epithelial neoplasms, cystadenoma, and benign cystic teratoma of germ cell origin, among others. Although many cysts are detected at routine physical examination, patients may be seen with acute or chronic pelvic pain, dysfunctional uterine bleeding, and abdominal or pelvic mass. All acute

General Ultrasonographic Characteristics of Cystic Ovarian Masses

Characteristic	Benign	Malignant
Size	<5–6 cm	>6 cm
Locules	Unilocular	Multilocular
Septa	Thin (2–3 mm)	Thick (>4 mm)
Internal echoes	Anechoic	Mixed echogenicity
	Homogeneous	Inhomogeneous
Inner wall structure	Smooth-walled	Papillarities
		Solid areas

(Courtesy of Thornton KL, DeCherney AH: *Yale J Biol Med* 64:599–606, 1991.)

events feature abdominal pain, often with peritoneal signs. However, most ovarian cystic masses present only with indolent symptoms referable to an enlarging pelvic mass.

Imaging.—Ultrasound is the most common imaging technique for these masses, and there have been several pathologic correlation studies. Benign cysts may tend to be smaller and unilocular and not to have thick septae. In one study, all totally anechoic lesions were benign (table). Sassone et al. recently developed a scoring system using transvaginal sonography with a specificity of 83% and sensitivity of 100%.

Laparoscopy.—Laparoscopy offers several advantages over traditional laparotomy. With advances in technique, laparoscopic aspiration is probably of no therapeutic value. It is, however, an integral part of the newer techniques. Cyst fenestration ensures histological examination of the lesion while allowing for permanent drainage and is useful in decreasing recurrence rate. In most cases of benign ovarian cysts, laparoscopic cystectomy is the treatment of choice. This is done by aspiration and fenestration of the cyst wall, followed by removal of the cyst wall from the ovarian cortex; closure appears unnecessary.

Discussion.—Laparoscopic surgery is becoming the main method of management for ovarian cysts, and ultrasonography is the most useful adjunct to preoperative management. Laparoscopy minimizes trauma to the tissue and keeps it moist, minimizing the formation of adhesions. It preserves the ovarian cortex and minimizes morbidity and recovery time. Almost all ovarian cysts will be managed this way as more gynecologists gain skill with the procedure.

▶ This is a thoughtful review of the laparoscopic management of ovarian cysts. The technique brings with it several problems that have not been resolved entirely. First is the issue of malignancy. Because malignant cysts or tumors must be removed intact and surgical staging must be performed, it is important to exclude malignancy before attempted laparoscopic management. This can be done with careful ultrasonic evaluation. Second, benign ovarian neoplasms must not be aspirated/fenestrated and left in situ. Fenestration is applicable only to simple/follicular and corpus luteum cysts. Because clinically significant cysts of this type cannot be confidently identified intraoperatively, frozen section is required. It is wrong to fenestrate (or biopsy) pathologic diagnosis or not to submit a specimen to pathology at all.—C.P. Morrow, M.D.

Videolaseroscopy for Oophorectomy

Nezhat F, Nezhat C, Silfen SL (Fertility and Endoscopy Ctr and Laser Endoscopy Inst of Atlanta)

Am J Obstet Gynecol 165:1323–1330, 1991 13–3

Introduction.—Operative laparoscopy is a safe, useful, cost-effective alternative to laparotomy in patients with benign pelvic disease. The variety of procedures possible is increasing. The results of 94 laparoscopic oophorectomies with videolaseroscopy performed in 76 patients were reviewed.

Methods.—The technique consists of a combination of high-resolution video imaging and high-power carbon dioxide laser applied to operative laparoscopy (Fig 13–2). The indications for the procedure included recurrent pain associated with endometriosis and adhesions in 17 patients, ovarian endometriomas in 40, prophylactic oophorectomy in 1, removal of the ovaries at the time of laparoscopically assisted vaginal hysterectomy in 15, and other indications in 3.

Results.—The procedure was completed with minimal blood loss and without major intraoperative or postoperative complications in all patients. Minor complications included abdominal wall ecchymosis in 2 patients and severe shoulder pain in 9. The procedure lasted 22–55 minutes, being shortest in the patient who required prophylactic oophorectomy. Those patients with laparoscopically assisted vaginal hysterectomy could be discharged 2 or 3 days after the procedure; the rest were discharged within 24 hours of the procedure, having an average hospital stay of 8.5 hours.

Conclusion.—Laparoscopic oophorectomy is a safe alternative to laparotomy, with all the advantages of outpatient surgery. Videolaseroscopy simplifies oophorectomy in the hands of an experienced operative laparoscopist.

▶ Laparoscopic oophorectomy has many potential uses. Some that come immediately to mind are prophylaxis in women with a family history of ovarian cancer; assisting oophorectomy in postmenopausal women who are undergoing vaginal hysterectomy or who have a small, apparently benign ovarian tumor; and removing the ovaries from women who have a postoperative diagnosis of endometrial carcinoma after hysterectomy without oophorectomy.—C.P. Morrow, M.D.

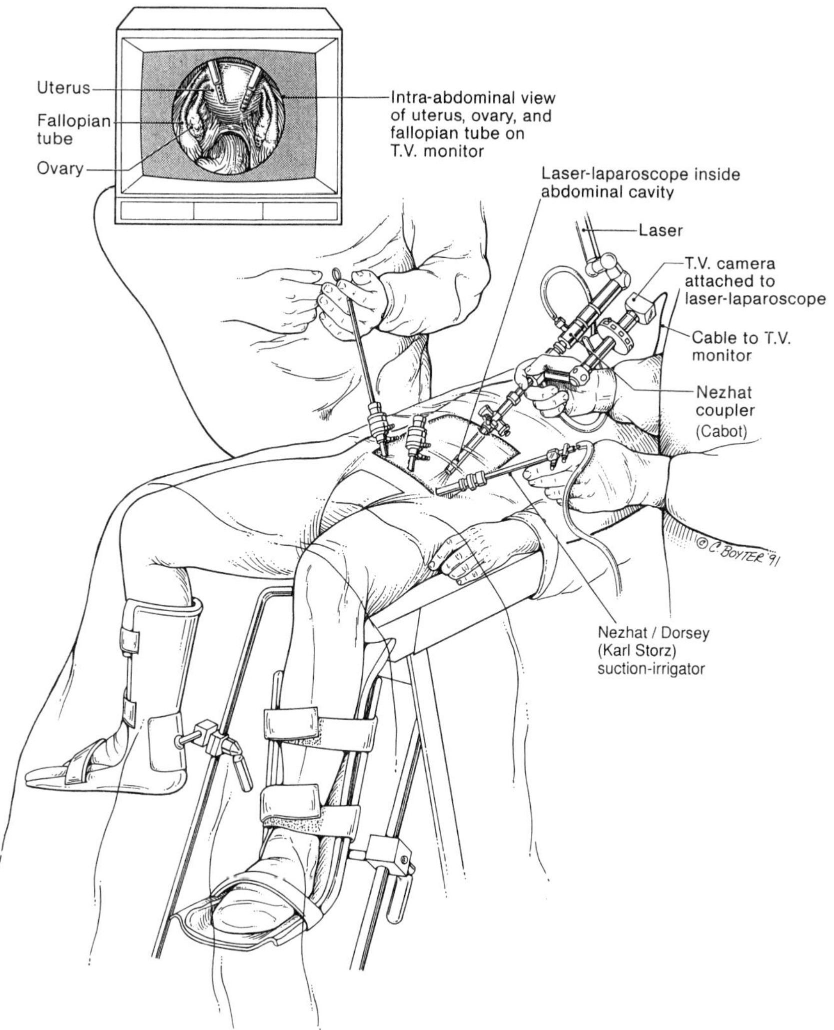

Fig 13–2.—Operating room setup. (Courtesy of Nezhat F, Nezhat C, Silfen SL: *Am J Obstet Gynecol* 165:1323-1330, 1991.)

A Randomised Trial Comparing Endometrial Resection and Abdominal Hysterectomy for the Treatment of Menorrhagia

Gannon MJ, Holt EM, Fairbank J, Fitzgerald M, Milne MA, Crystal AM, Greenhalf, JO (Royal Berkshire Hosp, Reading, England; Regional Technical College, Galway, Republic of Ireland)
BMJ 303:1362–1364, 1991 13–4

Surgery and Recuperation of Women

	Endometrial resection		Abdominal hysterectomy	
	Median (range)	Mean (95% CI)	Median (range)	Mean (95% CI)
Operating time (minutes)	30 (20-47)	30·5 (27·7 to 33·3)	50 (39-74)*	51·3 (48·4 to 54·2)
Hospital stay (days)	1 (1-3)	1·4 (1·2 to 1·6)	7 (5-12)*	7·1 (6·6 to 7·6)
Analgesia time (days)	0 (0-2)	0·2 (0 to 0·4)	7 (2-56)*	12·0 (6·8 to 17·2)
Recovery time (days)	16 (5-62)	21·3 (12·5 to 30·1)	58 (11-125)*	60·6 (47·0 to 74·2)
Return to work time (days)	14 (5-27)	14·9 (10·3 to 19·5)	64 (34-103)*	67·6 (55·8 to 79·4)

*$P < .001$.
(Courtesy of Gannon MJ, Holt EM, Fairbank J, et al: *BMJ* 303:1362–1364, 1991.)

Introduction.—Endometrial resection is an increasingly popular treatment for menorrhagia. It has many potential advantages over hysterectomy, but controlled trials have been lacking. A randomized controlled trial compared endometrial resection and abdominal hysterectomy in the treatment of menorrhagia.

Methods.—The subjects were 51 women with menorrhagia (median age, 40 years) who were awaiting abdominal hysterectomy. The women were randomized to receive either endometrial resection, performed by an experienced hysteroscopic surgeon, or abdominal hysterectomy, performed by 2 other gynecological surgeons. The 2 treatment groups were compared for length of operation, hospitalization, and recovery; cost of the operation; and short-term results.

Results.—The median operating times were 30 minutes for endometrial resection vs. 50 minutes for hysterectomy. The median hospital stays were 1 and 7 days, respectively. Recovery time was also shorter for endometrial resection than for hysterectomy, 16 vs. 58 days (table). The costs of the operations were £407 for endometrial resection vs. £1,270 for abdominal hysterectomy. Endometrial resection was repeated in 16% of the patients who did not have an acceptable improvement in symptoms, but none required hysterectomy during a mean follow-up of 1 year.

Conclusion.—Endometrial resection has many short-term benefits compared with abdominal hysterectomy in women with menorrhagia with no pelvic pathology. Endometrial resection is less expensive and less painful and has a shorter recovery time than hysterectomy. Longer follow-up in a greater number of patients is needed to establish the long-term efficacy and incidence of complications.

▶ At a time when cost-effectiveness is taking precedence over quality at any cost, this paper suggests that women with benign, uncomplicated menorrhagia should be treated by endometrial ablation (resection in this study). From the results, it seems that the ablation procedure is clearly superior, but there is only 1 year of follow-up, and 16% of the patients undergoing ablation had an unacceptable result. Although the cost of hysterectomy is triple that of ablation, hysterectomy is permanent and decisive. It also absolutely prevents the development of endometrial cancer. A lack of long-term results will not deter ablation from becoming the treatment of choice, but it is obvious that women undergoing endometrial ablation need long-term follow-up. This should to be part of the cost of the equation.—C.P. Morrow, M.D.

Self-Reported Long-Term Outcomes of Hysterectomy

Schofield MJ, Bennett A, Redman S, Walters WAW, Sanson-Fisher RW (Univ of Newcastle, Australia)

Br J Obstet Gynaecol 98:1129–1136, 1991 13–5

Background.—Hysterectomies are costly, major operations that are performed frequently. Women's perceptions of and satisfaction with the long-term outcomes of hysterectomy were investigated.

Methods.—A total of 236 women who had had a hysterectomy 2–10 years earlier were surveyed by telephone and postal questionnaire. These women were identified from a community survey in New South Wales, Australia. The main outcome measures were perceived benefits resulting from the hysterectomy, perceived physical and psychological problems resulting from the surgery, and satisfaction with care.

Results.—The most frequent benefit was relief from heavy bleeding, which was reported by 57% of the women; 32% reported that relief from heavy bleeding was the most important benefit. Most women said that their prehysterectomy symptoms had improved, but more than half reported having symptoms that they believed had worsened or been caused by the operation. Despite this, the respondents reported high levels of satisfaction with the procedure.

Conclusion.—Most of the women in this survey reported that relief from menstrual symptoms, such as excessive bleeding or pain, was the major reason they chose to undergo hysterectomy. These findings suggest a need for more closely examining decision-making about treatment for such menstrual symptoms.

▶ From this Australian study on patients' perception of the long-term (2–10 years) benefit obtained by hysterectomy, one gets the impression that the underlying purpose is to substantiate the authors' (or the governments') belief that many hysterectomies are being done without sufficient warrant. Nevertheless, although the question is worth investigating, it is seldom investigated. These authors found that 95% of the patients said they would make the same decision again, but 4% thought they were worse off after the operation. These are remarkably good results considering that more than half reported a worsening of symptoms or new symptoms consequent to the hysterectomy.—C.P. Morrow, M.D.

Effect of Hysterectomy on Anorectal and Urethrovesical Physiology

Prior A, Stanley K, Smith ARB, Read NW (Royal Hallamshire Hosp, Sheffield, England; Jessop Hosp for Women, Sheffield)

Gut 33:264–267, 1992 13–6

Background.—Women frequently date the onset of bowel and bladder dysfunction to the time of hysterectomy. However, there have been no prospective studies on the effect of total hysterectomy on anorectal and urethrovesical physiology.

Methods.—Twenty-six women were enrolled in a study of the association between vaginal or total abdominal hysterectomy and changes in anorectal and urethrovesical function. All the women were assessed before surgery and at 6 weeks and 6 months after surgery.

Findings.—There was a postoperative increase in both rectal and vesical sensitivity. The results were similar regardless of the type of hysterectomy. There were no significant changes in rectal or bladder compliance, and anal pressure and urethral pressure and length were not changed after surgery. Hysterectomy did not affect whole gut transit. Urinary

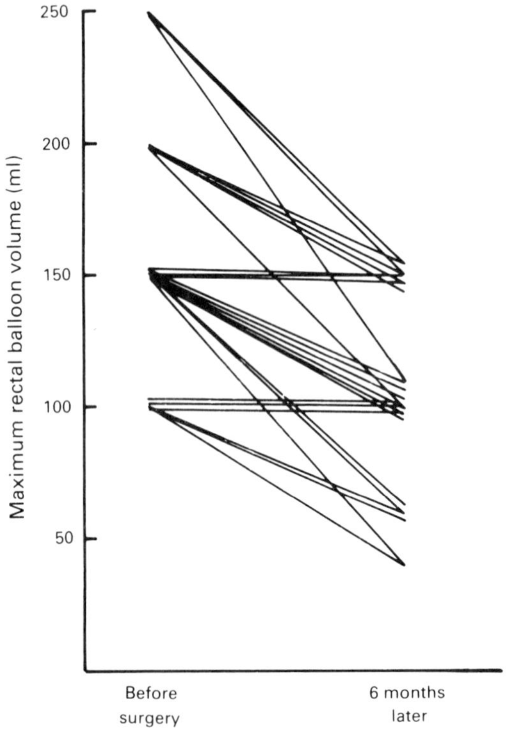

Fig 13–3.—Individual changes in maximum tolerated rectal balloon volume after hysterectomy. (Courtesy of Prior A, Stanley K, Smith ARB, et al: *Gut* 33:264–267, 1992.)

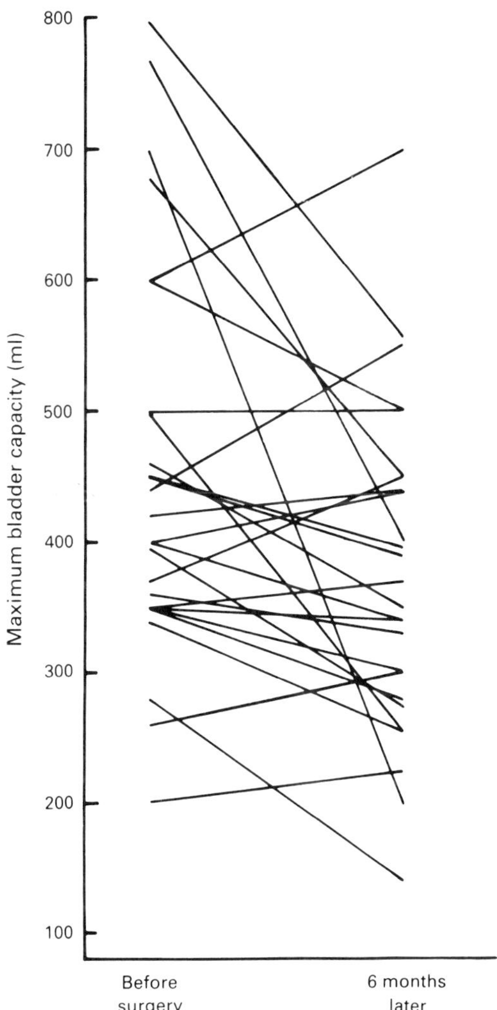

Fig 13–4.—Individual changes in maximum bladder capacity after hysterectomy. (Courtesy of Prior A, Stanley K, Smith ARB, et al: *Gut* 33:264–267, 1992.)

symptoms occurred de novo in 6 women, and gastrointestinal symptoms occurred in 2.

Conclusion.—Significant changes in rectal (Fig 13–3) and bladder (Fig 13–4) sensitivity occur after hysterectomy for benign disease. These changes appear to persist for at least 6 months. However, they are not always associated with urinary or gastrointestinal symptoms.

▶ It is not uncommon for patients to have new rectal and bladder complaints after hysterectomy for benign disease, and this study documents that there are measurable changes in the form of increased rectal and bladder sensitivity that last up to 6 months or longer postoperatively. The authors note that the changes are not typical of injury to the autonomic nerves, nor are they typical of trauma. Nevertheless, the latter seems to be the most likely explanation.—C.P. Morrow, M.D.

The Place of Oophorectomy at Vaginal Hysterectomy

Sheth SS (King Edward Mem Hosp; Sheth GS Med College, Bombay, India)

Br J Obstet Gynaecol 98:662–666, 1991 13–7

Objective.—Prophylactic oophorectomy in postmenopausal women undergoing hysterectomy is based on the late presentation of ovarian cancer and its poor response to treatment. A total of 740 women undergoing vaginal hysterectomy with attempted oophorectomy were compared with 700 others not having oophorectomy. Oophorectomy was offered to women who were postmenopausal or older than age 45 years, or to menstruating women older than 40 years of age with a history of ovarian neoplasm or a family history of ovarian cancer.

Observations.—Attempted oophorectomy was successful in 94% of cases. Operative success was influenced by tubo-ovarian disease and, less markedly, by obesity, uterine descent, uterine size, and vaginal access. An extra 11 to 20 minutes usually was required for oophorectomy. Thirty previously anemic patients required transfusion. No ureteral or bowel injuries resulted.

Conclusion.—Vaginal oophorectomy in conjunction with hysterectomy is a safe and reasonable procedure for the experienced surgeon. The ideal patient is a slim woman with adequate vaginal space and pliable soft tissues. The indications for oophorectomy are basically the same as at abdominal hysterectomy.

The Surgical Management of Vaginal Vault Prolapse

Creighton SM, Stanton SL (St George's Hosp, London)

Br J Obstet Gynaecol 98:1150–1154, 1991 13–8

Background.—Vaginal vault prolapse after hysterectomy is uncommon but can be very difficult to manage. Treatment is usually surgical. The surgeon must choose either a vaginal or abdominal route. The results of surgery for vaginal vault prolapse after hysterectomy in one patient series were reported.

Methods.—All 28 patients treated for vaginal vault prolapse between 1981 and 1990 at one center were reviewed retrospectively. The patients underwent a total of 33 operations. Twenty-three were colposacropexy, and 10 were a Zacharin procedure. Twenty-five of the women were seen within the past year.

Results.—The mean follow-up was 17.1 months for the colposacropexy and 33 months for the Zacharin procedure. The cure rates were 91% and 70%, respectively. The 2 most common complications were voiding difficulties and infection. Three cases of voiding difficulty developed after the Zacharin procedure, and 1 developed after colposacropexy. Two women needed removal of the Mersilene mesh after colposacropexy because of a persistent discharging sinus.

Conclusion.—In this series, the colposacropexy produced a better success rate. It is also a simpler procedure to perform. It has therefore become the procedure of choice at the center where the study took place. However, the procedure is also associated with a risk of infection that can necessitate supporting mesh removal.

▶ In the United States, approximately 15% of women in whom ovarian cancer develops have previously undergone hysterectomy, usually vaginal. Approximately two thirds of women in this study were older than 45 years of age when their hysterectomy was performed. Thus, one might conclude that routine oophorectomy done at the time of vaginal hysterectomy in the over-45 age group would reduce the incidence of ovarian cancer by 10%. Although routine removal of ovaries in postmenopausal women at the time of abdominal hysterectomy is considered a standard practice, removing the ovaries is widely ignored at vaginal hysterectomy in the same age group. Sheth (Abstract 13–7) addressed this discrepancy in his own practice and found that he was able to remove the ovaries with or without the tubes 95% of the time. No serious increase in operating time (10 to 20 minutes) or complications occurred. Ovarian removal at the time of vaginal hysterectomy should be taught in residency and performed whenever exposure makes it feasible in women of appropriate age.—C.P. Morrow, M.D.

▶ The Zacharin procedure rarely is used in this country but, as this article indicates, it may not be as good as the colposacropexy, a procedure which *is* used in this country. Unfortunately, the authors dismiss the sacrospinous ligament suspension as a blind procedure that can be complicated by bleeding from pudendal or sacral vessels and sciatic nerve injury. It probably is the best procedure overall for posthysterectomy vaginal vault prolapse—provided, of course, that the surgeon is trained in the technique.—C.P. Morrow, M.D.

Early Repair of Iatrogenic Injury to the Ureter or Bladder After Gynecological Surgery

Blandy JP, Badenoch DF, Fowler CG, Jenkins BJ, Thomas NWM (Royal London Hosp, London)

J Urol 146:761–765, 1991 13–9

Introduction.—Timing of surgery is an important matter for women who have a urinary tract injury in the course of hysterectomy. Early repair, if feasible, would be most welcome.

Patients.—Sixty-eight women were seen in 1970–1988 with urinary injury incurred during hysterectomy. Forty-three of them had ureteral injuries, whereas 25 had a vesicovaginal fistula. Thirteen of the latter patients were seen more than 6 weeks after hysterectomy. All patients with urine leakage received a diagnosis within 3 weeks of initial surgery.

Management.—A single injured ureter was reimplanted without tension using a Boari-Ockerblad flap. If both ureters were damaged, 2 Boari flaps were raised. An omental patch was used to cover the vaginal suture line after repairing a vesicovaginal fistula. If a large defect was present, half the bisected bladder wall was rotated down to fill the defect without tension.

Results.—None of the ureterovaginal fistulas recurred. Damage from renal obstruction was lessened in all instances; and there were no anastomotic strictures. One patient had detrusor instability after bilateral ureteral reimplantation. All patients with a vesicovaginal fistula had primary healing. In 1 patient, stress incontinence persisted and later was managed by colposuspension.

Implications.—These results call into question the usual view that iatrogenic urinary tract injuries occurring after gynecologic surgery should not be repaired until several months have passed. Vesicovaginal fistulas that follow a clean operation can be repaired at an early stage. Delay is, however, appropriate in patients with postpartum fistula.

▶ This is a fairly large series of ureteral fistulas reported from a referral center in London. All fistulas were repaired at the time of referral. There were 28 early referrals repaired within 6 weeks of injury. Based on 12 cases, the authors also recommend early repair of clean, uncomplicated vesicovaginal fistulas. None of the ureteral repairs were done by end-to-end ureteral anastomosis. Instead, all were reimplanted into the bladder. The authors did not manage any patients by means of stenting with or without percutaneous nephrostomy. The stent can be inserted with the help of ureteroscopy. This is the treatment of choice when possible, because it avoids a major operation. Early identification and referral will facilitate optimal management.—C.P. Morrow, M.D.

Iatrogenic Injuries to the Ureter During Gynecologic and Obstetric Operations

Neuman M, Eidelman A, Langer R, Golan A, Bukovsky I, Caspi E (Assaf Harofeh Med Ctr, Zerifin, Israel)

Surg Gynecol Obstet 173:268–272, 1991 13–10

Circumstance of Ureteral Injury

Surgical procedures	*No. of ureteral injuries*	
Abdominal hysterectomy		8
With Marshall-Marchetti	1	
With salpingo-oophorectomy	1	
Cesarean hysterectomy	3	
Cesarean sections		2
Salpingo-oophorectomy		4
Right	3	
Left	1	
Vaginal hysterectomy		2
With Marshall-Marchetti	1	
With bilateral salpingo-oophorectomy and ant. colporrhaphy	1	
Ant. colporrhaphy		1
Marshall-Marchetti		1
Total		18

Ant., Anterior.

Abbreviation: Ant, anterior.
(Courtesy of Neuman M, Eidelman A, Langer R, et al: *Surg Gynecol Obstet* 173:268–272, 1991.)

Background.—Complications from injury to the ureters during pelvic surgery are serious hazards. Data on 18 patients with iatrogenic injuries to the ureter during gynecological and obstetric surgery during a 30-year period were reviewed.

Patients.—The 18 patients ranged in age from 19 to 52 years. Injury occurred at abdominal hysterectomy in 44% of cases, adnexectomy in 22%, vaginal hysterectomy in 11%, and cesarean section in 11% (table). Ureteral injury was ligation of the ureter in 33% of cases, incision of the ureter in 17%, ureteral obstruction in 22%, and ureterovaginal fistula formation in 28%. Compound injuries occurred in 2 cases. In 77% of the patients, the injury was associated with attempts to achieve hemostasis, mostly in uterine and infundibulopelvic arteries. The presenting symptoms included urine leakage in 44%, pain in 33%, fever in 5%, and urosepsis in 12%.

Treatments and Outcomes.—Ureteral injury was recognized when it occurred in only 2 cases in which end-to-end anastomosis of the ureter was done. In the remaining patients, the injury was not recognized for 3 days to 8 months. Ureteroneocystostomy was done in 9 cases. Large ureteric segment injury required ureteroileocystostomy in 1. Ureteral stents were placed in 2 cases, and temporary percutaneous nephrostomy was used twice. The outcomes in 12 cases were good. Postoperative urinary tract calculi were recorded in 3 patients, and 2 patients had end-stage renal insufficiency. The incidence of ureteral injury progressively decreased during the 30-year period. The reduction in such injury during abdominal gynecologic and obstetric surgery was significant.

Conclusion.—Properly identifying and, when needed, isolating the ureter during surgery in which there is a risk is essential to reducing the incidence of ureteral injury. Patients who received a diagnosis at the time of the injury and were treated with end-to-end anastomosis had the best outcomes. Delayed diagnosis and treatment resulted in poor outcomes.

▶ The main message in this paper is the importance of early recognition of urinary tract injury in gynecological surgery. Patients who are most likely to have the urinary tract injured are those whose surgery has been difficult because of poor exposure, distorted anatomy, or bleeding (often all 3). In these cases, intraoperative testing of the integrity of the bladder and urinary tract and postoperative evaluation of the kidneys by ultrasound are helpful. If the patient has symptoms (urosepsis, flank pain, fever) postoperatively—even if the surgery wasn't difficult—the kidneys should be checked by ultrasound.—C.P. Morrow, M.D.

Optimum Duration of Surgical Scrub-Time

O'Shaughnessy M, O'Malley VP, Corbett G, Given HF (University College Hosp, Galway, Ireland)

Br J Surg 78:685–686, 1991 13–11

Objective.—What constitutes a good surgical scrub remains imprecisely understood. This study compared scrubbing with Hibiscrub (4% chlorhexidine gluconate) for 2, 4, and 6 minutes in 10 surgeons who were scheduled to perform clean abdominal operations. None had scrubbed in the past 24 hours.

Findings.—All scrub times led to significantly reduced hand bacterial colony counts at 1 hour, although there was a trend toward greater reductions after scrubbing for 4 or 6 minutes. No wound infections occurred, despite the lack of antibiotic coverage.

Conclusion.—A 4-minute scrub for the first case of the day and a 2-minute scrub for subsequent procedures are suggested.

▶ As the authors point out, the purpose of the surgical scrub is to remove dirt, grease, and transient resident bacteria. There are disadvantages to long scrub times, including skin trauma, dermatitis, greater water consumption, and wasted operating time. With the improved antiseptics that are available today, postscrub bacterial counts can be effectively reduced with a shorter scrub time. In this study, a 4-minute chlorhexidine scrub was as effective as the 6-minute scrub. The authors conclude that 4 minutes should be adequate for the first scrub of the day, and 2 minutes should be sufficient thereafter. These scrub times may not be applicable to Betadine or pHisoHex, because these agents do not produce an immediate or persistent reduction of the bacterial counts as adequately as 4% chlorhexidine does.—C.P. Morrow, M.D.

The Effect of Double Gloving on Frequency of Glove Perforations

Bennett B, Duff P (Univ of Florida College of Medicine, Gainesville)

Obstet Gynecol 78:1019–1022, 1991 13–12

Objective.—The frequency of glove perforation was determined during a 2-month period when obstetrical and gynecological surgeons were asked to double glove for all procedures. The gloves were tested by filling them with air and immersing them, and then by filling them directly with water.

Results.—Of the 441 sets of double gloves examined, 14% had holes in at least 1 of the 4 gloves and 6 sets had more than 1 perforation. Only 6 sets had perforations of both gloves at the same site. The thumb and index finger of the nondominant hand were most often perforated. Perforations were most frequent in major gynecological operations. Only one fifth of the perforations were recognized by the surgeon.

Suggestion.—In view of the findings and of the potential risk of HIV and hepatitis B infections, double gloving should be used in all obstetric and gynecologic surgery.

▶ There is no doubt that double gloving will reduce the frequency of glove perforations, which, in this study, are presumable used as a surrogate for needle sticks and the risk of innoculation with a dangerous virus, especially HIV. Such a procedure is also protection for the patient, because the surgeon can transmit the hepatitis and AIDS viruses by needle sticks. Most Ob/Gyn doctors don't operate on patients at high risk for these diseases. Nevertheless, at the very least we should determine which patients are at risk and use these protective measures. We should also be screened periodically to be sure we are not carriers.—C.P. Morrow, M.D.

Effects of Electrocautery on Midline Laparotomy Wound Infection

Kumagai SG, Rosales RF, Hunter GC, Rappaport WD, Witzke DB, Chvapil TA, Chvapil M, Sutherland JC (Univ Med Ctr, Tucson, Ariz)

Am J Surg 162:620–623, 1991 13–13

Background.—Techniques of wound creation and closure have important effects on healing. Electrocautery, at either the cutting (Ecut) or coagulating (Ecoag) current, may be used to incise the abdominal wall fascia. The healing of contaminated fascial wounds made by scalpel, Ecut, or Ecoag was compared in rats.

Methods.—A group of 57 Sprague-Dawley rats underwent a midline laparotomy incision using a surgical scalpel, Ecut, or Ecoag. After fascial closure with 4-0 interrupted nylon sutures, the animals were randomly assigned to receive contamination of the wound between the fascia and skin with *Escherichia coli* at a dose of 10^2, 10^5, or 10^7 organisms. When the animals died, or after 7 days, the investigators evaluated tensile

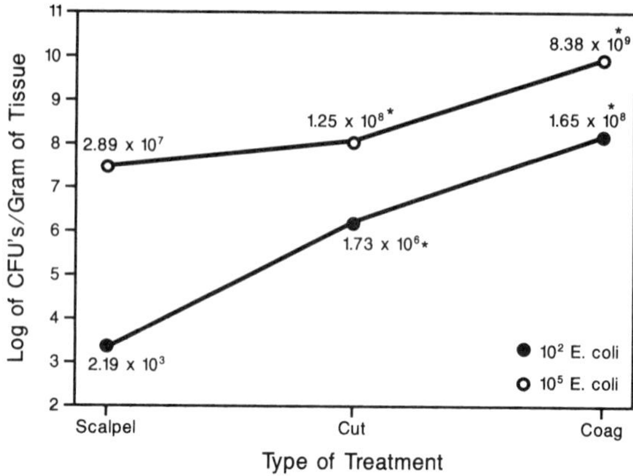

Fig 13–5.—Quantitative tissue cultures obtained at 7 days from animals inoculated with 10^2 and 10^5 organisms. (Courtesy of Kumagai SG, Rosales RF, Hunter GC, et al: *Am J Surg* 162:620-623, 1991.)

wound strength, blood cultures, and biopsy specimens of the fascia and incision.

Findings.—Incisions made with electrocautery showed significantly less tensile wound strength than incisions made with a scalpel. At the higher levels of *E. coli* inoculation, the tissue cultures showed more organisms in animals undergoing electrocautery incision (Fig 13-5). There was an inverse relationship between wound strength and *E. coli* concentration. Those animals that underwent electrocautery were also more likely to have bacteremia at 48 hours and to be dead at 7 days.

Conclusion.—Especially for contaminated wounds, the technique of incision of the abdominal fascia appears to affect wound healing. Intraperitoneal migration or lymphatic spread may explain the higher mortality and infection rate in the rats undergoing electrocautery. Complications such as these can be avoided by meticulous technique, judicious use of antibiotics, and enhancement of host resistance.

▶ Wound healing and wound infection are adversely influenced by many factors, including the patient's nutritional status, diabetes, obesity, uremia, chemotherapy, radiation therapy, hematoma, seroma, foreign body (suture), necrotic tissue, and bacterial contamination. Prophylactic antibiotics reduce the risk of wound infection. Kumagai et al. studied the effect of electrocautery vs. scalpel incision in an animal model. Their findings are consistent with studies reported over the years, i.e., that electrocautery causes more tissue injury than the scalpel. The increased tissue injury delays healing and increases the danger of infection if there is bacterial contamination of the wound. Electrocautery certainly can be used safely to open the abdomen, but it should not be used in the presence of patient factors that are associated with a high risk for delayed wound healing—unless permanent suture is used for closure. In addition, prophylactic antibiotics are indicated whenever bacterial contamination might occur.—C.P. Morrow, M.D.

Are Blood Cultures Effective in the Evaluation of Fever in Perioperative Patients?

Theuer CP, Bongard FS, Klein SR (Harbor-Univ of California Los Angeles Med Ctr, Torrance, Calif)

Am J Surg 162:615–619, 1991 13–14

Objective.—The value of blood culture in the perioperative period was examined by studying all cultures performed on adult surgical services in a 5-week period. A total of 364 cultures were available, representing 108 febrile events (with a temperature of 101.5°F or higher) in 72 patients lacking evidence of sepsis.

Findings.—All but 11% of the patients had undergone surgery before fever developed. Organisms were isolated in cultures from 9 patients, and 5 of these results represented pathogens. Two of these 5 patients had an identifiable source of bacteremia. The cost of identifying each of these 5 patients was $2,798. Neither the peak temperature nor the leukocyte count predicted positive cultures, but immune depression and the presence of an indwelling device were predictive. A positive result did not lessen morbidity or the risk of death in any instance.

Conclusion.—Blood cultures are not likely to be helpful in febrile adult perioperative patients who have no signs of sepsis.

▶ In a study from a surgical service, no cultures from 26 febrile events were positive on postoperative days 0–3, but cultures from 6 of 40 febrile events were positive on postoperative days 4–10. Other factors associated with a significant risk for positive blood culture were the presence of indwelling devices and clinical evidence for a site of infection. The authors make the point that blood cultures should not be obtained routinely from every febrile (> 101.5) postoperative patient; however, other factors need to be considered. There are certain dangers to needle sticks in addition to the added expense.—C.P. Morrow, M.D.

14 Gynecologic Urology

Urinary Incontinence in Women From 35 to 79 Years of Age: Prevalence and Consequences

Rekers H, Drogendijk AC, Valkenburg H, Riphagen F (Intl Health Found, Brussels; Univ of Rotterdam, The Netherlands)

Eur J Obstet Gynecol Reprod Biol 43:229–234, 1992 14–1

Purpose.—The reported prevalence of incontinence in nonhospitalized women in the United Kingdom, North America, and Scandinavia varies between 17% and 45%. Data on the prevalence of incontinence among women in the European continent have not been available. The prevalence and consequences of urinary incontinence in women living in the city of Zoetermeer in The Netherlands were studied.

Methods.—A questionnaire was mailed to 1,920 women between the ages of 35 and 80 years who were living in the community. Women who were living in residential homes for the elderly or receiving institutional care for other reasons were excluded from the survey. All completed questionnaires were computed and analyzed by using the BMDP statistical programs.

Results.—Completed questionnaires were returned by 1,299 women (67.7%), and 344 of them reported involuntary loss of urine. The prevalence of urinary incontinence was highest in the younger age groups (approximately 30%) and lowest in women aged 65–69 years (14.4%). The prevalence increased again to 25.6% in women aged 75–79 years. A total of 158 women with incontinence (45.9%) reported using protection against the loss of urine. Despite the fact that most women had had incontinence symptoms for years, only 28.2% had ever consulted a physician for their symptoms. Forty-three women (44%) with serious incontinence and 54 (22%) with minor incontinence had consulted a physician. The reason for not seeking medical help given by 87.6% of the women was that they considered their symptoms as not so serious. Fifty-three women indicated that either they did not want to talk about it, did not know who to talk to, or thought that other people could not help them.

Summary.—Urinary incontinence was present in 26.5% of Dutch women aged 35–80 years who were living in the community. Only 28.2% of the women who reported they were incontinent had ever sought medical consultation for their symptoms.

▶ This study from The Netherlands confirms surveys done in the United States, indicating that many women with urinary incontinence do not seek medical help. In this large series of noninstitutionalized women, more than 25% had urinary incontinence. Most of these incontinent women (72%) never sought medical help. These results indicate that almost 20% of women in this population have urinary incontinence and do not seek help. The results are even more disturbing because half these women used protection against their urine problem, i.e., the problem changed their life-style, and they still did not seek medical help. There were 3 major reasons for this: not wanting to talk about it, not knowing to whom to talk, and having the idea that other people could not help them.

The point of this work, as well as the surveys in the United States, is that women should be better educated about their urinary problems. They should be aware of the fact that incontinence is not necessarily a part of aging, that help is available, and that help does not necessarily indicate operation. Because women do not always "volunteer" this information, the physician should ask about urinary problems and offer help when needed.—A. Bergman, M.D.

Prevalence, Incidence and Correlates of Urinary Incontinence in Healthy, Middle-Aged Women

Burgio KL, Matthews KA, Engel BT (Univ of Pittsburgh; Natl Inst on Aging, Baltimore)

J Urol 146:1255–1259, 1991 14–2

Background.—Urinary incontinence is a common health problem among elderly individuals, especially among elderly women. Studies have shown that up to 49% of elderly individuals in the community have difficulty with urine control and up to 83% of nursing home residents have urinary incontinence. The prevalence, incidence, and correlates of urinary incontinence were assessed in a nonclinical, community-based sample of healthy, middle-aged women.

Study Design.—Of 2,405 women who were contacted by telephone as part of an ongoing prospective study of healthy premenopausal women, 2,138 (89%) agreed to be interviewed and 901 were actually interviewed. Only women aged 42–50 years who were not taking certain medications were included in the study. After the eligibility interview, 541 premenopausal nonpregnant women with a mean age of 47 years were entered into the study. The study participants were evaluated on 2 occasions approximately 3 years apart. Of 541 women who entered the study, 486 returned for the final clinic visit 3 years later.

Results.—At the final clinic visit, 41.6% of the women had never experienced involuntary urine loss, whereas 58.4% had experienced incontinence at some time, with 30.7% having incontinence on a regular basis at least once a month. After 3 years, the cumulative incidence of regular incontinence in previously continent women was 8%. Among those with regular incontinence, 64.9% had a urine loss volume of 1 or 2 drops, whereas 35.1% had to change their garments. In most of the women with incontinence, the onset was not associated with pregnancy or childbirth. Only 20.7% of those who ever experienced incontinence and 34% of those with regular incontinence wore some form of protection for urine loss, and only 19% of those who ever had incontinence and 25.5% of those with at least monthly incontinence sought treatment for incontinence. White race and a high body mass index were the only parameters identified as significant risk factors for urinary incontinence.

Conclusion.—Urinary incontinence is common among middle-aged women. Many women who would not take the initiative to inform their health care provider will acknowledge incontinence when asked.

▶ This is a very large, well-designed study on more than 500 patients with a 3-year follow-up. More than 50% of premenopausal middle-aged women had some degree of urinary incontinence, with more than 30% having incontinence on a regular basis. It is striking that less than 20% of women who have urinary incontinence to any degree and only 1 in 4 women with urinary incontinence on a regular basis sought treatment. Urinary incontinence is very common among middle-aged women, yet only few seek help. The physician should be aware of these numbers and ask about symptoms of urinary incontinence with evaluation for any other problem, because women do not volunteer this information. Public education should in part be the responsibility of health care providers.—A. Bergman, M.D.

Prazosin: A Neglected Cause of Genuine Stress Incontinence
Dwyer PL, Teele JS (Mercy Hosp for Women, Melbourne)
Obstet Gynecol 79:117–121, 1992 14–3

Background.—Prazosin is a common antihypertensive agent that reduces peripheral vascular resistance by selectively blocking α-1 adrenergic receptors on arteriolar smooth muscle. Alpha-1 adrenoceptor inhibition also relaxes smooth muscle in the urethra. All women at 1 clinic who had urinary incontinence and were receiving prazosin were studied to determine the incidence and cause of prazosin-related incontinence.

Urodynamic Diagnosis Related to Prazosin Ingestion in 1,335 Women Attending the Urodynamic Clinic

	Normal study	GSI	DI	GSI/DI	HB	VD
Women on prazosin	2 (3%)	39 (67%)	3 (5%)	11 (19%)	2 (3%)	1 (2%)
No prazosin	85 (7%)	663 (52%)	202 (16%)	175 (14%)	120 (9%)	32 (3%)
Significance (*P*)*	NS	<.05	<.05	NS	NS	NS

Abbreviations: GSI, genuine stress incontinence; *DI,* detrusor instability; *HB,* hypersensitive bladder; *VD,* voiding dysfunction; *NS,* not significant.
* Yates-corrected χ^2 test.
(Courtesy of Dwyer PL, Teele JS: *Obstet Gynecol* 79:117–121, 1992.)

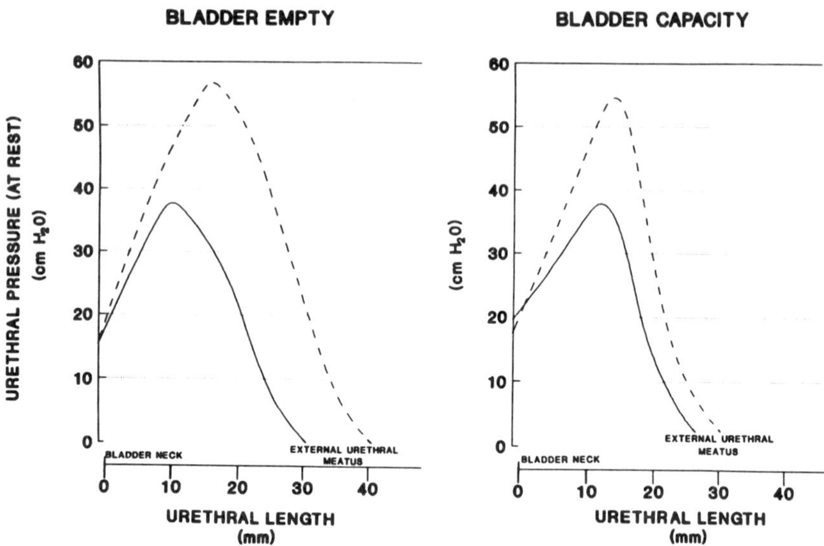

Fig 14–1.—The mean resting urethral pressure profiles before (*solid line*) and after (*dashed line*) prazosin withdrawal. Pressure measurements were made with the bladder empty and again at bladder capacity. (Courtesy of Dwyer PL, Teele JS: *Obstet Gynecol* 79:117–121, 1992.)

Methods and Findings.—Of the 1,335 women examined for urinary incontinence and other urinary symptoms between 1985 and 1990, 58 (4.3%) were taking prazosin. The incidence of genuine stress incontinence was 86.2% in those taking prazosin—significantly higher than in those not taking prazosin (incidence, 65.7%). Of the 45 women contacted, 25 had experienced improvement in their urinary incontinence or were cured after prazosin was withdrawn. All 25 of these women had stress incontinence. After prazosin withdrawal, there was a significant increase in functional urethral length, maximum urethral closure pressure, and abdominal pressure transmission to the urethra (table, Fig 14–1).

Conclusion.—Prazosin was found to be a frequently unrecognized cause of stress incontinence in women. Many of these women had unsuccessful and possibly unnecessary surgery.

▶ Investigating medications ingested by the patient is an important part of taking history in women with urinary incontinence. Various medications have significant effects on the lower urinary tract functions, and the physician should be well aware of this. The female urethra has many α-receptors, and α-sympathomimetic drugs have significant effects on the urethra. The α-sympathomimetic medications will cause contraction of the periurethral smooth muscles, whereas the α-blockers will relax them. Alpha-sympathomimetics (with or without estrogens) are among the better nonsurgical treatments for stress incontinence, whereas α-blockers can aggravate "borderline incontinence". Some women may be cured by switching α-blockers (usually taken for hypertension) to another antihypertensive medication.

This series emphasizes the very important clinical point of asking about drugs when taking history in incontinent women. This should not be a neglected cause. In this series, 25 of 45 women taking α-blockers had drug-related urinary incontinence. More disturbing is the fact that more than 50% of the women with drug-related urinary incontinence had an operation that was preventable. Any gynecologist who is considering an anti-incontinence operation should take a careful history, keeping in mind the effect of medications on the lower urinary tract.—A. Bergman, M.D.

Value of Urologic Investigation in a Targeted Group of Women With Recurrent Urinary Tract Infections

Nickel JC, Wilson J, Morales A, Heaton J (Queen's Univ, Kingston, Ont)

Can J Surg 34:591–594, 1991 14–4

Background.—Clinical studies suggest that excretory urography and cystoscopy are of no benefit in managing most women with a history of recurrent urinary tract infection (UTI). A 5-year study was done to determine the value of urological investigation in a select group of such women and to identify the risk factors that warrant such assessment.

Methods.—A total of 186 of 475 women with recurrent UTIs were prospectively targeted for assessment with cystoscopy and ultrasonography or excretory urography. The selection criteria were based on the degree of complicating factors. Selected women were required to be older than 16 years of age, to have had at least 3 UTIs in the preceding 12 months, and to have at least 1 of the following: gross hematuria during a UTI; persistent microscopic hematuria between UTIs; a history of pyelonephritis, diabetes, or an atypical presentation.

Findings.—Thirty-nine patients had significant abnormalities detected. Twenty of these patients needed surgery. There were no significant complications during any of the investigations. Four patients had previously unsuspected superficial transitional cell carcinoma of the bladder, and 5 had urinary tract calculi. In 5 of 6 patients discovered to have upper urinary tract obstruction, pyelonephritis or an atypical presentation was the primary indication. All 11 patients with lower urinary tract obstruction had urethral stenosis or stricture; all subsequently underwent urethral dilation. The remaining 12 patients had other abnormalities, including low-grade ureterovesical reflux confirmed by voiding cystourethrography.

Conclusion.—Cystoscopy and upper urinary tract assessment do appear to play a role in the management of selected women with UTIs. Some of these patients have significant abnormalities of the urinary tract that may be associated with recurrent UTIs. In the targeted population described, cystoscopy under local anesthesia and renal ultrasonography followed by excretory urography in only a few selected patients may be the most appropriate diagnostic approach.

▶ Thirty-nine of 186 patients with repeated urinary tract infections had significant abnormalities. Twenty of these patients needed surgery. The abnormalities included obstructive uropathy (upper or lower urinary tract), reflex, and even cancer. These are significant complications. This study demonstrates very clearly that some women with repeated urinary tract infections need a full urological evaluation including cystoscopy and x-ray studies.—A. Bergman, M.D.

Urodynamic Assessment and Lateral Urethrocystography: A Comparison of Two Diagnostic Procedures for Female Urinary Incontinence

Grischke E-M, Anton H, Stolz W, von Fournier D, Bastert G (Univ Women's Hosp, Heidelberg, Germany)

Acta Obstet Gynecol Scand 70:225–229, 1991 14–5

Introduction.—Lateral metallic-bead-chain urethrocystography provides information on urethrovesical anatomy in the diagnosis of stress incontinence. Urethrocystography, which simultaneously profiles urethral and bladder pressures, permits the diagnosis of urgency as well as stress incontinence. These 2 procedures were compared to determine their diagnostic relevance in 84 women who underwent urodynamic assessment and lateral chain urethrocystography. The patients included 6 without primary incontinence who were assessed for check-up purposes after surgery. Correlations between the 2 procedures were determined.

Results.—A urodynamic diagnosis of stress incontinence was associated with radiographic findings of rotational and vertical bladder neck descent (type Green I and II) in 91% of patients. Urodynamic findings of stress-urgency incontinence were associated with distortion of urethrovesical anatomy (type Green I and II) in 90% of patients. These radiological pathologies were found in 75% of patients with sensory urgency and in 53% of those with normal urodynamic findings. Of the 40 patients with bladder neck descent type Green II, 30 had urodynamic findings of stress incontinence. In addition, 73% of the patients with bladder neck descent type Green I also had urodynamic stress incontinence.

Conclusion.—Lateral urethrocystography had a 91% sensitivity but a low specificity for screening stress incontinence. The combination of this procedure with urodynamic and clinical examinations provides complementary information for the diagnosis and treatment of urinary incontinence.

▶ Lateral urethrocystography is an x-ray technique that exposes the patient to irradiation, is time consuming, and is not always easy for the patient.

Static urethrocystography has been shown to be of low specificity and to correlate poorly with the dynamic events of stress incontinence. Dynamic urethrocystography, especially when combined with pressure measurements, is very expensive and is indicated for selective cases, not as a screening test. This work finds lateral urethrocystography to be highly sensitive (91%), but of low specificity in evaluating urinary incontinence. A test with such a low specificity cannot serve as a screening test, especially because it is a quite complicated and expensive x-ray study. The role of x-ray in the evaluation of urinary incontinence should be reserved to a few selected indications and should not be used as a screening method of evaluation.—A. Bergman, M.D.

Usefulness of Urodynamic Investigations in Female Incontinence

De Muylder X, Claes H, Neven P, De Jaegher K (Clinique Saint Jean, Brussels)

Eur J Obstet Gynecol Reprod Biol 44:205–208, 1992 14–6

Purpose.—The role of urodynamic evaluation in the diagnosis of micturition disorders in female patients was studied prospectively.

Setting.—Clinical diagnosis and subsequent urodynamic findings were compared in 408 female patients with urinary incontinence. Detrusor instability was diagnosed if urethrocystometry demonstrated an increase in true detrusor pressure of 15 cm or more, whereas genuine stress incontinence was diagnosed when urinary incontinence occurred in the absence of detrusor contraction associated with an increase in intra-abdominal pressure.

Findings.—Of the 286 women with stress and/or urge incontinence, 79.7% had genuine stress incontinence, 16% had detrusor instability, and 4.2% had no objective evidence of incontinence (table). Moreover, among patients with pure stress incontinence, 28.2% had no genuine stress incontinence and 52% had detrusor instability. Although stress incontinence was a very sensitive predictor of genuine stress incontinence (94% sensitivity), it was not very specific (65%). Urgency and urge incontinence had limited sensitivity (62%) and specificity (47%) for detecting detrusor instability.

Conclusion.—The symptoms of stress and urge incontinence are rather poor predictors of micturition disorders in female patients. Although the symptom complex may give an index of suspicion on the nature of the functional disorder, it is not entirely reliable, and an accurate diagnosis is very difficult without full urodynamic investigation. Most female patients with urinary incontinence should undergo urodynamic evaluation, particularly those who are being considered for surgery of stress incontinence.

▶ A history of loss of urine only with stress—with no urinary urgency or frequency—is suggestive of stress urinary incontinence. Some physicians may apply the diagnosis of genuine stress incontinence and, perhaps, perform a surgical procedure when history of stress incontinence is "straight forward".

Comparison of History and Urodynamic Findings in 408 Patients Undergoing Multichannel Urodynamics

	History	Urodynamic diagnosis							
		GSI		DI		GSI & DI		CONT	
		n	%	*n*	%	*n*	%	*n*	%
Pure stress	170	69	41	36	21	53	31	12	7
Stress and urge	116	61	53	10	8	45	39	0	
Pure urge	122	8	7	86	70	6	5	22	18

Abbreviations: GSI, genuine stress incontinence; *DI*, detrusor instability; CONT, continent.
(Courtesy of De Muylder X, Claes H, Neven P, et al: *Eur J Obstet Gynecol Reprod Biol* 44:205–208, 1992.)

With such an approach, 28% of the patients in this series might have undergone an unnecessary procedure, and 50% might be worse or not improved after their operation. Most experts agree that history alone is insufficient to establish diagnosis of genuine stress incontinence; this study proves that point. Sophisticated and complicated urodynamic testing is not always available, and the minimum objective testing needed is unknown. Patients in this series who did not have stress incontinence had detrusor instability or no incontinence. Simple cystometry and the observation of loss of urine might have detected all of them. Sophisticated urodynamic testing should be reserved for the few patients with the combined problem of stress and detrusor instability incontinence.—A. Bergman, M.D.

Prevalence of Abnormal Urodynamic Test Results in Continent Women With Severe Genitourinary Prolapse

Rosenzweig BA, Pushkin S, Blumenfeld D, Bhatia NN (Univ of California, Los Angeles)

Obstet Gynecol 79:539–542, 1992 14–7

Introduction.—Prospective studies have shown that 15% to 80% of women with genitourinary prolapse have evidence of stress urinary incontinence after undergoing reduction of the prolapse in the urodynamic laboratory. However, the prevalence of detrusor instability or mixed urinary incontinence in women with severe prolapse has not been determined.

Patients.—Twenty-two women, aged 34–77 years, with severe genitourinary prolapse underwent complete urogynecological evaluation. Eighteen of the 22 were postmenopausal. Only those patients with prolapse of pelvic structures through the vaginal introitus and no symptoms of urinary incontinence (except for an occasional episode) were included in the study. Static and dynamic urethral pressure profiles were obtained with and without reduction of the prolapse with a properly fitting vaginal ring pessary.

Results.—Thirteen of the 22 women (59%) had an occult incontinence disorder on urodynamic testing; 4 had urine loss during cough pressure profiles after pessary placement, 4 had uninhibited detrusor contractions during retrograde medium-fill water cystometry, and 5 had both stress urinary incontinence and an unstable bladder. The remaining 9 women had no detectable urodynamic abnormality. Nine women (41%) had associated symptoms of frequency, nocturia, and urgency; 4 of the 9 had normal urodynamic test results and 5 had abnormal test results. Thus, associated symptoms were not helpful in distinguishing patients who had normal or abnormal urodynamic test results.

Conclusion.—Women with severe genitourinary prolapse may be at risk for uninhibited detrusor contractions. Urine loss in these patients may be masked in the presence of a prolapse.

► In this series, more than 50% of continent women with severe genitourinary prolapse had an "occult" urinary problem. The problem was "uncovered" with reduction of the prolapse. Clinical symptoms had a sensitivity of less than 50%, which has a lesser predictive value than "flipping a coin". Only 4 of 13 continent women with "occult incontinence" on urodynamics had a clinically observed loss of urine. Therefore, neither symptoms nor observation of urine loss are sensitive enough to predict who is at risk of having urinary incontinence post operatively. Urodynamic testing performed with cystocele reduction in these continent patients is probably the most sensitive way to identify "high risk" women, thus guiding the surgeon as to whether a "prophylactic" anti-incontinence procedure should be performed. Some women with severe pelvic relaxation may have "de novo" stress incontinence develop after their cystocele repair.—A. Bergman, M.D.

Use of Transvaginal Endosonography in the Evaluation of Women With Stress Urinary Incontinence

Johnson JD, Lamensdorf H, Hollander IN, Thurman AE (Fort Worth Urology Clin, Fort Worth, Tex)

J Urol 147:421–425, 1992 14–8

Background.—Uncomplicated stress urinary incontinence results from hypermobility of the bladder neck, which is caused by increased intra-abdominal pressure. Such hypermobility may be reliably assessed by transvaginal endosonography. Considerations of technique and findings in 279 women with genuine stress urinary incontinence were studied.

Technique.—The patient is placed in dorsolithotomy position with a comfortably full bladder. Using ultrasound guidance, a calcium alginate urethral swab is lubricated with lidocaine jelly and placed in the urethra, precisely at the bladder neck. The scanner is inserted in the distal vagina. The patient performs the Valsalva's maneuver which makes the bladder neck descend. The scanner is allowed to move with the bladder neck, with care taken not to support the neck with the transducer.

Observations.—Using this procedure, the bladder neck was seen to descend more than 1 cm in 271 of the 279 women. The average descent in 64 women without stress incontinence was .32 cm. Postoperative ultrasound examination in 89 patients who underwent bladder neck reconstruction showed a clear correlation between resolution of incontinence and stabilization of bladder neck mobility.

Discussion.—After bladder neck resuspension, this examination clearly demonstrates the benefits of the repair or documents its failure. If significant cystocele is seen, it may be difficult to locate the bladder neck sonographically; precision is increased by use of a calcium alginate swab placed as a marker exactly at the bladder neck.

► Ultrasound is now widely used in gynecology and is available in many offices. It has been proven helpful in assessing bladder-base mobility. One of the concerns in using a vaginal probe is preventing bladder-base mobility by the probe. The examining physician should be aware of this possibility and should keep the probe in the distal vagina only.

Vaginal ultrasound definitely has a role in assessing a patient with previous failures or patients with stress incontinence and no hypermobility of the bladder base by currently used tests. As a screening test, the simple "Q-tip test" can serve the same purpose at a lower cost. The authors used a cotton swab to locate the bladder base. No data is given on the correlation between the "cotton swab" test and ultrasound in assessing bladder base hypermobility. If the correlation is good, then the simple "cotton swab" test should serve as a screening test, and vaginal ultrasound should be reserved to the more complicated cases.—A. Bergman, M.D.

Symptom Analysis of Patients Undergoing Modified Pereyra Bladder Neck Suspension for Stress Urinary Incontinence: Pre- and Postoperative Findings

Kelly MJ, Roskamp D, Knielsen K, Leach GE, Bruskewitz R (Kaiser Permanente Med Ctr, Los Angeles; Univ of Wisconsin, Madison)

Urology 37:213–219, 1991 14–9

Introduction.—Although there are several procedures for the treatment of genuine stress urinary incontinence (SUI), accurate long-term outcome data have not been available. A retrospective chart review and patient interview were conducted to examine the outcome of a modified Pereyra bladder neck suspension (MPBNS) in patients with SUI who were followed up for at least 2 years.

Methods.—Only those patients with clinically proved urine loss from SUI who underwent complete urodynamic studies before operation were included in the analysis. Stamey's system was used to grade SUI. All patients meeting the selection criteria were contacted and interviewed by telephone. The follow-up ranged from 2 to 7.7 years; the median follow-up was 3.5 years. Any leakage attributable to SUI was rated as a surgical failure, and absence of any leakage with stress was rated as a surgical success.

Results.—Of 145 patients who met the inclusion criteria, 114 (79%) completed the follow-up interview. Analysis of the preoperative urinary symptoms revealed that 59% of the patients had urinary urgency before operation, and 59% had urinary frequency. After operation, the incidence of urgency symptoms decreased to 53% and the incidence of urinary frequency decreased to 52%. At follow-up, 58 patients (51%) reported having no SUI whatsoever. Examination of the 56 patients who reported postoperative SUI revealed that 54.5% of them had grade 1, 37.5% had grade 2, and 8% had grade 3 SUI. Overall, 76% of the patients stated that their subjective sense of urinary control was better or much better, 15% said it was the same, and 9% said it was worse or much worse. Thus, a total continence rate of 51% and a subjective success rate of 76% had been achieved at the time of follow-up. The subjective sense of postoperative urinary control correlated highly with the degree of postoperative SUI. Further examination of the data revealed that age, parity, weight, and previous anti-incontinence operations did not significantly affect the success rate.

Conclusion.—The persistent or de novo urgency symptoms after MPBNS were highly associated with postoperative stress leakage and subjective failure.

► This study correlates well with other reports on the long-term effect of needle suspension operation. The telephone follow-up of patients symptoms is less than optimal, and it may indicate only subjective success or failure, which does not always correlate with objective findings. However, the long-term follow-up in this study (median follow-up, 3.5 years; minimum follow-up, 2 years) indicates the efficacy of the procedure.

Fifty-one percent were subjectively cured by the procedure, and another 25% improved. In most studies, the objective findings are worse than the subjective results; therefore, the 24% subjective failure rate in this series may represent the higher objective failure rate of the procedure. Of interest is the fact that, in 23% of patients who failed their operation, recurrent incontinence was experienced more than 2 years' postoperatively. Because many incontinence operations attached soft tissues to soft tissues in the bladder neck suspension, perhaps 5-years' results are the real indicator of efficacy of an operative procedure.—A. Bergman, M.D.

Failure to Predict and Attempts to Explain Urinary Stress Incontinence Following Vaginal Repair in Continent Women by Using a Modified Lateral Urethrocystography

Borstad E, Skrede M, Rud T (Aker University, Oslo)

Acta Obstet Gynecol Scand 70:501–506, 1991 14–10

Background.—Continent women who have original repair for genitourinary prolapse are at a significant risk for urinary stress incontinence (USI). Whether women having USI after vaginal repair have certain specific preoperative anatomical features in common or whether the incontinence may be related to surgery was determined.

Methods and Findings.—Of 58 continent women undergoing urethrocystography before and 3 months after surgery for genitourinary prolapse, 16 (28%) had stress incontinence after the procedure. Preoperative radiological features were not useful in distinguishing those patients having incontinence from those who were still continent after surgery. Stress incontinence after a Manchester procedure for genital prolapse appeared to depend on an insufficient elevation of the bladder neck and a radical reduction of the cystocele. A parameter that combined 2 factors—percentage reduction of the cystocele minus the percentage elevation of the bladder neck—was significantly higher in women having stress incontinence than in those remaining continent (Figs 14–2 and 14–3).

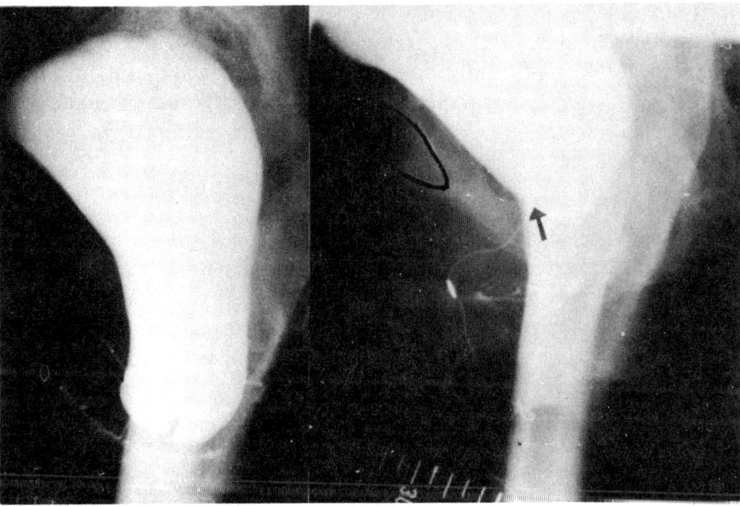

Fig 14–2.—Lateral urethrocysto-urethrograms performed preoperatively and postoperatively in a patient remaining continent after a Manchester procedure. A metric ruler was placed between the thighs to allow direct measurement on the roentgenographs. The urethra is visualized by a thin leaden thread, the external meatus is marked with a silver clip, and contrast dye indicates the bladder outlines. The bladder-neck is indicated by an *arrow*. (Courtesy of Borstad E, Skrede M, Rud T: *Acta Obstet Gynecol Scand* 70:501–506, 1991.)

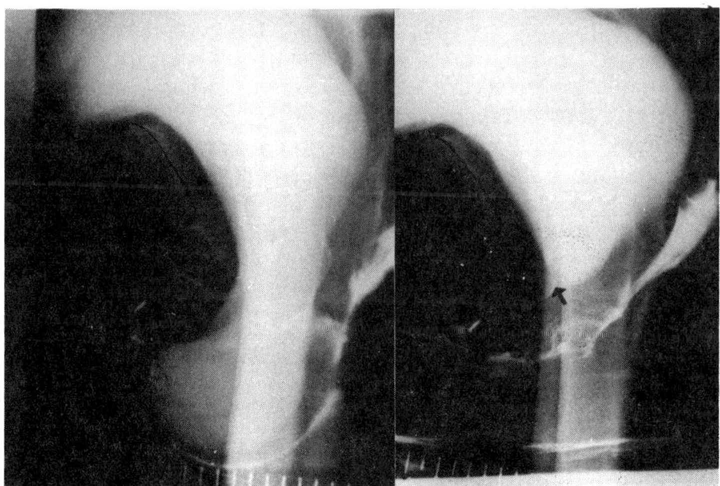

Fig 14–3.—Preoperative and postoperative lateral urethrocystograms of a patient with urinary stress-incontinence after a Manchester procedure. Same technique as in previous figure. (Courtesy of Borstad E, Skrede M, Rud T: *Acta Obstet Gynecol Scand* 70:501–506, 1991.)

Discussion.—As many as 25% of continent women have USI after a Manchester procedure is done for genital prolapse. A good elevation of the bladder neck, preferably combined with an adequate but not too tight reduction of the cystocele, seems important to avoid postoperative USI. Urethrocystography does not appear to be helpful in identifying women who will have USI after vaginal repair.

▶ The problem of stress incontinence developing after cystocele repair in previously continent women is of significant clinical importance. It is known that, although some continent women may have urinary sphincter incompetence, they stay continent because of the kinking effect on the urethra of a large cystocele; reducing the cystocele in continent women with sphincteric incompetence will uncover their problem resulting in postoperative stress incontinence (1). In this study, 28% of continent women had stress incontinence develop after their operation; this is an unacceptably high figure. Therefore, identifying women at high risk of having postoperative stress incontinence is of great clinical importance. This current paper tries to identify such women preoperatively.

Borstad et al.'s results indicate that x-ray studies are inadequate for this purpose. Their results are not surprising, because numerous studies have shown that "static" x-ray studies are not helpful in evaluation of urinary sphincter functions. A better method of preoperative evaluation of women with a large cystocele probably involves reducing the cystocele, filling their bladder to maximal capacity, and asking them to cough. The same manuever can be done while doing urodynamic testing. If simulating the operation by cystocele reduction results in a loss of urine or urodynamic evidence of weak sphincter, then these women need a "prophylactic" anti-incontinence procedure in addition to cystocele repair. In the absence of evidence of weak spincteric functions when reducing the cystocele, the surgeon should be aware not to "over correct" the prolapsed bladder and not to lift the bladder base higher than the urethrovesical junction (as suggested by the authors).—A. Bergman, M.D.

Reference

1. Bump RC, et al: *Obstet Gynecol* 72:291, 1988.

Transvaginal Ultrasonography and Urodynamic Evaluation After Suspension Operations: Comparison Among the Gittes, Stamey and Burch Suspensions

Kil PJM, Hoekstra JW, van der Meijden APM, Smans AJ, Theeuwes AGM, Schreinemachers LMH (Groot Ziekengasthuis, Hertogenbosch, The Netherlands; Catholic Univ Nijmegen, The Netherlands)

J Urol 146:132–136, 1991 14–11

Background.—Suspension operations are performed to elevate and fix the bladder neck, thereby relieving stress urinary incontinence. For purposes of patient selection and procedure evaluation, the bladder neck position and movement must be determined. Urodynamic evaluation and transvaginal ultrasonography were used to assess the results of the Gittes, Stamey, and Burch suspensions in 60 patients with stress urinary incontinence.

Methods.—Twenty-nine women underwent Burch colposuspension, 18 were treated with the Gittes method, and 13 were treated with the Stamey method. The 3 groups were comparable in age, duration of symptoms, parity, and preoperative urodynamic evaluation. Ultrasonographic evaluation that was performed after urodynamic investigation yielded information on the position of the bladder neck in relation to the symphysis.

Results.—The patients were evaluated at 3 months after operation and after a mean follow-up ranging from 10 to 39 months. The continence rates were similar for the 3 groups at 3 months (83% to 93%). Continence subsequently decreased, however, to 44% after the Gittes technique and to 69% after the Stamey procedure. Patients with Burch colposuspension retained a more durable continence rate (86%). Urodynamic evaluations revealed no significant differences among the 3 operations.

Conclusion.—The value of ultrasonography in providing information about the position of the bladder neck and base in patients with stress urinary incontinence has been confirmed. Urodynamic evaluation was of little use in evaluating results after suspension operations. The main factor concerning continence was the rotation angle and descent of the bladder neck.

▶ The main mechanism by which an incontinence operation restores continence is by suspension of the urethrovesical junction to a high retropubic position. Hertogs and Stanton (1) have shown that failure of an operation to cure genuine stress incontinence is often a result of failure to suspend the bladder neck in a high position. In evaluating women after operation when incontinence reoccurs, it is very important to know whether the failure is "functional" or "technical." "Functional failure" may be the presence of detrusor instability (either undiagnosed preoperatively or "de novo" postoperative development) or a failure occurring despite a well-suspended bladder; it should not be treated by a repeat bladder neck suspension. "Technical failure" occurs when bladder-base hypermobility still exists after surgery; it can be treated by another bladder neck suspension. Ultrasound is a readily available, good tool in evaluating bladder-base and urethrovesical junction (UVJ) mobility.

This study prospectively evaluates 3 operative procedures for stress incontinence. The abdominal procedure (Burch) was more successful in curing stress incontinence by more effectively suspending the urethrovesical junction to a high position. The vaginal procedures (Stamey and Gittes) were less effective in suspending the UVJ and resulted in higher failure rate in a long-term follow-up.

Vaginal ultrasound was very effective in the detection of postoperative bladder-base hypermobility, thus differentiating "functional" from "technical" failures. Although many gynecologists do not have a ready access to urodynamic centers, most have an easy access to sonograms. Vaginal ultrasonography is an important tool in evaluation of failed anti-incontinence operations, to assess bladder-base mobility, and to better estimate whether another bladder neck suspension is going to be beneficial to the patient.—A. Bergman, M.D.

Reference

1. Hertogs K, Stanton SL: *Br J Obstet Gynaecol* 92:1179, 1985.

Position and Mobility of the Urethrovesical Junction in Continent and in Stress Incontinent Women Before and After Successful Surgery

Carey MP, Dwyer PL (Univ of Melbourne; Mercy Hosp for Women, Melbourne)

Aust N Z J Obstet Gynaecol 31:279–284, 1991 14–12

Introduction.—Stress incontinence surgery is designed to elevate and fix the urethrovesical junction while maintaining the mobility of the surrounding tissues. The repositioning of the urethra should permit more complete transmission of intraabdominal pressure to the urethra, thereby creating a mechanical valve effect.

Methods.—The position and mobility of the urethrovesical junction were compared between 9 continent women and 27 women with genuine stress incontinence before and after successful surgery, using the Burch colposuspension or Stamey procedures. Each patient underwent lateral bead-chain urethrocystography (both at rest and straining) before and 3 months after surgery. The 9 controls also underwent urethrocystography and urodynamic assessment.

Results.—Both at rest and straining, women with genuine stress incontinence had significantly lower bladder neck positions than continent women did. At rest, but not with straining, these women also had urethrovesicular junctions significantly further from the posterior aspect of the symphysis pubis than did the continent women. The posterior urethrovesicular angles were similar in the 2 groups. After successful surgery in 25 patients, the urethrovesical junction was significantly higher, closer to the symphysis, and less mobile. The modified Burch colposuspension was associated with a higher final position than the Stamey procedure. Successful surgery resulted in significant narrowing of the posterior urethrovesical angle.

Conclusion.—Genuine stress incontinence in these patients was characterized by poor support of the bladder neck, with the urethrovesical junction lower and more distal to the urethrovesical junction than in continent women. Although suspension surgery can provide adequate repositioning and fixation of the urethrovesical segment, stress incontinence may persist, possibly because of postoperative development of poor intrinsic urethral function, detrusor instability, or overflow incontinence.

▶ This study, like the previous one (Abstract 14–11) emphasizes bladder-base and urethrovesical junction (UVJ) mobility as an important predisposing factor for development of stress urinary incontinence. Like the previous article, successful operation resulted in fixation of the UVJ in a high retropubic position. The authors used X-ray techniques to assess UVJ mobility. Like the previous study, the UVJ was fixed at a higher position after abdominal procedures compared with vaginal operations. An important clinical suggestion is made by the authors, i.e., while fixing the urethrovesical junction, the bladder base should be allowed some mobility so that the junction is not at the most dependent portion of the bladder during stress.—A. Bergman, M.D.

Pelvic Muscle Exercise for Stress Urinary Incontinence in Elderly Women

Wells TJ, Brink CA, Diokno AC, Wolfe R, Gillis GL (Univ of Rochester, NY; Univ of Michigan, Ann Arbor)

J Am Geriatr Soc 39:785–791, 1991 14–13

Introduction.—Stress urinary incontinence is the most common cause of urinary leakage in community-residing older women. Pelvic-muscle exercise (PME) and drug treatment with phenylpropanolamine (PPA), either alone or in combination with estrogen, appear to be effective in the treatment of stress urine loss. This clinical trial compared the effectiveness of PME and PPA in older community-living women with stress urinary incontinence.

Patients.—During a 4-year period, 338 women 55 to 90 years of age (mean age, 67.5 years) entered the study. A total of 72% of the women were incontinent daily, whereas 83% experienced large volume loss including pooling on the floor and 55% had experienced urine loss for more than 5 years. A diagnosis of urge incontinence was made when detrusor hyperactivity was present as demonstrated by uninhibited contractions of 15 cm or more of water during provocative cystometry. Women with both urethral incompetency and detrusor hyperactivity were given a diagnosis of mixed-type incontinence. Women who had urethral incompetency, either alone or in combination with detrusor hyperactivity, when stress was judged to be more dominant were randomly assigned to PME or PPA. The PME protocol consisted of 6 months of active pelvic-muscle exercise with monthly monitoring visits. No resistive practice device was used. Phenylpropanolamine was given in a dose of 50 mg daily for 2 weeks, increasing to twice daily for another 2 weeks if wetting continued by self-report.

Results.—On urodynamic studies, 284 women (84%) had urethral incompetency. Only 157 women entered the treatment phase, 118 of whom completed treatment. Fifty-four of 82 women assigned to PME completed treatment, for an attrition rate of 34%. Sixty-four of 75 women assigned to PPA completed treatment, for an attrition rate of 15%. The difference was statistically significant. Subjective improvement was reported by 77% of PME-treated women and 84% of PPA-treated women. The difference was statistically not significant. Objective examination revealed that the Digital Test for pelvic muscle strength was the only significant difference between treatment outcomes. Twenty-seven percent of PME-treated women and 14% of PPA-treated women became dry, and 21% of PME-treated women and 39% of PPA-treated women improved. Forty exercises per day were found to be an absolute minimum, but a goal of at least 80 exercises per day was likely to give improvement.

Conclusion.—Both PME and PPA are appropriate treatments for urinary stress incontinence in elderly women. However, adherence to treatment was better with PPA.

▶ Stress urinary incontinence is a major problem among older women living in nursing homes and other community facilities. In addition to PME exercises and PPA, small doses of vaginally administered estrogen also have proven to be effective in treating this disorder.—D.R. Mishell, Jr., M.D.

Assessment of Kegel Pelvic Muscle Exercise Performance After Brief Verbal Instruction

Bump RC, Hurt WG, Fantl JA, Wyman JF (Virginia Commonwealth Univ, Richmond, Va)

Am J Obstet Gynecol 165:322–329, 1991 14–14

Introduction.—Biofeedback via vaginal pressure measurements, electromyography, or digital palpation of pubococcygeus muscle tone has been advocated to facilitate the initiation of a Kegel exercise program in the treatment of urinary incontinence. However, most patients can perform Kegel exercises after only brief written or oral instructions. The efficacy of a brief verbal instruction on urethral sphincteric function during a Kegal contraction was assessed.

Methods.—A group of 47 women (mean age, 53.6 years) underwent a standardized urodynamic evaluation that included passive and dynamic urethral pressure profiles. After completion of the standard examination, a passive urethral pressure profile was repeated at a rate of 5 mm/second. Each patient was then asked to contract the muscles she would use if she was trying to keep from losing urine or trying to stop the stream after having started to urinate. Of the 47 patients, 28 had urinary incontinence as their major complaint. Of the 28, 14 had pure genuine stress incontinence, 4 had pure detrusor instability, 6 had mixed incontinence, and 4 had pure urethral instability. The other 19 women did not have incontinence.

Results.—A total of 28 patients (60%) had an effective Kegel effort, which was defined as a Kegel urethral pressure profile area equal to or greater than 120% of the passive urethral pressure profile area. However, 5 of these 28 patients achieved an effective Kegel effort with an appreciable increase in abdominal and vaginal pressure. Thus, only 23 (49%) of the patients had an ideal Kegel effort, which was defined as a significant increase in urethral pressure without a concurrent increase in vesical and abdominal pressure. No historic or urodynamic parameters could be found that reliably identified patients who were likely to have either an effective or ineffective Kegel effort.

Conclusion.—A simple verbal instruction alone is not adequate preparation for a patient starting a Kegel exercise program.

▶ The Kegel exercise was introduced by Arnold Kegel in the late '40s, with a reported success rate in curing stress urinary incontinence of more than 75% (1). These exercises have become popular again in the past few years, with a reported significant improvement or cure rate of more than 70%. However, these exercises require a devoted team that is willing to spend time in teaching the patient how to perform the exercise and a close follow-up to correct possible mistakes. A few of the mistakes may include tightening the wrong muscles or inadvertently creating a Valsalva maneuver. Good results from using the Kegel exercise can be expected only with good cooperation and a devoted team. This study proves that point in a very nice, prospective, urodynamic, objective way.

In a good and adequately performed Kegel exercise, urethral pressure should be increased with no change in abdominal pressure. This goal was achieved in less than 50% of the patients performing the Kegel exercise after brief verbal instruction. Verbal instruction with no follow-up is an inadequate way of instructing Kegel exercise, and results should be assessed only if the exercise is performed adequately.—A. Bergman, M.D.

Reference

1. Kegel A: *Am J Obstet Gynecol* 56:242, 1948.

Long-Term Effect of Pelvic Floor Exercises on Female Urinary Incontinence

Mouritsen L, Frimodt-Møller C, Møller M (Gentofte Hosp, Copenhagen)

Br J Urol 68:32–37, 1991 14–15

Background.—Research has shown that pelvic floor exercises have an effect on female urinary incontinence. Because no side effects have been reported, this conservative approach is recommended before surgery is considered. The results of a 3-month pelvic floor exercise program were analyzed to assess the permanent effect of this treatment on female stress incontinence.

Methods.—Seventy-six women who were incontinent and referred for surgery were enrolled in the exercise program, which was conducted by an experienced exercise physiotherapist. The patients were then followed up for 1 year.

Outcomes.—Thirty percent of the patients were cured, and 17% improved at the last assessment. Overall, surgery was avoided in 47% of the cases. No relapses occurred during follow-up. Those with mild incontinence benefited from intensified training; of these patients, 72% were cured. Those with severe incontinence and no immediate effect did not benefit from further exercise. Women with a positive hormone status and women of normal weight had significantly better cure rates. Subjective outcomes were confirmed by the 24-hour pad test.

Conclusion.—With an intensive pelvic floor exercise program, almost half of incontinent women may be cured or improved 1 year after the program is completed, thus avoiding surgery. For those in this series who were cured immediately after the exercises, the effect was permanent in 85%. Women with grades II or III incontinence who were subjectively unchanged or improved at their first assessment benefited only minimally from further exercises; such patients should be offered surgery at this time.

▶ This is another report on the beneficial effect of the Kegel exercises for women with urinary incontinence. The original Kegel series reported 70% favorable results (cure or significant improvement) in women with stress urinary incontinence. Later works confirmed these encouraging reports. In spite of the efficacy of this method, Kegel exercise did not gain popularity in the '60s and '70s, possibly because the exercise regimen requires a dedicated practitioner to work with the patient, and possibly because there is a lack of clear selection criteria for choosing women to participate in these programs. In the past few years, more centers report encouraging results of the Kegel exercise for women with urinary incontinence. This paper adds to our understanding about selecting women who are incontinent to participate in the Kegel exercise program. A 72% cure rate in women with mild incontinence, using a conservative approach, is a very good result. Poor results in women with grade II and III incontinence indicates which women should not undergo this program. In the presence of a motivated staff to teach and follow up performance, the Kegel exercise is a very reasonable alternative to surgery in a selected group of women.—A. Bergman, M.D.

Para-Urethral Collagen Implantation for Female Stress Incontinence
Eckford SD, Abrams P (Southmead Hosp, Bristol, England)
Br J Urol 68:586–589, 1991 14–16

Purpose.—Genuine stress incontinence (GSI) in women may be the result of bladder neck hypermobility, intrinsic urethral sphincter weakness, or both. A cross-linked collagen preparation was used for paraurethral injection to increase the urethral pressure in a series of women with GSI secondary to urethral sphincter weakness.

Patients.—Twenty-seven women, aged 34–79 years, with urodynamically confirmed GSI were entered into the study. Ten patients had previously undergone failed incontinence surgery. One month before paraurethral injection, patients underwent skin testing for hypersensitivity to collagen. Two patients had a positive response to the skin test and were excluded from the trial. The patients were evaluated by questioning and pad testing 1 month after the initial collagen injection. Those who had not become completely continent were retreated with a further collagen injection. Urodynamic evaluation was repeated 3 months after the last collagen injection.

Outcome.—Eighteen patients (72%) required retreatment after the initial collagen injection. Sixteen patients (64%) had complete cessation of GSI and 4 (16%) were improved, for an overall success rate of 80%. Collagen injection was successful in 9 of the 10 women (90%) who had had previous incontinence surgery and in 11 of the 15 women (73%) who had no previous surgery. A comparison of the urodynamic measurements obtained before and after collagen injection in the 16 symptomatically cured patients revealed an increase in maximum urethral closure pressure, a decrease in urine flow rate, and a decrease in the functional urethral length.

Conclusion.—Paraurethral injection of collagen appears to be a promising technique for the treatment of female GSI.

▶ Urinary incontinence persisting after operation for stress incontinence is a frustrating problem. One of the main reasons for a failed incontinence operation is detrusor instability (either as an undiagnosed preoperative finding or as a "de novo" postoperative phenomenon). After ruling out detrusor instability, diagnosis of stress incontinence should be established based on urodynamic testing. Once diagnosis of GSI is established, one should differentiate between "technical" and "functional" failures. "Technical" failures, i.e., when bladder-base hypermobility still persists after operation, are best treated by repeat operation to better support the bladder base. "Functional" failures are failures in spite of successful support to the bladder base. Women with "functional" failure of an incontinent operation are at high risk of failure of another incontinent operation, and they are good candidates for paraurethral collagen injections.

Paraurethral teflon injections were used in the '80s for similar conditions with reported good results. However, migration of teflon from the injection site and even pulmonary emboli prevented this method from gaining popularity. Recently, the GAX collagen was introduced with no reported problems of collagen migration.

The reported cure rate in this series is 53% with 20% improvement, for a 73% success rate in patients with no previous operation; this is almost as good as the cure rate associated with operative procedure. These results make this "office procedure" an attractive alternative to surgery. The authors report a 90% success rate in patients who had a previous incontinence surgery. These results are better than the cure rate reported after repeated operations. If these good results will hold in long-term follow-up, then paraurethral injection may become an excellent alternative to surgery in patients with previous failures. Currently, the main indication for paraurethral collagen injection should be limited to women with "functional" failure after incontinence surgery, i.e., stress incontinence in the absence of bladder-base hypermobility.—A. Bergman, M.D.

A 25-Year Experience With 519 Anterior Colporrhaphy Procedures

Beck RP, McCormick S, Nordstrom L (Univ of Alberta, Edmonton)

Obstet Gynecol 78:1011–1018, 1991 14–17

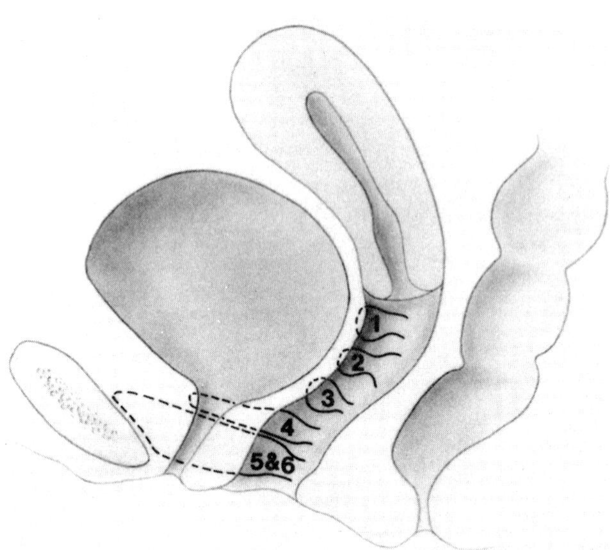

Fig 14–4.—Placement of the sutures in sagittal view. When tied, the fascia under the bladder base is plicated. Overcorrection of cystocele is avoided. When sutures 5 and 6, in the fascia under and around the urethra, are tied, the urethra is elevated more than the bladder base (and is tightened). (Courtesy of Beck RP, McCormick S., Nordstrom L: *Obstet Gynecol* 78:1011–1018, 1991.)

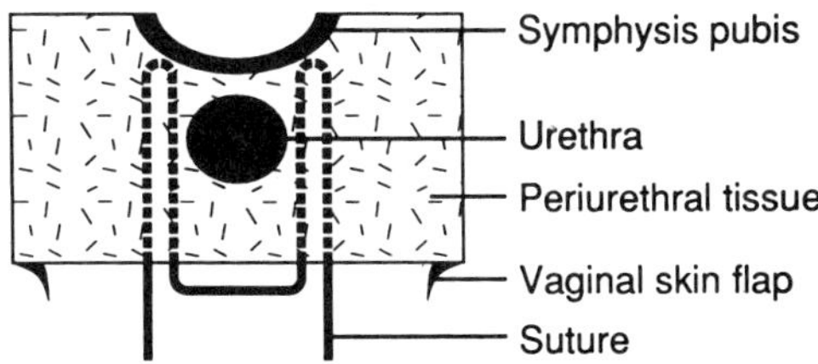

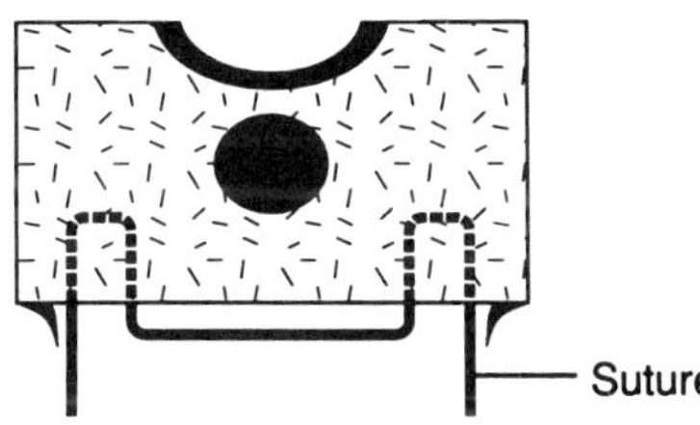

Fig 14–5.—Diagram illustrates correct (**A**) and incorrect (**B**) placement of sutures under and around the urethra. Correct placement of deep sutures close to the urethra tightens and elevates the urethra, whereas incorrect placement (too shallow and remote from the urethra) might correct prolapse, but produces minimal urethral tightening and elevation. (Courtesy of Beck RP, McCormick S., Nordstrom L: *Obstet Gynecol* 78:1011–1018, 1991.)

Background.—In the past decade, several studies have reported relatively unsatisfactory results with anterior colporrhaphy in the treatment of genuine stress urinary incontinence. One surgeon's 25-year experience with anterior colporrhaphy was reviewed (Figs 14–4, 14–5, 14–6).

Methods.—A total of 519 anterior colporrhaphies were reviewed to evaluate the treatment's efficacy in patients with genuine and mixed stress urinary incontinence. The incidence of new urinary incontinence after prolapse surgery, the incidence of new detrusor instability after incontinence and prolapse surgery, and the morbidity associated with anterior colporrhaphy were established.

Outcomes.—When a Kelly-Kennedy-type technique was modified to include a vaginal retropubic urethropexy, the cure rate in 194 patients with genuine stress incontinence increased from 75% to 94%. The surgical cure rate in patients with mixed incontinence was unsatisfactory (64%) in unselected cases. However, in selected cases, it was 84%, which was considered good. Previous surgery for incontinence, particularly more than 1 procedure, significantly decreased the cure rate for genuine stress incontinence. New incontinence after prolapse surgery developed in 11% of 1 subgroup. The postoperative incidence of new detrusor instability was 6%. Significant morbidity other than incontinence occurred in only 1% (table).

Conclusions.—Anterior colporrhaphy with vaginal retropubic urethropexy is the preferred initial operation for patients with genuine stress incontinence. These results compare favorably with other procedures, and

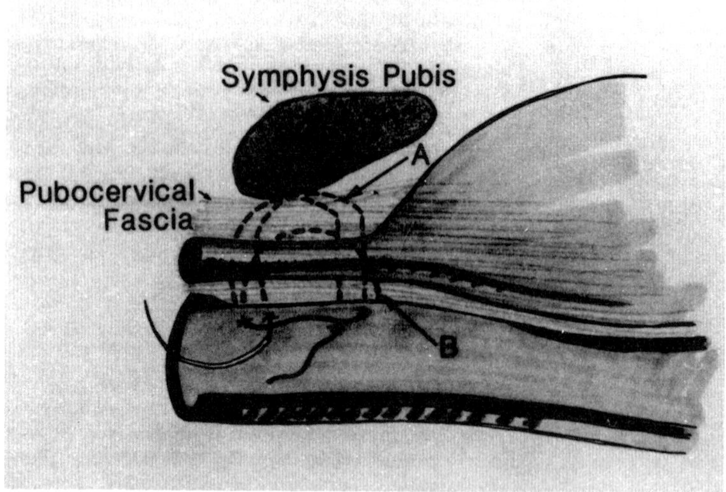

Fig 14–6.—Suture *A* shows proper placement of figure-of-eight suture in the pubocervical fascia lateral and close to the urethra. When tied, the suture plicates the fascia lateral to and under the urethra, elevating it. Suture *B* illustrates improper placement with respect to depth and direction. (Reprinted with permission from the American College of Obstetrics and Gynecologists. Courtesy of Beck RP, McCormick S: *Obstet Gynecol* 1982; 59:269; from Beck RP, McCormick S, Nordstrom L: *Obstet Gynecol* 78:1011–1018, 1991.)

the morbidity associated with this procedure is much lower than with abdominal retropubic procedures. In addition, vaginal prolapse, which often co-exists with stress incontinence, can be corrected simultaneously in the same operative field.

▶ This series reports a 75% cure rate of stress incontinence by anterior colporrhaphy using Kelly sutures and a more than 90% cure rate by the modified procedure. The first figure, the 75% cure rate, is the figure that is reported by other centers after anterior colporrhaphy and the Kelly procedure. The revised procedure includes the periosteum of the pubic bone in the suture, making it almost a Marshall-Marchetti-Krantz operation done vaginally. No wonder the results are better and a gynecologist performing the "standard" anterior colporrhaphy with Kelly sutures cannot expect similar results.

The authors' results were not as good when the patient had mixed incontinence. Other groups reported similar results. These findings indicate that some kind of urodynamic testing (cystometry as a minimal urodynamic workup) is required before any operation for stress incontinence. In mixed incontinence, these facts have to be discussed with the patient, because the cure rate is reduced significantly.

A third important point brought up in this article is the development of the "de novo" stress incontinence after prolapse surgery, which was 11% in 1 subgroup. This finding indicates that women with large cystocele should undergo some preoperative evaluation with cystocele reduction (preferred with

Treatment of Genuine Stress Incontinence With Anterior Colporrhaphy (N = 194)*

Result	Original technique (1965–1976)		Revised technique (1977–1990)	
	No. patients	Type of postoperative incontinence	No. patients	Type of postopera incontinence
Cured*	54 (75%)	0	111 (91%)	0
Improved	12 (17%)	6 GSI, 1 DI, 5 mixed	8 (7%)	4 GSI, 2 DI, 2 mixed
Failure	6 (8%)	1 GSI, 5 mixed	3 (2%)	2 GSI, 1 DI
Total	72 (100%)	18 (25%)	122 (100%)	11 (9%)

Abbreviations: GSI, genuine stress incontinence; *DI*, detrusor instability; and *mixed*, detrusor instability and genuine stress incontinence.
* $P = .003$ original vs. revised.
(Courtesy of Beck RP, McCormick S, Nordstrom L: *Obstet Gynecol* 78:1011–1018, 1991.)

a pessary) and a full bladder. If the patients lose urine on cough under these circumstances, some kind of "prophylactic" anti-incontinence procedure should be performed at the time of the cystocele repair.—A. Bergman, M.D.

Colpo-Needle Suspension for the Treatment of Urinary Stress Incontinence—A New Surgical Technique

Caspi E, Langer R (Assaf Haarofeh Med Ctr, Zerifin, Israel)

Br J Obstet Gynaecol 98:1183–1184, 1991 14–18

Introduction.—For the treatment of urinary stress incontinence, the Burch colposuspension, in which the anchoring site is the fixed Cooper's ligament, yields good results. In comparison, the transvaginal needle suspension of the bladder neck to the moving rectus muscles is easier to perform, with less postoperative morbidity, and entailing shorter hospital stays. A technique was developed that combines the anchoring of the bladder neck to the fixed ileopectineal ligaments, as in the Burch colposuspension, with a needle bladder neck suspension.

Technique.—The patient is placed in the lithotomy position, an 18F-gauge Foley catheter with 10-mL balloon is inserted, and a 4–5 cm transverse lower abdominal incision is made. The anterior rectus fascia is incised transversely, and the rectus muscles are separated at the midline. Longitudinal incisions in the anterior vaginal wall lateral to the bladder neck and urethra are made, with vaginal dissection around the bladder minimized. Triple helical bites are used to anchor monofilament prolene 1 gauge sutures. The sutures are passed suprapubically from the vagina using a Stamey needle, with one end passed through Cooper's ligament. The sutures on each side are tied firmly, bringing the paravaginal tissue in contact with the ileopectineal ligament. The vaginal and abdominal incisions are closed.

Results.—In 20 colpo-needle suspension procedures performed for women with genuine stress incontinence, there was no marked cystocele, uterine descent, or other uterine abnormalities requiring additional surgery. After 6–12 months of follow-up, all women were continent. The mean operating time was 38 minutes, with only 2 minor postoperative complications. The average hospital stay was 4.4 days. After an average of 7.1 days, spontaneous voiding was reestablished.

Conclusion.—The colponeedle technique seems to provide a simple, rapid procedure with excellent results. The risk of complications seems low, and the required hospitalization is short. Longer term follow-up and study of a larger sample are needed to validate these conclusions.

▶ One of the advantages of the retropubic abdominal procedures is that they anchor the endopelvic fascia to a firm structure, i.e., Cooper's ligament or the periosteum of the iliac bone. One of the advantages of the needle suspensions is that they are easier and quicker than most abdominal procedures.

However, the needle suspensions attach soft tissue to soft tissue, and these tissues may loosen with time. The group from Assaf Haarofeh introduces an interesting concept that combines the benefits of both needle suspension and retropubic procedures. The new technique anchors the helical endopelvic sutures to the firm Cooper's ligament, thereby avoiding the extensive perivesical dissection of the Burch procedure. The perivesical dissection of the Burch procedure results many times in significant bleeding. The average operative time of one half hour conforms with that of the needle suspensions. The short term results are promising, and it will be interesting to know the long-term effects of this procedure once the results are available—A. Bergman, M.D.

Adverse Urinary Symptoms After Total Abdominal Hysterectomy—Fact or Fiction?

Griffith-Jones MD, Jarvis GJ, McNamara HM (St James' Univ Hosp, Leeds, England)

Br J Urol 67:295–297, 1991 14–19

Objective.—Because hysterectomy has been proposed as the cause of various urinary symptoms, including urethral syndrome and stress incontinence, a prospective trial was undertaken to compare urinary symptoms after total abdominal hysterectomy with those occurring after dilatation and curettage (D & C).

Patients.—Eighty premenopausal women underwent hysterectomy and were compared with 78 others having dilatation and curettage alone. The groups were matched for age and parity.

Findings.—No urinary symptoms were more frequent after hysterectomy than after D & C, nor was the triad of frequency, urgency, and urge incontinence more common after hysterectomy (table). Stress incontinence was more frequent after D & C. Urgency and frequency did occur more often after hysterectomy, but it resolved within 3 months or less.

Conclusion.—Hysterectomy itself does not promote the occurrence of urinary symptoms, and it may actually protect against stress incontinence developing. These findings do not support the routine use of subtotal hysterectomy to prevent bladder and urethral dysfunction.

▶ Urinary symptomology unfortunately was assessed in this study by using a postoperative questionnaire instead of urodynamic testing and a personal interview. Nevertheless, the results agree with those of other studies indicating that hysterectomy without dissection of the bladder neck does not result in an increased incidence of urinary problems compared with a control group of women undergoing a dilatation and curettage.—D. R. Mishell, Jr., M.D.

Urinary Symptoms Before and After Hysterectomy and D & C

Symptom	*D & C (n=78)*		*Hysterectomy (n=80)*		*Chi-squared test*
	Before	*After*	*Before*	*After*	
Frequency	5	20	5	28	N/S
Nocturia	5	18	1	13	N/S
Urgency	3	21	6	27	N/S
Urge incontinence	2	15	5	25	N/S
Stress incontinence	1	25	4	16	$P<0.05$
Recurrent urinary tract infection	0	1	1	4	N/S
Voiding problems	2	7	0	5	N/S
Frequency, urgency + urge incontinence	1	9	3	8	N/S
Transient symptoms		8		22	$P<0.05$

(Courtesy of Griffith-Jones MD, Jarvis GJ, McNamara HM: *Br J Urol* 67:295–297, 1991.)

Single-Dose Compared With 3-Day Norfloxacin Treatment of Uncomplicated Urinary Tract Infection in Women

Saginur R, Nicolle LE, Canadian Infectious Diseases Society Clinical Trials Study Group (Ottawa Civic Hosp, Ont)

Arch Intern Med 152:1233–1237, 1992 14–20

Introduction.—Single-dose therapy for recurrent uncomplicated cystitis in women has many advantages, including compliance, less adverse antimicrobial effects, lower cost, and a possible decrease in the emergence of resistant organisms. However, studies of the efficacy of single-dose therapies have shown variable results, and the efficacy of single-dose therapy for this indication remains controversial. A prospective, randomized, double-blind study was designed to determine whether single-dose norfloxacin therapy is superior to 3 days of norfloxacin therapy in terms of efficacy and adverse effects.

Patients.—Of 219 nonpregnant women older than 18 years of age with acute uncomplicated urinary tract infection, 112 were randomly allocated to receive norfloxacin as a single 800-mg dose, and 107 received 400 mg of norfloxacin twice daily for 3 days. Clinical and laboratory evaluations were performed at baseline, 3 and 7 days after initiation of therapy, and 4 to 6 weeks after therapy. Complete data were available for 73 women who were single-dose recipients and 83 women who were treated with the 3-day regimen.

Results.—Women allocated to the 3-day regimen were significantly more likely to be bacteriologically cured at the 3- and 7-day follow-up visits than those allocated to single-dose therapy. At the 4- to 6-week follow-up visit, 57 (78%) single-dose recipients and 73 (88%) recipients of the 3-day dose regimen remained cured. The 2 regimens were equivalent for *Escherichia coli* infection, but single-dose therapy was significantly less effective for other organisms, primarily because of treatment failure in women with *Staphylococcus saprophyticus* infection.

Conclusion.—Three days of norfloxacin therapy is superior to single-dose therapy in the treatment of acute uncomplicated cystitis in women. Although the 2 regimens are equally effective for *E. coli* infection, single-dose therapy is ineffective for *S. saprophyticus.*

▶ Single-dose therapy has an advantage over the 3-day regimen because of better compliance by patients. It should be used if efficacy of the single dose is indeed as good as that of the 3-day treatment regimen. This well-conducted, multicenter study finds that, except for *E. Coli,* the 3-day regimen is superior to the 1-day treatment, and it should be the treatment chosen for uncomplicated acute urinary tract infections. The question still remains as to what the optimal length of treatment is if urinary culture indicating *E. Coli* infection is available.—A. Bergman, M.D.

15 Tumors

Cervix: Benign

The Efficacy and Safety of the Cytobrush During Pregnancy

Orr JW Jr, Barrett JM, Orr PF, Holloway RW, Holimon JL (Watson Clinic, Lakeland, Fla; Lakeland Regional Med Ctr, Fla)

Gynecol Oncol 44:260–262, 1992 15–1

Introduction.—The cytobrush reportedly increases the adequacy of cytological sampling in women of varying age, including those undergoing radiotherapy.

Methods.—The cytological findings obtained with the cytobrush were compared with those obtained with a cotton-tipped applicator in 300 pregnant women. Smears were obtained using a combination of a wooden spatula and cytobrush. A historic control group included 263 women who had been examined in the previous year.

Results.—Postabrasive spotting was frequent, but no patient required another visit after cytobrush examination. Adverse pregnancy events were similarly frequent in the patients and controls. The adequacy of smears, judged from the presence of endocervical cells, increased from 21% to 86%. The frequencies of abnormal smears were .8% using a cotton-tipped applicator and 1.8% using the cytobrush.

Conclusion.—The cytobrush is an effective means of obtaining adequate cervical cytological specimens during pregnancy, and its use in the antepartum period is safe.

▶ The cytobrush is becoming more popular for obtaining Pap smears, and one might properly ask whether it is safe to use in pregnancy, because it is a somewhat more aggressive instrument than the cotton-tipped applicator. The authors conclude that it is safe (which is not the same as saying that one could not rupture membranes or interrupt pregnancy with it), and that it also is more effective (judged by the rate of smears with endocervical cells). Unfortunately, this is not a randomized study, and the average gestational ages of the study groups are surprisingly different (13.4 vs. 19.1 weeks). In addition, the authors did not report the correlation between the abnormal smears and colposcopic findings. One would expect that the 2 methods would produce similar results, because nearly all the cervical dysplasias in this group of patients would be located on the ectocervix and accessible to the wooden spatula.—C.P. Morrow, M.D.

Clinical Significance of Hyperkeratosis on Otherwise Normal Papanicolaou Smears

Johnson CA, Lorenzetti LA, Liese BS, Ruble RA (Univ of Kansas Med Ctr, Kansas City, Kan)

J Fam Pract 33:354–358, 1991 15–2

Introduction.—Hyperkeratosis is commonly found on Pap smears, but its clinical importance remains uncertain.

Methods.—To determine the clinical significance of hyperkeratosis, 2,198 smears were reviewed, 184 of which demonstrated hyperkeratosis and no other pathologic findings. All but 1 of these patients had clinical data available which were compared with an age-matched control group with normal smears.

Results.—Patients with hyperkeratosis had significantly more infections by *Gardnerella vaginalis*, but they had fewer infections by *Chlamydia trachomatis* compared with the control group. Women with hyperkeratosis used a diaphragm more often. Inflammation was comparably frequent in the 2 groups. Colposcopy was performed in approximately half the patients with hyperkeratosis, and 28% of those examined had evidence of human papillomavirus or dysplasia. Hyperkeratosis was persistent in 1 of 14 patients followed up more than once.

Conclusion.—Patients with hyperkeratosis on a Papanicolaou smear should undergo follow-up colposcopy, including endocervical curettage, to detect associated pathology that may require treatment.

▶ The significance of hyperkeratosis on an otherwise normal Pap smear should be of interest to every gynecologist. In this study, the most important finding was the association with human papillomavirus and cervical intraepithelial neoplasia in 28% of the patients. This is a frequency to warrant routine colposcopy on this group of patients. (The authors recommendation for endocervical curettage is excessive; however, the article is written for family practitioners who presumably are not as skilled at colposcopy as are gynecologists.)—C.P. Morrow, M.D.

Long Term Follow Up of Women With Borderline Cervical Smear Test Results: Effects of Age and Viral Infection on Progression to High Grade Dyskaryosis

Hirschowitz L, Raffle AE, Mackenzie EFD, Hughes AO (Bristol Royal Infirmary; Southmead Hosp; Bristol Med School, Bristol, England)

BMJ 304:1209–1212, 1992 15–3

Objective.—Because an increasing number of women have borderline cervical smears, experience with 437 such women seen in 1981 was examined and compared with that of 437 age-matched control subjects with normal smear findings. The mean follow-up was 73 months for the women with borderline changes and 68 months for control subjects.

Findings.—High-grade dyskaryosis developed in 22.4% of the women with borderline cytological changes and in .9% of the control women. The risk of progression was highest for women aged 20–39 years. Human papillomavirus infection was initially diagnosed in 23% of the women with borderline changes, and significantly fewer of these women had high-grade dyskaryosis.

Implications.—Borderline change in a cervical smear increases the credability of progression to high-grade dyskaryosis. Women aged 20–39 years require especially close follow-up.

▶ This study from England deals with the significance of Pap smears showing minor nuclear abnormalities that could be caused either by inflammation or by early dysplastic changes; this group of patients does not warrant routine colposcopy but should have a repeat Pap smear at 6 months rather than at 12 months. During the mean follow-up of 6 years, 22% had high-grade dysplasia develop. This figure is similar to reports from the United States and emphasizes the importance of follow-up for this group of women.—C.P. Morrow, M.D.

Endocervical Glandular Atypia in Papanicolaou Smears

Goff BA, Atanasoff P, Brown E, Muntz HG, Bell DA, Rice LW (Massachusetts Hosp, Harvard Med School, Boston)
Obstet Gynecol 79:101–104, 1992 15–4

Introduction.—The importance of endocervical glandular atypia in a cervicovaginal Papanicolaou smear has not been established. To determine the incidence and clinical significance of endocervical atypia diagnosed on routine cytological cervical screening, 21,930 cervicovaginal smears were reviewed.

Results.—Of the 100 (.46%) patients with endocervical glandular atypia, follow-up data were available for 63. The follow-up smears were negative for at least 2 years in 7 patients, and biopsy specimens were negative in 15. There were endocervical polyps in 7 patients, endometrial hyperplasia in 2, mild dysplasia in 8, moderate dysplasia in 5, severe dysplasia in 6, squamous carcinoma in situ in 6, adenocarcinoma in situ in 5, and invasive adenocarcinoma in 2. In 12 women, smears showed endocervical atypia with features suggesting reactive atypia; 3 of these women had dysplasia. In 41% of the smears with endocervical atypia, there was co-existing squamous atypia or dysplasia (table).

Conclusion.—In as many as 50% of patients with endocervical atypia, there may be substantial cervical disease. In women with clinically important disease, atypical endocervical cells may be the first and only abnor-

Comparison of Smears Containing Endocervical Atypia With or Without Squamous Abnormalities

	Endocervical atypia only (*N* = 25)	Endocervical atypia with squamous atypia or dysplasia (*N* = 26)
Normal follow-up smears	3	3
Squamous metaplasia or chronic inflammation	4	6
Endocervical polyps	3	1
Endometrial hyperplasia	1	1
Mild dysplasia	1	7
Moderate dysplasia	1	2
Severe dysplasia	1	4
Squamous carcinoma in situ	4	2
Adenocarcinoma in situ	5	0
Adenocarcinoma	2	0
Clinically important cervical lesions	14 (56%)	15 (58%)

(Courtesy of Goff BA, Atanasoff P, Brown E, et al: *Obstet Gynecol* 79:101–104, 1992.)

mality. Further prospective studies on the importance of endocervical glandular atypia in smears are warranted.

▶ Although in this study endocervical glandular atypia (EGA) accounted for only .46% of Pap smears, from a referral perspective this finding seems to account for a disproportionate number of cases. In any event, if anyone doubted the significance of this finding, this report should make things clear. Twenty-two of 63 patients had premalignant lesions (excluding cervical intraepithelial neoplasia I), and 2 additional patients had invasive carcinomas, both of which were adenocarcinomas. Of the premalignant lesions, 17 were high-grade squamous intraepithelial lesions (SIL) and 5 were adenocarcinoma in situ (ACIS). There were 12 cases of EGA with reactive features, of which 3 had SIL; 25 cases with EGA only, of which 6 had SIL, 5 had ACIS, and 2 had adenocarcinoma; and 26 cases with EGA plus squamous atypia or dysplasia, of which 8 had SIL. The finding of EGA on a Pap smear is an indication for colposcopic evaluation and biopsy.—C.P. Morrow, M.D.

PCR-Detected Genital Papillomavirus Infection: Prevalence and Association With Risk Factors for Cervical Cancer

Rohan T, Mann V, McLaughlin J, Harnish DG, Yu H, Smith D, Davis R, Shier

RM, Rawls W (Univ of Toronto; McMaster Univ, Hamilton, Ont; Koffler Student Services Centre, Toronto; Wellesley Hosp, Toronto)
Int J Cancer 49:856–860, 1991 15–5

Background.—Epidemiological findings in cervical cancer support a causative role for a sexually transmitted infectious agent. The most likely candidates are human papillomavirus (HPV) types 6, 11, 16, and 18. Types 16 and 18 appear to dispose to higher-grade premalignant lesions and to cervical cancer itself.

Methods.—The polymerase chain reaction technique was used to detect HPV DNA in 105 women attending the University of Toronto Health Service clinic for routine reasons. The women provided a specimen of cervical cells and answered a questionnaire dealing with risk factors for cervical cancer. Nucleic acid from the cervical cells was screened with primers for HPV types 6, 11, 16, 18, and 33, as well as with an HPV consensus primer.

Findings.—The overall prevalence of HPV infection was 18%. The risk was significantly increased in those who had ever smoked cigarettes and subjects who usually had sexual intercourse during menstrual periods. These associations were independent of age at first sexual intercourse and the number of sexual partners. The risk of HPV infection was not related to the frequency of sexual intercourse, anal intercourse, or oral contraceptive use.

Interpretation.—At least some risk factors for cervical cancer may act by altering the risk of acquiring HPV infection.

▶ In this study of college students, 18% had evidence of genital HPV infection based on polymerase chain reaction testing of Pap smears. It is interesting that smokers were more likely to be HPV positive, because both HPV infection and smoking have been incriminated as etiological or risk factors for cervical carcinoma.—C.P. Morrow, M.D.

Systemic α-Interferon (Wellferon) Treatment of Genital Human Papillomavirus (HPV) Type 6, 11, 16, and 18 Infections: Double-Blind, Placebo-Controlled Trial

Yliskoski M, Syrjänen K, Syrjänen S, Saarikoski S, Nethersell A (Kuopio Univ Central Hosp, Kuopio, Finland; Wellcome Research Labs, Beckenham, England)
Gynecol Oncol 43:55–60, 1991 15–6

Introduction.—Genital human papillomavirus (HPV) infection is an important sexually transmitted disease. The natural history of these infections, which often are multicentric and recur after treatment, suggests that interferon therapy may be a logical approach.

Evaluation of Efficacy: 8th Week

Clinical response	Interferon group	Placet grouן
No. of patients evaluated	59	60
Complete response	8 (13.6%)	10 (16.7
Partial response	21 (35.6%)	14 (23.3
No response	30 (50.8%)	36 (60.0'
HPV DNA negative	29 (49.2%)	24 (40.0'

(Courtesy of Yliskoski M, et al: *Gynecol Oncol* 43:55–60, 1991.)

Study Design.—A double-blind, placebo-controlled trial of interferon was undertaken in 120 women whose Pap smears had shown changes consistent with HPV infection. The treatment and placebo groups each included 15 patients with lesions induced by each of the 4 HPV types (6, 11, 16, 18). Actively treated patients received 1.5×10^6 IU of interferon given subcutaneously 3 times in the first week, and twice this dose 3 times weekly for 6 additional weeks.

Results.—Side effects such as fever-chills, lethargy-fatigue, and headache occurred in 90% of the patients treated with interferon and in 53% of the placebo recipients. Fewer than one fifth of each group had a complete response after 8 weeks (table). There were no significant differences in response at 24 weeks and, after 1 year, approximately half the patients in each group had responded completely.

Conclusion.—Systemic interferon treatment did not significantly improve the outlook for patients in this study with genital HPV infection.

▶ This is a randomized, placebo-controlled study of the use of subcutaneous α-INF in the treatment of intraepithelial cervical HPV lesions documented by in situ hybridization. At 8 weeks, 50% of the INF group and 40% of the placebo group were HPV DNA negative, and at 1 year, 50% of both groups were free of disease. There was no significant difference in the remission rates for HPV types 6 and 11 compared with HPV types 16 and 18. These remission rates are not unlike the reported spontaneous remission rates indicating that α-INF used in this manner is entirely ineffective for treating cervical intraepithelial HPV, although it has been used successfully in the treatment of condylomata acuminata and juvenile laryngeal papillomatosis.—C.P. Morrow, M.D.

Dysplasia and the Natural History of Cervical Cancer: Early Results of the Toronto Cohort Study

Narod SA, Thompson DW, Jain M, Wall C, Green LM, Miller AB

Eur J Cancer 27:1411–1416, 1991 15–7

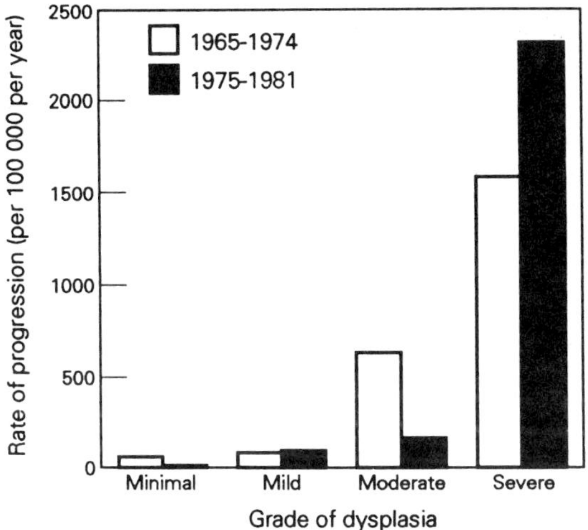

Fig 15–1.—Incidence of cervical malignancy among women with dysplasia by degree and calendar period. (Courtesy of Narod SA, Thompson DW, Jain M, et al: *Eur J Cancer* 27:1411–1416, 1991.)

Background.—An experience from a large laboratory in Toronto from 1962 to 1981 provides an unusual opportunity for reviewing preneoplastic abnormalities of cervical epithelium. The Toronto Cohort Study's early results on dysplasia and the natural history of cervical cancer were reported.

Methods and Findings.—A sample of 176,808 Papanicolaou smears was obtained from 70,236 women between 1962 and 1981. This sample was constructed from the records of a large cytopathology laboratory. Based on the distribution of the initial smear results, the prevalence of cervical dysplasia increased from 42.7 to 94.9 per 1,000 during the study period. The relative risks (RRs) for the manifestation of a malignancy in a subsequent cervical smear were 1.48 in those with minimal dysplasia, 3.42 in those with mild dysplasia, 20.9 in those with moderate dysplasia, and 71.5 in those with severe dysplasia. The initial severity of dysplasia for women in whom a malignancy developed was much more likely to be interpreted as moderate, with a RR of 5, or severe, with a RR of 42.3, than that for controls (Fig 15–1).

Conclusions.—These data support the notion that cervical dysplasia is indeed a risk factor for subsequent malignancy. Severe dysplasia is associated with the greatest risk.

▶ This is an interesting study reaffirming that cervical dysplasia, especially moderate and severe types, carries a very significant increased risk for the development of cervical carcinoma. What the RR for these entities means can be more readily seen from the incidence rates per 100,000 women per year: controls, 23.6; minimal dysplasia, 35; mild dysplasia, 81; moderate dysplasia, 498; and severe dysplasia, 1,706. Thus, the untreated patient with severe dysplasia on a Pap smear has nearly a 2% risk per year of having invasive cervical cancer.—C.P. Morrow, M.D.

The Management of Minor Degrees of Cervical Dysplasia Associated With the Human Papilloma Virus

Carmichael JA (Queen's Univ, Kingston, Ont)

Yale J Biol Med 64:591–597, 1991 15–8

Introduction.—Since the early 1980s, the number of patients with significant dysplasia referred to colposcopy clinics has decreased, whereas the number referred with minor degrees of cervical dysplasia associated with effects of the human papilloma virus (HPV) has increased. The findings in these women are almost always benign, with little evidence that they are at risk for greater dysplasia or invasive disease. The natural history of HPV-associated minor cervical dysplasia was studied.

Methods.—The study sample comprised 525 women whose colposcopic findings suggested mild-to-moderate cervical dysplasia. The women received no treatment and were followed up at 6-month intervals for up to 5 years. If the dysplasia progressed, patients were removed from follow-up and treated accordingly. If dysplasia regressed, the patients were referred back to the original physician to be followed with annual cytological examination.

Results.—At 6 months, 30.5% of the patients had regressed to a nondysplastic state; at 4½ years, this figure had increased to 77.3%. In another 7.8%, cervical dysplasia progressed (Fig 15–2). In 22 patients with

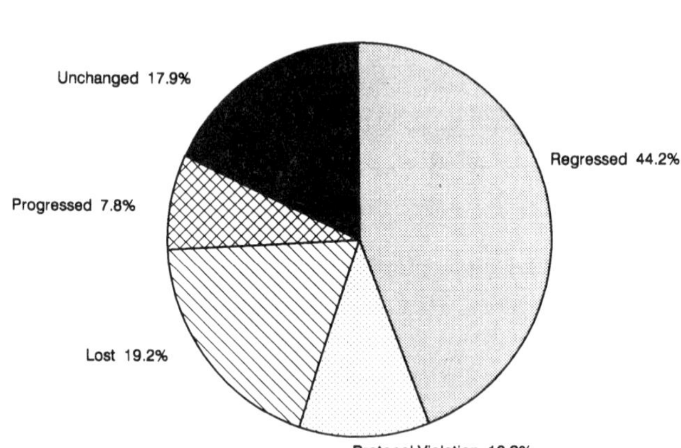

Fig 15–2.—Status of all patients 6 months after closure of the study. All patients were followed for 6–58 months, with a median follow-up of 30 months. Total patients = 525. (Courtesy of Carmichael JA: *Yale J Biol Med* 64:591–597, 1991.)

recurrent dysplasia of a minor degree, no invasive cancers have been diagnosed.

Conclusion.—Routine screening follow-up appears to be sufficient for patients with minor degrees or HPV-associated dysplasia. The great majority of these patients can be expected to regress to a nondysplastic state. For those who do progress screening will accurately identify the increased degree of dysplasia, allowing them to be referred for colposcopy and treatment as necessary.

▶ This paper documents that minor degrees of cervical dysplasia associated with HPV infection have a high rate of spontaneous regression after evaluation and biopsy. The practical implication of this is that cervical intraepithelial neoplasia I associated with HPV can be managed by observation and semiannual Papanicolaou smear with the expectation that most of these lesions will remit without therapy. This is particularly important for young women whose fertility might be compromised by therapy.—C.P. Morrow, M.D.

Endocervical Gland Involvement by Cervical Intraepithelial Neoplasia Grade III: Predictive Value for Residual and/or Recurrent Disease

Demopoulos RI, Horowitz LF, Vamvakas EC (New York Univ Med Ctr; Rita and Stanley Kaplan Cancer Ctr, New York)

Cancer 68:1932–1936, 1991 15–9

Background.—Carcinoma in situ or dysplasia persists in as many as 27% of patients who lack disease at the margins of cone-biopsy specimens. Microinvasive cancer can develop from both surface epithelium and endocervical glands.

Objective.—The risks of residual and recurrent disease were examined in 341 consecutive patients who received a cone-biopsy diagnosis of grade III cervical intraepithelial neoplasia (severe dysplasia and/or carcinoma in situ). The patients were followed through 1988.

Findings.—Ninety-six patients underwent hysterectomy within 8 weeks of cone biopsy. The presence of residual disease did not relate significantly to either positive margins or positive glands on cone biopsy. Recurrence developed in 12.7% of those women not undergoing hysterectomy. Multivariate analysis showed that both positive margins and positive glands correlated significantly with recurrent disease.

Conclusion.—A cone-biopsy finding of endocervical gland involvement by cervical intraepithelial neoplasia grade III denotes a potential for disease to recur in women who do not undergo hysterectomy.

▶ This study suggests that women undergoing cone biopsy for cervical intraepithelial neoplasia (CIN) 3 have a threefold increased risk for persistant/recurrent squamous neoplasia on follow-up if there is gland-duct involvement (GDI)—a risk nearly identical to that for women whose cone biopsy specimens have a positive margin. However, there are some peculiarities in this study. Among the 58 patients with positive GDI and negative margins, there were 11 recurrences (19%). Of these, 6 were CIN 1 and 3 were invasive. In addition, of the 96 patients with negative cone margins undergoing hysterectomy (all within 8 weeks postbiopsy), one third had residual CIN 3. This compares with 4 (2%) of 204 patients who did not undergo hysterectomy. The management of CIN has been predicated on the principle that the endocervical component is not multifocal. Although the evidence is inconsistent, the system nevertheless works very well. If GDI, as reported by Demopoulos et al., is an important risk factor for cone failure, then patients with this finding might warrant closer follow-up or even hysterectomy.—C.P. Morrow, M.D.

Comparison of Thermal Injury Zones in Loop Electrical and Laser Cervical Excisional Conization

Baggish MS, Barash F, Noel Y, Brooks M (State Univ of New York, Syracuse; Crouse Irving Mem Hosp, Syracuse, NY)

Am J Obstet Gynecol 166:545–548, 1992 15–10

Introduction.—Large-loop diathermy is an accepted approach to outpatient conization for cervical intraepithelial neoplasia, but thermal damage may make it difficult to assess the resection margins. The carbondioxide (CO_2) laser is an alternative to knife conization, and studies of many laser conizations have indicated very acceptable margins.

Objective and Methods.—Zones of thermal artifact were compared in 30 cervical conization specimens obtained by thin-loop electric excision and 30 others taken with the CO_2 laser, using a micrometer technique. Electrosurgery used a unit delivering 50 W of power. The laser conizations were done at 40 W of power with a .5-mm spot.

Findings.—The mean depth of coagulation at the ectocervical margin was .19 mm in thin-loop specimens and .16 mm in laser specimens. The thermal artifacts at the endocervical margin were .295 mm in thin-loop specimens and .14 mm in laser specimens. The extent of thermal injury did not significantly influence interpretations of marginal adequacy.

Conclusion.—Comparable cervical wounds are produced by electric conization using a thin-loop, high-frequency, low-voltage unit and by the high-power-density CO_2 laser. The electric method is simple and rapid.

▶ Because the loop technique for excision of cervical intraepithelial neoplasia seems destined to replace the laser, it is relevant to current clinical practice to evaluate the tissue damage from the loop compared with the laser. Baggish et al. find that the loop has a somewhat thicker zone of coagulation in the loop specimen, but the difference does not appear to be clinically significant. Of course, these are results achieved by experts. In the hands of the inexperienced, the cone specimen could easily be charred beyond the pathologic evaluation. Although it is easier to learn to use the loop than the laser, damaged specimens are still a very realistic concern. After learning to use the loop in the laboratory, each gynecologist should review the patient's tissue specimens with the pathologist until optimal specimens are routinely obtained.—C.P. Morrow, M.D.

Histological Differences Between Colposcopic-Directed Biopsy and Loop Excision of the Transformation Zone (LETZ): A Cause for Concern

Chappatte OA, Byrne DL, Raju KS, Nayagam M, Kenney A (St Thomas's Hosp, London)

Gynecol Oncol 43:46–50, 1991 15–11

Introduction.—Cytologic abnormalities require colposcopic examination of the cervix to determine the extent and severity of dysplasia. There is concern about the underestimation of cervical dysplasia in colposcopic biopsy specimens resulting in inadequate treatment. Colposcopic findings and colposcopic biopsy specimens were compared with the histology of loop excision of the transformation zone (LETZ) specimens.

Methods.—Colposcopic assessment and biopsy were performed on 100 women with abnormal cervical cytology. All were suitable for ablative therapy but were treated by LETZ on an outpatient basis.

Results.—There was poor agreement among the specimens, with identical degrees of dysplasia demonstrated in only 43% of patients. Colposcopic biopsy underestimated dysplasia in 16% of the patients and overestimated it in 41% compared with the LETZ specimens. Microinvasive carcinoma, which was missed by colposcopy and colposcopic biopsy, was diagnosed in 3 patients with LETZ histology.

Conclusion.—The disparity between histological findings is of great concern; LETZ should replace ablative therapy in the treatment of localized cervical dysplasia, and may obviate the need for pretreatment colposcopic biopsy. Also, LETZ limits the possibility of inadequate treatment and provides a method of audit for the colposcopist.

▶ The loop procedure is being promoted because it can be done in the office, because it is relatively inexpensive (compared with the laser or surgical cone biopsy) and, perhaps most importantly, because excision avoids the problem of treating unrecognized occult invasive cancer by local ablation. However, the frequency with which colposcopy-directed biopsy and endocervical curettage miss invasive cancer has not been clear. In this article, the authors found microinvasion in 3% of the patients undergoing loop excision for dysplasia. The discrepancy noted among the various degrees of dysplasia is of little clinical significance.—C.P. Morrow, M.D.

Treatment of Cervical Intraepithelial Neoplasia Using the Loop Electrosurgical Excision Procedure

Wright TC Jr, Gagnon S, Richart RM, Ferenczy A (Columbia-Presbyterian Med Ctr, New York; Chicoutimi Hosp, Chicoutimi, Quebec; McGill Univ, Montreal)

Obstet Gynecol 79:173–178, 1992 15–12

Introduction.—Outpatient ablation is an effective and very-well-accepted option for selected patients with cervical intraepithelial neoplasia (CIN). Loop electrosurgical excision offers a rapid and simple alternative to cryotherapy and laser ablation, and it allows diagnosis and treatment at a single session.

Technique.—Four-quadrant local anesthesia is administered after assessment of the cervix. Either a small-diameter rectangular loop electrode is used to remove the entire transformation zone (all CIN and all Schiller-negative areas) in multiple strips 4–7 mm deep or a large loop electrode is used to excise the transformation zone to a depth of 5–8 mm, in a single pass if possible. An attempt is made to remove the epithelium 4–5 mm beyond the point at which it becomes Schiller-negative. The base and edges of the crater are cauterized with the ball electrode. Endocervical curettage is done at the end of the procedure.

Experience.—Small loop electrodes were used in a majority of the 432 patients having outpatient electrosurgical excision. Discomfort was minimal, and fewer than 2% of the patients had bleeding after the procedure. Fewer than 1% had post-treatment stenosis. Eighty percent of the women treated with small loop electrodes were free of disease 4–48 months later, whereas 90% of those treated with large electrodes were free of disease after 6–12 months. Healing was similar to what is observed after laser ablation.

Conclusion.—Loop electrosurgical excision, in contrast to ablative treatments, provides a specimen for thorough histopathologic assessment. Large loop electrodes have been more than 90% effective in treating primary disease.

▶ Although the number of patients in this report is large (432), only 67 were treated with the large loop electrode for high-grade squamous intraepithelial lesion (CIN II and III). Of these, 91% were disease free at 6–12 months' follow-up. Delayed bleeding after large loop excision occurred in 15% of the authors' first 40 cases but was found in none of the following 117 cases because of the liberal application of Monsel's solution (paste) after achieving hemostasis with the ball electrode at the initial loop procedure. Otherwise, the authors report a very low frequency of post-loop complications. Only 2 of 141 patients had cervical stenosis develop. Apparently, none of the 243 patients with dysplasia was found to have invasion in the loop specimen. All patients had a pre-loop diagnosis of CIN or HPV lesion.—C.P. Morrow, M.D.

Cervix: Malignant

Cigarette Smoking and Cervical Cancer: Meta-Analysis and Critical Review of Recent Studies

Sood AK (Univ of North Carolina, Chapel Hill)

Am J Prev Med 7:208–213, 1991 15–13

Background.—Several reports have linked cigarette smoking with cervical cancer, but they have failed to correct for the confounding effects of other known risk factors. A meta-analysis of recent studies of the relationship between smoking and cervical cancer was reviewed.

Methods.—The literature from 1977 to 1990 was searched for case-control studies on the relationship between smoking and cervical cancer that included data on the number of cases and controls in various categories of smoking exposure. Nine such studies met these criteria; all 9 used similar definitions for cervical cancer and classification or smoking. Graphic methods were used to test for homogeneity before pooling the results.

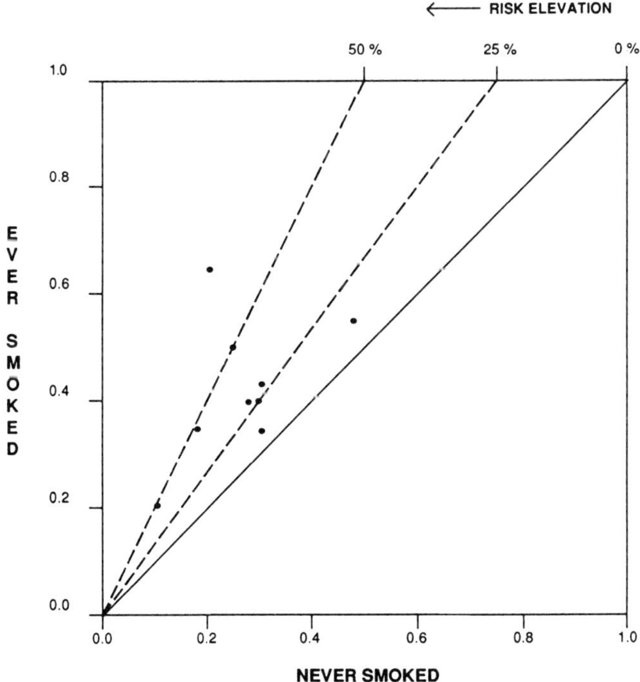

Fig 15–3.—The pooled cervical cancer rate in the ever-smoked group plotted on the vertical axis and the case rate in the control group plotted on the horizontal axis; the *solid diagonal line* shows equal rates, the *lower dotted line* shows a 25% increase in risk, and the *upper dotted line* shows a 50% risk elevation. (Courtesy of Sood AK: *Am J Prev Med* 7:208–213, 1991.)

Findings.—A consistent trend in risk was shown on graphic analysis (Fig 15–3). One atypical study was excluded from the rest of the analysis, although it showed results in the same direction. The crude data from the remaining 8 studies gave an odds ratio of 1.46 for ever having smoked. Including data from 5 studies that adjusted for factors including age and number of sexual partners, the weighted odds ratio was 1.42.

Conclusion.—Smoking may increase the risk of cervical cancer by 42% to 46%, even after adjustment for age and number of sexual partners. Future studies should address the concentration and effects of constituents of tobacco smoke and their metabolites in cervical mucus. In clinical practice, women who smoke may be followed more closely because of their increased risk of cervical cancer.

▶ As this meta-analysis indicates, cigarette smoking is associated with a nearly 50% increased risk for cervical carcinoma after adjusting for age and number of sexual partners. Thus, women who smoke but who have no other "high-risk" factors for cervical cancer should be followed by annual Pap smears like the high-risk patients. The American College of Obstetricians and Gynecologists and American Cancer Society recommendations for Pap screening intervals should be changed to include smoking in the definition of high risk.—C.P. Morrow, M.D.

Maternal and Fetal Outcome After Invasive Cervical Cancer in Pregnancy

Zemlickis D, Lishner M, Degendorfer P, Panzarella T, Sutcliffe SB, Koren G (The Hosp for Sick Children; Princess Margaret Hosp; Univ of Toronto, Toronto)

J Clin Oncol 9:1956–1961, 1991 15–14

Background.—The most common gynecological malignancy during the reproductive years is invasive carcinoma of the cervix. The effects of pregnancy on the course and survival of women with invasive cervical cancer were assessed.

Methods.—Forty women with invasive cervical cancer were compared with 89 nonpregnant women matched for age, calendar year of diagnosis, stage, and tumor type. The distribution of invasive cervical cancer stages in the pregnant women was compared with that in 1,963 women with invasive cervical cancer who were treated in the same 30-year period. This latter group consisted of women younger than 45 years of age who were registered at the same hospital. Pregnancy outcomes were assessed by comparing babies born to women with invasive cervical cancer with babies born to women of the same age who were not exposed to known teratogens or reproductive risks during pregnancy.

Findings.—Pregnant women with invasive cervical cancer had a 30-year survival rate identical to that of their matched controls. Women with invasive cervical cancer were 3.1 times more likely to receive a diagnosis of stage I disease. These women also had a significantly reduced chance of being diagnosed with stages III and IV cancer. The infants of women with cancer were comparable in gestational age and rates of prematurity with infants born to women without invasive cervical cancer; however, the former had lower birth weights than the latter. There were 2 (8%) stillbirths among the 24 pregnancies continuing to term, which was not significantly different from that for the general pregnant population of Ontario.

Conclusion.—Pregnancy per se does not seem to adversely affect the survival of women with invasive cervical cancer. Pregnant women are more likely to present with early disease because they have regular, pregnancy-related obstetric examinations. Pregnancy in such women has an increased risk for stillbirth, indicating the need for follow-up in a high-risk perinatal unit.

▶ It is good news that this study found no evidence that pregnancy per se adversely affects the survival of women with cervical cancer. It also is good news to learn that pregnant women who have cervical cancer are more likely to present with early stage disease. Unfortunately, this study, like all antecedent reports on this subject, does not actually prove that pregnancy has no adverse effect on cervical cancer outcome or that vaginal delivery is not deleterious. The problem is numbers, trimester, and stage. For example, of the 40-patient study group only, 27 patients received a diagnosis during pregnancy, and only 10 of these pregnancies went to term. The authors do not tell us how large a difference their sample size could detect: 5%, 10%, 20%? Nevertheless, we can reasonably assure our patients that the pregnancy per se is not deleterious with respect to cancer outcome. We cannot, however, be so sanguine about delivering a fetus or term infant through a cancerous cervix. Cesarean section is still tho route of choice for delivering of the pregnant woman with cervical cancer.—C.P. Morrow, M.D.

Stage III Ovarian Tumors of Low Malignant Potential Treated With Cisplatin Combination Therapy: A Gynecologic Oncology Group Study

Sutton GP, Bundy BN, Omura GA, Yordan EL, Beecham JB, Bonfiglio T (Indiana Univ Med School, Indianapolis; Roswell Park Mem Inst, Buffalo, NY; Univ of Alabama at Birmingham; Rush-Presbyterian St Luke's Med Ctr, Chicago; Univ of Rochester Med Ctr, Rochester, NY)

Gynecol Oncol 41:230–233, 1991 15–15

Introduction.—Ovarian epithelial tumors of low malignant potential (LMP) are neither benign nor malignant but they tend to recur or progress.

Methods.—Patients with International Federation of Gynecology and Obstetrics (FIGO) stage III ovarian cancer with less than 1 cm of residual disease were assigned to receive cisplatin plus cyclophosphamide, with or without doxorubicin. Of these 415 patients on review, 32 had LMP tumors.

Results.—Of the 32 patients, 13 had no residual disease after initial cytoreduction therapy. Cisplatin and cyclophosphamide only were administered to 20 patients, and 12 also received doxorubicin. Six of 14 second-look operations were negative. During a median follow-up of 32 months, only 1 patient died, and no cancer was found at autopsy. The other patients were alive a median of 30 months after treatment without clinical evidence of disease.

Conclusion.—Cisplatin-based chemotherapy is modestly active against stage III ovarian carcinoma of LMP, but serious toxicity is infrequent. The present patient who died in pancytopenia also received abdominal radiotherapy and melphalan. Cisplatin-based treatment cannot, however, be considered routine adjuvant therapy for patients with LMP ovarian tumors.

▶ Stage III LMP ovarian tumors carry an approximate 75% 5-year survival rate. It is still unclear whether chemotherapy can improve survival, although LMP tumors are well documented to respond to chemotherapy. In this Gynecologic Oncology Group study, 32 patients with optimal (< 1 cm residual) stage III LMP tumors received platinum-based chemotherapy. The results are difficult to interpret because 13 of the patients had no evidence of disease (NED) after initial surgery, and only half the total study group underwent second-look surgery. Of the 6 patients undergoing second look surgery who were NED at initial surgery, 4 had a negative second look, whereas only 2 of the 8 patients with residual disease after primary surgery who underwent second surgery were found to be free of disease.

In other words, based on second-look data, 2 of 6 patients who were negative at first operation were found to have progressed after 8 cycles of platinum-based chemotherapy, and only 2 of 8 patients with minimal residual disease after primary surgery who underwent second-look surgery were found to have a more complete surgical-pathologic response to 8 cycles of platinum-based chemotherapy. On the other hand, undoubtedly a reflection of the natural history of the disease, only 1 of the 32 study patients died (NED, treatment complication) and all others had NED clinically at a median follow-up of 32 months. Chemotherapy should be reserved for clinically progressive disease that is not amenable to surgical resection.—C.P. Morrow, M.D.

The Accuracy of Cervicovaginal Cytology in the Detection of Recurrent Cervical Carcinoma Following Radiotherapy

Shield PW, Wright RG, Free K, Daunter B (Royal Brisbane Hosp; Univ of Queensland, Brisbane, Australia)

Gynecol Oncol 41:223–229, 1991 15–16

Moving?

I'd like to receive my ***Year Book of Obstetrics and Gynecology*** without interruption.

Please note the following change of address, effective: ____________________

Name: ____________________

New Address: ____________________

____

City: ____________________ State: __________ Zip: __________

Old Address: ____________________

____

City: ____________________ State: __________ Zip: __________

Reservation Card

Yes, I would like my own copy of the ***Year Book of Obstetrics and Gynecology***. Please begin my subscription with the current edition according to the terms described below.* I understand that I will have 30 days to examine each annual edition. If satisfied, I will pay just $59.95 plus sales tax, postage and handling (price subject to change without notice).

Name: ____________________

Address: ____________________

City: ____________________ State: __________ Zip: __________

Method of Payment

❑ Visa ❑ Mastercard ❑ AmEx ❑ Bill me ❑ Check (in US dollars, payable to Mosby-Year Book, Inc.)

Card number ____________________ Exp date __________

Signature ____________________

LS-0907

*Your *Year Book* Service Guarantee:

When you subscribe to the ***Year Book***, we'll send you an advance notice of future volumes about two months before they publish. This automatic notice system is designed to take up as little of your time as possible. If you do not want the ***Year Book***, the advance notice makes it quick and easy for you to let us know your decision; and you will always have at least 20 days to decide. If we don't hear from you, we'll send you the new volume as soon as it's available. And, of course, the ***Year Book*** is yours to examine free of charge for 30 days (postage, handling and applicable sales tax are added to each shipment).

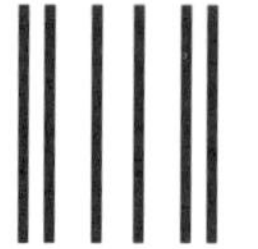

NO POSTAGE
NECESSARY
IF MAILED
IN THE
UNITED STATES

BUSINESS REPLY MAIL

FIRST CLASS MAIL PERMIT No. 762 CHICAGO, IL

POSTAGE WILL BE PAID BY ADDRESSEE

Chris Hughes
Mosby-Year Book, Inc.
200 N. LaSalle Street
Suite 2600
Chicago, IL 60601-9981

NO POSTAGE
NECESSARY
IF MAILED
IN THE
UNITED STATES

BUSINESS REPLY MAIL

FIRST CLASS MAIL PERMIT No. 762 CHICAGO, IL

POSTAGE WILL BE PAID BY ADDRESSEE

Chris Hughes
Mosby-Year Book, Inc.
200 N. LaSalle Street
Suite 2600
Chicago, IL 60601-9981

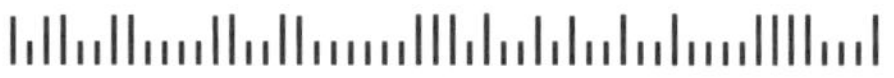

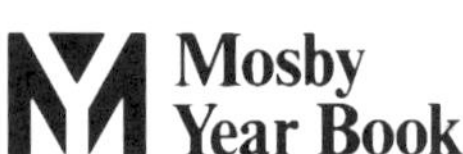

Dedicated to publishing excellence.

Introduction.—To determine whether cervicovaginal cytology accurately detects recurrent cervical cancer, 70 patients with confirmed recurrences after radiotherapy, with or without pelvic surgery, were studied. The specificity of testing was examined in a second group of 62 patients with a cytological diagnosis of persistent or recurrent cervical cancer after radiotherapy.

Results.—Recurrent cancer was diagnosed cytologically in 33% of the first 70 patients, and postradiation dysplasia was diagnosed in another 13%. The positive predictive value of a histological diagnosis of recurrent cancer after a positive cytology report was 98%. In one fourth of this group, the clinical signs of cancer were preceded by a cytological diagnosis of locally recurrent cancer. The recurrences were diagnosed cytologically a mean of 14.5 months after the completion of radiotherapy, and positive cytology preceded clinically evident recurrence by a mean of 6 months.

Conclusion.—Cytological smears are a valuable and inexpensive means of detecting locally recurrent cervical cancer or persistent cancer at an early stage. Cytology may give evidence of local recurrence before clinical signs or symptoms develop.

▶ The message in this report is that the importance of cervical/vaginal cytology in the follow-up of women treated by radiotherapy for cervical (or vaginal) carcinoma is local; an abnormal Pap smear is sometimes—if not frequently—the first indication of recurrent disease. In addition, it is invaluable in detecting postradiation squamous dysplasia. Topical estrogen cream applied nightly for 2–4 weeks will assist in evaluating the patient with a postradiation abnormal Pap smear.—C.P. Morrow, M.D.

Uterus

Body Mass at Different Ages and Subsequent Endometrial Cancer Risk

Levi F, La Vecchia C, Negri E, Parazzini F, Franceschi S (Univ of Lausanne, Switzerland; Istituto di Ricerche Farmacologiche "Mario Negri," Milan, Italy; Riferimonto Oncologico, Aviano, Italy)

Int J Cancer 50:567–571, 1992 15–17

Introduction.—Overweight and obesity are well-recognized risk factors for endometrial cancer. However, it is not clear whether nutritional and anthropometric factors early in life relate to the later risk of cancer.

Subjects.—The relationship between body mass index (BMI) at various ages and subsequent risk of endometrial cancer was examined in a multicenter case-control study that included 272 patients with histologically confirmed endometrial cancer and 571 control subjects with acute nonneoplastic disorders.

Findings.—The risk of cancer increased with increasing BMI in the third, fifth, and seventh decades of age. The risk estimates were higher at older ages. In women with normal BMI at the time cancer was diagnosed, there was no significant effect of past overweight. In those who were overweight at diagnosis a direct relationship with BMI was found at ages 20–29 years and 40–49 years.

Implications.—Overweight has a late stage effect on endometrial carcinogenesis. It seems important to avoid obesity in late middle and older age. The benefit could be greatest for those women who were overweight when younger.

▶ It is useful to know that the effect of obesity on the risk of endometrial carcinoma can be diminished or nullified by weight normalization, and that the longer a woman is obese, the greater the risk that she will have endometrial carcinoma develop.—C.P. Morrow, M.D.

Depot-Medroxyprogesterone Acetate (DMPA) and Risk of Endometrial Cancer

The WHO Collaborative Study of Neoplasia and Steroid Contraceptives

Int J Cancer 49:186–190, 1991 15–18

Introduction.—Women in more than 70 countries use depot-medroxy progesterone acetate (DMPA), generally in a dose of 150 mg given every 3 months for contraception.

Methods.—A case-control study was conducted to determine the risk of endometrial carcinoma associated with the use of this long-acting progestational contraceptive. Personal interviews were conducted with 122 women having confirmed endemetrial carcinoma and 939 control women.

Results.—The relative risk of endometrial cancer developing in women who had used DMPA at any time (but not for the *first* time in the year before diagnosis) was .21. All 3 DMPA-exposed women with endometrial cancer also had received estrogens premenopausally. Protection by DMPA appeared to last at least 8 years after its use ceased.

Conclusion.—Protection against endometrial carcinoma from DMPA is at least as great as that associated with combined oral contraceptives. Protection lasts some years after exposure to DMPA ends.

▶ This study supports the general belief that progestins do not increase the risk of endometrial carcinoma, but they most likely reduce the risk thereof. There are undesirable effects of DMPA, however. The associated is not readily reversible. It is also an anabolic agent, and many women experience an increased appetite and weight gain. Regarding a carcinogenic effect, the gynecological organ of greatest concern is the cervix. Some studies have suggested that progestins increase the risk for adenocarcinoma of the cervix, but the issue remains unresolved.—C.P. Morrow, M.D.

Increased Steroid Production by the Ovarian Stromal Tissue of Postmenopausal Women With Endometrial Cancer

Nagamani M, Stuart CA, Doherty MG (Univ of Texas, Galveston)

J Clin Endocrinol Metab 74:172–176, 1992 15–19

Objective.—In women with endometrial cancer, the ovarian stroma appears to secrete more steroids than in women without cancer. It is suggested that increased steroid secretion could contribute to the pathogenesis of endometrial cancer in postmenopausal women. Steroid production by isolated ovarian stromal tissues was studied in postmenopausal women with and without endometrial cancer, the effects of luteinizing hormone (LH) and insulin on ovarian steroid secretion also were investigated in these women.

Methods.—Ovarian stromal tissue from 18 postmenopausal women, 10 with and 8 without endometrial cancer, was obtained for investigation. All patients were at least 2 years postmenopausal. The investigations incubated the stroma either in medium alone or in medium with added LH, 50 ng/mL, or insulin, 500 ng/mL.

Results.—Stroma from the women with endometrial cancer secreted significantly more androstenedione, testosterone, and dehydroepiandrosterone (DHEA) than that from the women without cancer. There was no significant difference in progesterone or estradiol (Fig 15–4). With LH added to the medium, the release of androstenedione, testosterone, DHEA, and progesterone increased significantly. With insulin added to the medium, androstenedione was released from the stroma of the women with cancer but not from that of women without cancer.

Conclusion.—In postmenopausal women with endometrial cancer, androgen secretion by the ovarian stroma is significantly greater than in

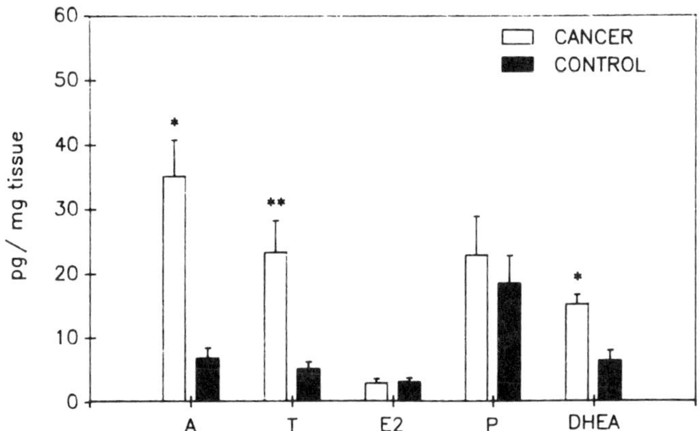

Fig 15–4.—Steroid production in vitro by ovarian stromal tissue of postmenopausal women with and without endometrial cancer (mean ± SE). *, $P < .001$, **, $P < .01$. (Courtesy of Nagamani M, Stuart CA, Doherty MG: *J Clin Endocrinol Metab* 74:172-176, 1992.)

postmenopausal women without cancer. Both LH and insulin may play an important role in this increase. These findings are in agreement with previous in vivo and histochemical studies.

▶ The endocrinology of endometrial carcinogenesis is complex and fascinating, as this paper attests. One of the most striking things about this study is that the patients with endometrial cancer (EC) weighed an average of 50 pounds more than the controls; 7 of 10 patients with EC were overweight. Unfortunately, the authors did not comment on the findings of the ovaries from the 3 normal-weight women with EC. Is the mechanism of endometrial carcinogenesis the same in normal/underweight women as in obese women? That is the question.—C.P. Morrow, M.D.

Endometrial Carcinoma in the Cancer Family Syndrome

Hakala T, Mecklin J-P, Forss M, Järvinen H, Lehtovirta P (Univ of Helsinki; Central Hosp of Central Finland, Jyväskylä)

Cancer 68:1656–1659, 1991 15–20

Introduction.—From 5% to 10% of patients with colorectal cancer have the cancer family syndrome (CFS). This syndrome is an important target of preventive efforts based on family screening.

Methods.—Data were reviewed on 26 women, treated for uterine adenocarcinoma in 1945–1988, who were from 19 CFS families. The formal criteria for CFS were met by 13 families. The mean patient age was 48 years. Histological differentiation was similar to that in a large control group. In 14 patients, there were 30 other malignancies, including 6 with several extra-endometrial lesions. Half the metachronous tumors were colorectal carcinomas.

Results.—The patients with endometrial cancer who had CFS had a 5-year survival rate of 73% compared with 68% for 442 control patients with endometrial carcinoma. Of 19 women with children, 9 had at least 1 child with cancer; 2 of the 9 had endometrial carcinoma alone.

Conclusion.—Endometrial carcinoma is a significant component of CFS. The proportion of patients with endometrial carcinoma who have hereditary disease remains unknown, and it is not clear whether hereditary endometrial carcinoma exists as an independent entity.

▶ The CFS criteria used in this study include (1) at least 3 relatives with colorectal cancer; (2) at least two consecutive generations affected; and (3) at least one of the colorectal cancers occurred before 50 years of age. Although the occurrence of endometrial carcinoma (EC) in 26 women from 19 families is impressive, the authors did not relate how many women in these families were at risk for the disease or what the expected number of cases would be. A total of 30 other malignancies were diagnosed in 14 women among the 26 with EC, the most common being gastrointestinal cancer (18 cases). Only 1 case of breast cancer and 2 cases of ovarian cancer were recorded in the EC study group. The average patient age at diagnosis of EC was 48.3 years compared with an EC control group average age of 61.8 years. The take-home lesson from this article is that, with respect to cancer, the family history of every patient is important. Patients with a family history of colorectal carcinoma need to be monitored more closely for the occurence of EC and colorectal cancer (and at an earlier age).—C.P. Morrow, M.D.

A Prospective, Randomized Comparison of the Pipelle Endometrial Sampling Device With the Novak Curette

Stovall TG, Ling FW, Morgan PL (Univ of Tennessee, Memphis)

Am J Obstet Gynecol 165:1287–1289, 1991 15–21

Background.—Endometrial sampling is an important diagnostic tool in gynecological practice. The Novak curette and vacuum aspirator have been found to be as accurate as curettage in histological results. The Pipelle endometrial suction curette, developed for endometrial sampling, is said to cause less patient discomfort. The 2 sampling devices were compared in a prospective, randomized trial.

Methods.—Patients with abnormal uterine bleeding were enrolled in the trial during a 2-year period. Those not wishing to participate and those who had a positive pregnancy test result were not included. A total of 149 had specimens obtained by the Pipelle curette and 126 by the Novak device. The 2 groups were similar in mean gravidity, parity, and menopausal status, although the Novak group had a higher mean age. Sample adequacy, pain associated with endometrial biopsy, and correlation of endometrial histological sampling with histologic findings after hysterectomy were compared.

Comparison of Endometrial Histological Results Between the Novak and Pipelle Groups

	Endometrial histologic finding			
Sampling method	*Endometritis*	*Hyperplasia*	*Proliferative or secretory*	*Insufficient tissue*
Pipelle (N = 149)				
No.	23	11	96	19
%	15.4	7.4	64.4	12.8
Novak (N = 126)				
No.	23	15	76	12
%	18.3	11.9	60.3	9.5

(Courtesy of Stovall TG, Ling FW, Morgan PL: *Am J Obstet Gynecol* 165:1287–1289, 1991.)

Findings.—Patients in the Novak biopsy group had a mean pain score of 4.36. Seventeen percent of that group reported severe pain. Those in the Pipelle group had a mean pain score of 3.21, with only 6.7% reporting severe pain. The pain scores were unaffected by menstrual day, gravidity, parity, or menopausal status. Tissue was insufficient in 12.8% of those in the Pipelle group and in 9.5% of those in the Novak group. Fifty patients eventually had hysterectomy. In 96%, the pathologic results at hysterectomy agreed with findings at endometrial sampling (table).

Conclusion.—The Pipelle endometrial suction curette appears to be as effective as the Novak device in providing adequate specimens for histological analysis. In addition, the Pipelle curette apparently causes less pain.

▶ It is unclear from the methods section of this paper how the specimen was obtained with the Novak curette, whereas the description for the Pipelle is quite specific. It probably makes a difference whether a syringe is used with the Novak Curette to create suction during the biopsy. It also probably is important to make several longitudinal passes with the instrument; this apparently was not done, the description stating merely that "the specimen was obtained from the fundal portion." (The fundus is the part of the uterus above the tubes. The authors surely meant corpus.) One cannot doubt that the larger instrument more frequently causes significant discomfort. The Pipelle curette may have an advantage in that it is more flexible. Also, because the diameter is smaller, the negative pressure probably is greater.

The problem with this study, as is true of most studies investigating these instruments (which the authors emphasize) is that the most important population is not studied. Only 10% of the patients evaluated were postmenopausal. If the purpose of the instrument is to evaluate normal endometrium, fine. However, if the goal is to find the best way for office diagnosis or exclusion of endometrial carcinoma, then the focus has to be on postmenopausal women. In this group of patients there will be more failed attempts, more inadequate specimens, and more wrong diagnoses. How effective are these instruments in detecting endometrial cancer in postmenopausal women?—C.P. Morrow, M.D.

Postmenopausal Bleeding From Unusual Endometrial Polyps in Women on Chronic Tamoxifen Therapy

Corley D, Rowe J, Curtis MT, Hogan WM, Noumoff JS, Livolsi VA (Univ of Pennsylvania; Lankenau Hosp, Philadelphia)

Obstet Gynecol 79:111–116, 1992 15–22

Introduction.—Postmenopausal bleeding from endometrial polyps in women given tamoxifen for breast cancer has been reported. Data on 4 patients with vaginal bleeding were reviewed.

Patients. —The women were aged 45–77 years; in all of them, infiltrating duct carcinoma of the breast was diagnosed. Treatment consisted of mastectomy and tamoxifen, 20 mg/day. All patients subsequently had vaginal bleeding. Endometrial polyps showed an edematous stroma. A prominent decidual reaction was noted in 2 patients; in the other 2, the stroma consisted of abundant fibrous tissue. There were foci of inflammatory cells, predominantly lymphocytes, and small areas of stromal necrosis. In all patients, the endometrial glands were cystically dilated and lined by plump columnar epithelium without marked cytological atypia. In 2 patients, there were abundant luminal secretions. In 3, there were areas of glandular crowding, suggesting focal adenomatous change. In 1 patient, a focus of adenocarcinoma was seen in the polyp stroma. In nonpolypoid endometrium from 2 patients, there was decidual reaction of the stroma and cystic dilation of some endometrial glands in 1. Cystic change and focal glandular crowding were noted in the endometrium not involved by polyp.

Conclusion.—Endometrial sampling should be considered before starting tamoxifen therapy and at different intervals during its use, even in asymptomatic patients. When vaginal bleeding occurs in a postmenopausal woman taking tamoxifen, endometrial sampling is important, because this symptom cannot be assumed to be the result of endometrial atrophy.

▶ The paradoxical effect of tamoxifen on the endometrium needs to be publicized to avoid overlooking endometrial hyperplasia and carcinoma in patients receiving long-term tamoxifen therapy. Whether periodic endometrial biopsy is warranted ultimately will depend on the actual frequency of endometrial carcinoma in these patients. At the very least, as the authors point out, uterine bleeding in this group of women must not be attributed to endometrial atrophy.—C.P. Morrow, M.D.

The New International Federation of Gynecology and Obstetrics Surgical Staging and Survival Rates in Early Endometrial Carcinoma

Gal D, Recio FO, Zamurovic D (Maimonides Med Ctr, State Univ of New York, Brooklyn)

Cancer 69:200–202, 1992 15–23

Background.—In 1988, the International Federation of Gynecology and Obstetrics (FIGO) published a new classification for the surgical staging of endometrial carcinoma. This new staging system was met with mixed reviews. A retrospective analysis of patients with clinical stage I endometrial adenocarcinoma who were undergoing primary surgery at 1 center was done to assess the new staging system and to determine whether it identifies a subset of patients with a better or poorer prognosis.

Comparison of Clinical and Surgical Stagings

Clinical stage	No. of patients	Surgical stage (%)							
		IA	*IB*	*IC*	*IIA*	*IIB*	*IIIA*	*IIIB*	*IIIC*
IA	62	22 (35)	23 (37)	6 (10)	—	—	6 (10)	1 (2)	4 (6)
IB	31	7 (23)	12 (39)	2 (7)	—	1 (3)	6 (18)	—	3 (19)
Total	93	29 (31)	35 (38)	8 (9)	—	1 (1)	12 (13)	1 (1)	7 (7)

(Courtesy of Gal D, Recio FO, Zamurovic D: *Cancer* 69:200–202, 1992.)

Methods.—The study included patients who were treated between 1979 and 1987. Sufficient surgical-pathologic data were available in 93 cases to allow reclassification based on the new FIGO system.

Findings.—Twenty-three percent of the patients were found surgically to have disease advanced beyond clinical stage I. The overall 5-year survival rate for the whole group was 90%; however, this rate was significantly better (98%) for patients with surgical stage I disease than for those with surgical stage III disease (60%). Survival did not differ significantly among patients with different substages within surgical stage I. The distribution of adjuvant therapy among the substages also did not differ significantly (table).

Conclusion.—Although the number of patients studied was relatively small, no statistical difference in survival rates was found for those with different surgical substage I. Patients with myometrial invasion in whom no nodal or peritoneal spread was found had survivals comparable to those without myometrial invasion. Further study will determine whether it is advantageous to disregard the substaging of patients with surgical stage I disease.

▶ This paper was selected because it compares clinical results for a group of patients using the old, clinical FIGO staging and the new, surgical FIGO staging. All patients had undergone aortic and pelvic node sampling and peritoneal cytology. As expected, the outcome was much better for surgical stage I vs. surgical stage III (both clinical stage I). The authors' suggestion that the subgroups of surgical stage I might all have the same prognosis, however, would not hold up in a large series of patients. For example, even with negative nodes and cytology, G3 cases with deep invasion have a poorer prognosis than G1 cases with no invasion.—C.P. Morrow, M.D.

The Significance of Squamous Differentiation in Endometrial Carcinoma: Data From a Gynecologic Oncology Group Study

Zaino RJ, Kurman R, Herbold D, Gliedman J, Bundy BN, Voet R, Advani H (Pennsylvania State Univ, Hershey; Johns Hopkins Univ, Baltimore, Md; Univ of Kansas, Wichita; LDS Hosp, Salt Lake City; Roswell Park Mem Inst, Buffalo, NY; et al)

Cancer 68:2293–2302, 1991 15–24

Background.—The biological importance of squamous differentiation in endometrial adenocarcinoma (AC)—found in approximately one fourth of tumors—is uncertain. Prognostic studies have suggested that the outlook for patients with adenoacanthoma (AA) is better than, the same as, or worse than that of AC. Part of the problem is semantic confusion between AA and adenosquamous carcinoma (AS).

Objective and Methods.—A histological study was carried out in 456 women with typical AC and in 175 others having typical AC with areas of squamous differentiation (SQ). The latter patients had been entered in a protocol study of stage I and II endometrial AC. Assessment of histological grade and invasion was done by the pathologist at the member institution and also at a highly structured review by Gynecologic Oncology Group pathologists.

Findings.—Differentiation of the squamous component paralleled that of the glandular component in most tumors. Carcinomas with SQ behaved similarly to typical AC, although not identically. Nodal metastasis was comparably frequent, but the presence of SQ correlated with better survival. Classifying tumors with SQ by the depth of myometrial invasion and by architectural grade of the glandular component was prognostically more helpful than merely distinguishing AA from AS. Patients whose tumors contained a squamous element had almost half the mortality to those with pure AC.

Recommendations.—The terms AA and AS should be replaced by the single term AC + SQ. Information on the architectural grade of glandular elements, the depth of invasion, and the presence of disease in the cervix will help in planning appropriate treatment.

▶ In this study, women with AS carcinoma were much more likely to have deep (greater than two thirds) myometrial invasion (53.7% vs. 24%), and women with AA were more likely to have greater than one third myometrial invasion (69.1% vs. 57%) than were women with adenocarcinoma without squamous elements. However, the correlation with the differentiation of the glandular component was such that there was no apparent independent effect of squamous differentiation on survival. The prognosis and treatment of endometrial carcinoma should be predicated on the grade of the glandular component, the depth of myoinvasion, etc. The presence of, or grade of, the squamous component apparently is not important.—C.P. Morrow, M.D.

Analysis of Complications in Patients With Endometrial Carcinoma Receiving Adjuvant Irradiation

Greven KM, Lanciano RM, Herbert SH, Hogan PE (Fox Chase Cancer Ctr, Philadelphia; Bowman Gray School of Medicine, Winston-Salem, NC)

Int J Radiat Oncol Biol Phys 21:919–923, 1991 15–25

Introduction.—Complications were analyzed in 310 patients with documented endometrial carcinoma who received adjuvant radiotherapy in 1970–1986; 48 patients had stage II and 1 had stage III disease. Radiotherapy was given preoperatively to 170 patients, postoperatively to 138, and at both intervals to 2.

Methods.—A 4-field technique was used in most patients given external beam treatment. The median dose to the whole pelvis was 4,140 cGy. In 75 patients, only intracavitary therapy was administered.

Results.—The median follow-up was 5.5 years, and the actuarial survival at 5 years was 78%. In 34 patients there were complications involving the rectum, small bowel, femoral head, or lower extremity edema. The 12 serious complications included degeneration in the femur/acetabular region in 4 patients and rectal or small bowel injuries in 9. Complications occurred more often in younger patients and in those given external radiotherapy.

Conclusion.—Pelvic irradiation clearly limits pelvic relapse in patients with endometrial cancer, but the risk-benefit ratio should be carefully considered before recommending adjuvant radiotherapy for controlling pelvic involvement.

▶ This paper reminds us that the decision to recommend external beam radiation therapy must carefully balance the risk of recurrence with the risk of complications. It is reasonable to accept that surgical stage (lymph node sampling) will increase the risk of radiotherapy; however, the trade-off is that fewer patients will see the whole pelvis radiation, and the finding of lymph node metastases easily justifies the risks attending the use of aggressive radiotherapy. The finding that the 4-field technique of external beam radiotherapy produced similar rates of complications when given pre- or postoperatively reinforces the validity of doing surgery first and selected radiotherapy postoperatively when the decision can be based on the final surgical-pathologic data.—C.P. Morrow, M.D.

Recurrence in Noninvasive Endometrial Carcinoma: Relationship to Uterine Papillary Serous Carcinoma

Lee KR, Belinson JL (Univ of Vermont, Burlington; Cleveland Clinic)
Am J Surg Pathol 15:965–973, 1991 15–26

Background.—Noninvasive uterine papillary serous carcinoma (UPSC) recently was described in endometrial polyps as a component of disseminated serous carcinoma. There also are reports of an increased rate of synchronous extrauterine tumors in patients with UPSC.

Series.—There were 28 recurrences among 227 consecutive patients with clinical stage I endometrial carcinoma who were operated on from 1978 through 1987. Slides from 98 patients lacking myometrial and vascular invasion were reviewed.

Findings.—Recurrences developed in 7% of the 98 patients with noninvasive lesions. Eleven other patients with noninvasive lesions and similar histological patterns did not have recurrent disease. The recurrences correlated closely with the presence of papillary serous carcinoma and also were associated with foci of clear cell carcinoma. Two of the 7 patients with recurrence had synchronous ovarian serous carcinoma.

Conclusion.—Recurrent endometrial cancer appears to correlate with the presence of pure UPSC in endometrial polyps, and this finding may be a marker for synchronous extrauterine serous carcinoma. Patients with UPSC should be carefully evaluated intraoperatively for extrauterine spread—even if frozen-section study fails to demonstrate myometrial invasion.

► As this paper documents, UPSC and, perhaps, papillary clear-cell carcinoma, carry a serious risk for recurrence and synchronous extrauterine primary cancers, even when they appear to be confined to the endometrium. We recommend complete surgical staging for these patients, including intracolic omentectomy. Even in the absence of extrauterine spread or myometrial invasion, postoperative adjuvant radiotherapy is indicated. Chemotherapy and hormone therapy appear to be ineffective.—C.P. Morrow, M.D.

A New Treatment for Endometrial Cancer With Gonadotrophin Releasing-Hormone Analogue

Gallagher CJ, Oliver RTD, Oram DH, Fowler CG, Blake PR, Mantell BS, Slevin ML, Hope-Stone HF (Royal London Hosp; Royal Marsden Hosp; St Bartholomew's Hosp, London)

Br J Obstet Gynaecol 98:1037–1041, 1991 15–27

Objective.—Endometrial cancer that recurs after surgery carries a poor outlook. A majority of afflicted patients have disease outside the pelvis. The antitumor efficacy of gonadotropin-releasing hormone (GnRH) analogs was examined in 17 patients with recurrent endometrial cancer, all of whom had symptomatic, progressive, and measurable disease.

Management.—Progesterone therapy was stopped at least a month before the start of analog treatment. Sixteen patients received monthly depot injections of 7.5 mg of leuprorelin, and 1 received 3.6 mg of gosterelin. Early in the study, 2 patients received tamoxifen as well.

Results.—Serum gonadotropins decreased to normal luteal-phase values within a month and remained suppressed for the duration of treatment. Six patients (35%) had a response, and 1 of them responded completely. Five patients were still in remission 7–30 months later, whereas 1 was lost to follow-up. All responders had previously failed both radiation therapy and progesterone therapy. Two other patients have had stable disease, whereas 8 have died of progressive disease. The median follow-up was 14 months.

Conclusion.—Treatment with a GnRH analogue is an effective, nontoxic approach to the treatment of recurrent endometrial cancer.

► This is a very interesting report, not only because of the practical implications for the treatment of progestogen-resistant recurrent/metastatic endometrial cancer, but also because the efficacy of GnRH analogue therapy is unexpected. As the authors point out, both progestogen and GnRH analog produce a reduction in gonadotropins and estrogens. Thus, they suggest that the success of GnRH analogue in treating endometrial cancer resistant to progestogen therapy is caused by a direct effect of the GnRH analogue on the cancer cells; however, the GnRH activity may result from a quantitative difference in the hormonal suppression effected by the 2 treatments.—C.P. Morrow, M.D.

Adenosarcoma of the Uterus: A Gynecologic Oncology Group Clinicopathologic Study of 31 Cases

Kaku T, Silverberg SG, Major FJ, Miller A, Fetter B, Brady MF (George Washington Univ, Washington, DC; Pennsylvania State Univ, Hershey, Pa; Univ of Colorado, Denver)

Int J Gynecol Pathol 11:75–88, 1992 15–28

Background.—Adenosarcoma of the uterus has benign or atypical glands and a sarcomatous stroma. It has been regarded as having low malignant potential, but some tumors have exhibited a very aggressive clinical course.

Series.—Thirty-one patients seen since 1979 with clinical stage I or II uterine adenosarcoma who underwent hysterectomy and staging laparotomy were studied. The mean patient age was 57.4 years. Six cases were reclassified as stage III after surgery. Pelvic lymph node metastases were found in 2 patients.

Pathologic Features.—Half the patients had no myometrial invasion, whereas 4 tumors extended into or through the outer third of the myometrium. Grossly, the tumors were polypoid or papillary masses. Microscopically, a bland or slightly atypical glandular component was associated with a sarcomatous stroma that usually was of low grade. Approximately half the tumors had a mitotic count exceeding 20 per 10 high-power fields.

Outcome.—Nine patients (30%) had recurrences, and 6 of them died of tumor after a mean follow-up of 38 months. Seventeen tumors were diagnosed as adenosarcoma with sarcomatous overgrowth, and 10 of them contained focal or extensive rhabdomyosarcoma. Both extrauterine spread and myometrial invasion correlated with an increased risk of recurrence. All 5 patients with metastases outside the pelvis died of disease.

Recommendation.—Staging laparotomy is indicated in women with clinical stage I and II adenosarcoma of the uterus.

▶ Uterine or cervical adenosarcoma can occur at any stage, but the average patient is postmenopausal. It initially was thought to be a tumor of low malignant potential, but it now appears that 25% of patients have relapses. Factors that are predictive of increases in recurrence are deep myometrial invasion, sarcomatous overgrowth, rhabdomyosarcoma and, of course, extrauterine spread at the time of diagnosis. Three of 19 stage I cases recurred (1 of 12 without sarcomatous overgrowth), and 2 of 9 reproductive-aged patients had recurrences of disease (1 in 7, stage I). The optimal treatment is unknown because of the rarity of the tumor; however, current recommendation includes surgical staging, modified or radical hysterectomy if the cervix is involved, and postoperative pelvic radiation or chemotherapy. If the tumor is extensive, preservation of the ovaries in the premenopausal woman is inadvisable.—C.P. Morrow, M.D.

Phase II Trial of Cisplatin as First-Line Chemotherapy in Patients With Advanced or Recurrent Uterine Sarcomas: A Gynecologic Oncology Group Study

Thigpen JT, Blessing JA, Beecham J, Homesley H, Yordan E (Univ of Mississippi, Jackson; Roswell Park Mem Inst, Buffalo NY; Univ of Rochester, Rochester, NY; Wake Forest Univ, Winston-Salem, NC; Rush-Presbyterian/St Luke's Med Ctr, Chicago)

J Clin Oncol 9:1962–1966, 1991 15–29

Background.—Mixed mesodermal sarcomas and leiomyosarcomas comprise 90% of uterine sarcomas. The use of cisplatin as first-line chemotherapy in patients with mixed mesodermal sarcoma and leiomyosarcomas of the uterus was studied.

Methods.—The Gynecologic Oncology Group includes more than 30 institutions, which contributed enough cases for phase II studies of chemotherapy in each of these 2 uterine sarcoma types. The 96 evaluable patients enrolled in the study had advanced or recurrent uterine sarcomas that no longer were controllable with surgery and radiotherapy. The patients had not received previous chemotherapy. Cisplatin, 50 mg/m^2, was given intravenously every 3 weeks.

Outcomes.—Of 63 patients with mixed mesodermal tumors, 5 responded completely, for a rate of 8%, and 7 responded partially, for a rate of 11%. Of 33 patients with leiomyosarcoma, 1 had a partial response, for a rate of 3%. The adverse effects were leukopenia in 23%,

Responses to Cisplatin

Response	Mixed Mesodermal Tumors (%)	Leiomyosarcoma (%)
CR	5 (8)	0 (0)
PR	7 (11)	1 (3)
Stable disease	32 (51)	18 (55)
Increasing disease	19 (30)	14 (42)
Total	63 (100)	33 (100)

(Courtesy of Thigpen JT, Blessing JA, Beecham J, et al: *J Clin Oncol* 9:1962–1966, 1991.)

nausea and vomiting in 73%, and mild azotemia in 42%. None of the patients had life-threatening toxicities (table).

Conclusion.—At the dose and schedule given, cisplatin had definite activity in patients with mixed mesodermal sarcomas who had no previous chemotherapy. However, cisplatin had little effect in patients with leiomyosarcoma.

▶ Until recently, oncologists have looked on uterine sarcomas as a single group of tumors from the point of view of therapy. This is another severely limited Gynecology Oncology Group study documenting that uterine leiomysarcomas and MMMT (carcinosarcomas) need to be evaluated and treated as biologically dissimilar tumors. The MMMTs are relatively sensitive to cisplatin, whereas the LMSs are quite resistant. This is probably also true of radiation therapy: LMS is more resistant to radiotherapy than is MMMT.—C.P. Morrow, M.D.

Ovary

Pooled Analysis of 3 European Case-Control Studies of Epithelial Ovarian Cancer: III. Oral Contraceptive Use

Franceschi S, Parazzini F, Negri E, Booth M, La Vecchia C, Beral V, Tzonou A, Trichopoulos D (Aviano Cancer Ctr, Aviano, Italy; Europëan Cancer Prevention Organization, Brussels; Inst for Pharmacological Research, Milan, Italy; London School of Hygiene and Tropical Medicine; Radcliffe Infirmary, Oxford, England; et al)
Int J Cancer 49:61–65, 1991 15–30

Background.—Many studies have confirmed a protective effect of combined oral contraceptives (OCs) against epithelial ovarian cancer. Protection increases with the duration of contraceptive use.

Objective.—Use of OCs was related to the risk of ovarian cancer in 3 hospital-based case-control studies carried out in Italy, the United Kingdom, and Greece. A total of 971 patients with cancer were compared with 2,258 controls younger than 65 years of age.

Findings.—Women who had used OCs at any time had a relative risk of ovarian cancer of .6 compared with those who had never used them. The protective effect was constant across age and parity levels. Protection appeared to increase with the duration of OC use; the relative risk in women who had last used OCs 15 years or more before diagnosis was .5. Among ever-users of OCs, women reporting first use before 25 years of age had an especially low risk for cancer.

Conclusion.—Protection against ovarian cancer appears to last at least 15 years after cessation of oral contraceptive use. It is possible that a protective effect is exerted at the early stages of carcinogenesis. A substantial number of deaths may be prevented by OC use. Ovarian cancer, along with breast cancer, must be considered in any risk-benefit assessment of OCs.

▶ There have been several studies reporting that OC use protects against the development of ovarian cancer, as does pregnancy. This meta-analysis provides some refinement of the data. The durability of the protective effect is greater than 15 years, and the greatest benefit is to women who used OC before age 25 (RR = .3) compared with after age 25 (RR = .8). Years of use is also influential (greater than or equal to 5 years, RR = .4; less than 2 years, RR = .76). If these studies are valid, during this decade we should see a decrease in the occurrence of ovarian cancer.—C.P. Morrow, M.D.

Tubal Sterilization, Hysterectomy, and the Subsequent Occurrence of Epithelial Ovarian Cancer

Irwin KL, Weiss NS, Lee NC, Peterson HB (Ctrs for Disease Control, Atlanta; Univ of Washington, Seattle)

Am J Epidemiol 134:362–369, 1991 15–31

Introduction.—Epithelial ovarian cancer may result from environmental agents that enter the peritoneal cavity through the vagina. If so, tubal sterilization and hysterectomy may block the ascent of potential carcinogens to the ovarian epithelium. In addition, the risk of ovarian cancer might be influenced by altered ovarian function consequent to tubal sterilization or hysterectomy.

Methods.—In a multicenter, population-based case-control study, data on 494 women with epithelial ovarian cancer diagnosed in 1980–1982 were compared with those of 4,238 control women accessed by random digit dialing.

Results.—The relative risk of ovarian cancer was .69 for women who had tubal sterilization, .55 for those who had hysterectomy, and .60 for those undergoing hysterectomy with unilateral oophorectomy. The lesser risk associated with tubal sterilization and hysterectomy lasted approximately 2 decades after surgery. The risk of cancer was least in women having hysterectomy/unilateral oophorectomy before 40 years of age.

Conclusion.—It is possible that the risk of ovarian cancer is lower in women who have had tubal sterilization or hysterectomy simply because there is an opportunity to screen for ovarian pathology at the time of surgery. Whether a biologic mechanism plays a role remains uncertain.

▶ The rationale for this study is partly based on the idea that ovarian carcinoma is related to the mesothelioma, and mesotheliomas are known to be caused by asbestos. In women, it has been proposed that talc, which chemically is very similar to asbestos, might be a cause of ovarian carcinoma because talc is known to gain access to the ovaries via the vagina. In fact, birefringent particles consistent with talc have been found in ovarian tumors, and previous epidemiological studies have suggested that women exposed to talc during infancy had an increased incidence of ovarian cancer (1). Furthermore, women who have undergone tubal sterilization or hysterectomy have a lower RR for ovarian carcinoma than controls.—C.P. Morrow, M.D.

Reference

1. Cramer DW, et al: *Cancer* 50:372, 1982.

Ovarian Cancer in Women With Prior Hysterectomy: A 14-Year Experience at the University of Miami

Sightler SE, Boike GM, Estape RE, Averette HE (Univ of Miami Med Ctr; Jackson Mem Hosp, Miami)

Obstet Gynecol 78:681–684, 1991 15–32

Introduction.—Ovarian cancer remains the leading cause of death from gynecological cancer. In most patients, the disease is diagnosed at an advanced stage. The 5-year survival rates have been less than 20% despite aggressive multimodality treatment. One effective approach to preventing this cancer is prophylactic oophorectomy in women undergoing hysterectomy for gynecological reasons.

Methods.—Among 755 women treated for ovarian cancer in 1977–1990 were 95 (12.6%) who previously had undergone hysterectomy and had cancer develop in 1 of the conserved ovaries. Both ovaries had been conserved in all but 1 of these women. The average age at hysterectomy was 43 years, and at the time of diagnosis of ovarian cancer, 60 years. Cancer developed in 13 women within 4 years of hysterectomy, in 6 of them within 18 months. More than two thirds of the women presented with stage III or stage IV disease.

Conclusion.—A policy of prophylactic oophorectomy at age 40 years and older would have prevented 5% of ovarian cancers in a combined literature series of more than 2,500 patients. If applied nationwide, such a policy might prevent the disease in more than 1,000 patients each year. Routine oophorectomy is recommended for all women older than 40 years who have undergone a hysterectomy. Prophylactic removal of the ovaries might also be considered in younger women undergoing pelvic surgery if high-risk factors are present.

▶ Among gynecologists in the United States, it has been standard practice for many years to remove routinely normal-appearing ovaries at the time of hysterectomy in women of peri- or postmenopausal age to prevent ovarian carcinoma. The recommended age at which prophylactic oophorectomy should begin does, however, vary. Most authorities favor age 45 years, but others, in agreement with this study, recommend age 40. Only rarely are later or earlier ages recommended.

Important issues other than ovarian carcinoma are also involved. The most significant issue involves the potential deleterious effects of castration. Even in the postmenopausal woman, the ovaries continue to have an endocrine function; however, for the premenopausal woman, castration without effective hormone therapy will increase the risk for osteoporosis and heart disease. Poor compliance with long-term estrogen therapy is a common problem among both the educated and the uneducated. The average patient who, at 40 years of age, has her ovaries removed and fails to take estrogen is probably at greater risk of an adverse outcome related to estrogen deficiency than a risk related to ovarian carcinoma. In my opinion, the earliest age at which "routine" prophylactic ovariectomy should be done is 45 years, unless the patient has a greater than average risk for the development of ovarian carcinoma: family history of ovarian cancer, previous ovarian epithelial neoplasm, infertility with "incessant ovulation".—C.P. Morrow, M.D.

Ovarian Cancer Screening in Asymptomatic Postmenopausal Women by Transvaginal Sonography

van Nagell JR Jr, DePriest PD, Puls LE, Donaldson ES, Gallion HH, Pavlik EJ, Powell DE, Kryscio RJ (Univ of Kentucky Med Ctr, Lexington)

Cancer 68:458–462, 1991 15–33

Objective.—Ovarian cancer remains the prime cause of death from gynecological cancer in the United States. The value of transvaginal sonography (TVS) in screening for ovarian cancer was examined in a series of 1,300 postmenopausal women who were examined from 1987 to 1991. All women were asymptomatic. Real-time ultrasonography was carried out using a 5-MHz vaginal transducer.

Findings.—Thirty-three women had abnormal ovarian morphology or size for longer than 1 month. The mean lesion diameter was 4 cm. Ovarian enlargement was apparent clinically in 10 of these women. All 27 women who were explored had tumors similar in size to that predicted

Ovarian Histological Condition in 27 Patients With Abnormal Transvaginal Sonography

Category	No.
Adenocarcinoma	3
Serous cystadenoma	14
Epithelial cyst	3
Leiomyoma	3
Hydrosalpinx	2
Endometrioma	1
Thecoma	1

(Courtesy of van Nagell JR Jr, DePriest PD, Puls LE, et al: *Cancer* 68:458–462, 1991.)

by TVS. Fourteen patients had serous cystadenomas and 3 had ovarian cancer, which was primary in 2 cases and metastatic from colon carcinoma in 1 (table). Women with a family history of ovarian cancer were at increased risk.

Conclusion.—Transvaginal sonography remains an experimental method, and its value in screening for ovarian cancer remains to be established. A multicenter trial is needed to compare TVS and serum CA-125 estimation with pelvic examination for detecting ovarian cancer.

▶ This is a relatively small but well-done study of transvaginal ultrasound (TVS) screening for ovarian cancer. All 1,300 women screened were postmenopausal, and 33 had abnormal scans (ovarian volume greater than 8 cm^3 or complex/solid areas). It is not completely clear how many patients had unnecessary laparotomies, but 18 of 27 had ovarian neoplasia. The 2 primary ovarian cancers, both of which were stage Ia, were not palpated at pelvic exam and had normal CA-125 values. All 5 ovarian cancers detected by Campbell et al. (1) in a screening of more than 5,000 women were also stage Ia. The prospect that TVS will prove to be cost effective for screening the general population is dim. However, it might very well be feasible for high-risk groups, especially women with a family history of ovarian cancer. Van Nagell et al. found the probability of finding a serous tumor in this group to be 4 times that of the other study patients.—C.P. Morrow, M.D.

Reference

1. Campbell S, et al: *BMJ* 299:1363, 1989.

Ultrasound Screening for Familial Ovarian Cancer

Bourne TH, Whitehead MI, Campbell S, Royston P, Bhan V, Collins WP (King's College School of Medicine and Dentistry, London; Royal Postgraduate Medical School, London)

Gynecol Oncol 43:92–97, 1991 15–34

Introduction.—There is a need for an effective means of detecting ovarian cancer before metastasis. Either multicenter trials are needed to assess potential screening measures, or women who are at high risk for the disease may need to be evaluated.

Study Plan.—Transvaginal ultrasonography was done to screen 776 asymptomatic women (age, 25 years and older) who had at least 1 close relative with ovarian cancer. In 87% of the patients, a first-degree relative was affected. The mean age was 51 years.

Outcome of Screening.—A group of 43 women (5.5% of those assessed) was referred for surgical investigation, and 39 underwent laparotomy. A total of 23 tumors were detected—including 3 primary ovarian cancers—for a prevalence of 3.9 per 1,000. All were International Feder-

Assessment Criteria for the Screening Procedure

Ovarian pathology	Detection rate (%)	Specificity (%)	Positive predictive value (%)	Odds*
Any mass	—	—	94.9*	18.6 to 1†
Any tumor	—	—	51.2*	1.0 to 1
Primary cancer	100	94.8	7.7	12 to 1‡

* Calculated from results of laparotomy.
† In favor of positive results on screening indicating the presence of each type of pathology; odds = positive value/(100 − positive predictive value).
‡ Against positive result on screening indicating the presence of each type of pathology; odds = positive predictive value/100 − positive predictive value).
(Courtesy of Bourne TH, Whitehead MI, Campbell S, et al: *Gynecol Oncol* 43:92–97, 1991.)

ation of Gynecology and Obstetrics (FIGO) stage Ia malignancies. No woman had ovarian cancer within a year of ultrasound study (table). The predictive value of a positive screen was 7.7%. The odds were 12 to 1 against finding primary ovarian cancer at exploration.

Conclusion.—The positive predictive value of transvaginal ultrasonography in this series of high-risk women exceeded that found in a previous population-based screening program, as did the prevalence of primary ovarian cancer.

▶ This study of transvaginal ultrasound screening of women with a family history of ovarian cancer suggests that it is worthwhile. Compared with screening of a more general population of women, the authors find a higher proportion with benign epithelial ovarian tumors (2.5% vs. .7%), a higher percentage with a positive screen (18% vs. 6%), a higher percentage with bilateral masses (48% vs. 11% of masses), and a significant increase in the predictive value of a positive screen (1 in 13 vs. 1 in 99). It is regrettable that the authors did not investigate the usefulness of the serum CA-125 determination, which may have increased the specificity of the ultrasonography. The highest false positive rate was observed in women who had previously undergone hysterectomy. Although the authors mentioned that ovarian cysts in some postmenopausal women disappeared on follow-up, no details were given.—C.P. Morrow, M.D.

Diagnosing the Correct Ovarian Cancer Syndrome

Trimble EL, Karlan BY, Lagasse LD, Hoskins WJ (Mem Sloan-Kettering Cancer Ctr, New York; Cedars-Sinai Med Ctr, Los Angeles)

Obstet Gynecol 78:1023–1026, 1991 15–35

Background.—As many as 10% of cases of ovarian cancer are ascribed to hereditary causes, but the most prominent risk factor in any individual is a positive family history of the disease. Lynch et al. found that familial ovarian cancer may be inherited as an autosomal dominant trait. At least 3 genotypes predispose to ovarian cancer: site-specific ovarian carcinoma; ovarian cancer in conjunction with breast cancer; and the Cancer Family Syndrome, which involves cancers of the colon, endometrium, and ovary.

Experience.—Four sisters were encountered whose maternal pedigree suggested a site-specific ovarian cancer syndrome. The paternal pedigree, however, closely accorded with the Cancer Family Syndrome. The primary cancers in the father's family included tumors of the colon, pancreas, bladder, ureter, and prostate. The sisters had endometrial, ovarian, and colon cancers.

Recommendations.—Screening for site-specific ovarian cancer includes estimation of CA 125, ultrasound study, and bilateral oophorectomy after the family is complete. For the breast/ovary syndrome, mammography and possible prophylactic mastectomy are in order. Colonoscopy and endometrial biopsy are necessary to screen for the Cancer Family Syndrome. Hysterectomy and bilateral oophorectomy may be done once childbearing is complete.

▶ This study alerts us to various familial cancer syndromes involving ovarian carcinoma. Its authors also emphasize that appropriate workup, follow-up, and counseling vary depending on the specific syndrome. The authors recommend prophylactic oophorectomy for women with any of the 3 syndromes after childbearing is complete, and they correctly call attention to the possibility of peritoneal carcinomatosis that may occur after oophorectomy and that mimics ovarian carcinoma. It is incumbent upon the gynecologist to request of the pathologist that those ovaries that are removed prophylactically be extensively sectioned, because the usual procedure for examining a normal-appearing ovary is to take a single section.—C.P. Morrow, M.D.

The Postmenopausal Palpable Ovary Syndrome: A Retrospective Review With Histopathologic Correlates

Miller RC, Nash JD, Weiser EB, Hoskins WJ (Uniformed Services Univ of the Health Sciences, Bethesda, Md)

J Reprod Med 36:568–571, 1991 15–36

Introduction.—Celiotomy is often indicated in women with the postmenopausal palpable ovary (PMPO) syndrome to rule out ovarian malignancy, but few data are available on the frequency of malignancy in these patients.

Methods.—Data on 20 patients with asymptomatic PMPO who were explored in 1982–1986 were reviewed retrospectively.

Results.—In 13 patients, there were ovarian neoplasms, and 3 had tumors that were either malignant or of borderline malignant potential. The latter patients had a lower mean parity than the others and had been postmenopausal for a longer time. The malignancy rate was 15% compared with 25% for a comparison group of women with adnexal masses larger than 5 cm. The clinical dimensions of the PMPO masses generally were smaller than the actual gross pathologic measurements.

Conclusion.—Further experience will determine whether pelvic examination, measurement of CA-125, or ultrasound study will be helpful in defining the risk of malignancy in patients with the PMPO syndrome.

▶ With the advent of ultrasound, the PMPO can be relegated to history. Nevertheless, it is of interest to know what the "palpable ovary" proves to be. For entry into this study, the patients were required to be asymptomatic, be more than 2 years postmenopausal, and have a palpable pelvic mass greater than 5 cm in diameter consistent with an enlarged ovary. Of the 20 patients in the study, 3 had malignant tumors, 9 had benign ovarian tumors, 4 had simple ovarian cysts, 1 had a pedunculated uterine leiomyoma, and 3 had a negative pelvis. In a group of similar asymptomatic postmenopausal women with masses greater than 5 cm in diameter, 25% were malignant. All postmenopausal women with asymptomatic palpable ovarian masses need ultrasonic and CA-125 evaluation. In the absence of malignant indicators, laparoscopy is indicated.—C.P. Morrow, M.D.

Risk Factors for Gestational Trophoblastic Disease: A Separate Analysis of Complete and Partial Hydatidiform Moles

Parazzini F, Mangili G, La Vecchia C, Negri E, Bocciolone L, Fasoli M (Istituto di Ricerche Farmacologiche "Mario Negri," Milan, Italy; Università di Milano, Italy; Inst of Social and Preventive Medicine, Lausanne, Switzerland)

Obstet Gynecol 78:1039–1045, 1991 15–37

Objective.—The risk factors for complete and partial hydatidiform mole were studied in a case-control series of 139 women with complete moles, 49 with partial moles, and 410 obstetric control subjects.

Findings.—The risk of mole decreased as the number of births increased, and the patients were more often nulliparous than the control women. The risk of both complete and partial mole was greater for women reporting spontaneous miscarriages. Infertility problems and difficulty in conceiving also were risk factors, but age at first pregnancy and induced abortion were not. Previous gestational trophoblastic disease increased the risk of both complete and partial mole, and a family history of disease was associated with complete mole. Smokers were at an increased risk. Women with blood group A who were married to group O men had an insignificantly increased risk of having mole (table).

Distribution and Corresponding Relative Risks for Cases and Controls According to Maternal and Mating Maternal/Paternal ABO Blood Groups: Milan, Italy, 1981–1990

	Complete mole	Partial mole	Control	Odds ratio (95% CI) Complete mole	Odds ratio (95% CI) Partial mole
Maternal blood group					
AB	6*	2	12	2.1 (0.8–5.7)	1.2 (0.3–5.7)
A	58	18	141	1.7 (1.1–2.6)	0.9 (0.5–1.7)
B	13	4	44		
O	38	25	168	Referent	Referent
Woman/partner					
All other combinations	90	40	303	Referent	Referent
Woman A/partner O	18	8	39	1.5 (0.9–2.7)	1.5 (0.7–3.5)

Abbreviation: CI, confidence interval.
* In some cases, the sum does not add up to the total because of the missing values.
(Courtesy of Parazzini F, Mangili G, La Vecchia C, et al: *Obstet Gynecol* 78:1039–1045, 1991.)

Conclusion.—The findings suggest that there are some similarities in the epidemiology of complete hydatidiform mole and partial mole.

▶ This study that the epidemiology of partial mole is similar to—or the same as—that of complete molar gestation, i.e., risk is increased in women with a history of spontaneous miscarriage, prior gestational trophoblastic diseases, and a family history of the disease. In addition, women with complete or partial mole were more often nulliparous and subfertile.—C.P. Morrow, M.D.

DNA Cytophotometry and Prognosis in Ovarian Tumors of Borderline Malignancy: A Clinicomorphologic Study of 80 Cases

Padberg B-C, Arps H, Franke U, Thiedemann C, Rehpenning W, Stegner H-E, Lietz H, Schröder S, Dietel M (Univ of Hamburg, Germany; Gen Hosp Hamburg-Wandsbek, Hamburg; Univ of Kiel, Kiel, Germany)
Cancer 69:2510–2514, 1992 15–38

Background.—Ovarian tumors of borderline malignancy (OTBM) are those epithelial ovarian neoplasms that show only some of the histological features of malignancy. The term embraces a wide range of biological behavior, including patients with continuous recurrence-free survival and those with rapidly fatal progression. In a series of OTBMs, DNA cytophotometry was performed.

Methods.—The study material comprised surgical specimens of 80 OTBMs, all of which underwent scanning DNA cytophotometry. Twenty-one of these tumors had diploid or euploid DNA histograms, whereas 59 had noneuploid or aneuploid patterns. The patients were followed up for at least 3 years and for a mean of nearly 7 years.

Log-Linear Model Illustrating the Associations Between DNA Pattern, Tumor Stage, and Prognosis of Ovarian Tumors of Borderline Malignancy

	Histogram types		
	I and II	***III and IV***	
FIGO stage			
$I_{a/b1}$ (early)	0/7	1/18	1/25
$I_{a/b2}$ and I_c-III (advanced)	0/14	10/41	10/55
	0/21	11/59	

Abbreviation: FIGO, International Federation of Gynecology and Obstetrics.
$P < .05$.
Numbers of cases of recurrent tumor/of patients at risk are stated for the respective groups.
(Courtesy of Padberg B-C, Arps H, Franke U, et al: *Cancer* 69:2510–2514, 1992.)

Results.—Eleven patients had recurrent disease, and 6 died. The DNA findings were correlated with the patients' postoperative course, as were a number of other morphological and clinical details, including age, stage of disease, histological findings, and extent of therapy. However, on statistical analysis, DNA content was found to be the only parameter that significantly affected prognosis (table). Of recurrent tumors and deaths resulting from tumor exclusively, all occurred in patients with noneuploid or aneuploid tumors. In contrast, none of the diploid or euploid tumors recurred.

Conclusion.—The prognosis of OTBM may be assessed profitably by DNA cytophotometry; the best application of this strategy is debatable. Tumors with diploid or euploid DNA histograms may be low-risk neoplasms that can be managed safely by conservative surgery.

▶ This study provides encouragement that one day those patients who have OTBMs that are destined to recur can be identified by testing the tumor tissue in the laboratory. Although the authors' results suggest that flow cytometry is the answer, a closer look at the data advises caution. All the cases that recurred did have an adverse histogram; however, all but 1 of the recurrences was in a patient with more advanced disease, mostly stage III. We do not need to know the histogram to recognize that these patients have a high risk for recurrence. Only 20% of patients with an adverse histogram had recurrence of disease.—C.P. Morrow, M.D.

Ovarian Metastases in Stage IB Carcinoma of the Cervix: A Gynecologic Oncology Group Study

Sutton GP, Bundy BN, Delgado G, Sevin B-U, Creasman WT, Major FJ, Zaino R (Indiana Univ, Indianapolis; Roswell Park Mem Inst, Buffalo, NY; George-

town Univ, Washington, DC; Univ of Miami; Med Univ of South Carolina, Charleston; et al)
Am J Obstet Gynecol 166:50–53, 1992 15–39

Objective.—The frequency of ovarian metastasis was examined in a series of 990 patients who underwent laparotomy had radical hysterectomy for clinical stage IB cervical carcinoma. The specific goal was to learn whether the risk is greater in adenocarcinoma and adenosquamous carcinoma than in squamous carcinoma of the cervix.

Findings.—Squamous lesions were seen in 77.9% of the patients, adenocarcinoma occurred in 12.2%, and adenosquamous carcinoma was seen in 8.2%. Ovarian involvement was found in .5% of the patients with squamous carcinoma and 1.7% of those with adenocarcinoma; the difference was not significant. All 6 women with ovarian metastases had other extracervical disease as well. Four of the 6 patients died of disease. Pelvic recurrences were not more frequent in patients with adenocarcinoma or adenosquamous lesions than in those with squamous carcinoma.

Recommendation.—It seems reasonable to conserve normal-appearing ovaries in young women having hysterectomy for cervical adenocarcinoma or adenosquamous carcinoma, as long as no other extracervical spread is identified. Also, the patient must accept a small risk of ovarian involvement going undetected.

▶ The issue of occult ovarian metastasis in cervical carcinoma is important because the ovaries usually are not removed in young women (younger than 45 years) undergoing radical hysterectomy. The results of this study are reassuring; however, the study does have some shortcomings. The ovaries were removed in only half the patients, and most of these women presumably were in the over-45 age group. Thus, it is of interest to note that, of the 6 patients with documented ovarian metastases, only one was older than 45 years of age. In other words, the patient population most likely to have ovarian metastases is the same population least likely to have the ovaries removed. Nevertheless, it seems to be a very safe procedure, especially in the absence of other metastases.—C.P. Morrow, M.D.

Borderline Epithelial Ovarian Tumors: A Review of 81 Cases With an Assessment of the Impact of Treatment

Manchul LA, Simm J, Levin W, Fyles AW, Dembo AJ, Pringle JF, Rawlings GA, Sturgeon JFG, Thomas GM (Princess Margaret Hosp, Toronto; Univ of Toronto)

Int J Radiat Oncol Biol Phys 22:867–874, 1992 15–40

Background.—For several reasons, including the lack of accepted pathologic criteria, the lack of understanding of the significance of intra-

Proportion of Relapses or Deaths in Relation to the Presence or Absence of Tumor Excrescences, Adhesions, Rupture, or Malignant Cells in Peritoneal Washings

		Proportion who died	Proportion who relapsed*
Excrescences	Absent	2/43	0/43
	Present	2/33	4/33
	Unknown	2/5	0/5
Adhesions	None	0/37	1/37
	Sharp	2/10	0/10
	Blunt	3/26	0/26
	Both	0/2	2/2
	Unknown	1/6	1/6
Peritoneal Cytology	Negative	1/18	0/18
	Positive	1/14	0/14
	Unknown	4/49	4/49
Tumour rupture	No	1/34	2/34
	Yes	3/20	2/20
	Unknown	2/27	0/27

* Relapse is defined as relapse or persistent disease.

(Courtesy of Manchul LA, Simm J, Levin W, et al: *Int J Radiat Oncol Biol Phys* 22:867–874, 1992.)

peritoneal implants, and the desire to limit the extent of surgery in young women, no consensus has been reached regarding the best management of borderline epithelial ovarian tumors. A series of women with borderline epithelial ovarian tumors was studied to assess their natural history, ascertain useful prognostic factors, and determine the value of adjuvant therapy.

Patients.—The study sample comprised 81 women with borderline epithelial ovarian tumors referred during a 21-year period. The mean patient age was 48 years. The presenting symptom was pain in 46% of patients, and 43% had a palpable pelvic mass. A total of 78% of patients had stage I and 11% each had stage II and III disease. Histological subtype was serous in 72% and mucinous in 28%. Peritoneal washings were done in 32 patients, with 14 patients showing malignant cells. Cyst rupture occurred in 25% of cases, surface excrescences in 40%, and adhesions in 46%, but none of these factors significantly affected recurrence rate or survival (table).

No adjuvant radiotherapy was given in 65 patients, whereas 11 had adjuvant radiation, 4 had adjuvant chemotherapy, and 1 had both. Therefore, no valid conclusions could be drawn about the effectiveness of adjuvant therapy. The 10-year overall survival (OS) was 85%, and the 10-year cause-specific survival was 96%. None of the patients with stage I disease died of their tumor; the 10-year OS was 90% in this group, and all but 2 patients received no adjuvant therapy. In more advanced stages, the 10-year OS was 75% and 10-year disease-free survival was 50%, regardless of the use of any adjuvant therapy.

Conclusion.—In patients with stage I borderline epithelial ovarian tumors, adjuvant therapy appears to be unnecessary. The current study can draw no conclusions about the need for adjuvant therapy in more advanced stages or about the adequacy of unilateral oophorectomy or ovarian cystectomy, because of the small numbers of patients. A multicenter tumor registry needs to be developed to provide a prospective database on these tumors.

▶ The title of this article is a little misleading because, as the authors state, they are unable to draw any conclusions about the impact of adjuvant therapy. It does, however, bring us up to date on the outcome of low malignant potential tumors with a well-analyzed study and a reasonably large number of patients. Although none of the 63 patients with stage I disease died of tumor, 2 are alive with disease (oddly, they are the only 2 who received adjuvant therapy). The 50% disease-free and 75% overall survival rates for the patients with stages II and III are noteworthy. It is important not to overtreat this group of patients in view of their relatively good prognosis, especially because an effective adjuvant therapy has not been determined.—C.P. Morrow, M.D.

Mucinous Ovarian Tumors With Pseudomyxoma Peritonei: A Clinicopathological Study

Kahn MA, Demopoulos RI (New York Univ Med Ctr, The New York Infirmary/Beekman Downtown Hosp, New York)

Int J Gynecol Pathol 11:15–23, 1992 15–41

Background.—Pseudomyxoma peritonei (PP) is rare. A study was done to compare mucinous ovarian tumors accompanied by PP with control tumors matched for histological diagnosis but not associated with PP for pathologic differences that may serve as useful prognostic indicators.

Methods.—Eight patients with mucinous ovarian tumors and PP were studied retrospectively. These patients were matched by their original ovarian tumor histology with 8 control patients with tumors but not PP. In each group, there were 4 benign tumors, 3 with low malignant potential, and 1 malignant.

Findings.—Compared with control tumors, case tumors more often showed cyst rupture, periovarian adhesions, mucinous lesions of the appendix, goblet cells, and tumor necrosis. All cases had pseudomyxoma ovarii containing mucinous epithelial cells. One control tumor showed pseudomyxoma ovarii but did not contain epithelial cells. The peritoneal mucin contained epithelial cells in all cases. Two cases displayed a change in histology 6 years after the original ovarian tumor surgery. One of these was not accompanied by PP until the first recurrence of the benign ovarian tumor.

Conclusion.—Pseudomyxoma ovarii with epithelial cells may presage the development of PP, malignant recurrence, or both. Additional studies with larger numbers of cases are needed to confirm whether cellular pseudomyxoma ovarii represents invasion.

▶ Pseudomyxoma peritonei is a strange phenomenon and is not well understood. This relatively large series of 8 cases sheds some light on the pathophysiology. For example, all cases had pseudomyxoma ovarii, i.e., the ovarian stroma was infiltrated by mucin-containing mucinous epithelial cells. The mucinous ascites also contains mucinous epithelial cells. This helps to explain the sometimes long-term benefit of removing the ascites; it actually is a form of tumor reductive surgery. The appendix was abnormal in half the cases (hyperplasia or carcinoma). A final observation is that 4 of the PP cases were associated with "benign" mucinous ovarian tumors.—C.P. Morrow, M.D.

The Accuracy of Frozen Section in the Diagnosis of Ovarian Neoplasms

Obiakor I, Maiman M, Mittal K, Awobuluyi M, DiMaio T, Demopoulos R (State Univ of New York–Health Science Ctr at Brooklyn; New York Univ Med Ctr)

Gynecol Oncol 43:61–63, 1991 5–42

Introduction.—The operative treatment of ovarian neoplasms in premenopausal women depends on the diagnosis based on frozen sections.

Methods.—To determine the accuracy of frozen-section diagnosis in women with suspected ovarian neoplasia, the results of 311 consecutive studies of ovarian masses performed in 1980–1989 were reviewed.

Results.—The final diagnosis was malignancy in 84 patients. The frozen-section diagnosis agreed with the final pathologic classification of benign or malignant masses in 94% of the patients, and it disagreed in 3.5%; 8 decisions were deferred. Most of the disagreements involved a frozen section diagnosis of benign epithelial tumor in which a lesion of low malignant potential was found on permanent section. Frozen-section diagnosis was 86% sensitive and 100% specific, with a negative predictive value of 95%. There were no false positive frozen-section diagnoses. Limited sampling often was responsible for a false negative result.

Conclusion.—In patients with a benign diagnosis based on frozen-section study, the omentum and peritoneum should be carefully evaluated at the time of surgery. A small number of patients may prove to have foci of borderline malignant change or focally invasive disease. A biopsy specimen should be obtained from any suspicious lesions.

▶ This article is a reminder that there are inherent limitations in frozen-section diagnosis. With regard to ovarian epithelial neoplasms, the gray zones between benign/borderline and borderline/malignant are most likely to give the pathologist difficulty. This is true to some degree because of sampling error. Rare and uncommon ovarian tumors are also more likely to be misdiagnosed by frozen section analysis. To avoid surgical errors based on an incomplete or mistaken intraoperative pathologic diagnosis, the surgeon can follow 3 general principles when operating on women of reproductive age: (1) perform cystectomy rather than ovariectomy (a must in the woman with only 1 ovary or with bilateral neoplasms); (2) if the neoplasms appear to be confined to the ovary (or ovaries—and at least 1 can be enucleated), do not perform a sterilizing procedure when the frozen-section diagnosis is malignancy; (3) always explore the abdomen completely (as if the tumor were malignant) and take peritoneal washings. Be sure to include a complete description of the operative findings in the dictated note.—C.P. Morrow, M.D.

Retroperitoneal Lymphatic Involvement With Epithelial Ovarian Tumors of Low Malignant Potential

Leake JF, Rader JS, Woodruff JD, Rosenshein NB (Johns Hopkins Hosp, Baltimore)

Gynecol Oncol 42:124–130, 1991 15–43

Introduction.—Retroperitoneal node involvement was evaluated in 171 patients in whom epithelial ovarian tumor of low malignant potential was diagnosed in 1979–1989. Of the patients, 34 underwent surgical staging including sampling of the retroperitoneal lymph nodes.

Tumor Characteristics.—The histology of the tumors was in 26 (76%) patients, mucinous in 7 (21%), and seromucinous in 1 (3%). Peritoneal implants were noninvasive in 11 of 13 patients. Half the patients had stage I disease, and 38% had stage III disease. Adjuvant treatment was given to 10 patients. The mean follow-up was 55 months.

Results.—Of 33 patients in whom the para-aortic nodes were sampled, 6 had positive findings. Of 12 patients, 2 had involved pelvic lymph nodes. Study of the retroperitoneal nodes led to upstaging in 6 of 27 patients with localized intraperitoneal disease. These patients were at a greater risk of relapsing than were those whose retroperitoneal nodes were negative for tumor. Nodal status did not, however, significantly influence survival in this series. The overall survival rate was 97%; no patient presently has evidence of disease.

Conclusion.—Retroperitoneal lymph node sampling at initial laparotomy may provide helpful prognostic information on patients with ovarian tumors of low malignant potential.

▶ Tumors of low malignant potential are important because they predominantly occur in women of reproductive age, are frequently diagnosed as carcinoma, and because even in the presence of metastases, the prognosis for the great majority of patients is excellent. In this study, 4 of 21 (19%) patients with disease apparently confined to the ovary (ovaries) had occult lymph node (aortic and/or pelvic) metastases. This frequency is higher than that reported for true ovarian carcinomas, but similar results for tumors of low malignant potential have been previously reported (1). Although adjuvant therapy may not be warranted in these cases because its efficacy remains in doubt, the information may be important, because patients with nodal metastases had a higher frequency or recurrence.—C.P. Morrow, M.D.

Reference

1. Yazigi R, et al: *Gynecol Oncol* 31:402, 1988.

Surgery Without Adjuvant Chemotherapy for Early Epithelial Ovarian Carcinoma After Comprehensive Surgical Staging

Monga M, Carmichael JA, Shelley WE, Kirk ME, Krepart GV, Jeffrey JF, Pater JL (Natl Cancer Inst of Canada, Queen's Univ, Kingston, Ont)

Gynecol Oncol 43:195–197, 1991 15–44

Introduction.—Because of the relatively few patients with early stage carcinoma of the ovary, it has been difficult to identify patients in whom the natural history is so good that adjunctive treatment is not warranted, and to determine what type of treatment would effect a good outcome in patients with unfavorable prognostic signs.

Methods.—In 1981–1987, 82 patients with cytology-negative stage IA–C ovarian carcinoma were enrolled in a study after surgical staging. The patients did not receive adjunctive treatment and were followed up for a mean of 4 years. None of the patients had extraovarian disease or a borderline malignancy.

Results.—Data on 39 patients with stage IA disease, 6 with IB disease, and 23 with stage IC tumors were reviewed. In 3 patients, there were recurrences, and 1 patient died. Only 1 patient with stage IA or IB disease had a recurrence. Neither adhesions nor rupture influenced the outcome.

Conclusion.—Carefully staged patients with stage I ovarian carcinoma and at least moderate differentiation can be monitored without adjunctive treatment. There should be no excrescences, and the results of cytologic study should be negative.

▶ This study asks whether surgical staging can safely be used to obviate the need for adjuvant therapy in early ovarian carcinoma. Patients with positive cytology, dense adhesions, and any evidence of extraperitoneal spread were excluded. Patients with intraoperative rupture, nondense adhesions, cytologically negative ascites, and grades 2 and 3 were included. Although surgical staging was required, this did not necessarily include retroperitoneal node sampling. Only 3 patients recurred, 2 of whom had clear cell carcinoma (2 of 16). Two (both clear cell) of the 3 recurrent cases were salvaged with chemotherapy.

The authors approach to management of early ovarian carcinoma is logical, with the exception that some of the categories of cases that are often considered high risk are too poorly represented in this study to conclude that it is safe to not treat. These include grade 3 cases (only 3) and cases with ascites (only 4). The clear cell cases probably should be routinely treated with adjuvant chemotherapy also (in this report 2 of 16).—C.P. Morrow, M.D.

Stage I Ovarian Epithelial Carcinoma: Survival Analysis Following Definitive Treatment

Lentz SS, Cha SS, Wieand HS, Podratz KC (Mayo Clinic and Found, Rochester, Minn)

Gynecol Oncol 43:198–202, 1991 15–45

Introduction.—More concerted cytoreduction efforts and the use of platinum-based cytotoxic regimens have resulted in most patients with ovarian epithelial carcinoma being free of clinically detectable disease within several months of diagnosis. Most are candidates for reassessment surgery. Survival analysis of patients with stage I disease shows variable 5-year survival rates (from 60% to 90%), indicating the need for caution in making significant treatment changes.

Methods.—Data on 55 patients treated for surgical stage I ovarian epithelial carcinoma in 1977–1986, in whom the lesion was optimally reduced and who had second-look laparotomy after selective adjuvant treatment, were reviewed to identify 1 or more subgroups at high risk for persistent or recurrent disease. Treatment was definitive, including surgical staging and adjuvant therapy in 51 (93%) patients and second-look laparotomy. The mean follow-up period from reassessment surgery was 94 months.

Results.—Treatment failures were found at second-look laparotomy in 6 (11%) patients and 5 (9%) other patients subsequently had recurrences after being declared disease free at second-look laparotomy. Pathologic analysis showed that grade and substage were important prognostic factors; 8 (89%) of the 9 deaths were associated with Broders grade 3 or 4 and/or stage IC. In the bivariate model consisting of patients with poorly differentiated stage IC lesions, 6 (43%) of 14 patients died of the disease, for a long-term survival rate that at best approximates the survival rate associated with optimally reduced stage III patients who are subjected to contemporary adjuvant treatment and second-look surgery.

Conclusion.—Intensive therapy, as used in advanced disease, is equally applicable to the high-risk stage I group identified in this study. Such therapy includes platinum-based chemotherapy, second-look laparotomy, and innovative salvage or investigational consolidation treatment.

▶ The data in this article reinforce previous data indicating that patients with poorly differentiated ovarian carcinoma or stage IC disease account for the majority of treatment failures in stage I. The frequency of recurrence was 38% for poorly differentiated tumors, accounting for two thirds of the deaths in the entire group (6 of 9). In this same group, 3 of 16 patients had a positive second-look laparotomy, whereas 5 of 38 stage IC patients had positive second-look laparotomy. Based on previously published data, we continue to recommend adjuvant therapy for patients with stage I ovarian carcinoma grade 2 or 3, or any grade (excluding borderline) with ascites, positive cytology, dense adhesions, or surface involvement. Because few of the patients in this report received platinum-based chemotherapy, the expected survival for patients with early stage, poorly differentiated ovarian cancer should be better than the 62% in this study.—C.P. Morrow, M.D.

Adjuvant Intraperitoneal Chromic Phosphate Therapy for Women With Apparent Early Ovarian Carcinoma Who Have Not Undergone Comprehensive Surgical Staging

Soper JT, Berchuck A, Clarke-Pearson DL (Duke Univ Med Ctr, Durham, NC)

Cancer 68:725–729, 1991 15–46

Introduction.—Approximately one third of women with epithelial ovarian carcinoma have disease that appears to be limited to the pelvis at the time of primary surgery. Surgery alone and combined surgery and pelvic radiotherapy have yielded survival rates of only 60% to 70% in patients with stage I disease, and rates of 40% to 50% in those with stage II disease.

Methods.—In 49 women with stage I or stage II ovarian cancer, chromic phosphate, 15 mci, was administered intraperitoneally as adjuvant treatment after primary surgery. Omentectomy was part of primary surgical treatment in 35 patients. Peritoneal washings or ascites were examined cytologically in 82% of patients.

Results.—Small bowel obstruction in 1 patient was the only significant toxicity. One fourth of the patients had recurrences after radiophosphorus therapy. Of 7 women with stage Ia grade 1 lesions, 1 had a recurrence. Survival adjusted for intercurrent deaths was 84% for patients with stage I and 86% for those with stage II disease. Disease-free survival was 79% for patients with stage I and 57% for those with stage II lesions.

Conclusion.—Radiophosphorus is not appropriate in women with apparent early stage epithelial ovarian cancer who have not been surgically staged. All such women should receive aggressive systemic treatment.

▶ The authors conclude from this study of patients with high-risk stage I and completely resected stage II disease that intraperitoneal ^{32}P is not adequate therapy for these patients when complete surgical staging has not been performed. Their conclusion is based on the relatively high frequency of recurrence (12 of 49) and the site of recurrence: of 12 patients with recurrence, 7 recurred extraperitoneally, predominantly in the lymph nodes. However, patients with early ovarian cancer who have been optimally staged and have been found to have negative nodes may not be good candidates for ^{32}P therapy, because they will surely have more extensive adhesions and, therefore, an increased risk of complications from intraperitoneal therapy.—C.P. Morrow, M.D.

Morbidity and Mortality Associated With Primary and Repeat Operations for Ovarian Cancer

Venesmaa P, Ylikorkala O (Helsinki Univ, Finland)

Obstet Gynecol 79:168–172, 1992 15–47

Introduction.—Even primary surgery for ovarian cancer carries substantial morbidity, and an increasing number of women are having repeat exploration. Recent operations include pelvic and para-aortic lymphadenectomy, which may increase the risk of complications.

Series.—The risk of complications was examined in 536 women who, in 1977–1990, had 472 primary and 299 repeat operations for ovarian cancer. Primary surgery was considered optimal, with no more than 2 cm

Characteristics of 472 Primary and 299 Repeat Operations in Relation to Operative Complications

	Primary	*P*	Repeat
Stage at presentation			
I–II	208		130
III IV	264		169
No. of operations	472		299
Age	58 ± 14		53 ± 16
Complications			
Blood loss >1000 mL	98 (21%)	<.001	9 (3%)
Fever	20 (4%)	<.01	3 (1%)
Urinary tract infection	86 (18%)	<.001	27 (9%)
Bowel complication	34 (7%)	NS	17 (6%)
Wound complication	14 (3%)	NS	3 (1%)
Thromboembolism	10 (2%)	<.05	1 (0.3%)
Mortality	5 (1%)	NS	0

Abbreviation: NS, not significant.
Note: Data are presented as no. (%) or mean ± 1 SD.
(Courtesy of Venesmaa P, Ylikorkala O: *Obstet Gynecol* 79:168–172, 1992.)

of residual tumor, in 63% of cases. A large majority of repeat procedures were done to determine the tumor status.

Results.—Blood loss exceeding 1L occurred in 21% of the primary operations and in 3% of the repeat operations (table). Urinary tract infection was twice as frequent after primary as after repeat surgery, but it was not related to the extent of disease. Bowel complications were more frequent when primary surgery was suboptimal or merely exploratory. There were 5 deaths after primary surgery and none after repeat surgery.

Conclusion.—Operations for ovarian cancer—especially repeat procedures—were generally well tolerated in this series, and they should not be avoided out of a fear of complications. Lymphadenectomy is justified if it enhances survival.

▶ The morbidity associated with primary and secondary surgery for ovarian carcinoma will naturally depend upon the extent of disease, the aggressiveness of the surgery, the surgeons' judgment and skill, etc.; therefore, the data in this paper have to be interpreted with caution, particularly with regard to the absolute numbers and percentages. However, the point of the paper is that second-look surgery for ovarian carcinoma is attended by substantially less morbidity than is initial surgery. In terms of the risk of surgery, this becomes an important consideration for the elderly, those with important medical problems, and those who will require tumor reductive surgery. Considering the low likelihood of benefit from tumor reductive surgery after platinum failure, extensive surgery (with its risks of complications) is seldom warranted anyway.—C.P. Morrow, M.D.

Long-Term Survival in Ovarian Cancer: Mature Data From The Netherlands Joint Study Group for Ovarian Cancer

Neijt JP, ten Bokkel Huinink WW, van der Burg MEL, van Oosterom AT, Willemse PHB, Vermorken JB, van Lindert ACM, Heintz APM, Aartsen E, van Lent M, Trimbos JB, de Meijer AJ (Utrecht Univ Hosp, Utrecht, The Netherlands; Netherlands Cancer Inst, Amsterdam; Daniël den Hoed Kliniek, Rotterdam; Univ Hosp, Antwerp, Belgium; Groningen Univ Hosp, Groningen, The Netherlands; et al)

Eur J Cancer 27:1367–1372, 1991 15–48

Background.—There have been few reports on long-term survival in patients with advanced ovarian cancer. The experience with 2 studies of advanced epithelial ovarian cancer was updated.

Methods.—The 2 studies, begun in 1979 and 1981, included 377 patients. The subjects in the first study were randomized to receive hexamethylmelamine, cyclophosphamide, methotrexate, and 5-fluorouracil (Hexa-CAF), or cyclophosphamide, hexamethylmelamine, doxorubicin, and cisplatin for 5 days (CHAP-5). In the second study, the patients received either CHAP-5 or cyclophosphamide and cisplatin on 1 day (CP).

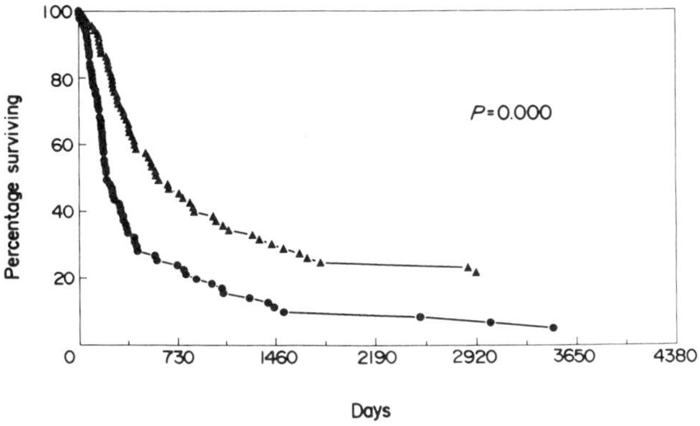

Fig 15–5.—Progression-free survival after treatment with Hexa-CAF or CHAP-5. *Solid triangle* indicates CHAP-5 (92 entered; 62 progressed); *filled circle* indicates Hexa-CAF (93 entered; 77 progressed). (Courtesy of Neijt JP, ten Bokkel Huinink WW, van der Burg MEL, et al: *Eur J Cancer* 27:1367–1372, 1991.)

In the first study, patients who failed to respond to Hexa-CAF were given a cisplatin-containing regimen. Patients in the first study were followed up for a median of 9.5 years, and those in the second study were followed for a median of 7.7 years.

Results.—The 10-year survival rates were 9% for patients initially treated with Hexa-CAF and 21% for those treated with CHAP-5 (Fig 15–5). The 8-year survival rates were 21% for patients with CHAP-5 and 23% for CP. Fifty percent of the Hexa-CAF group who were still alive at 10 years had had progressive disease successfully treated with cisplatin. In both studies, of the patients who achieved complete pathologic remission, approximately 60% were alive at 5 years and 40% at 10 years. Of those patients who had microscopic disease at second-look surgery, 35% survived for 5 years. At 5 years, nearly half the patients with grade I tumors were still alive, and at 10 years, 30% were alive; for other grades, these survivals were halved.

Conclusion.—Cisplatin-containing chemotherapy regimens can increase the 5- and 10-year survival rates in patients with advanced ovarian cancer by more than 10%. Cyclophosphamide/cisplatin appears to be the best regimen for the treatment of these cancers.

▶ The good news from this report is that progress is being made in the treatment of advanced ovarian carcinoma. The addition of platinum has boosted the long-term survival by 10 percentage points. The bad news is, of course, that the progress is slow and occurs in small increments. Perhaps taxol will add another 10% to the cure rate.—C.P. Morrow, M.D.

Taxol: An Important New Drug in the Management of Epithelial Ovarian Cancer

Markman M (Mem Sloan-Kettering Cancer Ctr, New York; Cornell Univ, New York)

Yale J Biol Med 64:583–590, 1991 15–49

Introduction.—In several trials, taxol, a product obtained from the bark of the Pacific yew, has exhibited substantial activity in patients with cisplatin-resistant ovarian cancer. The agent has produced unique side effects that may relate to stabilization of microtubules.

Clinical Trials.—Taxol has been administered by infusion in nearly a dozen phase 1 clinical trials. Antineoplastic activity has been found in melanoma, leukemia, non–small-cell lung cancers, and tumors of the stomach, colon, breast, and head/neck region, as well as in ovarian cancer. Hypersensitivity reactions were frequent in early trials when the drug was infused rapidly. Neutropenia is a dose-limiting toxic effect. Sensory neuropathy and asymptomatic bradycardia also have occurred. Intraperitoneal taxol therapy appears to be a possibility.

Resistant Ovarian Cancer.—Antineoplastic activity has been observed in several heavily pretreated patients with ovarian cancer. Even tumors that are resistant to cisplatin-based therapy have responded to intravenously administered taxol. A trial of combined taxol and cisplatin therapy has begun.

▶ This drug has received a lot of notice in the press, partly because of its activity against ovarian cancer (a disease that has caught the attention of the press), partly because the drug is in limited supply, and partly because obtaining it from the Pacific yew tree is an environmental issue. Unfortunately, the publicity given to the drug in popular magazines has raised the expectations of recovery beyond reason among thousands of women in this country who have recurrent ovarian carcinoma. It is, in fact, a very exciting discovery, because it appears not to have cross-resistance to platinum in ovarian carcinoma. Some women with ovarian cancer resistant to platinum have had a dramatic and sustained remission with taxol, but relapse is the rule. The drug is not curing any of these patients. The results of taxol as a first-line agent in combination with platinum are not yet available. If taxol is to be a savior of patients with ovarian cancer, it will have to be in the previously untreated group. Watch the headlines.—C.P. Morrow, M.D.

Simultaneous Carcinoma Involving the Endometrium and the Ovary: A Clinicopathologic, Immunohistochemical, and DNA Flow Cytometric Study of 18 Cases

Prat J, Matias-Guiu X, Barreto J (Autonomous Univ of Barcelona)

Cancer 68:2455–2459, 1991 15–50

Objective.—The findings were reviewed for 18 women who had carcinomas involving both the endometrium and ovary. Nuclear DNA content was estimated by flow cytometric study in 13 cases.

Findings.—Nine cases were classified as separate primary tumors, and the other 9 were classified as a uterine primary with ovarian metastasis or an ovarian primary with uterine metastasis. In 7 of the 9 cases of independent primary tumors, there were different immunohistochemical profiles in the ovarian and uterine lesions. In contrast, similar staining features were present in only 4 of the 9 metastatic cases. Aneuploid stemlines in the endometrial and ovarian tumors differed in 5 cases of independent primaries and in 1 case of metastasis.

Conclusion.—Immunohistochemical methods and DNA flow cytometry may be of some help in distinguishing between independent and metastatic tumors of the endometrium and ovary; however, the distinction still rests largely on traditional clinicopathologic criteria.

▶ Simultaneous ovarian and endometrial tumors are relatively common, and they sometimes present a dilemma to the pathologist and clinician. When the endometrial tumor is well differentiated and noninvasive, or only superficially invasive, the 2 lesions are independent primaries, even though the histology may be identical (and often is). When the uterine tumor is extensive and the ovarian lesions have the typical appearance of a metastatic tumor, the situation is clear. When the 2 tumors are histologically dissimilar (e.g., mucinous ovarian tumor) the situation also is clear. Occasionally, however, the endometrial and ovarian tumors are of the same histology (endometrioid) and are well-developed cancers. These usually are independent primaries. This is no idle exercise, because the prognosis for stage III uterine carcinoma is undoubtedly worse than the prognoses for simultaneous stage I ovarian and stage I uterine cancer. Both DNA ploidy and hormone receptor analysis can assist in differentiating those various situations.—C.P. Morrow, M.D.

Gestational Trophoblastic Disease

Risk Factors for Epithelial Ovarian Tumours of Borderline Malignancy

Parazzini F, Restelli C, La Vecchia C, Negri F, Chiari S, Maggi R, Mangioni C (Istituto di Ricerche Farmacologiche "Mario Negri," Milan, Italy; Univ of Lausanne, Switzerland)

Int J Epidemiol 20:871–877, 1991 15–51

Background.—Borderline ovarian tumors account for 10% to 15% of malignant ovarian tumors in the epithelial category. A case-control study was conducted in the greater Milan area of Northern Italy to obtain further data on the epidemiology of borderline ovarian tumors.

Methods and Results.—Ninety-one women with histologically confirmed borderline ovarian tumors were compared with 273 control subjects hospitalized for acute nongynecological, hormonal, or neoplastic disease. Women with 3 or more births had a relative risk (RR) of .6 compared with nulliparas; however, this finding was nonsignificant statistically. The risk of borderline tumors increased (also nonsignificantly) with older age at first birth. Compared with women who first gave birth at 24 years of age or younger, women having their first children between the ages of 25 and 29 years and at 30 years or older had RRs of 1.3 and 1.7, respectively. There was no significant relationship between borderline ovarian cancer and age at menarche, menopausal status, or lifelong menstrual patterns. Women with borderline ovarian tumors tended to have a later age at menopause than those without such tumors, but this trend was nonsignificant. Ten percent of the cases and 25% of the controls reported using oral contraceptives. Compared with those who had never used oral contraceptives, the multivariate RR for those who had ever used oral contraceptives was .3. The risk decreased with duration of use to .2 in users for 2 years or more.

Conclusion.—This study provides evidence of similarities between borderline and invasive ovarian tumor epidemiology. It found a substantial protection by oral contraception on the 2 histological subtypes, a possible protective effect of high parity and of early age at first birth, and an increased risk in women with late age at menopause, although it found no substantial relationship with age at menarche. These findings may be interpreted within the framework of the "incessant ovulation" hypothesis in ovarian carcinogenesis, in which ovulation or "ovulatory cycles" are the relevant exposure that defines the incidence of the neoplastic lesions, thereby suggesting an epidemiological continuum between various grades of malignancy of epithelial ovarian neoplasms.

▶ It is of interest to know that ovarian tumors of low malignant potential (LMP) are epidemiologically similar to their frankly malignant counterparts (i.e., pregnancy and use of oral contraceptives protect, whereas nulliparity and late age at first birth increase the risk). Unfortunately, the authors did not investigate the familiality of these LMP tumors. Others have reported that there is no aggregation of ovarian LMP tumors in families (1).—C.P. Morrow, M.D.

Reference

1. Schildkraut JM, Thompson WD: *Am J Epidemiol* 128:456, 1988.

A Flow Cytometric Study of 137 Fresh Hydropic Placentas: Correlation Between Types of Hydatidiform Moles and Nuclear DNA Ploidy

Lage JM, Mark SD, Roberts DJ, Goldstein DP, Bernstein MR, Berkowitz RS
(Brigham and Women's Hosp; Harvard School of Public Health, Boston)

Obstet Gynecol 79:403–410, 1992 15–52

Background.—Placental hydrops is a spectrum of pathologic conditions that includes hydropic abortus, partial hydatidiform mole, and complete hydatidiform mole. There are clinically significant prognostic differences between hydropic entities, and past studies have identified pathologic and cytogenetic differences among them.

Study Plan.—A total of 142 hydropic placentas were studied. Thirty-nine percent of them were complete moles; 35% were partial moles; and 26% were hydropic abortuses. The DNA ploidy was estimated by flow cytometric analysis in 137 cases.

Findings.—Nearly three fourths of the hydropic abortuses were diploid, and 11% were triploid. Ninety percent of partial moles were triploid or nearly so. A total of 43% of the complete moles were tetraploid, 4% were polyploid, and 2% were triploid. Tumor persisted in one third of the cases of complete mole and in 12% of partial moles. Tetraploid moles were associated with higher initial β-human chorionic gonadotropin levels than diploid moles, but not with a greater risk of persistent tumor. A majority of patients with persistent tumor achieved remission with single-agent chemotherapy.

Discussion.—Greater heterogeneity of DNA content was found in molar gestations in this study than has been previously reported. Nuclear DNA ploidy was not an independent predictor of persistent complete mole.

► Nuclear ploidy has been measured in numerous benign, premalignant, and malignant conditions, with the expectation that clinical behavior could be more accurately predicted by this means than by currently available methods of histopathologic analysis. Unfortunately, the results have been disappointing in all but a few instances, e.g., breast cancer. Thus, where the technique could be of greatest value to the clinician, it has most often proved to be of marginal or no value. To cite a few examples: dysgerminoma, granulosa cell tumor, ovarian tumors of low malignant potential, and well-differentiated endometrial carcinoma. In this study of pathologic placentas, flow cytometry comes up short again. The method was unable to predict which molar gestations would behave in a malignant fashion or to distinguish the hydropic abortus, which presumably has no increased risk for gestational trophoblastic disease (GTN), from the partial or classic moles, which have a very significant risk of subsequent GTN.—C.P. Morrow, M.D.

Results With the EMA/CO (Etoposide, Methotrexate, Actinomycin D, Cyclophosphamide, Vincristine) Regimen in High Risk Gestational Trophoblastic Tumors, 1979 to 1989

Newlands ES, Bagshawe KD, Begent RHJ, Rustin GJS, Holden L (Charing Cross Hosp, London)

Br J Obstet Gynaecol 98:550–557, 1991 15–53

Introduction.—The efficacy and safety of EMA/CO chemotherapy were examined in an open study of 148 consecutive patients referred in a 10-year period with high-risk gestational trophoblastic tumor, 76 of whom had not previously received chemotherapy.

Patients.—Of the patients, 27 were treated after a nonmolar miscarriage, 53 after term delivery, and 68 after a hydatidiform mole. Risk status was based on age (younger or older than 39 years), the chorionic gonadotropin level, the size of the largest tumor mass, and the number and site of metastases.

Results.—The remission rate was 82% for previously untreated patients and 89% for those previously given chemotherapy. The overall survival rate was 85%. Within 3 weeks of starting chemotherapy, 10 previously untreated patients died of extensive disease. Adding cisplatin salvaged 9 of 11 patients who became drug resistant. Complete remission was achieved with salvage surgery alone in 7 of 8 patients. Of 8 patients who relapsed after EMA/CO therapy, 6 achieved a sustained remission after further chemotherapy and/or surgery. Complications were acceptable, although acute myeloid leukemia developed in 1 patient. Menses usually returned within a few months of treatment. No fetal anomalies occurred.

Conclusion.—Presently, EMA/CO therapy is the preferred treatment for patients with high-risk gestational trophoblastic tumor. Salvage surgery is helpful for those who become drug resistant.

▶ This is good news, indeed, that 82% of World Health Organization–designated high-risk gestational trophoblastic tumors can be cured with EMA/CO chemotherapy, a combination regimen developed by the authors at Charing Cross. Similar results were obtained in treating patients who had received prior chemotherapy. Half the patients dying of gestational trophoblastic tumors died of very extensive disease within 3 weeks of initiating chemotherapy. Death usually resulted from pulmonary insufficiency or brain metastases. It is of interest that 9 of 11 patients in whom resistance to EMA/CO developed were salvaged by the addition of *cis*-platinum. Thus, it appears that the optimization of EMA/CO chemotherapy for gestational trophoblastic tumors will require the addition of *cis*-platinum.—C.P. Morrow, M.D.

Vulva/Vagina

Laser Vaporization of Grade 3 Vaginal Intraepithelial Neoplasia

Hoffman MS, Roberts WS, LaPolla JP, Fiorica JV, Cavanagh D (Univ of South Florida at Moffitt Cancer Ctr and Research Inst, Tampa)

Am J Obstet Gynecol 165:1342–1344, 1991 15–54

Introduction.—A variety of treatments have been used for vaginal intraepithelial neoplasia. The results of laser vaporization performed for grade 3 disease in 26 patients in 1984–1990 were reviewed. Hysterectomy was previously performed in 20 patients, in 10 because of cervical neoplasia. Vaginal neoplasia had been treated previously in 10 patients.

Methods.—A carbon dioxide laser was introduced under colposcopic guidance, and the lesions were vaporized to a depth of 1–2 mm, including at least a 1-cm margin of normal-appearing mucosa. The procedure was performed on an outpatient basis unless other measures were necessary.

Results.—In 11 (42%) patients, vaginal neoplasia recurred after a mean of 22 weeks; 3 of them had invasive cancer at the time of recurrence. Invasion was seen on a biopsy specimen at the time of laser treatment in 1 patient who subsequently underwent radiotherapy. In 14 patients, there was no evidence of disease after a mean follow-up of 117 weeks.

Conclusion.—Laser vaporization alone is not adequate treatment for grade 3 vaginal intraepithelial neoplasia in the region of the vaginal cuff scar. However, it could be combined with excision of the cuff scar region.

Upper Vaginectomy for In Situ and Occult, Superficially Invasive Carcinoma of the Vagina

Hoffman MS, DeCesare SL, Roberts WS, Fiorica JV, Finan MA, Cavanagh D
(Univ of South Florida, Tampa)

Am J Obstet Gynecol 166:30–33, 1992 15–55

Introduction.—Vaginal intraepithelial neoplasia usually is diagnosed during the workup of an abnormal Papanicolaou smear. A wide range of treatments has been used, including local excision, partial or total vaginectomy, radiation therapy, laser vaporization, and topical administration of 5-fluorouracil.

Patients.—Upper vaginectomy was performed in 32 patients with grade 3 vaginal intraepithelial neoplasia. All but 1 had undergone a prior hysterectomy, 25 for cervical neoplasia. Fourteen patients had previously been treated for vaginal intraepithelial neoplasia.

Results.—Nine patients (28%) were found to have invasive cancer. Four of the other 23 patients (17%) had recurrent vaginal neoplasia after a mean interval of 78 weeks; 1 had superficial invasion at the time of recurrence. Nineteen patients were free of disease for a mean of 152 weeks. One patient with invasive disease died. There were few serious operative complications.

Conclusion.—Upper vaginectomy is the preferred treatment for grade 3 vaginal intraepithelial neoplasia involving the vaginal apex near a vaginal cuff scar. Whether this procedure is also indicated for superficially invasive vaginal cancer remains to be established.

▶ The message in these papers is important: laser vaporization of squamous dysplasia in the region of the vaginal cuff scar is risky, both in terms of treatment failure and in terms of missing the diagnosis of associated, clinically inconspicuous, invasive carcinoma. Vaginal intraepithelial neoplasms (VAIN) have a proclivity for the vaginal apex—particularly the "dog ears" created at the vaginal angles by hysterectomy. Surgical excision is the preferred treatment to minimize treatment failure and to assure that invasive carcinoma will not be overlooked. As the authors suggest, laser vaporization of the more distal portion of an extensive lesion can be combined with surgical excision, thereby minimizing the trauma and vaginal shortening. However, particularly in postmenopausal women, the colposcopic interpretation of VAIN can be difficult (as these papers attest). Optimal estrogen stimulation of the vaginal mucosa (e.g., vaginal extrogen cream applied nightly for 2–4 weeks) with Lugol's staining is the best way to delineate the extent of VAIN, and it should be considered essential to adequate evaluation.—C.P. Morrow, M.D.

Identification of Risk Factors for Diethylstilbestrol-Associated Clear Cell Adenocarcinoma of the Vagina: Similarities to Endometrial Cancer

Sharp GB, Cole P (Univ of Tennessee, Memphis; Univ of Alabama, Birmingham)

Am J Epidemiol 134:1316–1324, 1991 15–56

Background.—The daughters of women who took diethylstilbestrol (DES) during pregnancy have a significantly increased risk of clear cell adenocarcinoma of the vagina and cervix developing. Whether some of the major risk factors for endometrial cancer are also risk factors for vaginal clear cell adenocarcinoma was determined in DES-positive women.

Methods.—This epidemiological case-control study included 106 women with clear cell adenocarcinoma of the vagina and 447 women without cancer. Both case and control subjects had been exposed to DES in utero.

Number of DES*-Positive Cases and Controls, According to Dichotomized Adolescent Body Mass Indexes and Heights, United States 1971–1983

Characteristic	Cases	Controls	Crude relative risk	95% confidence interval	Adjusted relative risk‡	95% confidence interval
Shorter/thinner§	3	101	1.0		1.0	
Taller/thinner	17	105	5.4	1.74–17.09	3.5	0.90–13.72
Shorter/more obese	17	103	5.6	1.78–17.39	2.9	0.76–11.19
Taller/more obese	31	112	9.3	3.31–26.25	7.4	2.13–25.54

* *DES,* diethylstilbestrol.

Body mass indexes were 13.7–19.2 kg/m² for "thinner" subjects and 19.3–33.30 kg/m² for "more obese" subjects. The heights of "shorter" subjects were 134–161 cm, and the heights of "taller" subjects were 162–180 cm. Analysis was restricted to 74 cases diagnosed at age 16 years or later and interviewed within 10 years of diagnosis.

‡ Adjusted for year of birth, socioeconomic status (maternal education: < 12, 12, or ≥ 13 years), and week of initial maternal DES exposure (1 through 12 or ≥ 13).

§ Reference category.

(Courtesy of Sharp GB, Cole P: *Am J Epidemiol* 134:1316–1324, 1991.)

Findings.—Controlling for age, socioeconomic status, and time during gestation of initial DES exposure, a significantly increased risk of this cancer was found in women who were taller or heavier than their peers at 14 and 15 years of age. The relative risk of clear cell adenocarcinoma of the vagina for women in the highest tertile for height (compared with those in the lowest tertile) was 2.5. A similar comparison of body mass revealed a relative risk of 2.8. Trend tests showed that both factors had significant dose-response relationships with risk of this cancer. The DES-positive patients who were interviewed more than 10 years after diagnosis were also significantly thinner than those cases interviewed less than 7 years after diagnosis, thereby suggesting that adolescent adiposity level is associated with survival for women with this cancer (table).

Conclusion.—Increased adiposity and height in adolescence seem to be strong, independent, but not interactive, risk factors for the development of vaginal clear cell carcinoma in women exposed to DES in utero. Moderately obese and tall women appear to be at greater risk than thinner, shorter women. Height and body mass are also risk factors for endometrial cancer.

▶ The results of this study are interesting, not only because they identify a subpopulation of DES-exposed females who are at an increased risk for cervical/vaginal clear cell carcinoma, but also because the factors associated with the increased risk (increased height and weight) are also risk factors for endometrial carcinoma. These factors are associated with higher plasma levels of estradiol. It is also notable that patients with non–DES-associated cervical adenocarcinoma are epidemiologically similar to patients with endometrial cancer.—C.P. Morrow, M.D.

Dysplastic Vulvar Nevi

Blickstein I, Feldberg E, Dgani R, Ben-Hur H, Czernobilsky B (Kaplan Hosp, Rehovot, Israel)

Obstet Gynecol 78:968–970, 1991 15–57

Introduction.—As many as 3% of all melanomas involve the female genitalia, a high frequency considering the limited size of this area and the rarity of solar exposure. In only 2 patients has a dysplastic nevus been reported at this site.

Methods.—Eighteen pigmented vulvar lesions were excised in about 500 parturients seen in 1985–1990. Of the lesions, 3 proved to be dysplastic nevi. All of the women, aged 21–30 years, had multiple nevi on the torso and extremities; 2 had features of dysplastic nevus syndrome. Only 1 of the 3 women was aware of the vulvar lesion, although all the nevi were brown or black and greater than 5 mm in diameter. None of the women had evidence of malignant melanoma.

Results.—The compound nevi exhibited active junctional nests in the dermoepidermal region, with some atypical nuclei and pleomorphism. Some nests were surrounded by delicate fibrous tissue.

Conclusion.—Vulvar dysplastic nevi may be more common than was previously thought. All pigmented genital lesions more than 5 mm in diameter or those with irregular borders or variegated pigmentation deserve definitive histological diagnosis.

▶ The question of which pigmented vulvar lesions should be excised has never been answered satisfactorily, but this study puts the focus on dysplastic, rather than juctional, nevi. The dysplastic nevus clearly carries a significant risk for malignant transformation; it is relatively easy to identify and should be removed prophylactically. In addition, the common nevus and any pigmented lesion that darkens, grows, or becomes symptomatic should be removed. Although it sometimes is recommended that all pigmented lesions of the vulva be excised routinely, this surely is excessive. The majority of pigmented vulvar lesions are either lentigenes or garden variety nevi.—C.P. Morrow, M.D.

Carcinoma of the Vulva: Epidemiology and Pathogenesis
Crum CP (Brigham and Women's Hosp, Boston)
Obstet Gynecol 79:448–454, 1992 15–58

Background.—Vulvar squamous carcinoma, an uncommon neoplasm, afflicts a spectrum of women. It has been associated with granulomatous vulvar diseases, human papillomaviruses (HPVs), and chronic inflammatory disorders of the vulva. The epidemiological, histopathologic, and viral data supporting the division of invasive vulvar carcinomas into distinct subsets were reviewed.

Discussion.—Existing data suggest the hypothesis that vulvar carcinoma comprises at least 2 distinct subsets. One appears to be related to sexual factors (HPV). In the other, the pathogenesis remains largely undefined (table). Associations have been established between vulvar carcinoma, syphilis, and chronic granulomatous diseases; however, syphilis and other granulomatous diseases may simply be markers for sexual activity unique to the women in studies establishing the association. The cloning of numerous HPV DNA types from genital lesions in the past 15 years has provided much information linking HPV to a spectrum of genital lesions, including genital warts, vulvar intraepithelial neoplasia, and invasive cancers. Papillomaviruses provide the strongest direct connection between vulvar cancer and sexually transmitted disease. The absence of HPV DNA in most vulvar cancers found in older women suggests that the potential epidemiological heterogeneity of vulvar carcinomas needs to be reassessed. Few studies have addressed the possibility that there is a distinct subset of vulvar carcinomas in older women that is unrelated to sexual factors.

A Proposed Model for Vulvar Carcinoma

	Group I	Group II
Age	Relatively younger (35–65)	Older (55–85)
Previous condyloma	Common	Uncommon
Previous STD	Common	Uncommon
Preexisting lesion	VIN (carcinoma in situ)	Vulvar inflammation Lichen sclerosus Hyperplasia
Co-factors in development	Age Immune status Viral integration	Vulvar "atypia" Mutated host genes?
Histopathology of tumor	Intraepithelial-like (basaloid) or poorly differentiated	Keratinizing Well differentiated
Cervical neoplasia	High association	Low association
Smoking*	High incidence	Low incidence
HPV nucleic acids	Frequent (>60%)	Seldom (<15%)

Abbreviations: STD, sexually transmitted disease; *VIN,* vulvar intraepithelial neoplasia; *HPV,* human papillomavirus.

* This variable is included because of its association with vulvar intraepithelial neoplasia and carcinomas that coexist with the disease. Its significance is not clear, and causation is not established.

(Courtesy of Crum CP: *Obstet Gynecol* 79:448–454, 1992.)

Conclusion.—Evidence suggests that a substantial proportion of vulvar carcinomas afflicting American women may not be related to a venereally transmitted agent. Studies that integrate the various disciplines are needed to place HPV in proper perspective. Strategies need to be developed to identify those women who are at risk for vulvar carcinomas unrelated to this virus.

▶ Although this article may not have much clinical value, the authors present an interesting clinical observation: HPV probably is not the etiological agent for all vulvar squamous carcinomas. The accompanying table presents the distinguishing characteristics of HPV-associated and non–HPV-associated vulvar carcinoma. The latter occurs in older women on a background of lichen sclerosus. It would be a disservice to these women to invoke the sexually transmitted disease theory in discussing vulvar carcinoma with these patients.—C.P. Morrow, M.D.

Minimally Invasive Vulvar Carcinoma: An Indication for Conservative Surgical Therapy

Kelley JL III, Burke TW, Tornos C, Morris M, Gershenson DM, Silva EG, Wharton JT (Univ of Texas, MD Anderson Cancer Ctr)

Gynecol Oncol 44:240–244, 1992 15–59

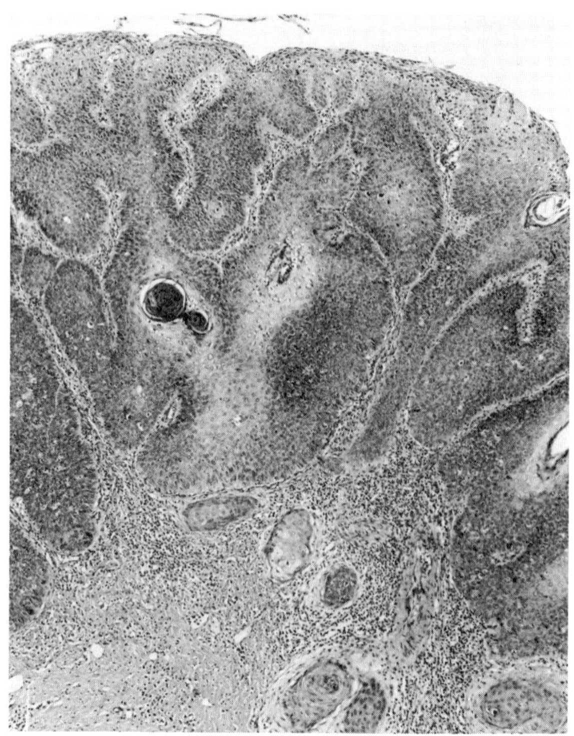

Fig 15–6.—Squamous carcinoma in situ with small detached nests of invasive carcinoma (maximum depth of invasion, less than 1 mm).

(Courtesy of Kelley JL III, Burke TW, Tornos C, et al: *Gynecol Oncol* 44:240–244, 1992.)

Introduction.—It may be possible to treat squamous carcinoma of the vulva with 1 mm or less of stromal invasion with local resection without inguinal node dissection. An optimal patient group with minimally invasive tumors was studied to determine whether groin dissection could safely be deleted.

Methods.—A retrospective review of data on 255 patients with stage I and II vulvar carcinoma identified 24 patients with minimally invasive carcinoma. In all 24 patients, charts were reviewed in detail, and the diagnoses were confirmed pathologically. The preoperative diagnosis was preinvasive disease in 7 patients, stage I disease in 10, stage II disease in 7, and associated vulvar carcinoma in situ in 15. Local excision was performed in 2 patients, radical wide excision in 11, hemivulvectomy in 5, radical vulvectomy in 6, and unilateral or bilateral inguinal node dissection in 11.

Results.—Life-table survival at 5 years was 89%. Dysplasia recurred in 4 (17%) patients, and 4 (17) had invasive recurrence; 1 invasive recurrence was in an inguinal node in a patient who had been treated by hemivulvectomy and negative ipsilateral superficial node dissection. According to univariate analysis, there were no significant associations between recurrence and age, symptom duration, margin status, location, International Federation of Gynecology and Obstetrics (FIGO) stage, or co-existing vulvar intraepithelial neoplasia (Fig 15–6).

Conclusion.—Large areas of co-existing dysplasia and variable gross appearances make it difficult to apply FIGO staging criteria to lesions with minimal focal invasion. Wide or radical wide excision of lesions with "high-risk" carcinoma in situ or those with 1 mm or less of stromal invasion on biopsy specimens is adequate treatment. If final pathologic review shows deeper invasion, a selective lymph node dissection can be performed. These patients should be closely monitored with colposcopy and biopsy.

▶ In this retrospective study of 24 patients with vulvar carcinoma and no greater than 1 mm of invasion, 4 patients had "recurrent carcinoma" 2–7 years post-treatment. Only 1 of these is clearly recurrent as distinguished from a new lesion. This patient had an ipsilateral groin dissection done as part of the initial procedure. The authors are correct in recommending surgical therapy for the primary lesion (without treatment to the groin nodes) for women with squamous carcinoma limited to 1 mm of invasion. It is important that the specimen be thoroughly examined microscopically to be sure there is no lymphovascular space invasion and that there is no area of deeper invasion. Attentive follow-up is important, because vulvar carcinoma tends to be multifocal and asynchronous. Although it may be true that more radical therapy will produce slightly fewer "recurrences," the morbidity is unacceptable. The superficial node dissection has been discredited by Gynecologic Oncology Group clinical studies (1). When vulvar carcinoma is more invasive than 1 mm or when there is left ventricular systolic index, both the superficial and the deep groin nodes should be dissected.—C.P. Morrow, M.D.

Reference

1. Gynecologic Oncology Group: *Obstet Gynecol* 79:490, 1992.

16 Infections

Diverging Gonorrhea and Syphilis Trends in the 1980s: Are They Real?

Gershman KA, Rolfs RT (Ctrs for Disease Control, Atlanta)

Am J Public Health 81:1263–1267, 1991 16–1

Background.—Reported cases of both gonorrhea and syphilis decreased in the early 1980s; however, since 1986, incidence of syphilis has increased whereas the incidence of gonorrhea continues to decrease. The recent spread of syphilis has been associated with drug use. It is not clear whether the diverging national trends mask a contemporaneous increase in both diseases.

Study.—In addition to reviewing reports of gonorrhea and primary and secondary syphilis in the United States for the period from 1981 to 1989, gonorrhea screening results from 6 states for 1985–1989 were examined. In addition, reports of both diseases by census tract in Rochester, New York during 1986 to 1989 were reviewed.

Findings.—Both gonorrhea and syphilis decreased in incidence in the United States from 1981 to 1985. Subsequently, gonorrhea decreased by

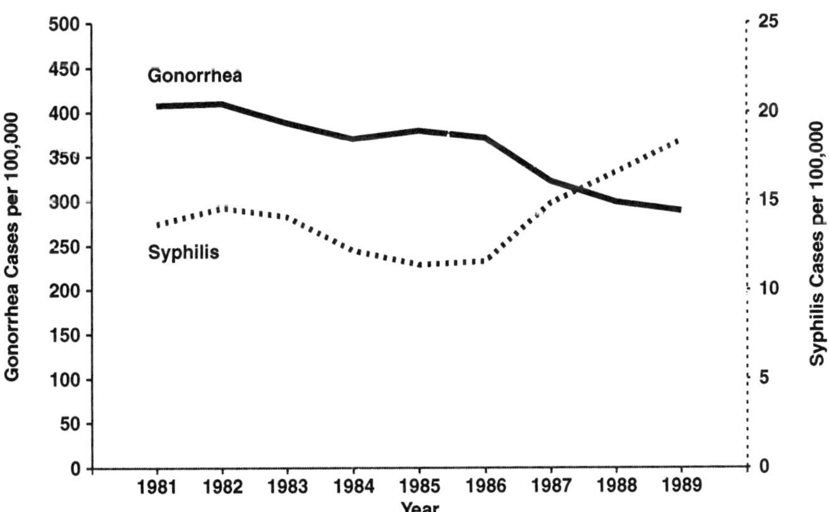

Fig 16–1.—Trends in incidence of gonorrhea and primary and secondary syphilis, United States, 1981 to 1989. (Courtesy of Gershman KA, Rolfs RT: *Am J Public Health* 81:1263-1267, 1991.)

22%, whereas the incidence of syphilis increased by 59% (Fig 16–1). In whites, gonorrhea decreased by 48% in 1986–1989, and syphilis decreased by 11%. Gonorrhea decreased by 50% in Hispanics and, at the same time, syphilis decreased by 27%. In blacks, however, gonorrhea decreased by only 13%, whereas the incidence of syphilis increased by 100%. The incidence of gonorrhea decreased or was stable in 45 states, whereas syphilis rates increased in 22 states; in 18 of these 22 states, gonorrhea decreased or remained unchanged. Trends were quite similar in 6 states where syphilis increased when the years 1986 and 1989 were compared for gonorrhea screening results in women.

Conclusion.—There appears to be a true decrease in the incidence of gonorrhea. Blacks exhibit a simultaneous increase in the incidence of syphilis for reasons that remain unclear.

▶ Even though the number of cases of syphilis in the United States is increasing while gonorrhea is decreasing, gonorrhea is much more prevalent, as is shown in Figure 16–1. The incidence of syphilis in 1989 in the United States was approximately 1 in 5,000 people, whereas that for gonorrhea was 1 in 300. The initial infection of syphilis, like that of HIV infection, is relatively indolent; therefore, many people with either of these 2 infections usually do not seek medical treatment by clinicians. Therefore, it is important to screen for these diseases by the appropriate diagnostic studies in anyone infected or exposed to other sexually transmitted diseases.—D.R. Mishell, Jr., M.D.

Use of Nonoxynol-9 and Reduction in Rate of Gonococcal and Chlamydial Cervical Infections

Niruthisard S, Roddy RE, Chutivongse S (Queen Saovbha Mem Inst, Bangkok; Thai Red Cross Society, Bangkok; Chulalongkorn Univ, Bangkok, Thailand; Family Health Intl, Research Triangle Park, NC)

Lancet 339:1371–1375, 1992 16–2

Objective.—In a single-blind randomized field trial, the efficacy of the spermicide nonoxynol-9 (N-9) for the prevention of cervical infections with *Chlamydia trachomatis* and/or *Neisseria gonorrhoeae* was studied in women at high risk for these diseases.

Treatment.—A total of 343 women recruited from massage parlors in Bangkok, Thailand, who had intercourse with multiple partners each day and who were without evidence of sexually transmitted infection, were studied. In a random fashion, 186 women used condoms and N-9 and 157 used condoms and a placebo (vaginal lubricant insert) every time vaginal intercourse took place. Compliance with condom use was similar in both groups.

Outcome.—Overall, N-9 reduced the rate of cervical infection by 25%, the reduction being largest (40%) in women using N-9 for more

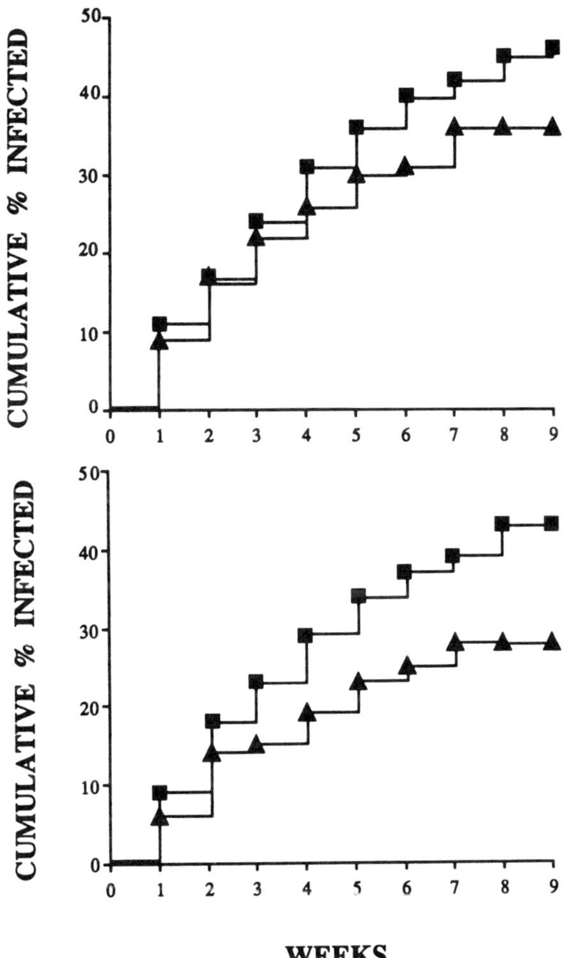

Fig 16–2.—Life table curves for overall use (**upper**) and 75% compliance (**lower**) showing the cumulative percentages of women with gonococcal and chlamydial cervical infection, N-9 users vs. placebo users. *Filled squares*, placebo, *filled triangles*, N-9. Log-rank test, *P* = .07 (**upper**), *P* = .04 (**lower**). (Courtesy of Niruthisard S, Roddy RE, Chutivongse S: *Lancet* 339:1371–1375, 1992.)

than 75% of their coital acts. The 9-week cumulative event rates of infection were 36 per 100 for women using N-9 and 46 per woman for women using placebo, and 28 per 100 and 42 per 100, respectively, in women with 75% compliance; these differences were significant (Fig 16–2). There was a greater than 90% probability that N-9 use provided a protective effect against cervical infection; however, the protection offered by condoms was greater than that for N-9. The rate of yeast vulvovaginitis or genital ulcers did not differ significantly in both groups, but women using N-9 reported more symptomatic irritation than placebo users.

Conclusion.—The use of vaginal N-9 spermicide reduces the rate of cervical infection among high-risk women, particularly among those with greatest compliance. Its use with condoms appears to be a better strategy than condoms alone only for protection against gonococcal and chlamydial cervical infection.

▶ This study shows that, even with frequent (but not constant) use of condoms during sexual intercourse with multiple partners, an N-9 containing spermicide further reduces the rate of cervical infection with chlamydia or gonorrhea. Thus, women at risk for contacting these sexually transmitted pathogens should be advised to use a spermicide, especially if their sexual partner does not use a condom.—D.R. Mishell Jr., M.D.

Barrier Contraceptives and Sexually Transmitted Diseases in Women: A Comparison of Female-Dependent Methods and Condoms

Rosenberg MJ, Davidson AJ, Chen J-H, Judson FN, Douglas JM (Health Decisions Inc, Chapel Hill, NC; Univ of North Carolina; Dept of Public Health, Denver; Univ of Colorado Health Sciences Ctr, Denver, Colo)

Am J Public Health 82:669–674, 1992 16–3

Purpose.—Most efforts to control sexually transmitted diseases (STDs) have emphasized condoms to the virtual exclusion of other barrier methods. The effects of 3 popular forms of barrier contraceptives on the prevalence of STDs and other vaginal infections were evaluated retrospectively.

Setting.—The charts of 4,162 women who made 5,681 visits to a large urban STD clinic were reviewed. Condom use was reported at 18% of

Risk of Clinical Outcome for Users of Contraceptive Sponge or Diaphragm as Compared with Users of Condoms

Outcome	Odds ratio Crude	Odds ratio Adjusted*	95% Confidence interval
Gonorrhea	0.28	0.45	0.22-0.92**
Trichomoniasis	0.24	0.33	0.17-0.64**
Chlamydia	0.33	0.84	0.25-2.81
Bacterial vaginosis	1.03	0.88	0.59-1.31
Candidiasis	1.60	1.62	1.15-2.28**

* Adjusted for age, race, number of sexual partners in previous month, number of new partners in previous month, total lifetime partners, symptoms, reason for visit, and history of chlamydia, gonorrhea, or trichomoniasis.

** $P(2) < .05$.

(Courtesy of Rosenberg MJ, Davidson AJ, Chen J-H, et al: *Am J Public Health* 82:669–674, 1992.)

visits, diaphragm use at 4%, contraceptive sponge use at 2%, and no barrier (tubal ligation or no contraceptive) at 76%. *Chlamydia trachomatis* was the most prevalent infection, followed by *Candida* (12.2%), *Neisseria gonorrhoeae* (11.9%), *Trichomonas vaginalis* (11.1%), and bacterial vaginosis (10.7%).

Findings.—Compared with women who used no contraceptive or with tubal ligations, women who used sponge and diaphragm had at least 65% lower rates of infection with *N. gonorrhoea* and *T. vaginalis*, condom users had 34% and 30% lower rates, respectively. Both sponge and diaphragm users had lower rates of *C. trachomatis* infection, whereas condom users showed no reduction in the prevalence of chlamydia. Compared with women who relied on their partner's use of condoms, women who used contraceptive sponge or diaphragm had significantly lower rates of gonorrhea and trichomoniasis (table). Candidal infections were more common in diaphragm users, whereas bacterial vaginosis occurred with similar frequency in all groups.

Implications.—Efforts to help control STDs should be oriented more toward women. Female-dependent barrier methods provide a greater extent of protection against STDs than do condoms. Furthermore, the discrepancy between the high levels of condom efficacy in previously reported studies and these findings may be the result of different frequencies of use, with condoms more often used improperly and/or intermittently.

▶ This observational study provides information indicating that, among certain populations at high risk for acquiring sexually transmitted disease, the diaphragm may be more effective in preventing transmission of certain pathogens (particularly gonorrhea) than the condom. This is because of more constant use of the former, rather than the latter, barrier contraceptive. This data, combined with the information in Abstract 16–2 indicates that women with multiple sexual partners should be encouraged to use a diaphragm together with a spermicide because of poor compliance with condom usage among their sexual partners.—D.R. Mishell, Jr., M.D.

Pelvic Inflammatory Disease: Trends in Hospitalizations and Office Visits, 1979 Through 1988

Rolfs RT, Galaid EI, Zaidi AA (Ctrs for Disease Control, Atlanta)
Am J Obstet Gynecol 166:983–990, 1992 16–4

Objective.—Pelvic inflammatory disease is not a reportable condition. The recent trends in pelvic inflammatory disease occurrence, current antibiotic therapy, and use of surgical procedures for pelvic inflammatory disease were described.

Setting.—Data from the National Hospital Discharge Survey for 1979 to 1988 were obtained to assess the trends in hospitalization for pelvic

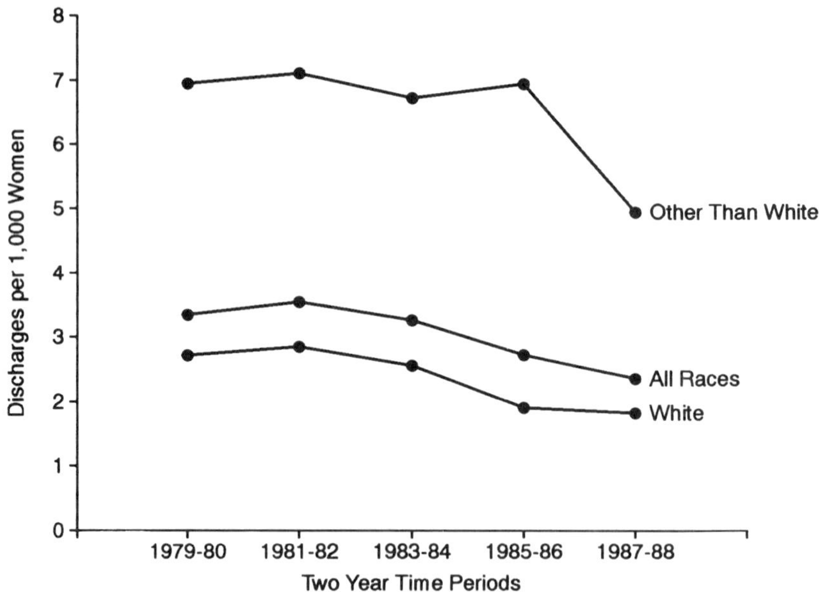

Fig 16–3.—Trends in hospitalization for acute pelvic inflammatory disease among white and other-than-white women in United States from 1979 to 1988. Acute pelvic inflammatory disease refers to ICD-9 codes designating acute disease or unspecified duration of disease. Rates are presented as 2-year means. (Courtesy of Rolfs RT, Galaid EI, Zaidi AA: *Am J Obstet Gynecol* 166:983–990, 1992.)

inflammatory disease. Data from the National Disease and Therapeutic Index for 1979 to 1989 were reviewed to evaluate trends in office visits.

Findings.—For women aged 15–44 years, a mean of 167,800 women were hospitalized each year for acute pelvic inflammatory disease and 80,750 were hospitalized for chronic pelvic inflammatory disease, for a rate of 3.03 and 1.46 per 1,000 women, respectively. Nearly 400,000 first visits were made each year to private physicians' offices, for a rate of 7.1 and 7.3 per 1,000 for acute and chronic disease, respectively. Women aged 20–24 years and women of other-than-white race had the highest mean hospitalization and visit rates for acute disease. Although the rate of initial office visits did not change in this time period, hospitalization rates decreased by 36% and 40% for acute and chronic disease, respectively, and they decreased similarly for both racial groups (Figs 16–3 and 16–4). Hospitalization rates decreased least, and in 1987 to 1988, they were highest for women 15–19 years of age. The rate for office visits remained stable.

Surgery was performed less frequently for acute (42%) than for chronic (90%) disease, with 36% and 63%, respectively, undergoing a procedure involving organ removal. Laparoscopy was performed in 12% and 19%, respectively, with little change over time. However, the use of ultrasonography increased significantly over the study period. The mean hospital stay did not change. One antimicrobial drug was prescribed in

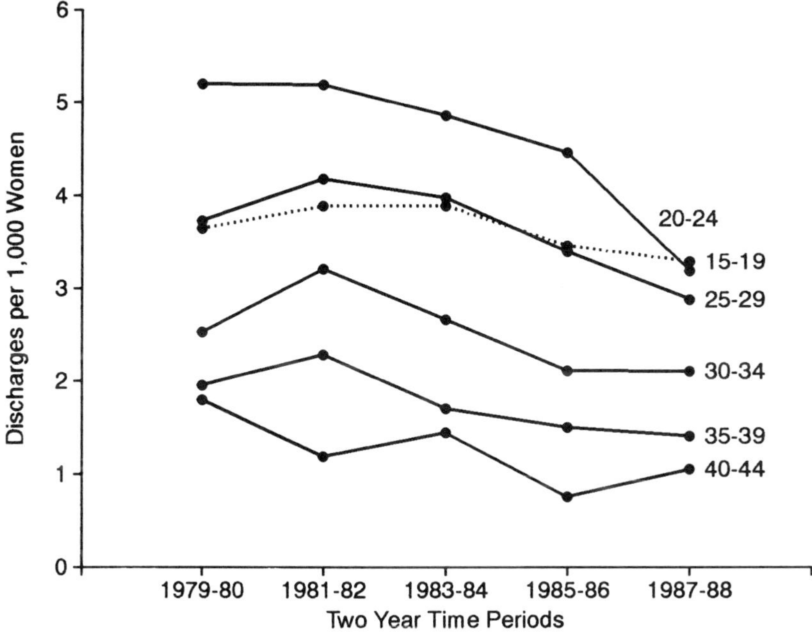

Fig 16–4.—Trends in hospitalizations for acute pelvic inflammatory disease in United States from 1979 to 1988, by 5-year age groups. Acute pelvic inflammatory disease refers to ICD-9 codes designating acute or unspecified-duration disease. Rates are presented as 2-year means. (Courtesy of Rolfs RT, Galaid EI, Zaidi AA: *Am J Obstet Gynecol* 166:983–990, 1992.)

87% of office visits and 2-antibiotic combination in 21%. The proportion of women receiving a drug effective against *Chlamydia trachomatis* increased significantly over time.

Implications.—The reductions in hospitalizations for pelvic inflammatory disease may reflect a decrease in incidence, changes in physician hospitalization practices, and in the spectrum of severity of pelvic inflammatory disease.

▶ Although the rate of hospitalization for pelvic inflammatory disease decreased in the United States from 1979 to 1988, the rate of initial office visits was unchanged. This dichotomy was probably the result of earlier diagnosis and more rapid and effective treatment, especially because clinicians became more aware of the clinical manifestations of chlamydial infection during this time. It is disconcerting to learn that a surgical procedure was performed on one third of women 15–19 years of age who were hospitalized for acute pelvic inflammatory disease and two thirds of those in the 40–44 year age range. One third of the women undergoing a surgical procedure for acute disease had 1 or more organs removed, whereas 30% had a therapeutic operation without organ removal and only 17% had a diagnostic operative procedure. It is hoped this high incidence of therapeutic operative procedures is not occurring at present in the United States.—D.R. Mishell, Jr., M.D.

Self-Reported Pelvic Inflammatory Disease in the United States, 1988

Aral SO, Mosher WD, Cates W Jr (Ctrs for Disease Control, Atlanta)

JAMA 266:2570–2573, 1991 16–5

Introduction.—In 1982, pelvic inflammatory disease (PID) was frequent in American women of reproductive age, especially in blacks, women aged 30 and older, and formerly married women.

Methods.—Data on self-reported PID were acquired from the National Survey of Family Growth, Cycle IV, undertaken in 1988, to identify changes in those women who reported PID in 1982–1988.

Findings.—All earlier findings were replicated. Data for 1988 showed that PID is more common in women with 2 or more sex partners than in those with a single lifetime partner, and that it is more frequent in women reporting a history of sexually transmitted disease (STD). Being black increased the chance of having self-reported PID by 50%. Racial differences in risk factors are shown in the table. The number of lifetime sex partners, current age, and a history of STD were risk factors for both white and black women.

Discussion.—Pelvic inflammatory disease remains widely prevalent in American women. Preventing lower genital tract infection is critical in avoiding PID and its complications. Black women appear to increase their risk disproportionately when they have more than a single lifetime sex partner. The effect of formerly being married was more evident in white than in black women.

Factors Associated With Self-Reported Pelvic Inflammatory Disease by Race

	White	Black
No. of lifetime sexual partners	X	X
Current age	X	X
Race	X	X
History of sexually transmitted diseases	X	X
Vaginal douching	X	...
Age at first intercourse	X	...
Marital status	X	...

Note: by logistic regression, $P < .01$; $\chi^2 = 403.3$ for all races, 267.7 for whites, and 60.7 for blacks; $df = 8$ for all races, 7 for whites, and 7 for blacks.

(Courtesy of Aral SO, Mosher WD, Cates W Jr: *JAMA* 266:2570–2573, 1991.)

▶ In contrast to other studies investigating the association of risk factors and the development of acute salpingitis, this study used a nonselected, nationally representative sample of women. The risk factors shown in the table have been previously identified, but they still should be used when counseling women about the methods to prevent this serious disease and its resultant sequelae.—D.R. Mishell Jr., M.D.

Pelvic Inflammatory Disease: Findings During Inpatient Treatment of Clinically Severe, Laparoscopy-Documented Disease

Livengood C III, Hill GB, Addison WA (Duke Univ, Durham, NC)

Am J Obstet Gynecol 166:519–524, 1992 16–6

Objective.—Previous studies have shown that clinical examination in patients with suspected pelvic inflammatory disease (PID) has a diagnostic specificity of 65% or less. Furthermore, the diagnostic criteria for clinically severe PID are not well defined. The relationship between clinically severe PID and laparoscopic diagnosis and grading was assessed, the relative efficacy and safety of 2 antibiotic treatment regimens were evaluated, and therapeutic success and failure were defined.

Patients.—Thirty-three women with a clinical diagnosis of severe PID made up the study sample. To be eligible for study inclusion, patients had to have 1 or more of the following clinical signs: significant peritonitis, vomiting or paralytic ileus, temperature of 39°C or greater, white blood cell count greater than 20,000/mm^3 or less than 4,000/mm^3, postural hypotension, adnexal fixation or mass, or disease persistence or progression after 72 hours or more of outpatient antibiotic therapy. All patients underwent laparoscopic examination under general anesthesia. Based on the laparoscopic findings, PID was classified as mild, moderate, or severe. Severe PID was defined as the presence of an inflammatory mass. Patients with documented PID were then randomly assigned to intravenous (IV) therapy with 600 mg of clindamycin given every 6 hours, either with 2 gm of cefamandole given every 6 hours, or 100 mg of doxycycline plus 10 ml of 4% sodium bicarbonate alternating with placebo every 6 hours to achieve double blinding. Antibiotic therapy was discontinued upon discharge. All patients were contacted 10 days after discharge to inquire about subjective signs of PID relapse.

Results.—Of 33 patients with a clinical diagnosis of PID, 23 (70%) had PID documented at laparoscopy. Based on laparoscopic grading, 10 patients (44%) had mild PID, 6 (26%) had moderate PID, and 7 (30%) had severe PID. Eleven patients were treated with cefamandole and clindamycin, and 12 received doxycycline and clindamycin. Both regimens were 100% effective, and there was no difference in terms of response to therapy between the 2 regimens. Subjective relapse did not occur. The number of days of drug therapy until response was not associated with initial clinical sign score, temperature of 38°C or greater, white blood cell count of 10,000/mm^3 or greater, pelvic mass on physical examination, or old adhesions on laparoscopy. However, days to response were significantly associated with laparoscopic grading of disease severity.

Conclusion.—Clinical diagnosis and grading of severe PID has poor specificity. Laparoscopic grading of PID severity seems accurate. Both antibiotic regimens are effective. Postdischarge antibiotic therapy is not necessary.

▶ This study confirms earlier data indicating that the clinical diagnosis of PID—even when severe enough to require hospitalization—is only accurate about two thirds of the time. Although performing routine laparoscopic diagnostic evaluation for all women suspected of having PID is not cost effective, this procedure is advisable in all women without the typical clinical findings of salpingitis, especially if the findings are consistent with the diagnosis of appendicitis. In this study, the authors found that the absence of cervical motion and adnexal tenderness upon performance of a bimanual pelvic examination was the best indicator of an adequate clinical response to therapy. If these signs are still present, therapy should be continued. This pelvic "stress test" has been used in our institution for many years, and continuing antibiotic therapy and bed rest until adnexal and cervical tenderness disappears has reduced the incidence of recurrence of symptoms and readmission in the first weeks after discharge.—D.R. Mishell, Jr., M.D.

Long-Term Sequelae of Acute Pelvic Inflammatory Disease: A Retrospective Cohort Study

Safrin S, Schachter J, Dahrouge D, Sweet RL (Univ of California, San Francisco)

Am J Obstet Gynecol 166:1300–1305, 1992 16–7

Objective.—Acute pelvic inflammatory disease (PID) is associated with substantial morbidity, economic costs, and risk of long-term sequelae. The frequency and predictors of the long-term sequelae of PID were determined.

Patients.—A computerized medical record search identified 140 women who had been discharged during 1985 with a diagnosis of PID, salpingitis, or tubo-ovarian abscess. All 140 charts were extracted for baseline characteristics. Between April 1988 and March 1989, repeated attempts were made to locate these 140 women. Those who could be located were interviewed by telephone using a standardized questionnaire.

Results.—The chart review revealed that 55 (39%) women had a history of PID. Of these women, 27 had had 1 prior episode, and 28 had had 2 or more prior episodes. Cervical, endometrial, or tubal specimens yielded *Neisseria gonorrhoeae* in 63 (50%) of 127 women and *Chlamydia trachomatis* in 32 (27%) of 118 women examined for these pathogens.

Fifty-one women (36.5%) were interviewed at a median interval of 37.5 months after the index PID episode. Two women refused, and 87 could not be traced. Seventeen women (40%) met the definition of involuntary infertility. Univariate and multivariate analysis identified a previous history of PID, young age at the time of first sexual intercourse, and 2 or more days of abdominal or pelvic pain before admission as risk factors for involuntary infertility. Twelve women (24%) had chronic pelvic pain for 6 months or more after hospitalization; of these women, 9 sought medical attention for the pain and 4 were treated with antibiotics. A history of PID was statistically associated with chronic pelvic pain after treatment. Twenty-two women (43%) had 1 or more episodes of PID after the index episode at a median of 2.1 months after admission. A history of PID before the index episode was statistically associated with PID recurrence. Of the 25 women (48%) women who had a subsequent pregnancy, 2 (2.4%) had an ectopic pregnancy after the index episode of PID. The risk factors for ectopic pregnancy could not be established because of the small numbers involved.

Conclusion.—The high frequency of long-term sequelae—in spite of hospitalization for close observation and parenteral antimicrobial therapy—suggests that further studies are needed to more accurately assess the incidence of predictors of these sequelae.

▶ With current antimicrobial therapy, the risk of dying of acute salpingitis is nearly nonexistant. Nevertheless, the high incidence of sequelae of this disease, including infertility (40%), chronic pelvic pain (24%), and high rate of recurrence (43%) remains a major health problem. Because the rate of recurrence steadily increases with the number of episodes (from 30% with 1 episode to 50% with 2, to 70% with 3 episodes), perhaps prophylactic use of antibiotics during menses in the first year after hospital discharge should be offered to women with recurrent episodes of acute salpingitis.—D.R. Mishell, Jr., M.D.

US-Guided Transvaginal Drainage of Pelvic Abscesses and Fluid Collections

van Sonnenberg E, D'Agostino HB, Casola G, Goodacre BW, Sanchez RB, Taylor B (Univ of California, San Diego Med Ctr)

Radiology 181:53–56, 1991 16–8

Objective.—Ultrasound was used as an aid to inserting needles and catheters transvaginally in 14 women who had a variety of deep pelvic fluid collections and were symptomatic. Thirteen patients were treated for both diagnosis and cure, whereas 1 had a diagnostic procedure only. The most frequent indications for drainage were fever and sepsis, and the most common specific lesion was a tubo-ovarian abscess.

Management.—All patients but 1 received antibiotics. Drainage was achieved with an 18- to 22-guage needle in 7 patients and with a catheter in 6. Sonography was performed transvaginally in 12 patients and transabdominally in 2. Transvaginal studies were done in either the ultrasound suite or in a fluoroscopy room using a portable ultrasound unit. All collections were evacuated as completely as possible.

Results.—Transvaginal ultrasound frequently was the best procedure because of the proximity of fluid to the vagina. A mean of 71 mL of fluid was removed. Only 5 patients had positive cultures. In 11 cases, transvaginal drainage precluded the need for surgery. Two patients had a tubo-ovarian phlegmon removed after the transvaginal procedure. There were no major complications. The catheters were left in place for approximately a week on average.

Conclusion.—Ultrasound-guided transvaginal drainage is an effective and safe approach to remove pelvic abscesses and fluid collections. There is no radiation exposure, and the method is less expensive than CT-guided procedures.

▶ Drainage of fluid in the pelvis can now be safely accomplished by placing a needle or catheter into the cul-de-sac through the vaginal wall, using the guidance of vaginal probe ultrasonography. Use of this technique may avoid the need for a major surgical procedure in the treatment of tubo-ovarian abscess. More importantly, it may preserve ovarian function.—D.R. Mishell, Jr., M.D.

Percutaneous Drainage of Tubo-Ovarian Abscesses

Casola G, vanSonnenberg E, D'Agostino HB, Harker CP, Varney RR, Smith D
(Univ of California, San Diego)

Radiology 182:399–402, 1992 16–9

Background.—Although percutaneous drainage is an established procedure for the treatment of abscesses, it is not generally used to treat tubo-ovarian abscesses (TOAs). However, some studies have suggested that percutaneous drainage is an alternative to surgery. The techniques for and physicians' experience with percutaneous drainage of TOAs were evaluated.

Methods.—A total of 27 TOAs in 16 patients ranging in age from 14 to 40 years were studied. In each case, the abscess failed to defervesce, despite an average of 5 days of intravenously administered ampicillin, gentamicin, and clindamycin. Ultrasound detected 26 of the abscesses, with appearances ranging from cystic to solid masses; CT detected the other abscess. Guidance for drainage was achieved with CT in 21 cases, endovaginal ultrasound in 4, and transabdominal ultrasound in 2. The abscesses were approached transgluteally in 11 patients, transvaginally in 6, and through the anterior abdominal wall in 10. At the time of drainage and during hospitalization, the catheters were irrigated with small amounts of saline.

Results.—The clinical response was good in 15 of 16 patients. Twenty-two collections decreased in size on follow-up ultrasound examination. The mean duration of drainage was 6 days, and the mean amount of fluid drained was 59 mL. An average of only 5 mL was drained when needle aspiration alone was done. Two patients had the complication of sciatica, and 1 had transient bacteremia. The abscess recurred in 2 patients at 3 and 4 months after drainage; 1 had bilateral salpingectomy, and the other had total abdominal hysterectomy and bilateral salpingo-ophorectomy.

Conclusion.—Percutaneous drainage probably should be preferred to surgery for TOAs in which medical therapy fails. Transvaginal drainage can be done with the use of endovaginal ultrasound. This route was used whenever possible. Needle aspiration can be done in abscesses smaller than 3–4 cm.

▶ The development of transvaginal and transabdominal ultrasonography has simplified and made safer the technique of placement of catheters into a TOA. Previously, when women with these abscesses failed to respond to antibiotic therapy, it was necessary to perform a bilateral salpingo-ophorectomy, usually with hysterectomy. With the technique of transvaginal or percutaneous drainage of the abscesses, it is now possible to avoid castrating many of these young women.—D.R. Mishell, Jr., M.D.

A Comparison of Single-Dose Cefixime With Ceftriaxone as Treatment for Uncomplicated Gonorrhea

Handsfield HH, McCormack WM, Hook EW III, Douglas JM Jr, Covino JM, Verdon MS, Reichart CA, Ehret JM, Gonorrhea Treatment Study Group (Seattle–King County Dept of Public Health; Univ of Washington, Seattle; City of New York Dept of Health; State Univ of New York Health Sciences Ctr, Brooklyn; Baltimore City Health Dept; et al)

N Engl J Med 325:1337–1341, 1991 16–10

Background.—Because of the increase in penicillin- or tetracycline-resistant *Neisseria gonorrhoeae*, the recommended treatment for uncomplicated gonorrhea is a single dose of intramuscular ceftriaxone. Cefixime is a new, orally administered cephalosporin that has excellent activity against *N. gonorrhoeae* and is suitable for single-dose administration. Oral administration may be more convenient than intramuscular administration, and it reduces the frequency of needle use in a population at risk for infection with HIV. In a multicenter study of men and women with uncomplicated gonorrhea, the efficacy of oral cefixime was compared with intramuscular ceftriaxone.

Methods.—In an unblinded, multicenter trial, 209 men and 124 women with uncomplicated gonorrhea were randomized to receive a single dose of either 400 mg or 800 mg of oral cefixime, or 250 mg of intramuscular ceftriaxone.

Results.—The cure rate was 96% in patients receiving the 400-mg dose of cefixime, 98% in patients receiving 800 mg of cefixime, and 98% in patients receiving ceftriaxone. All 3 regimens were effective independent of the antimicrobial resistance of the isolates. Pharyngeal infection was eradicated in 20 of 22 patients, but *Chlamydia trachomatis* infection persisted in at least half the infected patients in each treatment group.

Conclusion.—A single dose of 400 or 800 mg of cefixime administered orally appears to be as effective as the currently recommended regimen of 250 mg of ceftriaxone given intramuscularly. Cefixime should be followed with a regimen effective against C. *trachomatis.*

▶ This well-done study indicates that a single oral dose of cefixime is as effective as a single injection of ceftriaxone in the treatment of gonorrhea in men and women, and that both agents were more than 95% effective. Both drugs were effective in treating gonococcal isolates, which demonstrated antimicrobial resistance. Because cefixime is less expensive than ceftriaxone and does not have to be given by injection, use of cefixime may become the preferred initial treatment of gonococcal infection. The incidence of gastrointestinal side effects was significantly greater with the 800-mg dose of cefixime than with the 400-mg dose; however, the frequency of side effects was similar between the lower doses of cefixime and ceftriaxone. Therefore, a single 400-mg dose of cefixime is recommended.—D.R. Mishell, Jr., M.D.

Comparative Evaluation of Clindamycin/Gentamicin and Cefoxitin/Doxycycline for Treatment of Pelvic Inflammatory Disease: A Multi-Center Trial

The European Study Group (Centre Hospitalier Intercommunal de Villeneuve, St Georges, France; Rudolf-Virchow Hosp, Berlin, Germany; Krankenhaus am Urban, Berlin, Germany

Acta Obstet Gynecol Scand 71:129–134, 1992 16–11

Background.—One treatment recommended by the Centers for Disease Control for pelvic inflammatory disease (PID) is intravenous clindamycin plus gentamicin or tobramycin, followed by oral clindamycin given for a total of 10 to 14 days. This randomized, multicenter trial compared the clinical utility of this treatment with that of a cefoxitin-doxycycline combination.

Methods.—The prospective, open-label study took place at 10 centers. The subjects were 170 women aged 15–51 years who needed hospital treatment for acute PID. One group received clindamycin, 900 mg administered intravenously every 8 hours, and gentamicin, 2 mg/kg followed by 1.5 mg/kg, administered intravenously every 8 hours for at least 4 days. After intravenous therapy, 450 mg of clindamycin was given orally every 6 hours for 10 days. The other group received cefoxitin, 2 g

	Clinical Outcome	
	Clindamycin-Gentamicin (N = 60)	Cefoxitin-Doxycycline (N = 55)
Clinical success	52/60 (87%)	46/55 (84%)*
Clinical failure	7/60 (12%)	9/55 (16%)
Side effect failure	1/60 (1%)	0

* Not significant (Fisher's exact test).
(Courtesy of The European Study Group: *Acta Obstet Gynecol Scand* 71:129–134, 1992.)

intravenously every 6 hours, plus doxycycline, 100 mg given intravenously every 12 hours, for a minimum of 4 days. This was followed by 100 mg of doxycycline administered orally every 12 hours for 10 days. An unsatisfactory response was defined as no change or worsening of signs and symptoms during the first 2–3 days of treatment.

Results.—Approximately two thirds of each group was judged eligible for efficacy assessment. Eighty-seven percent of the clindamycin-gentamicin group and 84% of the cefoxitin-doxycycline group had a satisfactory response (table). Seven patients in the former group and 9 in the latter failed treatment; 1 patient in each group required surgery. The proportion of patients with side effects was similar, the most common side effects being gastrointestinal, such as glossitis, nausea, vomiting, diarrhea, and anal discomfort.

Conclusion.—For women with PID, clindamycin-gentamicin treatment appears to have a similar cure rate to cefoxitin-doxycycline. The 2 regimens also have similar rates of eradication of *Chlamydia trachomatis* and *Neisseria gonorrhoeae* when either or both are present. Without long-term follow-up, effects on fertility, ectopic pregnancy, and recurrent infection cannot be assessed.

▶ There are several satisfactory inpatient antibiotic treatment regimens that can adequately treat the signs and symptoms of acute salpingitis. This study indicates that a regimen of cefoxitin and doxycycline is as effective as the regimen of clindamycin and gentamicin for the treatment of acute salpingitis. It remains to be determined whether the prevalence of the sequelae of acute salpingitis leads to infertility and/or ectopic pregnancy differs between these 2 regimens. Until studies indicating that one of these regimens is superior to the other in terms of the sequelae of salpingitis are done, it would appear best to use the less costly of these 2 regimens, considering the total cost of intravenous administration as well as the cost of the drug.—D.R. Mishell, Jr., M.D.

A Comparison of Three Rapid Chlamydial Tests in Pregnant and Nonpregnant Women

Ferris DG, Martin WH (Med College of Georgia, Augusta)

J Fam Pract 34:593–597, 1992 16–12

Purpose.—It is difficult to detect cervical *Chlamydia trachomatis* infections on the basis of symptoms or physical findings alone. Chlamydia trachomatis culture is considered the criterion standard of comparison; however, the reported sensitivity of a culture of a single endocervical specimen is only 67% to 77%. The sensitivity of 3 commercially available rapid enzyme immunoassay (EIA) tests to detect C. *trachomatis* cervicitis was evaluated.

Methods.—Endocervical samples from 506 women (age, 18–35 years) seeking routine gynecological medical care at 1 of the study sites were invited to participate in the study. The tests used in this study were Abbott TestPack Chlamydia and Kodak Surecell Chlamydia (which were previously evaluated but subsequently modified) and a new solid-phase sandwich EIA kit (Unipath Clearview Chlamydia) that was not previously available. To control for variability, all tests were performed according to the manufacturers' specifications by one medical technologist who was blinded to the culture results.

Results.—Forty-seven women had positive chlamydial cultures. The overall prevalence of C. *trachomatis* cervicitis was 9.3%. One third of the patients (33.8%) were pregnant. The majority (95.6%) of women who had less than 10 leukocytes per high-power field on a vaginal wet-mount preparation did not have C. *trachomatis* infection. Conversely, 88.2% of the women infected with C. *trachomatis* had more than 10 leukocytes per high-power field. None of the women who used barrier contraceptive methods had C. *trachomatis* infection, whereas 10.1% of the women who used nonbarrier or no contraception had chlamydial cervicitis.

The Clearview and Surecell EIAs both had a sensitivity of 85.1%. Clearview had a specificity of 98.5%, and Surecell had a specificity of 99.3%. TestPack had a sensitivity of only 66%, but it had a specificity of 99.8%; it failed to detect disease in approximately one fifth of the women who were infected and who were correctly identified by the other 2 EIAs. Surecell performed best in the pregnant group, with a sensitivity of 95.8% and a specificity of 99.3%. Clearview performed best in the nonpregnant group, with a sensitivity of 82.6% and a specificity of 98.7%. TestPack had a specificity of 75% in the pregnant group and 56.5% in the nonpregnant group.

Conclusion.—Both the Clearview and Surecell chlamydial EIAs perform well, particularly for pregnant women.

▶ Because the results of culture of *C. trachomatis* take several days to be made available, in certain clinics with a high-risk population and a low rate of follow-up, rapid EIAs may be more suitable and cost effective. This study shows the accuracy of 3 rapid chlamydia tests in pregnant and nonpregnant women. Each of the tests require a varying amount of time and dexterity to perform the procedure. Therefore, training with positive and negative controls should be performed before using the results for clinical decisions. Perhaps just counting the number of leukocytes observed microscopically in the discharge could be used to decide whether to treat with a week of tetracycline.—D.R. Mishell, Jr., M.D.

Ingestion of Yogurt Containing *Lactobacillus acidophilus* as Prophylaxis for Candidal Vaginitis

Hilton E, Isenberg HD, Alperstein P, France K, Borenstein MT (Long Island Jewish Med Ctr, New Hyde Park, NY)

Ann Intern Med 116:353–357, 1992 16–13

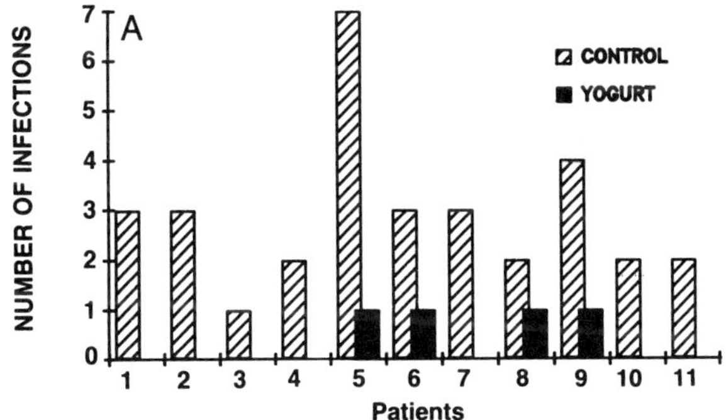

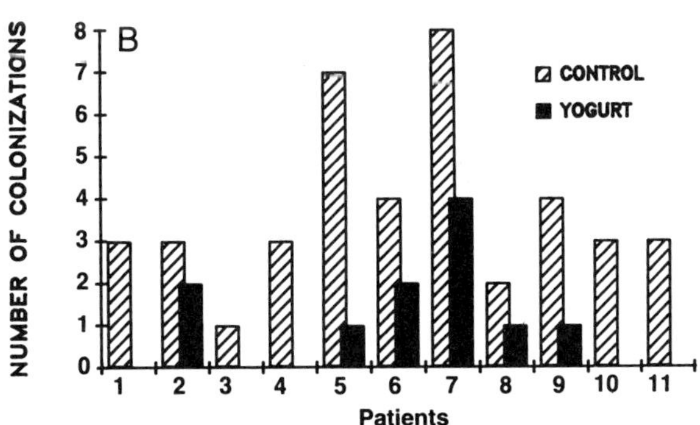

Fig 16–5.—*Candida* infections and colonizations. **A,** number of *Candida* infections per 6 months in individual patients. **B,** number of colonizations per 6 months in individual patients. (Courtesy of Hilton E, Isenberg HD, Alperstein P, et al: *Ann Intern Med* 116:353–357, 1992.)

Effect of Yogurt on Candidal Infections and Colonizations

Variable	Control Arm	Yogurt Arm	*P* Value†
Infections per 6 months, *n*	2.54 ± 1.66	0.38 ± 0.51	< 0.001
Colonizations per 6 months, *n*	3.23 ± 2.17	0.84 ± 0.90	0.001
Examinations in which infection was detected, %	0.33 ± 0.19	0.13 ± 0.19	0.002

All values are expressed as mean ± SD.
† Calculated by paired *t*-test.
(Courtesy of Hilton E, Isenberg HD, Alperstein P, et al: *Ann Intern Med* 116:353–357, 1992.)

Introduction.—Many patients with chronic vulvovaginal candidal infections fail treatment with current therapies. Some reports have suggested that systemic prophylaxis can be effective, including anecdotal reports of topical and systemic administration of yogurt. A trial was done to determine whether eating yogurt containing *Lactobacillus acidophilus* could prevent vaginal candidiasis.

Methods.—Thirty-three women with recurrent and microbiologically confirmed vulvovaginal candidal infection were recruited for the cross-over study. The patients were randomized to eat yogurt, 8 ounces/day, for 6 months and then to eat no yogurt for 6 months, or vice versa. The yogurt chosen yielded more than 10^8 colony-forming units of *Lactobacillus acidophilus* per mL.

Results.—Only 13 women completed the protocol. Twelve were excluded for protocol violations, 10 of whom had been started on the no-yogurt arm. Another 8 women who began on the yogurt arm did not wish to complete the study because of clinical improvement. Per 6-month period, the mean number of infections was 2.54 in the no-yogurt arm vs. .38 in the yogurt arm (Fig 16–5, table). The mean numbers of positive colonizations were 3.23 and .84 per 6 months, respectively. Symptomatic relief was reported by all patients who began on the no-yogurt arm and were crossed over to the yogurt arm.

Conclusion.—Ingestion of *L. acidophilus*-containing yogurt appears to decrease both candidal colonization and infection in women with recurrent infections. The gastrointestinal strain of *L. acidophilus* appears to colonize the patient's vaginal tract.

► This is a novel, well-tolerated approach to managing the vexing problem of recurrent vaginal yeast infection. Eating 8 ounces of yogurt a day may be preferable to applying medications directly into the vagina whenever symptoms of candidal vaginitis occur.—D.R. Mishell, Jr., M.D.

Treatment of Candidal Vaginitis: A Prospective Randomized Investigator-Blind Multicenter Study Comparing Topically Applied Econazole With Oral Fluconazole

Osser S, Haglund A, Weström L (Univ Hosp of Lund, Sweden; Univ Hosp of Malmö, Sweden; Univ Hosp of Linköping, Sweden; Univ Hosp of Umeå, Sweden; Central Hosp of Norrköping, Sweden; et al)

Acta Obstet Gynecol Scand 70:73–78, 1991 16–14

Introduction.—Candidal vulvovaginitis has traditionally been treated with topical application of antimycotic agents. Fluconazole is a new agent designed for the systemic treatment of genital mycoses, including yeast fungi. The efficacy of a topically applied vaginal econazole depot tablet was compared with that of orally administered fluconazole prospective, multicenter, single-blind clinical trial.

Patients.—During a 7-month period, 258 women with a clinical diagnosis of candidal vaginitis were randomly allocated to a topically administered 150-mg econazole vaginal depot tablet or an orally administered 150-mg fluconazole capsule, both of which were given as a single dose. Follow-up visits were scheduled 7–10 days after the recruitment visit (RV), 28–35 days after the RV, and 80–100 days after the RV. Clinical failure was defined as persistence of the symptoms and clinical signs of candidal vaginitis from one visit to the next, and clinical recurrence was defined as the reappearance of symptoms after a symptom-free interval.

Results.—Of 235 evaluable women, 121 received fluconazole and 114 received econazole. At the 28- to 35-day visit, the clinical and mycological cure rates were significantly higher in women treated with the oral fluconazole tablet than in those given the econazole vaginal tablet. The cumulative cure rates at the 3-month visit were 51.2% in fluconazole-treated women and 39.5% in econazole-treated women; however, the difference was statistically not significant. There was no significant difference in cure rates at the 7- to 10-day visit. The side effects with either drug were minor. When asked about their preference for either topical or oral therapy, 68.3% of the women given fluconazole preferred oral treatment and 38.8% of those given econazole preferred topical treatment.

Conclusion.—Orally administered fluconazole is a simple and effective alternative to the topical treatment of acute candidal vaginitis.

► Vaginal yeast infection is a common problem that is difficult to irradicate because of the high rate of recurrent infection. Some recently marketed imidazoles and triazoles have been shown to be effective when given topically for 1–3 days instead of the traditional 7-day therapy. Although systemic administration of midazoles may be associated with serious side effects, administration of the oral triazole, fluconazole, that was used in this study is not associated with liver toxicity and does not affect serum lipids. Therefore, clinicians may elect to use this agent for some women who prefer oral to vaginal therapy, because it appears to be as effective as the vaginally administered agent.—D.R. Mishell Jr., M.D.

Comparison of Different Metronidazole Therapeutic Regimens for Bacterial Vaginosis: A Meta-Analysis

Lugo-Miro VI, Green M, Mazur L (Univ of Texas, Houston)

JAMA 268:92–95, 1992 16–15

Introduction.—Bacterial vaginosis (BV) is the most prevalent form of vaginitis, and metronidazole currently is the drug recommended for treatment. A regimen of 500 mg twice a day for 7 days currently is recommended, but the optimal dosage and duration have not yet been established. A meta-analysis was conducted to determine whether there is a metronidazole regimen that is best in regard to rates of cure and recurrence.

Methods.—A literature search was performed to find clinical trials comparing different oral metronidazole regimens that included diagnostic criteria for BV and criteria to detect cure to treatment. Only 16 of the 52 articles identified evaluated different metronidazole regimens, and only 10 met the inclusion criteria; the rest were nonrandomized studies or reports of personal experience. The 10 studies provided a total population of 1,203 patients.

Findings.—The patients could be categorized into 4 treatment groups: group A included 413 patients treated with a single 2-g dose; group B, 193 patients treated with a single 2-g dose for 2 days; group C, 317 patients treated for 5 days with 400 mg given 2 or 3 times per day; and group D, 280 patients treated for 7 days with 500 mg given twice a day or 400 mg administered 3 times a day. The groups showed no significant differences in cure rates, with analysis having a 99% chance of detecting such a difference if one existed (table). Five studies evaluated the patients for recurrent disease; again, no significant differences in cure rate were found.

Cure Rates After the First Follow-up Evaluation

	Group A Single Dose (n=413)	Group B Single Dose Twice (n=193)	Group C 5 d (n=317)	Group D 7 d (n=280)
Cured	351	169	274	244
Not cured	62	24	43	36
Cure rate, %	85	87	86	87

Overall difference among groups was not significant. $\alpha = .05$; $P = .78$.
(Courtesy of Lugo-Miro VI, Green M, Mazur L: *JAMA* 268:92–95, 1992.)

Conclusion.—To increase compliance, decrease side effects, and lower cost, a single dose of metronidazole should be given as treatment for BV. This treatment has proven equally effective as longer regimens. The cure rate is no different between patients whose sexual partners are and are not treated; treatment of the male partner has not been shown to be beneficial.

▶ This compilation of data from several epidemiological studies by a statistical technique called meta-analysis indicates that it is no more beneficial to treat BV with metronidazole for 5–7 days than to use a single treatment of 2 g of the drug. Because compliance is better and cost is less with the single-dose therapy, it should become the treatment of choice. As has been previously shown, no benefit is derived from treatment of the male partner.—D.R. Mishell, Jr., M.D.

Bacterial Vaginosis: Treatment With Clindamycin Cream Versus Oral Metronidazole

Schmitt C, Sobel JD, Meriwether C (Wayne State Univ, Detroit)

Obstet Gynecol 79:1020–1023, 1992 16–16

Background.—Presently, bacterial vaginosis is treated with orally administered metronidazole, which usually is curative but has unpleasant side effects. Clindamycin, which is highly active against anaerobic bacteria, may be a useful alternative.

Objective and Methods.—Orally administered metronidazole and intravaginal clindamycin cream were compared in a double-blind study of 61 women with bacterial vaginosis. Women were assigned to use 2% vaginal clindamycin cream (5 g daily) for 1 week plus placebo tablets, or 500 mg of metronidazole given twice daily plus a placebo cream.

Results.—Twenty-five women assigned to clindamycin therapy and 23 given metronidazole were evaluable. The overall cure rates were 72% for the clindamycin-treated group and 87% for the metronidazole-treated group. Three clindamycin-treated women and 2 women who were given metronidazole had symptomatic yeast vaginitis. Symptomatic bacterial vaginosis recurred in approximately one fifth of each group within 4 weeks of treatment, and another one fifth of each group had asymptomatic bacterial vaginosis. Symptomatic *Candida* infection developed in 6 women in the clindamycin group and in 5 women in the metronidazole group. Three patients in each group withdrew because of side effects.

Conclusion.—Orally administered metronidazole and clindamycin in vaginal cream form are comparably effective in treating bacterial vaginosis. Use of the cream can eliminate the systemic side effects caused by orally administered metronidazole.

▶ Although the initial cure rates of the 2 agents used in this study were statistically insignificant, the study's small sample size may have prevented the 72% cure rate with clindamycin from being significantly different from the 87% cure rate with metronidazole. Larger studies are necessary before claims of equivalent efficacy achieved using clindamycin and metronidazole for the treatment of bacterial vaginosis can be considered valid. Until then, it would be preferable to continue to use metronidazole as the drug of choice and to consider clindamycin cream an alternative when metronidazole cannot be tolerated because of its side effects.—D.R. Mishell, Jr., M.D.

Comparison of Female to Male and Male to Female Transmission of HIV in 563 Stable Couples

European Study Group on Heterosexual Transmission of HIV (European Centre for the Epidemiological Monitoring of AIDS, France; Universita di Bologna, Italy; Athens School of Hygiene, Greece)

BMJ 304:809–813, 1992 16–17

Objective.—A European multicenter cohort study was undertaken to estimate the risks of heterosexual transmission of HIV infection.

Subjects.—A total of 563 couples from 9 European countries were enrolled. The study group included 156 female index patients with 159 male partners, and 400 male index patients with 404 female partners. Most index subjects were intravenous drug users or former drug users. Couples had been together for a median of 3 years.

Female-to-Male Transmission.—All male contacts who were HIV positive had had unprotected vaginal intercourse with index women. The risk of transmission correlated with both the clinical state and the T4-cell count of the index subject. Infection occurred in 42% of the contacts of women with advanced HIV infection (odds ratio = 17.6). Infected contacts had had longer relationships. Human immunodeficiency virus seropositivity also correlated with sexual contact during menses (odds ratio = 3.4).

Male-to-Female Transmission.—The risk of transmission to female contacts correlated with advanced HIV infection (odds ratio = 2.7), anal sex (odds ratio = 5.1), and contacts older than 45 years (odds ratio = 3.9). Couples with at least 2 of these factors had a 54% risk of disease transmission. The crude male-to-female transmission rate was 20% compared with 12% for female-to-male transmission.

Implications.—Heterosexual transmission of HIV infection does not depend on high-risk sexual practices. Any factor impairing the integrity of the genital mucosa, whether traumatic, infectious, or hormonal, may increase the risk of transmission.

▶ This interesting study demonstrates not only the overall risk of transmission of HIV by sexual intercourse with male or female infected sexual partners, but also the factors that increase the risk of such transmission. It is important to note that, in this study, none of the 24 sexual partners who had always used condoms during sexual relations became infected. Also, sexual transmission of the virus *did* occur among couples who did not practice anal sex or had intercourse during menses, provided they did not consistently use condoms. Therefore, the risk factors for transmission are relative, not absolute.—D.R. Mishell, Jr., M.D.

Man-To-Woman Sexual Transmission of the Human Immunodeficiency Virus: Risk Factors Related to Sexual Behavior, Man's Infectiousness, and Woman's Susceptibility

Lazzarin A, Saracco A, Musicco M, Nicolosi A, Italian Study Group on HIV Heterosexual Transmission (Univ of Milan, Italy; Dept of Epidemiology and Med Informatics, Milan; Columbia Univ, New York)

Arch Intern Med 151:2411–2416, 1991 16–18

Background.—Heterosexual intercourse is not in itself sufficient for transmission of HIV. Some co-factors probably influence the likelihood of transmission. These may include sexual behavior and duration of risk, infectiousness, and host susceptibility. A prospective cross-sectional study was performed on women who were steady sexual partners of HIV-infected men to evaluate the risk factors for HIV transmission.

Methods.—The study sample comprised 368 women at 16 centers. Each woman was the steady sexual partner of an HIV-infected man; none of the women were previously known to be infected. Human immunodeficiency virus antibody testing revealed that 99 women 27.7% were positive. Data were gathered from review of the men's medical records and interviews with the women. For each risk factor investigated, the crude odds ratios (ORs) were calculated.

Findings.—According to multiple logistic regression analysis, factors negatively associated with transmission of HIV infection were the woman's awareness of her partner's infection, use of condoms, and use of oral contraceptives. Odds ratios were .2, .3, and .5, respectively, (table). Women who had intercourse more than twice a week and those exposed to HIV for 2–5 years had an increased risk, with respective ORs of 2.4 and 3.5. Transmission was more common in couples who had anal sex (OR, 2.8), women who reported vaginitis (OR, 4.9), women who had genital warts (OR, 33.3), and women who used intrauterine devices (OR, 3.1). Risk was associated with a CD4+ cell count of lower than 400 per mm^3 in the infected men. The women's awareness of their partners' HIV status increased condom use but did not result in a lower frequency of sexual intercourse or avoidance of anal sex.

Conclusion.—Heterosexual transmission of HIV appears to be affected by the frequency of intercourse and the use of condoms. Anal sex

Risk Factors for Man-to-Woman Sexual Transmission of HIV: Analysis by Multiple Logistic Regression

	Odds Ratio	95% CI
Risk duration, y		
<1	1	...
1-5	3.5	1.8-6.7
>5	0.8	0.3-2.1
Weekly frequency of sexual intercourse, >2	2.4	1.2-4.9
Condom use		
Never	1	...
Sometimes	0.7	0.3-1.6
Often or always	0.3	0.1-1.0
Anal sex	2.8	1.3-6.3
Man's $CD4^+$ cell count $\leq 400/mm^3$	4.9	2.1-11.2
Man with AIDS	1.4	0.4-4.7
Awareness of man's infection	0.2	0.0-1.1
History		
Syphilis or genital herpes	1.4	0.2-8.8
Genital warts	33.3	4.5-244.1
Vaginitis	4.9	2.4-10.2
Intrauterine device use	3.1	1.4-7.1
Oral contraceptive use	0.5	0.3-1.0

Abbreviation: CI, confidence interval.
(Courtesy of Lazzarin A, Saracco A, Musicco M, et al: *Arch Intern Med* 151:2411-2416, 1991.)

is an important mechanism of HIV transmission. The woman's awareness of her partner's seropositivity is an important preventive factor. Oral contraceptives may decrease risk, whereas use of an intrauterine device appears to increase risk.

▶ With the steadily increasing incidence of AIDS among heterosexual individuals, the findings of this study provide important information for patient counseling. Several other studies have shown that an average of only 15% of women who are regular sexual partners of HIV-infected men acquire the infection, and the chance of a woman becoming infected after a single exposure to an infected male is very low. Thus, heterosexual intercourse is a necessary—but not sufficient—condition for transmission of the HIV virus. The factors that reduce the frequency of transmission include use of condoms and oral contraceptives, and avoidance of anal intercourse. Use of condoms is the greatest factor for preventing HIV transmission. Women with vaginitis or genital warts should have these conditions treated if their sexual partners are infected with HIV to possibly reduce the risk of transmission.—D.R. Mishell, Jr., M.D.

Intravenous Immunoglobulin Therapy for Toxic Shock Syndrome

Barry W, Hudgins L, Donta ST, Pesanti EL (Univ of Connecticut, Farmington; Dept of Veterans Affairs Med Ctr, Newington, Conn)

JAMA 267:3315–3316, 1992 16–19

Objective.—Treatment of toxic shock syndrome traditionally has relied on maintaining hemodynamic and respiratory function and antibiotic treatment. There have been no reported attempts to supplement these measures with neutralization of the responsible toxins. A case of a woman with toxic shock syndrome, which was caused by a toxin-producing strain of *Streptococcus pyogenes* that responded to intravenous immunoglobulin (IVIG) after showing no response to conventional therapy, was presented.

Case Report.—Woman, 32, was admitted to the hospital with sore throat, fever, nausea, vomiting, diarrhea, and diffuse macular rash. Vital signs were temperature, 38.9°C; pulse, 120 beats per minute and regular; blood pressure, 88/60 mm Hg; and respirations, 20 to 24 per minute. The patient had a fine morbilliform, blanching rash over her trunk and proximal limbs. She was started on vigorous fluid resuscitation and oxacillin sodium, 2 g, administered intravenously every 4 hours, and aztrenonam sodium, 2 g, administered intravenously and followed by 1 g given every 12 hours. However, the hypotension was uncorrected and the tachypnea began to worsen. The patient's fingertips were a dusky red, and she complained that they were exquisitely tender. The respiratory rate increased to 40 breaths per minute in the intensive care unit. Arterial blood while the patient breathed 60% oxygen by mask showed a pH of 7.41, Pco_2 of 25 mm Hg, and Po_2 of 134 mm Hg. Her chest radiograph revealed worsening interstitial edema. The next day, cultures showed large amounts of group A β-hemolytic *S. pyogenes* organisms. Penicillin G, 2 million units administered intravenously every 4 hours, was started, and IVIG, .4 g/kg, was given over 6 hours in an attempt to reverse the patient's toxic state. Her condition was notably improved in the next 12 hours. The tachypnea and fingertip pain resolved, and her dyspnea improved subjectively along with improvement in arterial blood gas measurements.

Discussion.—Treatment with IVIG is associated with quick improvement in respiratory status, reversal of vasospastic changes in the fingers, and cessation of progressive subcutaneous edema. These benefits probably result from neutralization of the *S. pyogenes* toxin by infused antibodies.

► Although a single case report does not have the validity of a series of reports, the dramatic improvement noted with intravenous immunoglobulins after failure to improve with large doses of intravenous antibiotics is noteworthy and warranted selection of this abstract. Perhaps such therapy may be lifesaving in other instances of severe toxic shock syndrome.—D.R. Mishell, Jr., M.D.

17 Endocrinology

Inhibin Concentrations Throughout the Menstrual Cycles of Normal, Infertile, and Older Women Compared With Those During Spontaneous Conception Cycles

Lenton EA, de Kretser DM, Woodward AJ, Robertson DM (Jessop Hosp for Women, Sheffield, England; Monash Univ, Melbourne, Australia)

J Clin Endocrinol Metab 73:1180–1190, 1991 17–1

Introduction.—Previous studies have shown that plasma inhibin levels are detectable throughout the normal menstrual cycle. Inhibin profiles were obtained during menstrual cycles of women with 2 normal and 2 abnormal types of cycles.

Methods.—Plasma immunoreactive inhibin levels were measured daily in 7 women with spontaneous conception cycles, in 8 women with apparently normal nonconception menstrual cycles, in 7 infertile women with luteal phase defects, and in 6 perimenopausal women. Daily luteinizing hormone (LH), follicle stimulating hormone (FSH), progesterone, and estradiol plasma levels were also measured.

Results.—During the follicular and early luteal phases of the normal nonpregnant cycles, the inhibin levels were significantly greater than those in spontaneous conception cycles. After implantation, inhibin levels increased to levels in excess of those seen at any time in the nonconception cycles (Figs 17–1 and 17–2). Whereas progesterone levels increased within 24 hours of the first detectable increase in human chorionic gonadotropin, inhibin levels did not increase until 3 days later. After this point, inhibin levels increased serially and in parallel with progesterone levels. Levels of LH and FSH were markedly suppressed after implantation. In cycles with luteal phase defects, follicular and early luteal inhibin levels were also greater than those in conception cycles, but this difference was only significant in the midfollicular phase. Follicular phase inhibin levels in perimenopausal cycles were lower than those in normal menstrual cycles and cycles with luteal phase defects, but they were not distinguishable from those in conception cycles. Perimenopausal estradiol levels were significantly lower during the early follicular phase, whereas follicular and luteal FSH levels were significantly greater than those during conception cycles. The FSH and estradiol levels around menstruation in perimenopausal cycles showed a far closer temporal association between FSH and estradiol than between FSH and inhibin.

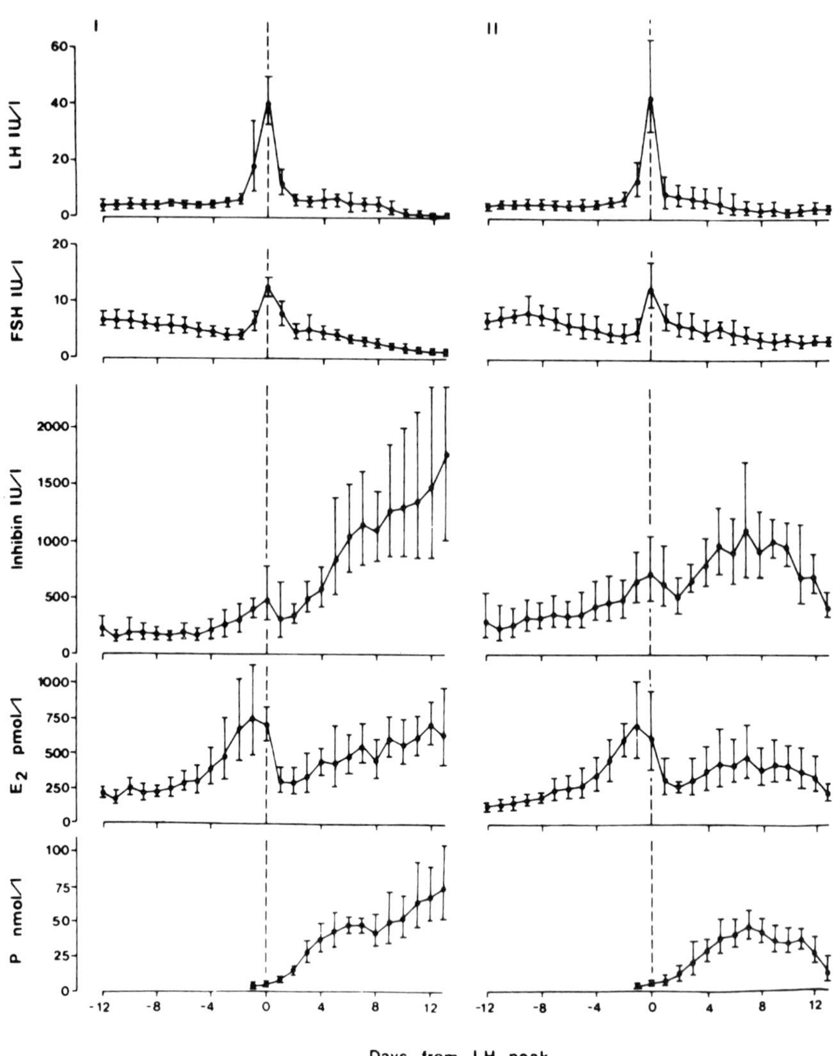

Fig 17–1.—Geometric mean concentrations (and 68% confidence intervals) of LH, FSH, inhibin, estradiol (E_2), and progesterone (*P*) in groups I (spontaneous conception cycles) and II (apparently normal nonconception cycles). (Courtesy of Lenton EA, de Kretser DM, Woodward AJ, et al: *J Clin Endocrinol Metab* 73:1180–1190, 1991.)

Conclusion.—Inhibin levels increase and decrease throughout the menstrual cycle in a manner similar to, but at specific times significantly different from, that of estradiol and progesterone. Inhibin is a peptide of granulosa cell origin that may be an indicator of the follicular pool size during the early stage of the cycle. Furthermore, there is no clear evidence of a negative feedback relationship between inhibin and FSH. In

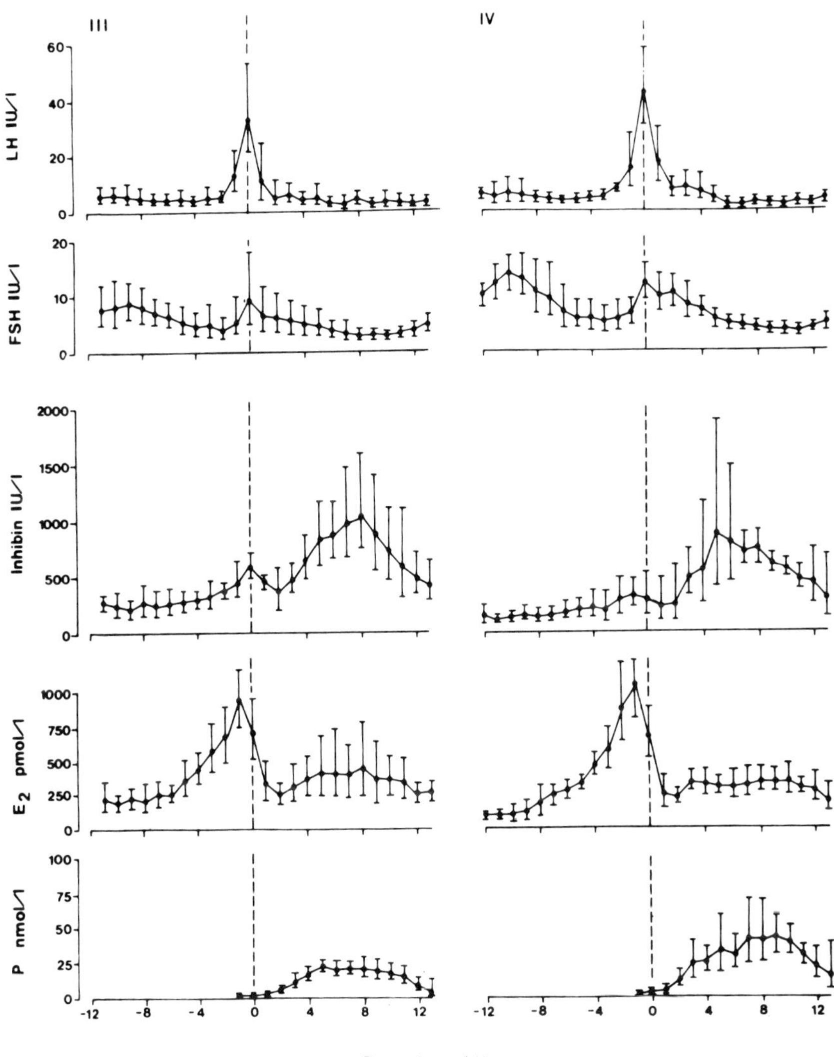

Fig 17–2.—Geometric mean concentrations (and 68% confidence intervals) of LH, FSH, inhibin, estradiol (E_2), and progesterone (*P*) in groups III (infertile women with defective luteal phases) and IV (regularly cycling women older than 40 years). (Courtesy of Lenton EA, de Kretser DM, Woodward AJ, et al: *J Clin Endocrinol Metab* 73:1180–1190, 1991.)

the early follicular phase, estradiol seems to be a better candidate for this role.

▶ Inhibin is a peptide hormone produced by granulosa cells during the follicular phase of the cycle and in the corpus luteum during the luteal phase. The authors have developed an assay for measurement of this hormone in serum and have enhanced our understanding of this recently isolated hormone. Inhibin is detectable in the serum throughout the normal menstrual cycle; there are 2 peaks—one at midcycle and the other in the midluteal phase. The levels are about twice as high in the midluteal phase as in the follicular phase, which indicates that the corpus luteum is a major source of inhibin in the human.—D.R. Mishell, Jr., M.D.

The Return of Postpartum Fertility Monitored by Enzyme-Immunoassay for Salivary Progesterone

Bolaji II, Tallon DF, Meehan FP, O'Dwyer EM, Fottrell PF (University College, Galway, Ireland)

Gynecol Endocrinol 6:37–48, 1992 17–2

Objective.—More knowledge of the events involved in returning postpartum ovarian function is needed before lactational amenorrhea can be fully exploited as a means of regulating fertility. Relatively few attempts have been made to identify the return of fertility by salivary steroid determinations.

Methods.—A solid-phase enzyme immunoassay for estimating salivary progesterone and estrone uses horseradish peroxidase as the label. Thirty postpartum women with uneventful singleton term deliveries were studied. Twenty of them elected to breast-feed their infants. Daily progesterone profiles were recorded, and ovulation was inferred from a sustained increase to above 251 pmol/L.

Results.—The mean duration of breast-feeding was 84 days. Eighty percent of lactating women and all those who did not lactate began menstruating within a year of giving birth. Initial menses occurred after 57 days in the nonlactating women and at 123 days in those who were breast-feeding. Seven lactating women (35%) ovulated before the first menses. The mean interval from delivery to initial ovulation was 88 days in the lactating women and 65 days in those who did not lactate. No woman ovulated in the first month after delivery. The peak salivary levels of progesterone, but not estrone, increased progressively from the first cycle to the second and later cycles.

Conclusion.—The acceptability of frequent saliva sampling and the availability of a rapid assay for salivary progesterone make this a convenient means of monitoring the return of fertility after delivery.

▶ Nearly all women who nurse their infants post partum and do not use any supplemental feedings will not ovulate during the first 6 months post partum as long as they remain amenorrheic. However, most nursing women in urban areas introduce some form of supplemental feeding before the infant is 6 months old and then are at risk for ovulation and conception. Because approximately 30% of the initial menses are preceded by ovulation, the possibility of conception occurring before menses resumes is not uncommon. Unfortunately, detecting an increase in progesterone will also occur after ovulation is instituted; therefore the value of daily progesterone measurement appears to be of little benefit.—D.R. Mishell, Jr., M.D.

Total Body Bone Density in Amenorrheic Runners

Myerson M, Gutin B, Warren MP, Wang J, Lichtman S, Pierson RN Jr (Columbia Univ, New York)

Obstet Gynecol 79:973–978, 1992 17–3

Purpose.—Amenorrhea secondary to endurance training was thought to be reversible upon reduction of training. It is now believed that amenorrhea-associated hypoestrogenemia contributes to bone loss similarly as in the menopause, and that bone mass may not be completely replaced upon the resumption of menses. Using dual-photon absorptiometry, total body bone mineral content and total body bone mineral density, as well as regional bone mineral density were measured in 13 amenorrheic runners, 13 eumenorrheic runners, and in 12 sedentary controls, all ranging in age from 21 to 35 years.

Methods.—The runners had run at least 40 km per week for at least the past 3 years. Amenorrheic runners reported that they had had fewer than 3 menstrual periods in the past year; the mean duration of amenorrhea was 4.2 years.

Results.—Eumenorrheic runners were significantly heavier than amenorrheic runners, but there was no significant difference in the percentage of body fat between the 2 groups of runners. Amenorrheic women had significantly lower estradiol and progesterone values than eumenorrheic women. Both groups of runners had similar estimated lifetime calcium intakes. The amenorrheic runners had significantly lower total body bone densities and total bone mineral contents in the trunk and spinal regions of the body than eumenorrheic runners, and they had values similar to those of the sedentary controls. After adjusting for body weight, the differences in total bone density and bone mineral content were no longer statistically significant, but values for the lumbar spine approached significance, with controls greater than eumenorrheic runners and the latter greater than amenorrheic runners.

Conclusion.—The benefit of running plus adequate estrogen levels result in higher bone mineral densities in eumenorrheic runners, whereas the benefit of running in amenorrheic runners is counteracted by the negative effect of hypoestrogenemia. The lower bone densities in amenorrheic runners appear to be proportional to their lower body weight.

▶ Estrogen deficiency leads to increased rates of bone resorption and osteoporosis in young women as well as postmenopausal women. Weight-bearing exercise does not prevent this bone loss, and because it is difficult to increase rates of bone formulation, the osteoporosis is usually not reversible.

For this reason, amenorrheic runners should be advised to take estrogen to reduce their risk of fractures.—D.R. Mishell Jr., M.D.

Evidence for Existence of Immunoglobulins That Block Ovarian Granulosa Cell Growth ***in Vitro*****. A Putative Role in Resistant Ovary Syndrome?**

van Weissenbruch MM, Hoek A, van Vliet-Bleeker I, Schoemaker J, Drexhage H (Academic Hosp of the Vrije Universiteit, Amsterdam; Erasmus Univ, Rotterdam, The Netherlands)

J Clin Endocrinol Metab 73:360–367, 1991 17–4

Background.—Among women with premature ovarian failure (POF), some have premature depletion, or atresia, of the follicles, and some have immature follicles. The latter condition is generally referred to as "resistant ovary syndrome". Immunoglobulin G (IgG) may block the trophic action of follicle-stimulating hormone (FSH) in many patients with POF.

Patients and Findings.—Serological studies were performed in 26 patients with POF, aged 18–38 years. In 5 patients, IgG obtained from their own serum blocked the stimulatory action of FSH on rat granulosa cell DNA synthesis. For each patient, blocking was optimal at different IgG concentrations. Concentrations of antihuman IgG of 10^{-3} or more

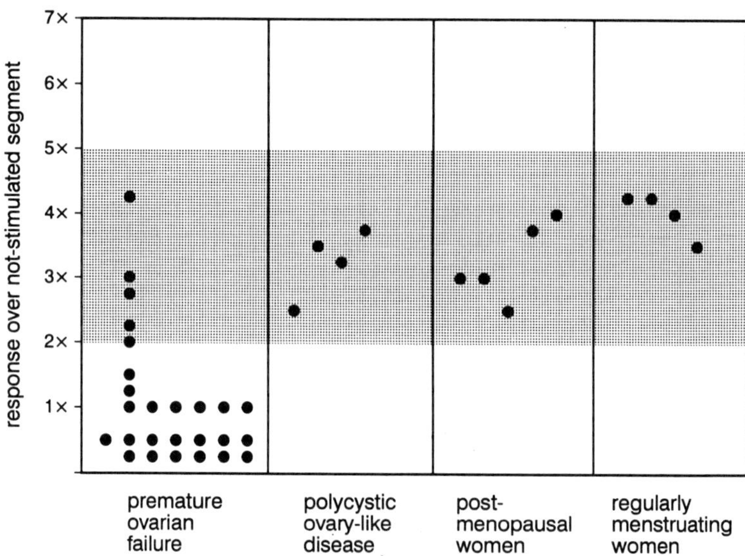

Fig 17–3.—The optimal growth blocking effect on FSH-induced DNA synthesis exerted by IgG preparations from patients with POF (n = 26). The minimal growth effect of the control subjects was also included. The *shaded area* represents the range of value with .5 units/L pituitary FSH. None of the control IgGs showed blocking effects. (Courtesy of van Weissenbruch MM, Hoek A, van Vliet-Bleeker I, et al: *J Clin Endocrinol Metab* 73:360–367, 1991.)

neutralized the blockade. In in vitro studies of rat ovarian segments, none of 13 IgG preparations obtained from controls blocked DNA synthesis, whereas 81% of the preparations from the POF group did (Fig 17–3). Fourteen of these 21 patients had resistant ovary syndrome, 12 proven by biopsy and/or intermittent response to gonadotropin treatment; specific diagnostic data were lacking in the other 7. In the 5 women who were negative for ovarian blocking IgGs, lack of follicles was the predominant finding.

Conclusion.—Immunoglobulin G may block FSH-stimulated granulosa DNA synthesis in approximately 80% of patients with POF. Further studies are needed to ascertain the exact prevalence of this finding, but it provides further evidence that immune mechanisms are involved in many cases of POF.

▶ The results of this study indicate that a high proportion of young women with POF have the resistant ovary syndrome, and that this syndrome is associated with an abnormality of their immune system. If these results are confirmed, the presence of increased levels of an IgG that blocks FSH activity in vitro may be used to establish a diagnosis of resistant ovaries without the necessity of performing an ovarian biopsy. In contrast to premature ovarian failure caused by a lack of ovarian follicles, which cannot be treated, this cause of premature ovarian failure may be able to be treated with corticosteroids or intermittent gonadotropin-releasing hormone.—D.R. Mishell Jr., M.D.

Effect of Estrogen Replacement Therapy on Bone Mineral Content in Girls With Turner Syndrome

Mora S, Weber G, Guarneri MP, Nizzoli G, Pasolini D, Chiumello G (Univ of Milan, Italy)

Obstet Gynecol 79:747–751, 1992 17–5

Introduction.—Osteoporosis is a common complication of Turner syndrome. Because estrogen deficiency is closely associated with osteoporosis, it is postulated that lifelong estrogen deficiency maybe the cause of osteopenia in Turner syndrome.

Study Design.—The prevalence of osteoporosis was assessed in 49 untreated patients with Turner syndrome. The effect of estrogen replacement therapy on bone mineralization was studied in 27 patients who started replacement therapy before or after 12 years of age and in 9 patients who were followed up prospectively for a mean 3.17 years. Bone mineral content was measured by single-photon absorptiometry at the distal third of the right radius.

Results.—In untreated patients, radial bone mineral content was below the 95% normal confidence interval in 89.8% of the patients (Fig 17–4). Bone mineral content correlated positively with weight and body

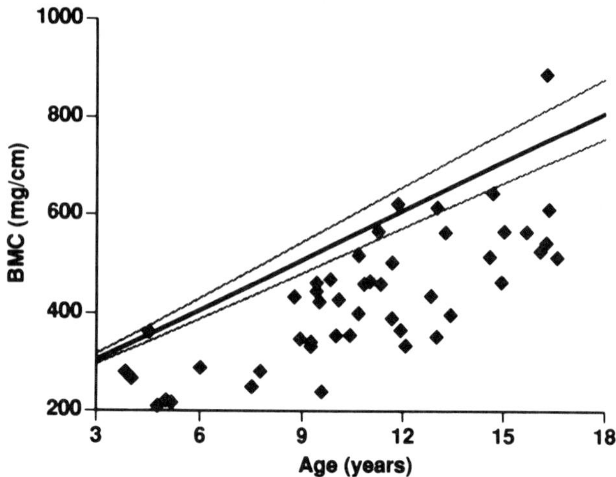

Fig 17–4.—Bone mineral content (BMC) values of 49 untreated patients with Turner syndrome, plotted against the normal BMC curve ± 95% confidence interval (*dotted lines*). (Courtesy of Mora S, Weber G, Guarneri MP, et al: *Obstet Gynecol* 79:747–751, 1992.)

mass index, and the Δ in bone mineral content correlated inversely with patients' ages. Estrogen replacement therapy was started in 16 girls before and in 11 girls after 12 years of age. The mean bone mineral content Δ in the early-treated group was significantly less than that in the late-treated group. Likewise, in patients followed up prospectively after estrogen replacement therapy, bone mineral content Δ values changed significantly during the first 2 years of treatment. However, bone mineral content did not normalize during the replacement therapy.

Implications.—Estrogen deficiency per se is not the primary cause of osteoporosis in young girls with Turner syndrome. Estrogen replacement therapy prevents further decreases in bone loss, but it fails to normalize the low bone mineral content. Early treatment is preferable to preserve bone mineral content in these patients.

▶ Estrogen deficiency at any time of life leads to increased rates of bone resorption without affecting rates of bone formation. Administering estrogen to women with estrogen deficiency will reduce the rates of bone resorption to the normal range without increasing the rate of bone formation. Therefore, it is possible to prevent osteoporosis by administering exogenous estrogen (as shown in this study); however, it is not possible to completely reverse the process once bone loss has occurred. The same effects of estrogen deficiency and estrogen replacement occur postmenopausally.—D.R. Mishell Jr., M.D.

Clinical History and Outcome of 59 Patients With Idiopathic Hyperprolactinemia

Sluijmer AV, Lappöhn RE (Academisch Ziekenhuis Groningen, The Netherlands)

Fertil Steril 58:72–77, 1992 17–6

Purpose.—There is little information on the natural history of hyperprolactinemia, and there have been very few long-term prospective studies of the idiopathic form of the disease. A long-term follow-up study was done to gain more insight into the clinical course of idiopathic hyperprolactinemia.

Patients.—The subjects were 59 women who had hyperprolactinemia with no demonstrable cause. Ten chose to refrain from medical treatment (group 1); 33 had been treated with bromocriptine but were drug free for at least 6 months before final follow-up (group 2); and 16 were receiving drug treatment throughout the study period (group 3). The median follow-up was 78 months. In group 1, prolactin (PRL) levels increased in 7 patients, but 7 were symptom free at final follow-up. The final PRL levels and symptoms were no different between women who had and had not been pregnant. In group 2, normal PRL levels were achieved by 28 patients, and 20 conceived during treatment. The mean PRL decreased significantly after delivery and lactation, and it normalized in 13 cases. Overall, there were no significant deteriorations in serum PRL. In the 7 patients with persistent disease, postpartum pituitary imaging was normal. Altogether in group 2, 21 women had normal PRL values at final follow-up, 2 had a decrease of more than 50%, and

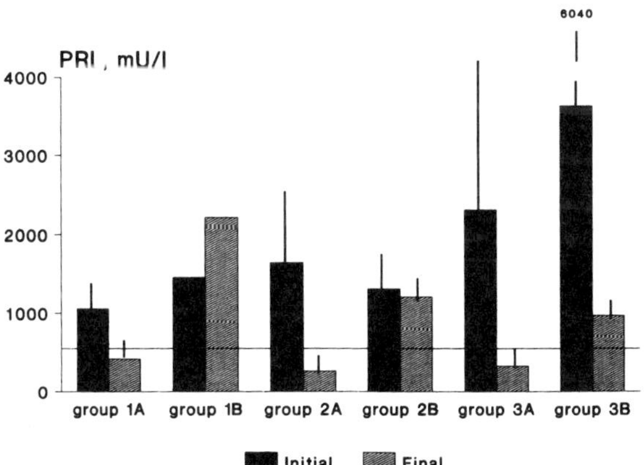

Fig 17–5.—Initial (*darkly shaded bar*) and final (*lightly shaded bar*) prolactin (PRL) levels (means ± standard deviation) in idiopathic hyperprolactinemia. The *horizontal line* represents the upper normal level of serum PRL. *Group 1* (n = 10): no treatment. *IB:* 2 patients using oral contraceptives. *Group 2:* ever treated patients. 2A (normal final PRL): n = 21; 2B (PRL still high): n = 12. *Group 3:* 16 patients still using dopaminergic drugs at final exam. A (normal final PRL): n = 13; *B* (PRL still high): n = 3. (Courtesy of Sluijmer AV, Lappöhn RE: *Fertil Steril* 58:72–77, 1992.)

10 had no change. All but 1 patient in group 3 had a regular menstrual cycle with normal midluteal progesterone values. In all 3 groups, the PRL levels either decreased or were unchanged in all patients but 1 (Fig 17-5). Findings of repeat pituitary imaging studies were normal. Proportions of women who did and did not get pregnant were similar in groups 1 and 2.

Conclusion.—Patients with idiopathic hyperprolactinemia appear to seldom—if ever—progress to prolactinoma. The condition seems to be self-limiting, with a course that is unaffected by administration of dopaminergic drugs or by the occurrence of pregnancy. The need for treatment in these patients is doubtful. In this study, only group 1 illustrates the natural course of the disease.

▶ The results of this longitudinal study indicate that it is not necessary to treat idiopathic hyperprolactinemia unless the subject: (1) wishes to ovulate; (2) is bothered by galactorrhea; or (3) has low estrogen levels, which may cause osteoporosis. In the latter instance, estrogen can be given, instead of bromocriptine; however, bromocriptine should be given for the first 2 problems. If the initial pituitary imaging is normal, there is no need to repeat this examination.—D.R. Mishell, Jr., M.D.

Long-Term Effects of Time, Medical Treatment and Pregnancy in 176 Hyperprolactinemic Women

Crosignani PG, Mattei AM, Severini V, Cavioni V, Maggioni P, Testa G (Univ of Milano, Italy)

Eur J Obstet Gynecol Reprod Biol 44:175–180, 1992 17–7

Background.—Because of the widespread use of medical treatment for hyperprolactinemia, there is little knowledge of its natural evolution. Changes in prolactin (PRL) concentrations were followed in hyperprolactinemic women who were undergoing medical treatment, were pregnant, or were "just waiting," to evaluate the independent effects of treatment, pregnancy, and time in this condition.

Methods.—A total of 176 women with hyperprolactinemia were observed for a mean of 45 months. They had a mean basal PRL level of 97 ng/mL. Eighty-seven women had CT evidence of pituitary tumors; the most common clinical presentation was amenorrhea. Prolactin-reducing treatment was given in 107 patients. Forty-six had a normal sella, and 61 had prolactinoma. They were treated with a variety of drugs, and doses were tailored for most women to achieve normoprolactinemia. Seventy-three women became pregnant, in most cases as a result of the medical treatment. Finally, 38 patients were followed up for a mean of 19 months with no pregnancy or other relevant endocrine factor. Serum PRL levels were categorized as unchanged, which could include an increase or a decrease of less than 50%; halved, which indicates a decrease of at least 50% but levels still greater than 20 ng/mL; and normalized, with levels 20 ng/mL or less.

Results.—The initial PRL concentrations were 79 ng/mL for the 89 patients with functional hyperprolactinemia and 87 ng/mL for those with pituitary adenoma; the final PRL concentrations were 52 and 87 ng/mL, respectively. Levels became normal in 26% of "functional" patients, halved in 16%, and doubled in 8%. In patients with adenoma, the PRL levels normalized in 12%, halved in 21%, and doubled in 10%.

After 1 or more cycles of treatment, PRL became normal in 17% of functional patients, halved in 20%, and doubled in 4%. For the prolactinoma group, these figures were 10%, 13%, and 10%, respectively. In the pregnant women, PRL decreased significantly only in those women with a normal sella, becoming normal in 36% of the functional patients, halved in 21%, and increased in only 5%. For pregnant patients with prolactinoma, the PRL levels normalized in 17%, halved in 24%, increased in 10%. In the "just waiting" group, no significant changes were seen in either subgroup, nor were there any changes in the sella. Analysis showed that there were significantly more normalized or improved patients in the pregnancy group. Dopaminergic treatment yielded a lesser but still significant cure rate in functional patients only.

Conclusion.—Medical treatment seems to reduce PRL concentrations in 35% of functional patients and 20% of those with microadenoma. The most active PRL-reducing agent is pregnancy, with improvement in 50% of idiopathic cases and 40% of patients with adenoma. "Functional" hyperprolactinemia is improved preferentially by both pregnancy and medical treatment.

► The results of this Italian study are in agreement with the Dutch study reported in Abstract 17–6 for patients with functional hyperprolactinemia. In addition, the results of this study show that many women with microadenoma also develop markedly decreased and/or normal prolactin levels over time, with an increased likelihood of this happening if they become pregnant. Thus, these results indicate that pregnancy is a beneficial, not deleterious, event for women who have a prolactin secretory pituitary microadenoma, and that serial pituitary imaging is unnecessary after the diagnosis of a microadenoma or functional hyperprolactinemia is established.—D.R. Mishell, Jr., M.D.

Pituitary Enlargement With Suprasellar Extension in Functional Hyperprolactinemia Due to Lactotroph Hyperplasia: A Pseudotumoral Disease

Peillon F, Dupuy M, Li JY, Kujas M, Vincens M, Mowszowicz I, Derome P (Hôpital Pitié-Salpêtrière, Paris; Hôpital Foch, Suresnes, France; Hôpital Necker; Paris; Hôpital Lariboisière, Paris)

J Clin Endocrinol Metab 73:1008–1015, 1991 17–8

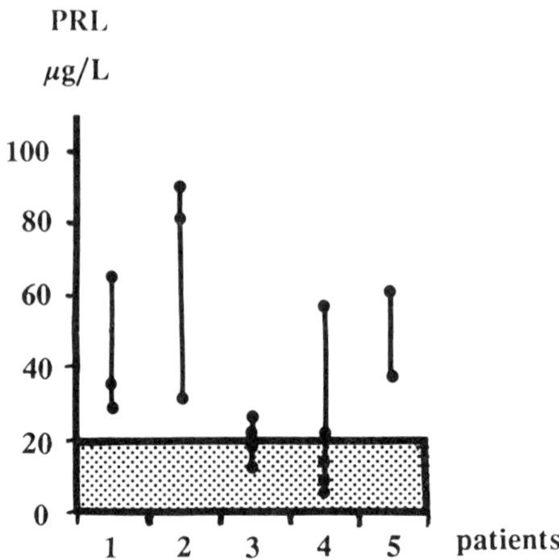

Fig 17–6.—Basal plasma PRL in the 5 patients with functional hyperprolactinemia. Each point (*circles*) corresponds to assays performed in the same patient at different intervals. The normal basal plasma PRL level is less than 19 μg/L. (Courtesy of Peillon F, Dupuy M, Li JY, et al: *J Clin Endocrinol Metab* 73:1008–1015, 1991.)

Introduction.—In addition to the well-documented prolactin (PRL)-secreting adenomas, there exists a large spectrum of functional hyperprolactinemic states. Data were reviewed on 5 women with functional hyperprolactinemia in whom a PRL-secreting adenoma was suspected because of an enlarged pituitary gland on CT or MRI, but in whom no adenoma was found at operation.

Methods.—Of the 5 patients, aged 21–38 years, 4 had oligomenorrhea with or without galactorrhea and 1 had amenorrhea with galactorrhea; 2 patients complained of infertility. Basal serum PRL levels were determined in the morning after an overnight fast and 15 minutes of rest, 2–6 times per patient, on different days for each patient.

Results.—All 5 patients had basal plasma PRL values ranging from slightly increased to high, but repeated sampling also showed normal values in 2 of them (Fig 17–6). However, all 5 patients had a large PRL response to thyrotropin-releasing hormone. On plain skull films and hypocycloidal polytomography, the sella turcica was normal in size. There was no reduction in thickness of the cortical bone and no pathologic double contour of the floor. In contast, the CT or MRI scans of all 5 patients showed an intrasellar mass with suprasellar extension. All patients were operated on by the transsphenoidal route, but no pituitary adenoma was found. Surgical biopsy specimens were obtained from 4 patients, and 3 biopsy specimens showed lactotroph hyperplasia.

Conclusion.—This study demonstrates the existence of a new syndrome of pseudotumoral functional hyperprolactinemia, which may mimic a PRL-secreting adenoma on CT or MRI scans.

► Lactotroph hyperplasia is a cause of hyperprolactinemia, and it may be misinterpreted as a prolactin-secreting adenoma when sensitive pituitary imaging techniques are used. Because the natural history of prolactin secretory microadenomas is benign, as reported in Abstracts 17–6 and 17–7, their treatment should be medical, with bromocriptine, rather than surgical removal. Even the uncommon large macroadenomas, which can cause blindness by compression of the optic stalk, are best treated initially with bromocriptine.—D.R. Mishell Jr., M.D.

Women With Polycystic Ovary Syndrome Wedge Resected in 1956 to 1965: A Long-Term Follow-Up Focusing on Natural History and Circulating Hormones

Dahlgren E, Janson PO, Johansson S, Mattson L-Å, Lindstedt G, Crona N, Knutsson F, Lundberg P-A, Odén A (Sahlgrenska Hosp, Göteborg, Sweden; Östra Hosp, Göteborg)

Fertil Steril 57:505–513, 1992 17–9

Objective.—The reported prevalence of polycystic ovary syndrome (PCOS) among women of child-bearing age varies from 3.5% to 7.5%. A hormonal imbalance in women with PCOS is well documented. Whether this imbalance in women with PCOS continues into and after the menopause was investigated.

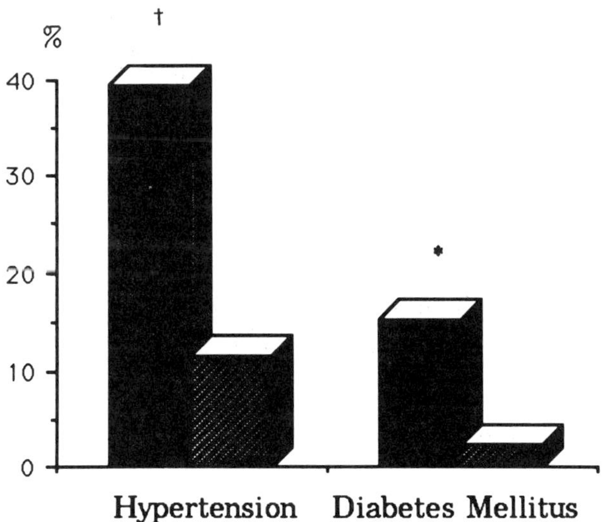

Fig 17–7.—Prevalence of hypertension (medically treated) and manifest diabetes mellitus in 33 subjects with PCOS and 132 referents. *Filled bars* show subjects with PCOS; *striped bars* show referents. Statistical comparisons were made between women with PCOS and referents. The differences were considered significant at $^*P \leq .05$ and $^\dagger P \leq .001$. (Courtesy of Dahlgren E, Janson PO, Johansson S, et al: *Fertil Steril* 57:505–513, 1992.)

Methods.—The study population consisted of 49 women with histopathologically confirmed PCOS who had undergone either ovarian resection or oophorectomy for benign disease between 1956 and 1965. Thirty-eight of the 49 women showed typical histopathologic findings. Thirty-three women with PCOS, who were aged 40–59 years at the time of the study, completed a questionnaire; 30 of them underwent a physical examination. A total of 132 age-matched referents selected from a population study of women completed a questionnaire, and 120 of them underwent a physical examination.

Results.—The mean age at menarche of the women with PCOS was 14 years, which was not statistically different from that in the referents. The duration of the menstrual period in menstruating women was 7.9 days for women with PCOS and 5.5 days for referents. Women with PCOS reported irregular periods more often than did referents. At the time of the study, 30.4% of the women with PCOS and 56.4% of the referents had entered the menopause. Hysterectomy had been performed in 21% of the women with PCOS and in 7% of the referents. None of the women had atypia or malignant cells in the vaginal smear. Infertility, hirsutism, and oligomenorrhea were more common among women with PCOS. Women with PCOS had a marked increase in the prevalence of central obesity, higher basal serum concentrations of insulin, and a higher prevalence of diabetes mellitus and hypertension than referents (Fig 17–7).

Conclusion.—The typical hormonal profile found in younger women with PCOS remains into and after menopause. Perimenopausal women with PCOS have an increased prevalence of hypertension and diabetes mellitus in addition to the classic symptoms of anovulation, hirsutism, and infertility.

▶ This paper is of interest because it is the first cohort follow-up study of women with PCOS until age of menopause. The problems of obesity, hypertension, and diabetes, as well as significantly increased concentrations of serum testosterone in the PCOS group, indicate that these women are at increased risk of having cardiovascular disease and should be counseled accordingly. The low incidence of endometrial atypia and malignancy in this group may be the result of increased premenopausal use of oral contraceptives because of irregular menses. Young women with PCOS are at increased risk of having endometrial hyperplasia and adenocarcinoma develop.—D.R. Mishell, Jr., M.D.

Peripheral Androgen Blockade Versus Glandular Androgen Suppression in the Treatment of Hirsutism

Carmina E, Lobo RA (Università di Palermo, Palermo, Italy; Univ of Southern California)
Obstet Gynecol 78:845–849, 1991 17–10

Objective.—Hirsutism in women has been attributed to increased peripheral androgen metabolism. The clinical efficacy of dexamethesone was compared with that of spironolactone in the treatment of hirsutism in women, and whether serum markers of ovarian, adrenal, or peripheral androgen production may be helpful determinants of treatment was determined.

Treatment.—Twenty hyperandrogenic women with hirsutism were treated for up to 2 years. Based on their sensitivity to dexamethasone, as assessed by a short-term dexamethasone suppression test, 11 women were treated with dexamethasone, .37 mg/day, and 9 received spironolactone, 100 mg/day, for at least 1 year. Thereafter, the 11 patients treated with dexamethasone were treated with the combination of dexamethasone and spironolactone for an additional year. Hirsutism was assessed using a modified Ferriman-Gallwey score.

Outcome.—For the patients treated with dexamethasone, the androgen levels were suppressed into the normal range, but the Ferriman-Gallwey scores decreased modestly by only 20%, although this decrease was significant. In contrast, for the patients treated with spironolactone, serum androgen levels did not change significantly; however, the Ferriman-Gallwey scores decreased significantly (by 47%). Thus, for both groups, the clinical responses after treatment did not correlate with changes in androgen levels. For the patients treated with a combination of dexamethasone and spironolactone, serum androgen levels were not significantly different from the levels obtained after dexamethasone treatment alone, but the Ferriman-Gallwey scores improved markedly.

Conclusion.—These data support the concept that peripheral androgen metabolism is the primary determinant of hirsutism in women. Measurement of serum androgen levels is not helpful in predicting the response to therapy.

▶ Women who are bothered by excessive hair growth do not care whether treatment reduces serum androgen levels. They want the treatment to decrease the amount of hair. The results of this study show that spironolactone, an agent that peripherally acts to decrease androgen action at the target organ more effectively decreases hair growth than dexamethasone, an agent that decreases androgen production, in a group of women with increased androgen levels. Spironolactone is also the best treatment for women with hirsutism and normal serum androgen levels, an entity that was previously called "idiopathic hirsutism" but is now known to be caused by an increased androgen metabolism in the target tissue. It usually is best to administer spironolactone with an estrogen-dominant oral contraceptive to prevent irregular bleeding and increase sex hormone–binding globulin (SHBG) levels.

Increasing SHBG keeps more serum testosterone bound and inactive and less serum in the unbound biologically active form.—D.R. Mishell, Jr., M.D.

Treatment of Hirsutism in Women With Flutamide

Marcondes JAM, Wajchenberg BL, Minnani SL, Samojlik E, Luthold WW, Kirschner MA (Hospital das Clinicas, Sao Paolo, Brazil; Newark Beth Israel Med Ctr, New Jersey)

Fertil Steril 57:543–547, 1992 17–11

Background.—Previous research has shown that cyproterone acetate given alone as a single monthly intramuscular dose was effective in the treatment of hirsute women. The clinical efficacy of a pure nonsteroidal antiandrogen, flutamide, was assessed in the treatment of hirsute women.

Methods.—Nine females, aged 17–33 years, were treated. Their hirsutism ranged from moderate to severe. Each woman was given flutamide, 250 mg, 3 times daily for 3 months. No estrogens were co-administered.

Results.—Seven patients had clinical improvement in the degree of their hirsutism. Their Ferriman-Gallwey scores decreased from a mean of 28.1 to 24.5. Two patients with eumenorrhea became oligomenorrheic. One became amenorrheic during treatment, and another woman with oligomeorrhea became amenorrheic while receiving flutamide therapy. Altogether, 4 of the 9 patients had menstrual cycle deterioration. Except for dry skin in 2 cases, no other serious side effects occurred. After 3 months of treatment, no significant changes were seen in any of the serum androgens or in the measured or calculated testosterone fractions. Basal luteinizing hormone and follicle-stimulating hormone levels were normal before and after therapy.

Conclusion.—Flutamide appears to affect hirsutism without influencing any of the hormonal parameters studied. More detailed, longer term trials are warranted.

▶ The treatment of hirsutism is a problem in the United States because the antiandrogen cyproterone acetate, which is successfully used to treat excess hair growth throughout the world, is not available here. A combination of a low-progestin-dose oral contraceptive plus spironolactone is frequently effective, but trials of other agents, such as the antiandrogen flutomide, are certainly warranted.—D.R. Mishell, Jr., M.D.

Experience With the First 250 Endometrial Resections for Menorrhagia

Magos AL, Baumann R, Lockwood GM, Turnbull AC (Royal Free Hosp, Lon-

don; John Radcliffe Hosp, Oxford, England)
Lancet 337:1074–1078, 1991 17–12

Background.—Transcervical resection of the endometrium (TCRE) is a hysteroscopic method of endometrial ablation similar to transurethral resection of the prostate. Using the electrocautery loop of a resectoscope (an instrument used for removal of submucous fibroids), the entire thickness of the endometrium is excised. The efficacy of the technique for the management of menorrhagia was evaluated in the first 250 consecutive endometrial resections performed on 234 patients.

Patients.—Sixteen patients had repeat procedures. The women's mean age was 42.3 years; 210 women were parous. The mean cycle length was 26.4 days, and the mean menstrual period was 8.4 days; 213 had been treated medically for menorrhagia. In all but 5 patients, the indication for surgery was abnormal menstruation; most women chose TCRE as an alternative to hysterectomy, and in 16, TCRE was considered medically preferable. In 170 women, menstruation was primarily heavy; in 70, it was heavy and painful; in 4, it was frequent, prolonged, or continuous; and in 1 it was painful. The only patient who was postmenopausal had menorrhagia while taking hormone replacement therapy.

Results.—In 238 cases, hysteroscopic surgery was successfully completed; in 11 cases, total resection was not possible. The principal complication was uterine perforation, which occurred in 4 patients. The few minor complications included postoperative hemorrhage, nausea, and infection. Two hundred three patients were followed up from 3 months to 2½ years. Fewer than 10% of the patients had no improvement in their periods. Most had lighter, shorter, and less painful periods. From 27% to 42% of patients achieved amenorrhea, and the satisfaction rate was more than 80%. Three patients who had repeat resections later underwent hysterectomy.

Conclusion.—Endometrial resection was beneficial whether or not menorrhagia was accompanied by dysmenorrhea, whether or not danazol was given preoperatively, and whether or not myomectomy was done at the same time. However, the results were less satisfactory in younger than in older women. Partial resection was less effective than total resection in improving menstrual symptoms, but patient satisfaction was higher after the first 6 postoperative months with partial than with total resection.

▶ Endometrial ablation with electrocautery by a resectoscope or rollerball, as well as by laser, is being used instead of hysterectomy for women with menorrhagia who have minimal or no uterine pathology and fail to respond to medical management with increasing frequency. Because this technique has only been used for a few years, it is extremely important to determine what the long-term effects of such therapy are. This large study of a consecutive group of patients with 3 months to 2½ years' follow-up after ablation provides useful information regarding this relatively short period of follow-up. However, as the authors state in the final sentence of their manuscript, the long-term results need to be assessed by life-long monitoring of these patients, and the value of the procedure needs to be compared with that of hysterectomy.—D.R. Mishell, Jr., M.D.

A Comparative Study of Danazol and Norethisterone in Dysfunctional Uterine Bleeding Presenting as Menorrhagia

Bonduelle M, Walker JJ, Calder AA (Glasgow Royal Infirmary, Glasgow, Scotland)

Postgrad Med J 67:833–836, 1991 17–13

Introduction.—Norethisterone and danazol are widely used in the treatment of primary menorrhagia. The efficacy of norethisterone has not been documented. In contrast, there is published evidence that danazol is effective. The efficacy and safety of norethisterone and danazol in the control of primary menorrhagia were compared in a randomized, open study.

Patients.—Thirty patients who received a diagnosis of dysfunctional uterine bleeding presenting as menorrhagia were entered into the study on the basis of clinical selection criteria. All patients had undergone physical examination and dilatation and curettage within the preceding 3–12 months to exclude underlying pathology. Fifteen patients were randomized to 3 treatment cycles with danazol, 200 mg, given once daily, and 15 were randomized to 3 cycles of treatment with norethisterone, 5 mg, taken 3 times daily from day 19 to 26. Six patients were subsequently excluded from analysis. Eight patients withdrew from the study, 4 in each treatment group. Bleeding intensity scores were obtained from daily scores assigned on a descriptive scale.

Results.—Bleeding intensity scores were significantly lower with danazol than with norethisterone for the third menses. Compared with baseline values, bleeding scores and the number of pads or tampons used were significantly improved with danazol, but not with norethisterone. The patients' overall assessments of their condition and of the efficacy of treatment showed no significant differences between the 2 treatments. However, during treatment, patients assessed their blood loss to be significantly less with danazol than with norethisterone. Two patients reported voice changes during norethisterone therapy. Seven norethisterone-treated patients and 8 danazol-treated patients complained of weight gain during treatment, but only 4 patients actually had gained more than 3 kg at the end of the study.

Conclusion.—Danazol is more effective than norethisterone in controlling menorrhagia.

▶ The medical treatment of menorrhagia caused by ovulatory dysfunction bleeding (without uterine pathology) is difficult. Effective methods of treatment include low-dose combination oral contraceptives, high doses of progestins, nonsteroidal anti-inflammatory agents, danazol, and GnRH analogs. Although this study indicates that a single 200-mg tablet of danazol is more effective than high doses of a progestin, danazol is expensive and has androgenic side effects. A combination of low-dose oral contraceptives and 500 mg of mefenamic acid given 3 times daily during menses is an effective initial therapy for this condition.—D.R. Mishell, Jr., M.D.

Effects of Mefenamic Acid on Menstrual Hemostasis in Essential Menorrhagia

van Eijkeren MA, Christiaens GCML, Geuze HJ, Haspels AA, Sixma JJ (Univ Hosp Utrecht, The Netherlands)

Am J Obstet Gynecol 166:1419–1428, 1992 17–14

Objective.—Prostaglandin synthesis inhibitors are the drugs of choice for essential menorrhagia. Studies have shown that these agents diminish menstrual blood loss by 30% to 50%. Although their mechanism of action is still poorly understood, an effect on menstrual hemostasis is assumed. The effects of prostaglandin synthesis inhibitors on menstrual hemostasis in essential menorrhagia were examined.

Patients.—Of 11 women scheduled for hysterectomy because of menorrhagia and whose menstrual blood loss exceeded 80 mL, 6 were randomly allocated to receive 500 mg of mefenamic acid 3 times daily, starting 5 days before the expected next menstruation. The other 5 patients were given placebo 3 times daily. The patients continued taking the tablets until menstrual bleeding had stopped. Menstrual blood loss was measured again, and 5 days before the next menstruation, the patients started to use the same tablets as during the study period. Vaginal or abdominal hysterectomy was performed with the patient under general anesthesia during the first 24 hours of menstruation. Light and electron microscopy were used for morphological and morphometric studies of the extirpated uteri.

Results.—The mean menstrual blood loss measured before the start of therapy did not differ between the 2 groups. In the mefenamic acid-treated patients, blood loss decreased by a mean of 40%; in 5 of them, menstrual blood loss decreased to within the normal range. Macroscopic examination showed dark red blood-engorged areas in all 11 uteri. Endometrial height did not differ between the 2 groups. However, the total number of vessels seen in light microscopy was significantly reduced in mefenamic acid-treated patients compared with placebo-treated patients. The uteri of women treated with mefenamic acid had fewer vessels without a hemostatic plug, their plugs were further transformed, their platelets were more firmly interdigitated and more degranulated, and more empty balloons and fibrin fibers were observed compared with the uteri of placebo-treated women. Menstrual blood loss in placebo-treated patients correlated positively with the number of both occlusive and nonocclusive hemostatic plugs. There were no differences between the 2 groups with respect to the diameters of the total number of vessels.

Conclusion.—Mefenamic acid appears to improve platelet aggregation and degranulation and increase vasoconstriction. How mefenamic acid causes further transformation of hemostatic plugs and increases vasoconstriction remains to be determined.

▶ One prostaglandin, thromboxane, increases hemostasis, whereas another, prostacycline, inhibits hemostasis. It is unclear why prostaglandin synthesis inhibitors, which should inhibit synthesis of both these prostaglandins, effectively reduce menstrual blood loss. Nevertheless, administration of mefenamic acid, the prostaglandin inhibitor, during the menses of women with ovulatory dysfunctional bleeding (as well as those with intrauterine device-induced menorrhagia) will decrease the amount of blood loss significantly and may also avoid the need for hysterectomy or endometrial ablation in women with menorrhagia and no anatomical uterine pathology.—D.R. Mishell, Jr., M.D.

The Combination of a Depot Gonadotrophin Releasing Hormone Agonist and Cyclical Hormone Replacement Therapy for Dysfunctional Uterine Bleeding

Thomas EJ, Okuda KJ, Thomas NM (Newcastle Gen Hosp, Newcastle-upon-Tyne, UK)

Br J Obstet Gynaecol 98:1155–1159, 1991 17–15

Background.—In theory, long-term therapy with a gonadotropin-releasing hormone (GnRH) agonist could be combined with cyclical hormone replacement therapy (HRT) to treat dysfunctional uterine bleeding by reducing menstrual loss while nullifying the hypoestrogenic side effects and bone demineralization. Whether a combination of a depot GnRH agonist and cyclical HRT reduces menstrual blood loss was determined.

Methods.—In this open, observational study, menstrual blood loss before, during, and after 3 months' treatment was compared. Blood loss was measured objectively. The participants were 20 women complaining of regular, heavy menstrual loss in whom no cause could be found. Each received depot goserelin combined with cyclical HRT.

Results.—Pretreatment menstrual blood loss ranged from 23 to 397 mL, with a median of 68 mL. Only 40% of the women had a greater than 80 mL loss per period. In the 3 treatment cycles, median blood loss was 30 mL, 16 mL, and 17 mL, respectively. There was a significant reduction in the median length of menstruation and the number of towels or tampons used per period in the third treatment cycle. The number of women complaining of dysmenorrhea, premenstrual symptoms, flooding, and clot passage also decreased significantly. Seventeen women reported hot flushes. Eighteen were completely satisfied with the treatment and would have continued it for more than 12 months.

Conclusion.—The combination of a depot GnRH agonist and cyclical HRT is a successful means of treating dysfunctional uterine bleeding. It also was well accepted. The main side effect—host flushes—occurred very infrequently, although they were severe in 2 cases. The occurrence of flushes in spite of the HRT suggests that the higher dose of estrogen, 2 mg, may be better in the future.

► Ovulatory dysfunctional uterine bleeding (heavy regular bleeding episodes without anatomical pathology) is difficult to treat medically. It is a frequent cause of hysterectomy when it occurs in women who have completed childbearing. The treatment described in this abstract is effective but expensive. Therefore, initially, it is best to try a combination of low-dose oral contraceptives combined with a nonsteroidal anti-inflammatory agent during the days of menstrual bleeding. This regimen also is effective, but it is associated with less expense than a GnRH agonist.—D.R. Mishell, Jr., M.D.

Nafarelin for Endometriosis: A Large-Scale, Danazol-Controlled Trial of Efficacy and Safety, With 1-Year Follow-Up

Doswell L, for the Nafarelin European Endometriosis Trial Group (Syntex Research, Palo Alto, Calif; Syntex Pharmaceuticals International, Maidenhead, Berkshire, England)

Fertil Steril 57:514–522, 1992 17–16

Background.—In a previous study, the gonadotropin-releasing hormone agonist analogue (GnRH-a) nafarelin acetate was found to be as effective as danazol in the treatment of endometriosis. The efficacy and safety of nafarelin and danazol for the treatment of endometriosis were further investigated.

Methods.—A total of 307 patients with laparoscopically diagnosed endometriosis were enrolled in a randomized, double-blind, double-dummy study. Nafarelin was given to 206, and danazol was given to 101. Treatment lasted for 6 months. Each patient used intranasal nafarelin, 200 μg, twice a day, and oral placebo capsules given 3 times a day or 200-mg danazol capsules given 3 times a day plus a placebo intranasal spray.

Results.—Endometriosis growth and symptoms improved significantly during treatment in both groups. After therapy, the symptoms returned, but their severity was less than at baseline. The group treated with danazol had an increase in mean body weight. Although serum glutamic oxaloacetic transaminase increased in both groups, it increased significantly

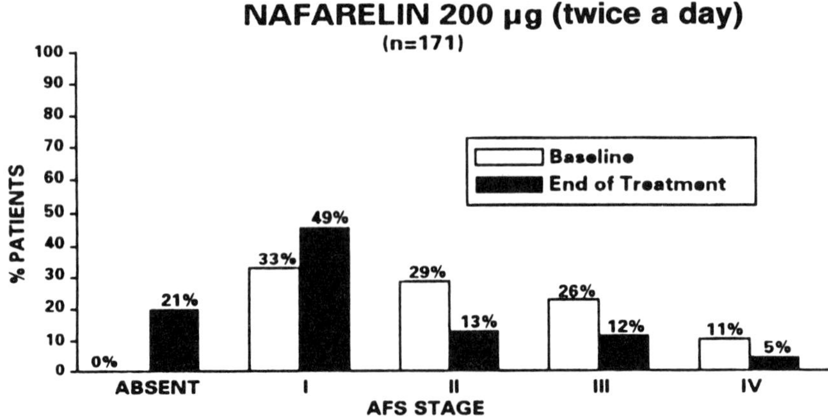

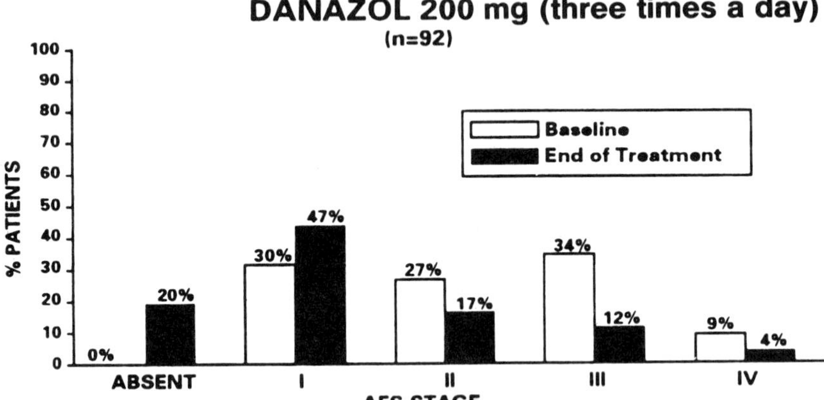

Fig 17–8.—Distribution of patients by American Fertility Society (AFS) stage at admission and end of 6-month treatment. The stages of AFS are 0 (absent, score = 0), I (minimal, 1–5), II (mild, 6–15), III (moderate, 16–40), and IV (severe, > 40). The difference between baseline and end of treatment was significant ($P < .001$, McNemar's test) within each treatment group with respect to the proportion of patients improving at least 1 stage. (Courtesy of Doswell L, for the Nafarelin European Endometriosis Trial Group: *Fertil Steril* 57:514–522, 1992.)

more in the danazol users. More nafarelin recipients had hot flushes (Figs 17–8 and 17–9).

Conclusion.—Nafarelin was therapeutically equivalent to danazol in the treatment of endometriosis, as demonstrated in the improvement rate of the laparoscopic score, American Fertility Society stage, total symptom severity score, and total symptom severity category. Although the physiological effects of nafarelin therapy are rapidly reversible, the treatment effects linger, leaving many patients asymptomatic or much improved as long as a year after the treatment has stopped.

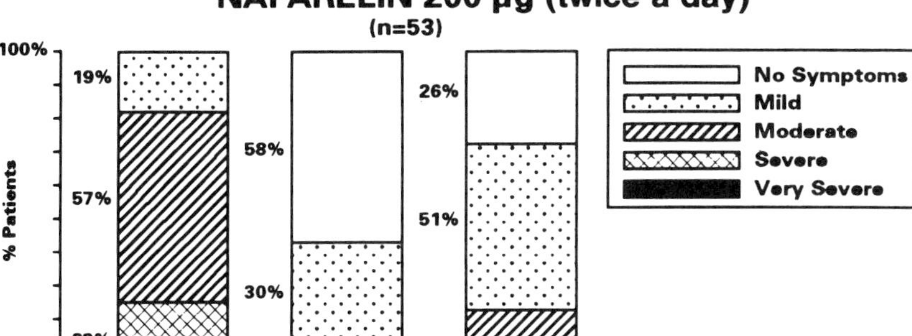

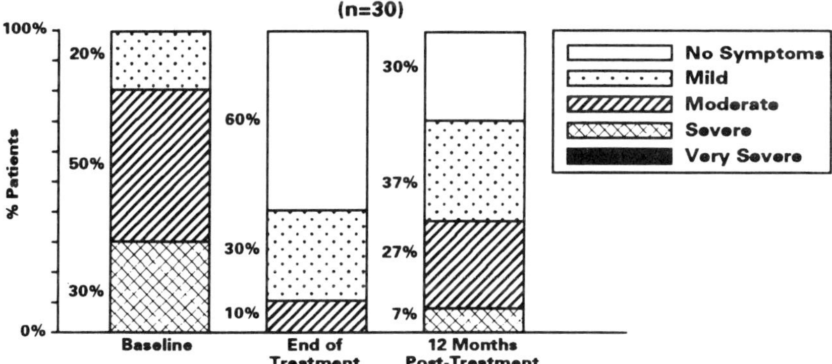

Fig 17–9.—Total symptom severity among patients completing 12-month follow-up. Total symptom severity score is the sum of 5 separate symptom scores from absent (0) to severe (3) on a 4-point scale. The differences from admission and from end of treatment to 12 months post-treatment were significant ($P < .001$, McNemar's test) within each treatment group with respect to the proportion of patients improving by at least 1 severity category. (Courtesy of Doswell L, for the Nafarelin European Endometriosis Trial Group: *Fertil Steril* 57:514–522, 1992.)

▶ Because they have less androgenic side effects than danazol, the use of GnRH agonists has become more popular than the use of danazol in the treatment of pelvic pain and dysmenorrhea associated with endometriosis. Clinicians should be aware that neither agent is approved for the treatment of infertility associated with endometriosis, because neither drug has been found to have higher pregnancy rates than placebo when given to infertile women with endometriosis.—D.R. Mishell, Jr., M.D.

Cholesterol Fractions and Apolipoproteins During Endometriosis Treatment by a Gonadotrophin Releasing Hormone (GnRH) Agonist Implant or by Danazol

Lemay A, Brideau N-A, Forest J-C, Dodin S, Maheux R (St Francois d'Assise Hosp, Laval Univ, Quebec

Clin Endocrinol 35:305–310, 1991 17–17

Background.—Several steroid-dependent gynecological conditions may respond to therapy with gonadotropic-releasing hormone (GnRH) agonist formulations. The gonadotroph is downregulated, thereby preventing the release of adequate luteinizing hormone and follicle-stimulating hormone. The effects of GnRH agonist and danazol on cholesterol fractions and subfractions and apolipoproteins were compared.

Methods.—Thirty-nine patients aged 22–37 years with endometriosis confirmed by laparoscopy entered the study. None had endometriosis severe enough to require surgery within the next 6 months. Twenty-six patients were randomized to receive the GnRH agonist goserelin, and 13 were randomized to treatment with danazol. Goserelin (3.6 mg) was injected under the skin of the lower abdominal wall every 29th day; danazol was given in the recommended maximum dosage (2 × 400 mg/day). Treatment was evaluated for 6 months.

Results.—At 1-month follow-up, the serum levels of estradiol were maintained in the menopausal range with goserelin and in the early follicular phase range with danazol. The patients in the goserelin group had significant increases of high-density lipoprotein-cholesterol (HDL-C) (31.4%), HDL_2-C (24.6%), and HDL_3-C (45.7%); changes in low-density lipoprotein-cholesterol (LDL-C), ApoA-1, and ApoB were not significant. Danazol increased LDL-C (10.5%) and ApoB (29%) and signifi-

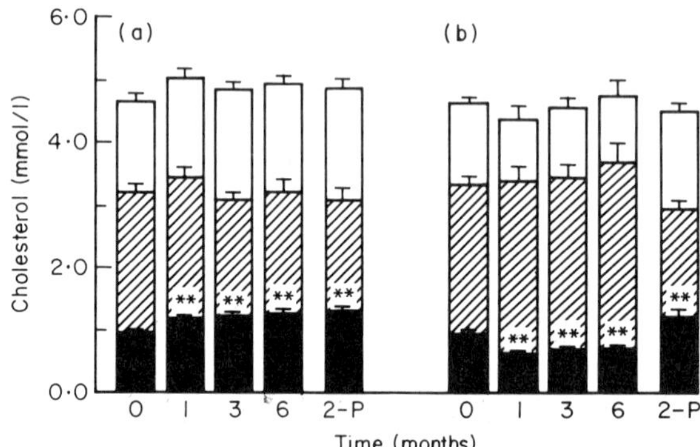

Fig 17–10.—Mean ± standard error of mean serum concentrations of total cholesterol (*open areas*); LDL-C *striped areas*, and HDL-C (*filled areas*) before treatment (0), at months 1, 3, and 6 of treatment, and at month 2 of post-treatment (2-P) (**a**) with goserelin; (**b**) with danazol. **$P < .01$ from pretreatment. (Courtesy of Lemay A, Brideau N-A, Forest J-C, et al: *Clin Endocrinol* 35:305–310, 1991.)

cantly decreased HDL-C (23.9%), HDL_2-C (56.6%), and ApoA-1 (35.6%). Overall, total cholesterol and LDL-C did not significantly change in either group. At 6 months, however, HDL-C had increased 31.4% with goserelin treatment and decreased 23.9% with danazol (Fig 17–10).

Conclusion.—Cholesterol metabolism is favorably affected by GnRH agonist treatment in patients with endometriosis. Although the adverse changes caused by danazol are temporary, this drug probably should not be used for prolonged treatment or in patients with increased baseline levels of cholesterol.

▶ This study confirms the fact that danazol has an adverse effect on serum lipoproteins, increasing the deleterious LDL-C and decreasing the beneficial HDL-C. For this reason, it is possible that prolonged use of this agent for 1 year or more may accelerate the development of atherosclerosis. It is unclear why the GnRH agonist treatment increased HDL-C in this study because it has been shown that, at the time of the menopause, when endogenous estrogen levels decrease, the HDL-C levels also decrease. Oral estrogen replacement reverses this pattern.—D.R. Mishell, Jr., M.D.

Danazol-Induced Hepatocellular Adenomas: A Case Report and Review of the Literature

Kahn H, Manzarbeitia C, Theise N, Schwartz M, Miller C, Thung SN (City Univ of New York)

Arch Pathol Lab Med 115:1054–1057, 1991 17–18

Introduction.—Danazol rarely has been implicated in the development of primary liver tumors. Only 2 cases of benign and 2 cases of malignant hepatocellular tumors associated with the use of danazol have been reported. In these previous cases, the women had received the drug for 2 to 4 years (table). The case report of a patient in whom multiple hepatocellular ademonas developed 6 months after the patient started danazol therapy was reviewed.

Danazol-Induced Liver Tumors

Source, y	Patient No./Sex/Age,y	Lesions	Daily Dosage, mg/Duration
Buamah,[2] 1985	1/F/49	HCC	200/2 y
Weill et al,[4] 1988	2/F/30	HCC	400/4 y
Middleton et al,[5] 1989	3/F/35	HCA	600/3 y
Fermand et al,[6] 1990	4/F/43	HCA	600-400/4 y
Present case	5/F/39	HCAs	600/6 mo

Abbreviations: *HCC*, hepatocellular carcinoma; *HCA*, hepatocellular adenoma.
(Courtesy of Kahn H, Manzarbeitia C, Theise N, et al: *Arch Pathol Lab Med* 115:1054–1057, 1991.)

Case Report.—A 39-year-old white woman was admitted with sudden onset of right upper quadrant abdominal and epigastric pain. A sonogram obtained the next morning revealed a large mass in the right lobe of the liver. The patient had used oral contraceptives for 8 months 20 years before admission. For the last 6 months before admission, she had been treated with danazol, 600 mg/day, to reduce fibroid tumors of the uterus. She underwent resection of the right-lobe liver mass. Pathologic examination was consistent with hepatocellular adenoma.

Remark.—This is believed to be the first case in which multiple hepatocellular adenomas were discovered after only 6 months of danazol therapy.

▶ Although a causal association between danazol use and development of liver adenomas in this patient cannot be established with certainty, an association between development of these liver tumors and ingestion of other anabolic and androgenic steroids is fairly well documented. There have been 4 other cases in the literature documenting liver adenomas developing in women who had been taking danazol for 2–4 years. Therefore, clinicians should be aware that hepatic adenomas can develop in women taking danazol, and they should palpate the right upper quadrant of the abdomen periodically in such women to determine whether a mass is present. If upper abdominal pain develops while the patient is taking danazol, a liver scan should be performed. Perhaps women who receive danazol for more than 1 year should have periodic liver scans performed in addition to periodic liver function tests.—D.R. Mishell, Jr., M.D.

18 Menopause

The Normal Menopause Transition

McKinlay SM, Brambilla DJ, Posner JG (New England Research Inst, Watertown, Mass)

Maturitas 14:103–115, 1992 18–1

Background.—Women in the United States and other western countries live an average of 75–80 years, which is approximately 30 years beyond the cessation of their menses. Despite this life expectancy, little is known about the normal range of experience concerning menopause. A large and comprehensive cohort study of mid-aged women provided, for the first time, stable estimates of parameters in the normal menopause transition.

Subjects.—A cohort of 2,570 women aged 45–55 years was selected from a random cross-section of 8,050 women who responded to mailed questionnaires. The cohort was made up of women who had menstruated in the preceding 3 months (defined as premenopausal) and had not undergone removal of the uterus and/or ovaries. The prospective study consisted of 6 telephone interviews at 9-month intervals during a 5-year follow-up with excellent retention of the subjects. A subset of the cohort consisted of women who were premenopausal rather than perimenopausal at baseline. Perimenopause was defined as 3–11 months of amenorrhea at 1 contact or increased menstrual irregularity at 1 contact, followed by more such irregularity or 3–11 months of amenorrhea at the next contact. Covariates include age, education, parity, body mass index, and current cigarette smoking.

Findings.—The estimated median age at last menstrual period was between 50 and 52 years in previous studies compared with 51.3 years from the baseline survey sample. The median age from the inception of perimenopause was 47.5 years, and the length of the perimenopausal transition was estimated at nearly 4 years. Current smoking was the only variable that affected menopause transition timing. Smokers tended to have an earlier and shorter perimenopause. The duration of perimenopause was associated with increased physician consultations and might be associated with the rate of hot flash reporting. The rates for symptoms showed an increase in perimenopause and a compensatory decrease in the postmenopause.

Conclusion.—For the first time, data is available on the entire transmenopausal process in a general, community-dwelling, representative sample of women. One important finding is that nearly 10% of women cease menstruating abruptly without perimenopause. This study is valuable because of the low rates of hormone therapy among the study population. As hormone therapy is increasingly prescribed in perimenopause, it will be difficult to replicate this study.

▶ Estrogen production by the ovary does not abruptly stop at the time of menopause. Instead, ovarian estrogen production gradually decreases during a period of several years. During this time, production of ovarian estrogen and circulating estrogen levels usually fluctuate, which leads to menstrual irregularity and the development of hot flushes before the menopause. If uterine bleeding occurs frequently, low-dose oral contraceptives can be used to cause regular bleeding episodes during this perimenopausal transition. If bleeding occurs at prolonged but irregular intervals and is heavy, then administration of a progestin for the first 10 days of each calendar month can be used to induce regular withdrawal bleeding before administration of sequential estrogen-progestin replacement therapy.—D.R. Mishell, Jr., M.D.

Early Menopause in Long-Term Survivors of Cancer During Adolescence

Byrne J, Fears TR, Gail MH, Pee D, Connelly RR, Austin DF, Holmes GF, Holmes FF, Latourette HB, Meigs JW, Strong LC, Myers MH, Mulvihill JJ (Natl Cancer Inst, Bethesda, Maryland; Information Management Services, Rockville, Md; California State Dept of Health Services, Emeryville; Univ of Kansas, Kansas City; Univ of Iowa, Iowa City; et al)

Am J Obstet Gynecol 166:788–793, 1992 18–2

Introduction.—The outcome of cancer during childhood or adolescence has improved greatly in the past 20 years. The first report on the

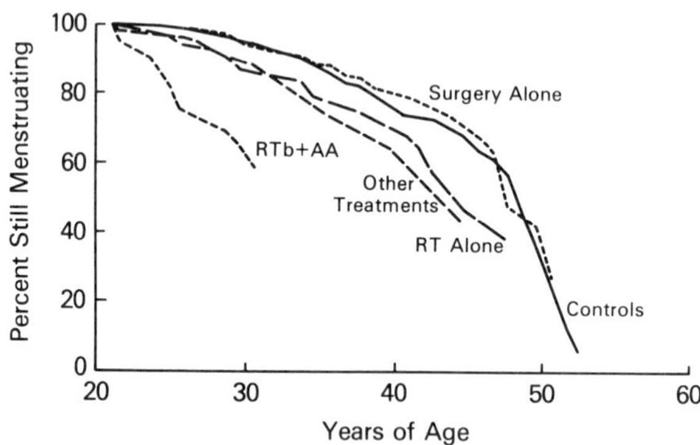

Fig 18–1.—Proportion still menstruating among cancer survivors who received their diagnosis between ages 13 and 19, grouped by type of treatment received compared with proportion of controls still menstruating (Kaplan-Meier curves). Survivor and control cohorts only. *RTb + AA*, Radiotherapy below diaphragm plus alkylating agents. (Courtesy of Byrne J, Fears TR, Gail MH, et al: *Am J Obstet Gynecol* 166:788–793, 1992.)

risks for early menopause among long-term survivors of adolescent cancer was reviewed.

Patients.—A total of 1,067 women in whom cancer was diagnosed before 20 years of age, who were at least 5-year survivors, and who were menstruating after 21 years of age were interviewed. Self-reported menopause status, classified as well by treatment received, was compared with that in 1,599 control women.

Outcome.—Of the 1,048 survivors, 94 (9%) had reached menopause by age at cohort entry. Compared with controls, women given their diagnosis after 12 years of age were significantly more likely to become menopausal at an earlier age, whereas women given their diagnosis before 12 years of age were not at greater risk, except for women with Hodgkin's disease. Of those with cancer diagnosed between the ages of 13 and 19 years, the risk of menopause was 4 times greater than in controls by ages 21 to 25, and it decreased at later ages. The greatest increase in risk was among women in their early 20s, who were treated with both radiation below the diaphragm and alkylating agents (RTb + AA) (relative risk [RR]= 27.39). The risk was also increased significantly among women treated with alkylating agents alone (RR, 9.17) and those treated with radiation alone (RR, 3.66). The menopausal rate for women treated with surgery alone (RR, 1.12) did not differ significantly from that of control women. The median age at menopause was 32 years for women treated with RTb + AA compared with 44 years among women treated with radiotherapy alone or other therapies (Fig 18–1).

Conclusion.—The risk for early menopause is substantial among long-term survivors of adolescent cancer who are still menstruating by 21 years of age. Considering the increasing use of radiation and chemotherapy and the continued trend toward delayed childbearing, these women should be advised of their smaller window of fertility.

▶ This study provides useful information regarding duration of ovarian function for counseling young women treated for malignancy. It is interesting that women treated with chemotherapy before puberty (while the ovary is quiescent) were less likely to have ovarian damage than women treated after cyclic ovarian function had been initiated.—D.R. Mishell, Jr., M.D.

Estrogen Improves Psychological Function in Asymptomatic Postmenopausal Women

Ditkoff EC, Crary WG, Cristo M, Lobo RA (Univ of Southern California School of Medicine, Los Angeles)

Obstet Gynecol 78:991–995, 1991 18–3

Background.—Estrogen treatment has been suggested to improve mood and psychological function in postmenopausal women. This notion is controversial, however, because previous studies involved heterogeneous groups of subjects, were not double-blind, and included women experiencing somatic symptoms relieved by estrogen treatment. The effects of placebo and conjugated equine estrogens on psychological function in asymptomatic postmenopausal women were compared in a randomized double-blind study.

Methods.—Estrogen doses of .625 and 1.25 mg were tested in the 3-month study. The participants were 36 asymptomatic women, aged 45 to 60 years. The Minnesota Multiphasic Personality Inventory-168, the Profile of Adaptation to Life, and the Beck Depression Inventory were used to assess psychological function. Memory was evaluated using the Wechsler Adult Intelligence Scales, which measure digit span and digit symbol.

Findings.—All subjects were psychologically well adjusted. Both the income management scale of the Profile of Adaptation to Life and the Beck Depression Inventory improved in the estrogen groups, but these findings were not related to dose. Memory was not significantly affected.

Conclusion.—The direction of the changes in several of the scores of the Minnesota Multiphasic Personality Inventory suggested a trend of beneficial effects of estrogen treatment in this series of patients. Estrogen therapy may indeed improve the quality of life of postmenopausal women, even when they are symptom free.

► Several previous studies have suggested that estrogen replacement therapy is a mood elevator for postmenopausal women. This well-done study provides confirmation of the fact that estrogen replacement improves the mood of women who receive it. The women in this study did not believe they were depressed, but their mood still increased. For postmenopausal women who suffer symptoms of depression, estrogen replacement should be the initial form of therapy.—D.R. Mishell, Jr., M.D.

Estrogen Use and Depressive Symptoms in Postmenopausal Women

Palinkas LA, Barrett-Connor E (Univ of California, San Diego, La Jolla)

Obstet Gynecol 80:30–36, 1992 18–4

Background.—Several studies suggest that estrogen replacement therapy has antidepressant effects, but these studies were conducted mainly in selected cohorts. The potential antidepressant effects of estrogen replacement therapy were evaluated in a community-based sample of postmenopausal women.

Setting.—Using the Beck Depression Inventory, depressive symptoms during the previous 2 weeks were assessed in 1,190 women 50 years and older from Rancho Bernardo, California. Of these, 24.7% were current estrogen users. Categorical depression was defined as scores of 13 or higher on the Beck Depression Inventory. The mean depressive symp-

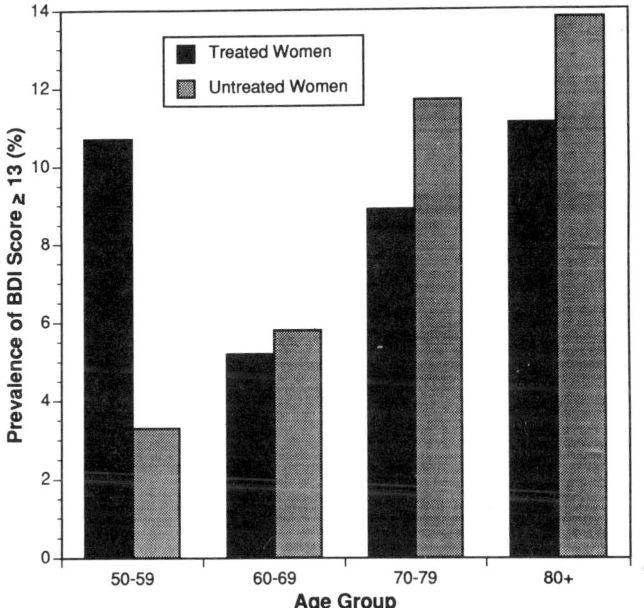

Fig 18–2.—Prevalence of Beck Depression Inventory scores of 13 or greater by age and hormone replacement therapy status. (Courtesy of Palinkas LA, Barrett-Connor E: *Obstet Gynecol* 80:30-36, 1992.)

tom scores did not differ among women taking estrogen with progestin, unopposed estrogen, or conjugated equine estrogen.

Findings.—Overall, the prevalence of depressive symptom scores of 13 or higher was 9%. Overall age-adjusted mean depressive symptom scores and the proportion of women with categorical depression did not differ significantly between current users and nonusers of estrogen. However, among women aged 50–59 years, current users had a significantly higher rate of categorical depression and higher mean depressive symptom scores than untreated women of the same age (Fig 18–2). In addition, treated women at 50–59 years of age were twice as likely to use antidepressants as were untreated women. After age 60, the mean depressive symptom scores and rates of categorical depression increased significantly in untreated women, but not in treated women. Similar effects were noted when depressive symptom measures were stratified by the number of years since the last menstrual period (LMP) (Fig 18–3). By 21 years after the LMP, treated women had a significantly lower mean depressive symptom score than did untreated women; however, the prevalence of categorical depression was increased among current users whose LMP was within 10 years.

Implications.—The greater depressive symptoms in current users of estrogen replacement therapy aged 50–59 years may reflect treatment selection bias, because more symptomatic depressed climacteric women

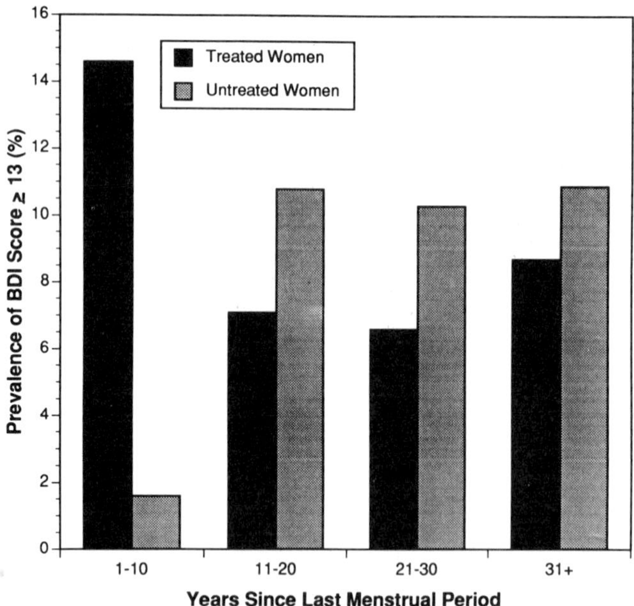

Fig 18–3.—Prevalence of Beck Depression Inventory scores of 13 or greater by years since last menstrual period and hormone replacement therapy status. (Courtesy of Palinkas LA, Barrett-Connor E: *Obstet Gynecol* 80:30–36, 1992.)

seek treatment. Furthermore, the reduced risk after 60 years of age may reflect a long-term benefit of estrogen replacement or selective discontinuation of estrogen by depressed women. Estrogen therapy provides relief of physical symptoms that can cause psychological distress.

▶ The results of this cross-sectional study showing decreased symptoms of depression among women older than 60 years who are taking estrogen replacement than among estrogen nonusers is in agreement with the randomized, blinded, prospective study of Ditkoff et al. (Abstract 18–3), as well as studies by Dennerstein et al. and Campbell and Whitehead. It appears that, after the perimenopausal years, estrogen acts as a mood elevator. This effect is another reason, in addition to the prevention of osteoporosis and atherosclerosis, for all postmenopausal women to receive estrogen replacement.—D.R. Mishell, Jr., M.D.

Postmenopausal Hormone Replacement Therapy Prevents Central Distribution of Body Fat After Menopause

Haarbo J, Marslew U, Gotfredsen A, Christiansen C (Univ of Copenhagen, Glostrup Hosp, Glostrup, Denmark)

Metabolism 40:1323–1326, 1991 18–5

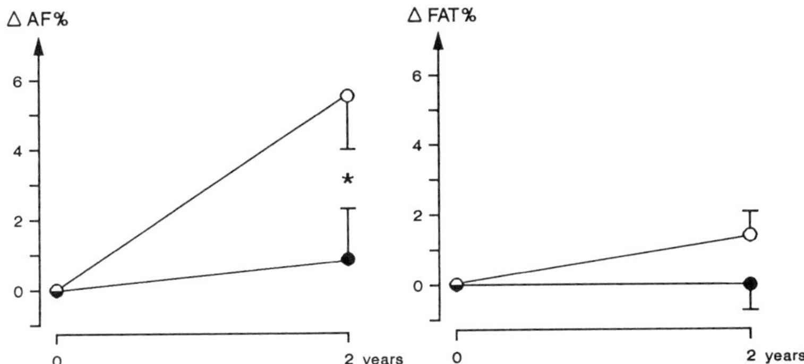

Fig 18–4.—Change in abdominal fat percentage (AF%) and total body fat percentage (FAT%) in the estrogen-progestogen group (*filled circles*) and placebo group (*open circles*). $^{*}P < .05$. (Courtesy of Haarbo J, Marslew U, Gotfredsen A, et al: *Metabolism* 40:1323–1326, 1991.)

Background.—The central distribution of body fat is an independent predictor of cardiovascular disease in women. Estrogen may be partly responsible for the peripheral distribution of body fat in premenopausal women; thus, menopause may induce a more central distribution of the body fat, thereby contributing to the increased risk of cardiovascular disease after menopause. The effect of menopause and hormone replacement treatment on body composition in early postmenopausal women was determined in a randomized prospective, controlled study.

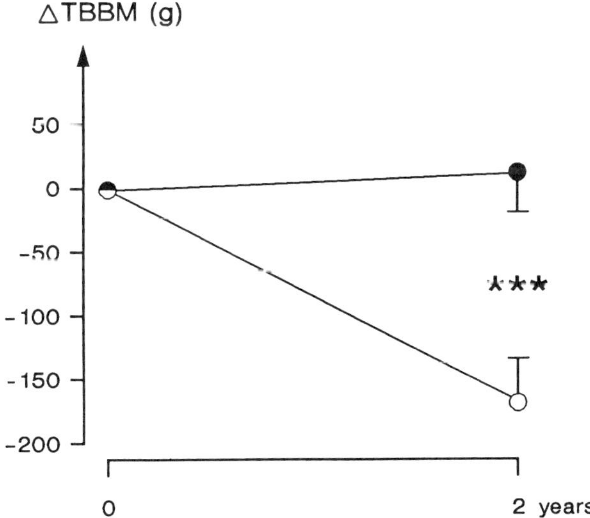

Fig 18–5.—Change in total body bone mineral in the estrogen-progestogen group (*filled circle*) and placebo group (*open circle*). $^{***}P < .001$. (Courtesy of Haarbo J, Marslew U, Gotfredsen A, et al: *Metabolism* 40:1323–1326, 1991.)

Method.—Seventy-five Danish postmenopausal women, aged 45 to 55 years, who had become menopausal 6 months to 3 years previously, were blindly assigned to treatment with 2 mg of estradiol valerate continuously combined with 1 mg of cyproterone acetate or sequentially combined with 75 μg levonorgestrel placebo. Sixty-two women, or 83%, completed the 2-year study.

Results.—All 3 groups were well matched. No significant differences in body composition were noted. The 2 hormone replacement groups were pooled thereafter. The abdominal fat percentage was virtually unchanged in the estrogen-progestogen group, and it increased significantly in the placebo group (Fig 18–4). Total body fat percentage tended to increase in the placebo group and was unchanged in the estrogen-progestogen group. Lean body mass tended to decrease in the placebo group, and it remained the same in the estrogen-progestogen group. The latter group also had unchanged total body bone mineral values, which were reduced significantly in the former (Fig 18–5).

Conclusion.—This study suggests that hormone replacement treatment prevents increases in abdominal fat that occur after menopause. Combined estrogen-progestogen therapy also appears to prevent bone loss after menopause and may maintain the premenopausal relationship between lean body mass and fat mass.

▶ These investigators have found another reason why estrogen replacement should be administered to all postmenopausal women without contraindications to its use. Perhaps some of the reluctance of most women to use estrogen replacement can be overcome if their physician informs them that estrogen will prevent a 5% increase in abdominal fat that will occur in 2 years if they do not take estrogen replacement.—D.R. Mishell, Jr., M.D.

Prevention of Postmenopausal Osteoporosis: A Comparative Study of Exercise, Calcium Supplementation, and Hormone-Replacement Therapy

Prince RL, Smith M, Dick IM, Price RI, Webb PG, Henderson NK, Harris MM (Sir Charles Gairdner Hosp, Nedlands, Australia; King Edward Mem Hosp for Women, Subiaco, Australia)

N Engl J Med 325:1189–1195, 1991 18–6

Background.—There is a high prevalence of bone fractures among women with osteoporosis. This represents a major public health problem for which prevention is critical. A double-blind, placebo-controlled, randomized study was conducted to compare the effects of 3 approaches to the prevention of osteoporosis: exercise, calcium supplementation, and hormone-replacement therapy.

Methods.—The study sample comprised 120 postmenopausal women (mean age, 56 years) with distal forearm bone density values less than

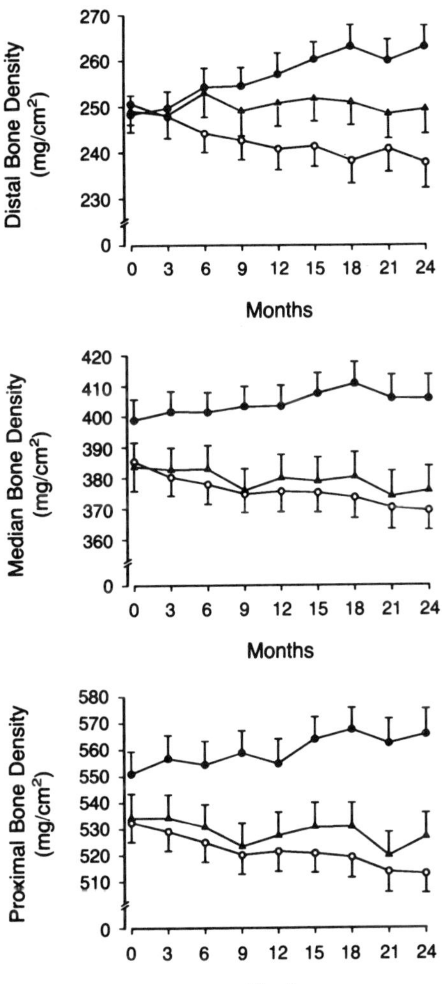

Fig 18–6.—Effects of the 3 interventions on bone density at distal, median, and proximal forearm sites during the 2-year study period. *Open circles* indicate exercise group; *solid triangles,* the exercise-calcium group; and *solid circles,* the exercise-estrogen group. The values shown are means ± SE for all women remaining in each group at the time indicated. After 2 years, there were 35 women remaining in the exercise group, 36 in the exercise-calcium group, and 32 in the exercise-estrogen group. (Courtesy of Prince RL, Smith M, Dick IM, et al: N *Engl J Med* 325:1189–1195, 1991.)

290 mg/cm². Forty-one women were assigned to an exercise program; 39 to exercise plus calcium lactate-gluconate, 1 g/day; and 40 to exercise plus medroxyprogesterone acetate, 2.5 mg/day, and estropipate, .625 mg/day for 1 month, followed by 1.25 mg day for the rest of the 2-year study period. Bone density at 3 forearm sites and indexes of calcium metabolism were measured periodically throughout the study, and symptom

scores were recorded (Fig 18–6). For comparison, a control group of 42 women with normal bone density was also followed.

Results.—The control group and the exercise group both lost significant bone at the distal forearm site; −2.7% and −2.6% of baseline per year, respectively. This compared with a decrease of −.5% in the exercise-calcium group and an increase of 2.7% in the exercise-estrogen group. At the median forearm site, bone loss was significantly less in the exercise-calcium group than in the exercise group, and it increased in the exercise-estrogen group. Forty-seven percent of the women in the exercise-estrogen group experienced breast tenderness, compared with only 20% of the other 2 treatment groups. Among women in the exercise-estrogen group who had not had hysterectomy, 52% had vaginal bleeding at some point, compared with 11% in the exercise group and 12.5% in the exercise-calcium group.

Conclusion.—Exercise and calcium supplementation or estrogen-progesterone replacement can slow or prevent bone loss in postmenopausal women with low bone density. Estrogen replacement is more effective in increasing bone mass than calcium supplementation, but it is also associated with more side effects. Osteoporosis may be prevented by bone-density screening and appropriate intervention.

▶ The dose of estrogen used in this study was greater than the amount recommended to prevent bone loss, .626 mg; therefore, the frequency of breast tenderness was greater than that which would occur with the physiological replacement dose of estrogen. Nevertheless, the results confirm what has been shown in numerous other studies, namely that estrogen replacement is much more effective than calcium supplementation and/or exercise in the prevention of bone loss and the reduction in the incidence of osteoporotic fractures postmenopausally.—D.R. Mishell, Jr., M.D.

Treatment of Postmenopausal Osteoporosis With Calcitriol or Calcium

Tilyard MW, Spears GFS, Thomson J, Dovey S (Univ of Otago, Dunedin, New Zealand)

N Engl J Med 326:357–362, 1992 18–7

Background.—The decrease in calcium intake and fractional intestinal absorption of calcium with increasing age may be factors in the pathogenesis of osteoporosis. Calcitriol (1,25-dihydroxyvitamin D_3) has been used to treat osteoporosis because of its ability to increase gastrointestinal absorption of calcium and to stimulate osteoblastic and osteoclastic activity in the skeleton. However, clinical trials of calcitriol therapy have produced conflicting results. Women with postmenopausal osteoporosis were studied in a randomized, 3-year trial to determine the effect of calcitriol on the incidence of vertebral fractures and to examine the safety of calcitriol in comparison with calcium supplementation.

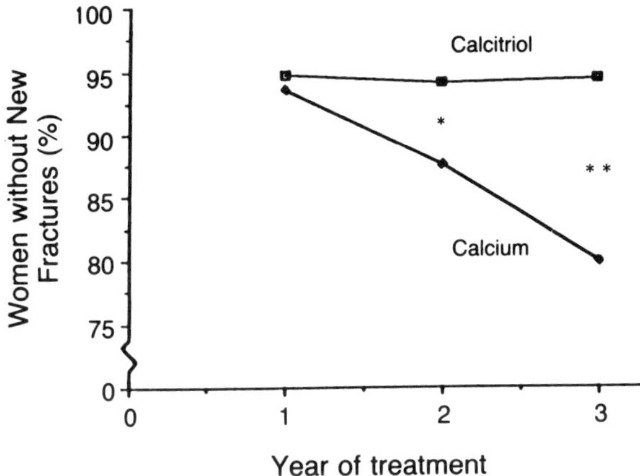

Fig 18–7.—Proportion of women in the calcitrol and calcium groups who did not have new vertebral fractures during the 3 years of study. In the comparisons of the treatment groups, a *single asterik* denotes $P < .01$, and a *double asterik* denotes $P < .001$. (Courtesy of Tilyard MW, Spears GFS, Thomson J, et al: *N Engl J Med* 326:357–362, 1992.)

Patients.—A total of 622 fully ambulatory postmenopausal women aged 50–79 years were enrolled in the study. The women had all sustained 1 or more vertebral compression fractures; new vertebral fractures were detected by annual lateral roentgenography of the spine. None of the women were taking estrogen for the treatment of osteoporosis. The women were randomized into a group of 314 who received calcitriol and a group of 308 who received calcium gluconate. Of the 622 women who were enrolled, 515 completed 1 year of treatment, 476 completed 2 years, and 432 completed 3 years.

Findings.—The women who received calcitriol and who had 5 or fewer vertebral fractures at base line had a significant reduction in the rate of new vertebral fractures during the second and third years of treatment compared with the women who received calcium. The calcitriol group had 11 peripheral fractures (including the hip, wrist, forearm, or other site) in 11 women, compared with 24 peripheral fractures in 22 women in the calcium group (Fig 18–7). Occurrence of side effects in the 2 groups was not significantly different. The most common side effect was gastrointestinal symptoms, usually nausea.

Conclusion.—Women randomized to receive calcitriol had a threefold reduction in the rate of new vertebral fractures compared with the women who received calcium. The effect of calcitriol was evident only after 2 years in the trial and only in those women who had mild-to-moderate osteoporosis. At a dosage of .25 μg twice a day, calcitriol had no important side effects, and it significantly reduced the rate of new vertebral fractures.

▶ Osteoporosis by itself is asymptomatic, but the fractures caused by osteoporosis can be debilitating or even fatal. A major advantage of this study is that fracture incidence, rather than bone density, was used as the parameter of treatment efficacy. For women with established mild-to-moderate osteoporosis, administration of calcitrol significantly reduces the occurrence of new vertebral fractures. Of course, it is much better to prevent or delay the development of osteoporosis by encouraging all postmenopausal women to receive estrogen replacement.—D.R. Mishell, Jr., M.D.

Low-Dosage Micronized 17β-Estradiol Prevents Bone Loss in Postmenopausal Women

Ettinger B, Genant HK, Steiger P, Madvig P (Kaiser Permanente Med Care Program, Oakland, Calif; Univ of California, San Francisco; Hologic, Inc, Waltham, Mass)

Am J Obstet Gynecol 166:479–488, 1992 18–8

Purpose.—Bone loss in women can be prevented or slowed by estrogen replacement. Studies have suggested that most patients can be protected by half the customary dosage of conjugated estrogen taken with calcium. A double-blind, randomized study used a dose-ranging design to test the degree of protection against bone loss resulting from micronized 17 β-estradiol.

Methods.—The subjects were 63 women, aged 40 to 58 years, who were within 5 years of menopause. The subjects were randomized to receive placebo or active treatment with micronized 17 β-estradiol, in doses of .5, 1, or 2 mg. Pills were given in a cyclic regimen on 23 of 28 days for 18 months. Oyster shell calcium also was given to increase calcium intake to more than 1,500 mg/day.

After this first phase of the study, the women enrolled in an open study of 1 mg of micronized 17 β-estradiol given for 25 days per month. Those with an intact uterus also were given medroxyprogesterone acetate, 10 mg per day, for the last half of the month. Usual diet was continued, but one third of subjects were randomized to stop taking calcium. Efficacy was assessed by quantitative CT to measure spinal trabecular bone mass; spinal dual-photon absorpimetry and radial single-photon absorpimetry also were done.

Results.—The subjects complied with treatment very well. All 3 treatment groups showed significant improvement in spinal trabecular bone density; the placebo group had a mean annual loss of 5% (Fig 18–8). Other bone density measurements tended in the same direction but were not significant. Greater increases in spinal trabecular bone density were seen in the 2 higher-dose groups. The mean menopause symptom score was unchanged in the placebo group but was reduced significantly in all 3 active treatment groups.

Forty-one women also completed phase 2. The women who stopped taking calcium supplements had an average daily dietary calcium intake similar to that in phase 1. The annual increase in spinal trabecular bone

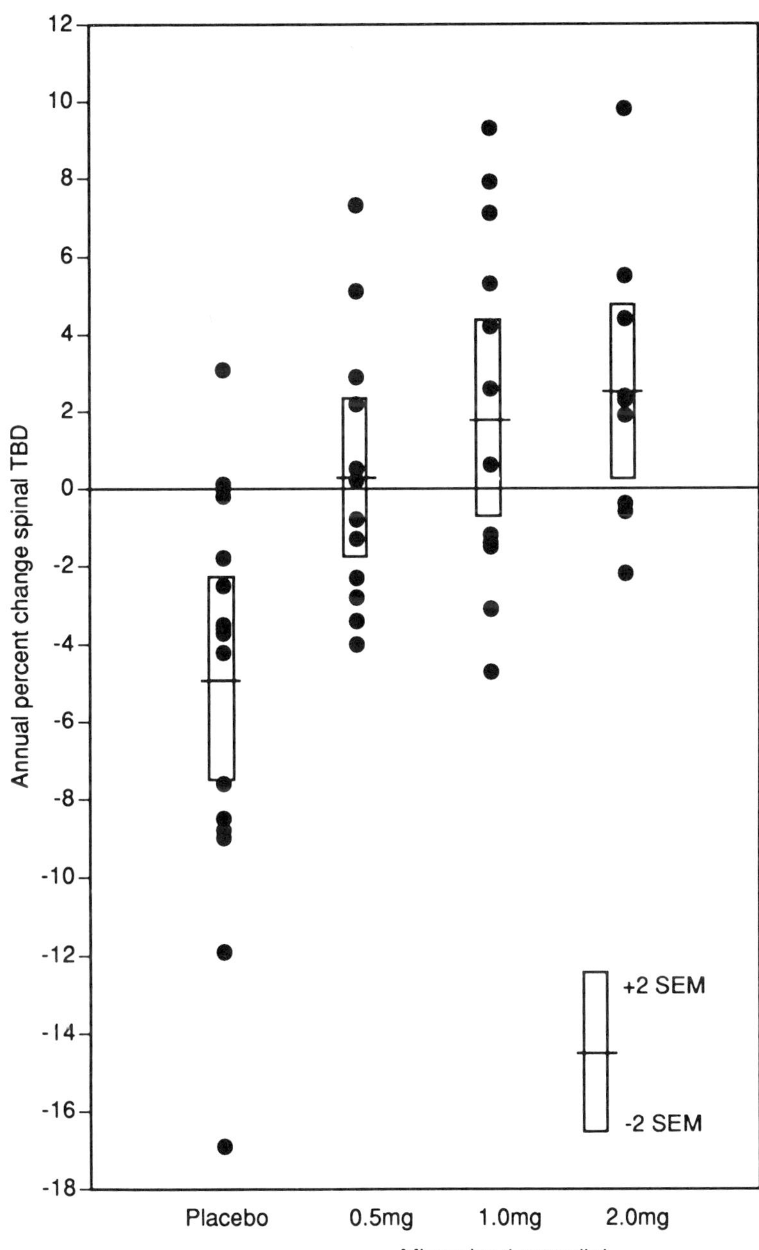

Fig 18–8.—The changes in mean (±2 SEM) annual percentage and each subject's spinal trabecular bone density (*TBD*) in 46 postmenopausal women given micronized estradiol (phase 1). All subjects received calcium supplements. (Courtesy of Ettinger B, Genant HK, Steiger P, et al: *Am J Obstet Gynecol* 166:479–488, 1992.)

density during this phase was 2%, with a significant positive correlation between total calcium intake and change in spinal trabecular bone density.

Conclusion.—At a dose range of .5 to 2 mg, micronized 17 β-estradiol has a continuous skeletal dose-response effect. At a dose of 1 mg, calcium intake appears to positively modify the skeletal response. No skeletal effects are detected for medroxyprogesterone, 10 mg/day, given for 12 days per month in the current study.

▶ For asymptomatic postmenopausal women, it has previously been determined that the minimal physiological replacement dose of conjugate equine estrogens that will prevent bone loss is .625 mg. A similar dosage of estrone sulfate also is necessary to prevent bone loss. Only .5 mg of micronized estradiol is necessary to prevent bone loss, but the lowest available dosage of this product is 1 mg, which also completely prevents postmenopausal bone loss. The results of this study suggest, but do not prove, that calcium supplementation is beneficial for women taking postmenopausal estrogen replacement. Other studies, however, indicate that calcium supplementation is unnecessary for women taking adequate dosages of estrogen, provided they ingest at least 500 mg of calcium daily in their diet.—D.R. Mishell, Jr., M.D.

The Effects of Plasma Estradiol Levels on Increases in Vertebral and Femoral Bone Density Following Therapy With Estradiol and Estradiol With Testosterone Implants

Garnett T, Studd J, Watson N, Savvas M, Leather A (King's College Hosp, London; Lister Hosp, London)

Obstet Gynecol 79:968–972, 1992 18–9

Background.—Percutaneous estradiol (E2) implants are used for estrogen replacement therapy. Cross-sectional studies have shown that E2 implants prevent postmenopausal bone loss, and it has been suggested that E2 implants are more effective than oral estrogen therapy. However, E2 implants are often given with testosterone (T). Whether T confers any additional bone-sparing effect was determined.

Patients.—The study was performed with 75 healthy postmenopausal women recruited from outpatient clinics. Of 50 women who requested hormone replacement therapy, 25 were randomly allocated to implants containing 75 mg of E2 alone and 25 to implants containing 75 mg of E2 and 100 mg of T. The implants were inserted in the subcutaneous fat of the anterior abdominal wall under local anesthesia every 6 months. Women with an intact uterus received norethindrone acetate, 5 mg/day, for the first 10 days of each calendar month. The 25 women who did not want hormone therapy served as controls. Bone density was measured at the lumbar spine, femoral neck, Ward triangle, and trochanteric and intertrochanteric regions at baseline and at 1 year.

Results.—At the end of the 1-year study, bone density at the lumbar spine had decreased by 1.8% in the control group, whereas it had increased by 7.8% in women treated with E2 alone and by 6.3% in women treated with E2 plus T. Bone density at the femoral neck had decreased by 3% in the control group and increased by 4% in both the E2 and the E2 plus T treatment groups. Bone density at the Ward triangle decreased by 3.5% in the control group and increased by 7.3% in the E2 group and by 5.6% in the E2 plus T group. There were no significant differences in bone density at any of the sites measured between women given E2 alone and those receiving E2 plus T. The increase in bone density was not associated with chronologic age, menopausal age, or initial bone density; however, bone density was significantly correlated with serum E2 levels after 1 year of hormone replacement therapy.

Conclusion.—The addition of T to an estrogen replacement regimen confers no additional bone-sparing effect in postmenopausal women.

▶ The high continuous amounts of E2 administered in this study resulted in mean E2 serum levels of approximately 150 pg/mL, which are several-fold higher than the E2 levels in the follicular phase of normal menstrual cycles, approximately 50 pg/mml. This amount of estrogen appears to increase bone density over time. Others have shown that oral estrogen, even in large amounts (1.25 mg of conjugated equine estrogen) does not increase bone density. Whether the increased bone density with high-dose estradiol implants will reduce the fracture rate in women with established osteoporosis has not been determined.—D.R Mishell, Jr., M.D.

Postmenopausal Estrogen Therapy and Cardiovascular Disease: Ten-Year Follow-Up From the Nurses' Health Study

Stampfer MJ, Colditz GA, Willett WC, Manson JE, Rosner B, Speizer FE, Hennekens CH (Harvard Med School and Brigham and Women's Hosp; Harvard School of Public Health)

N Engl J Med 325:756–762, 1991 18–10

Background.—The influence of exogenous hormones on the risk of cardiovascular disease has long been debated. Two studies came to opposite conclusions concerning the benefits of estrogen use in the risk of coronary disease. The results for coronary disease and stroke from a 10-year follow-up of a large cohort were assessed.

Methods.—A cohort of 48,470 postmenopausal women, aged 30–63 years, was followed up. These women were participants in the Nurses' Health Study, and they did not have a history of either cancer or cardiovascular disease at enrollment. During 337,854 person-years of follow-up, there were 224 strokes, 405 cases of major coronary disease, and 1,263 deaths from all causes.

Relative Risk of Cardiovascular Disease Among Current and Former Postmenopausal Hormone Users, as Compared With Those Who Never Used Postmenopausal Hormones

Group†	No. of Person-Years	Major Coronary Disease		Fatal Cardiovascular Disease		Total Stroke		Ischemic Stroke		Subarachnoid Hemorrhage	
		No. of cases	RR (95% CI)	No. of cases	RR (95% CI)	No. of cases	RR (95% CI)	No. of cases	RR (95% CI)	No. of cases	RR (95% CI)
No hormone use	179,194	250	1.0	129	1.0	123	1.0	56	1.0	19	1.0
Current hormone use	73,532										
Adjusted for age	—	45	0.51 (0.37–0.70)	21	0.48 (0.31–0.74)	39	0.96 (0.67–1.37)	23	1.26 (0.78–2.02)	5	0.80 (0.30–2.10)
Adjusted for age and risk factors	—		0.56 (0.40–0.80)		0.61 (0.37–1.00)		0.97 (0.65–1.45)		1.46 (0.85–2.51)		0.53 (0.18–1.57)
Former hormone use	85,128										
Adjusted for age	—	110	0.91 (0.73–1.14)	55	0.84 (0.61–1.15)	62	1.00 (0.74–1.36)	34	1.14 (0.75–1.74)	12	1.42 (0.70–2.90)
Adjusted for age and risk factors	—		0.83 (0.65–1.05)		0.79 (0.56–1.10)		0.99 (0.72–1.36)		1.19 (0.77–1.86)		1.03 (0.47–2.25)

Note: Relative risk determined after adjustment for age and multiple risk factors.

Abbreviations: RR, relative risk; *CI*, confidence interval.

*Women with no hormone use served as the reference category in this analysis. The risk factors included in the multivariate models were age (in 5-year categories), cigarette smoking (none, former, current [1-14, 15-24, and ≥ 25 cigarettes per day]), hypertension (yes, no), diabetes (yes, no), high serum cholesterol level (yes, no), parental myocardial infarction before the age of 60 years (yes, no), Quetelet index (in 5 categories), past use of oral contraceptives (yes, no), and time period (in 5 2-year periods).

(Courtesy of Stampfer MJ, Colditz GA, Willett WC, et al: *N Engl J Med* 325:756-762, 1991.)

Results.—After adjustment for age and other risk factors, the overall relative risk of major coronary disease in women currently taking estrogen was .56. Women with natural or surgical menopause had a significantly reduced risk. The duration of estrogen use appeared to have no effect, independent of age. The relative risk for current and former estrogen users compared with women who had never used estrogen was .89 for total mortality and .72 for mortality from cardiovascular disease. When current users were compared with those who had never used estrogen, the risk of stroke was .97, with no marked differences according to type of stroke (table).

Conclusion.—Current estrogen use is associated with a reduced incidence of coronary heart disease and mortality from cardiovascular disease in postmenopausal women. However, it is not associated with any change in the risk of stroke.

▶ There have been 15 other prospective studies comparing the effect of postmenopausal estrogen on cardiovascular disease, and all but 1 have found estrogen use to have a significantly protective effect. Although this study was not randomized, it is the largest and most carefully performed prospective study, and the results should solidify the belief that estrogen use retards the development of coronary atherosclerosis. Because cardiovascular disease is the major cause of death of postmenopausal women, use of estrogen postmenopausally prolongs a woman's lifespan substantially.—D.R. Mishell, Jr., M.D.

Effects of Estrogen Replacement Therapy on Serum Lipid Values and Angiographically Defined Coronary Artery Disease in Postmenopausal Women

Hong MK, Romm PA, Reagan K, Green CE, Rackley CE (Georgetown Univ, Washington, DC)

Am J Cardiol 69:176–178, 1992 18–11

Introduction.—Coronary artery disease (CAD) is the most common cause of death of women, but it generally occurs only after menopause. This has led to the suggestion that estrogen replacement therapy could confer cardioprotection. The lipid values and angiographic findings in women who were and were not receiving estrogen replacement therapy were studied.

Methods.—Ninety consecutive postmenopausal women undergoing diagnostic coronary angiography for chest pain were studied. Stenosis of 25% or more in 1 or more major coronary artery system(s) was considered to indicate CAD. Eighteen patients were taking estrogen.

Findings.—The mean ages were 58 years in the estrogen group and 63 years in the no-estrogen group. Body mass index and traditional cardiac risk factors were likewise different, but none of these differences attained significance. The estrogen group had a significantly higher mean high-density lipoprotein (HDL) cholesterol level and a significantly lower ratio of mean total to HDL cholesterol. The no-estrogen group had a higher mean low-density lipoprotein cholesterol level and a lower triglyceride level, but these differences were nonsignificant. Of the women who were not taking estrogen, 68% had CAD, compared with 22% of those who were taking estrogen. Thus, the odds ratio of CAD in a patient taking estrogen was .13. The strongest independent predictor of CAD was absence of estrogen use; the only other significant predictor was total/HDL cholesterol ratio.

Conclusion.—Estrogen use in postmenopausal women may decrease the risk of CAD, increase the HDL cholesterol level, and decrease the total/HDL cholesterol ratio. Because all patients were undergoing elective angiography, they represent neither postmenopausal women in the general population nor those with CAD.

▶ The findings of this study increase the steadily growing body of evidence that indicates that postmenopausal estrogen replacement retards the acceleration of coronary atherosclerosis in postmenopausal women. Many of the recent articles supporting this conclusion have appeared in journals, such as this one, which internists read. Therefore, our colleagues in internal medicine are now becoming convinced that estrogen replacement is good for the health of postmenopausal women, and many of them are now initiating postmenopausal estrogen therapy instead of stopping the treatment gynecologists have begun.—D.R. Mishell, Jr., M.D.

Estrogen Replacement Therapy and the Risk of Venous Thrombosis

Devor M, Barrett-Connor E, Renvall M, Feigal D Jr, Ramsdell J (Univ of California; San Diego School of Med, La Jolla)

Am J Med 92:275–282, 1992 18–12

Objective.—Many physicians believe that estrogen replacement therapy causes thrombophlebitis, and they will not use it for women at risk. However, there are few clinical data to support this association. The relationship between estrogen and thrombophlebitis, including other presumed thrombotic risk factors, was analyzed in a case-control study.

Methods.—The subjects were identified by examination of admissions of women, aged 45 years or older, during an 8-year period. A total of 121 women with a discharge diagnosis of thrombophlebitis, deep venous thrombosis, pulmonary embolism, or other venous thrombosis were thus identified. Two controls were identified for each patient, for a total of 236 participants. Subjects and controls were matched for age within 5 years, admission date within 1 year, admitting service, and method of payment. The mean patient age was 65.4 years.

Findings.—Estrogen use was reported by 5.1% of the subjects and 6.3% of controls. In all subjects and most controls, the hormones used were conjugated estrogens. The odds ratio for estrogen use as a risk factor for acute venous thrombosis was .79. Excluding those patients with a history of thrombosis and their matched controls, the odds ratio was .58; excluding patients younger than 50 years of age, the odds ratio was .69. Among the 74 patients with thrombosis on admission, the odds ratio was 1.12, and excluding "other venous thrombosis" cases—which usually are iatrogenic—the odds ratio was 1.35. Even when all indeterminate cases were considered estrogen users and all indeterminate controls were considered nonusers, the odds ratio was 1.29.

Conclusion.—There appears to be no significant relationship between estrogen replacement therapy and risk of significant venous thrombosis, even in the presence of known risk factors for thrombosis. This series is sufficient to detect a potential twofold increase in risk.

▶ The pharmacological dose of estrogen in the older high-dose oral contraceptive increased levels of clotting factors in the circulation and was associated with an increased risk of both venous and arterial thrombosis. However, the smaller physiological dose of estrogen used for hormone replacement postmenopausally does not cause an increase in levels of clotting factors and, as shown in this abstract, it is not associated with an increased risk of venous thrombosis. The product labeling for estrogen replacement states that it is only contraindicated in women with a history of thrombophlebitis associated with the use of estrogen.—D.R. Mishell, Jr., M.D.

Progestagen Supplementation of Exogenous Estrogens and Risk of Endometrial Cancer

Voigt LF, Weiss NS, Chu J, Daling JR, McKnight B, van Belle G (Univ of Washington, Seattle)

Lancet 338:274–277, 1991 18–13

Background.—The increased risk of endometrial cancer resulting from administration of estrogen has led many to recommend concurrent use of a progestagen, which counters endometrial proliferation. Few data, however, are available on the effect of exogenous progestagen when used as a supplement to noncontraceptive estrogen.

Series.—This population-based case-control study included 158 incident cases of endometrial cancer diagnosed in women aged 40–64 years in the period 1985–1987. The patients were interviewed in person by trained personnel. Controls were recruited by random phone dialing.

Observations.—Women who had used exogenous estrogen at any time, but not progestagen, had a threefold greater risk of endometrial cancer developing than did those who never had used either hormone. The risk increased after 3 years of estrogen use and subsequently in-

Risk of Endometrial Cancer Associated With Use of Estrogens (for at Least 3 Years) and Progestagens

—	No (%) of cases*	No (%) of controls	OR (95% CI)†
No hormone	78 (72)	132 (85)	..
Oestrogen only	43 (19)	11 (7)	5·7 (2·5–12·8)
Any progestagen‡	13 (9)	13 (8)	1·6 (0·6–3·9)
< 10 days/month	7 (6)	4 (3)	2·4 (0·6–9·3)
Time between reference and last use:			
≤1 yr	4 (3)	3 (2)	
>1 yr	3 (3)	1 (1)	
≥10 days/month	6 (4)	9 (6)	1·1 (0·4–3·6)
Time between reference and last use:			
≤1 yr	5 (3)	6 (4)	
>1 yr	1 (1)	3 (2)	

* Percentages standardized to age distribution of controls.
† Adjusted for age (continuous), parity (continuous), and Quetelet's index (continuous).
‡ All progestagen use was for 6 months or longer.
(Courtesy of Voigt LF, Weiss NS, Chu J, et al: *Lancet* 338:274–277, 1991.)

creased. Estrogen users who had also used a progestogen for at least 4 months had a relative risk of only 1.3. The relative risk was .9 for women using progestagen for 10 or more days a month. Women who used a progestagen as well as estrogen for longer than 3 years had a relative risk below 2 (table). When a progestagen was used at least 10 days a month, there was no excess risk relative to nonusers.

Conclusion.—The risk of endometrial cancer associated with unopposed estrogen use is substantially reduced by concomitant use of a progestagen for 10 or more days a month.

▶ There is a paucity of well-performed epidemiological studies such as this to determine the effect of adding a progestin to estrogen replacement therapy for postmenopausal women. Although the dosage and type of progestin was not investigated in this study, the conclusion that use of a progestin for a least 10 days a month eliminated increased the risk of endometrial cancer associated with long-term unopposed estrogen replacement is reassuring. It agrees with the results of the few earlier studies that have also investigated the effect of progestin supplementation. It is important to note that the addition of a progestin does not prevent the development of endometrial cancer. Use of a progestin only reduces the increased risk associated with unopposed estrogen.—D.R. Mishell, Jr., M.D.

Endometrial Histology and Bleeding Patterns After 8 Years of Continuous Combined Estrogen and Progestogen Therapy in Postmenopausal Women

Leather AT, Savvas M, Studd JWW (Kings College Hosp, London)
Obstet Gynecol 78:1008–1010, 1991 18–14

Background.—The main obstacle to hormone replacement therapy is probably the return of vaginal bleeding resulting from the cyclic progestogen that is given to prevent pathologic endometrial conditions. Continuous use of combined estrogen and progestogen has enabled postmenopausal women to avoid monthly bleeding and progestogen side effects. The long-term safety of this treatment is not known, however.

Methods and Findings.—The endometrial histology and bleeding patterns of 38 patients (of an original group of 52 who completed 1 year of treatment) receiving treatment (1 conjugated equine estrogen in combination or 17 norethindrone daily) for up to 10 years and 3 others who had a hysterectomy before 10 years of treatment were reviewed. The mean duration of combination therapy use was 8 years. Six women had episodes of breakthrough bleeding after attaining amenorrhea; all 6 had an endometrial curettage at the time of the bleeding episode. Two of these women had atrophic endometria; 2, endometrial polyps; and 2, adenocarcinoma. The adenocarcinomas were diagnosed at 2 and 4.5 years. The women with adenocarcinoma had a hysterectomy; the 4 women with benign endometria later became amenorrheic again. Each woman with persistent amenorrhea had atrophic endometrium on the curettage done for the study, irrespective of their pretreatment biopsy.

Conclusion.—Continuous combined estrogen and progestogen is an effective treatment for avoiding withdrawal bleeding in postmenopausal women. However, there have been no reports on the safety of this treatment in the long term. The current report is the first study of the effect of many years' treatment with this combination on the endometrium, and it is the only report of the development of endometrial adenocarcinoma.

▶ One of the major reasons why women with uteri do not wish to receive hormone replacement therapy is that the cyclic administration of a progestin produces monthly uterine bleeding in 80% of women using this regimen. The bleeding episodes are sufficiently annoying so that many women discontinue the use of all hormonal replacement with its associated health benefits. In an effort to increase compliance with the hormonal replacement regimens, many clinicians are using a continuous uninterrupted treatment regimen whereby the estrogen and progestin are given together once a day every day. As shown in this study, most women remain amenorrheic for many years, and all amenorrheic women had atrophic endometria. If bleeding does occur, the possibility of carcinoma exists and appropriate diagnostic studies need to be performed. Women receiving sequential progestin therapy can also have endometrial cancer develop. It is important for clinicians to remember that the addition of a progestin does not eliminate the risk of endometrial cancer. Progestin use only eliminates the increased risk of endometrial cancer caused by use of estrogen alone.—D.R. Mishell, Jr., M.D.

Intrauterine Release of Levonorgestrel: A New Way of Adding Progestogen in Hormone Replacement Therapy

Andersson K, Mattsson L-Å, Rybo G, Stadberg E (East Hosp, Göteborg, Sweden)

Obstet Gynecol 79:963–967, 1992 18–15

Introduction.—Progestogens can be administered locally in the uterine cavity. Whether an intrauterine device (IUD) releasing levonorgestrel can protect the endometrium from proliferation and reduce uterine bleeding in perimenopausal women when combined with oral estradiol was determined, and this therapy was compared with conventional cyclic estrogen-progestogen therapy.

Study Design.—Forty perimenopausal women were randomly assigned to 1 of 2 estrogen-progestogen regimens. One group was treated cyclically for 3-week periods with 2 mg of estradiol (E2) valerate; during the last 10 days, 250 μg of levonorgestrel was added. The other group received a daily oral dose of 2 mg of E2 valerate and had a 20-μg/24-hour levonorgestrel-releasing IUD. Treatment was given for 12 months.

Outcome.—Subjective complaints related to estrogen deficiency were equally reduced in both treatment groups. All women treated cyclically bled regularly during the study period (Fig 18–9). In contrast, bleeding disturbances were reduced gradually in the IUD group, and 15 of 18

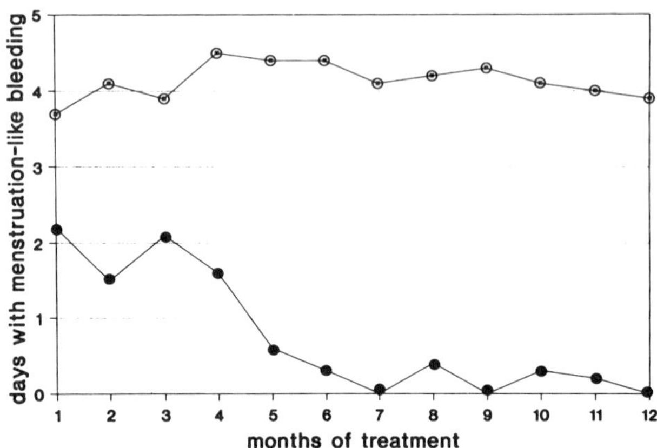

Fig 18–9.—The mean number of days with menstruation-like bleeding each month in perimenopausal women (N = 37) during 12 months of hormone replacement therapy. One group (*open circles*) was treated cyclically in 3-week periods with 2 mg of E2 valerate a day and 250 μg of levonorgestrel for the last 10 days. Another group (*filled circles*) was treated with 2mg of E2 valerate a day without interruption and had a 2-μg/24-hour levonorgestrel-releasing IUD inserted. (Courtesy of Andersson K, Mattsson L-Å, Rybo G, et al: *Obstet Gynecol* 79:963–967, 1992.)

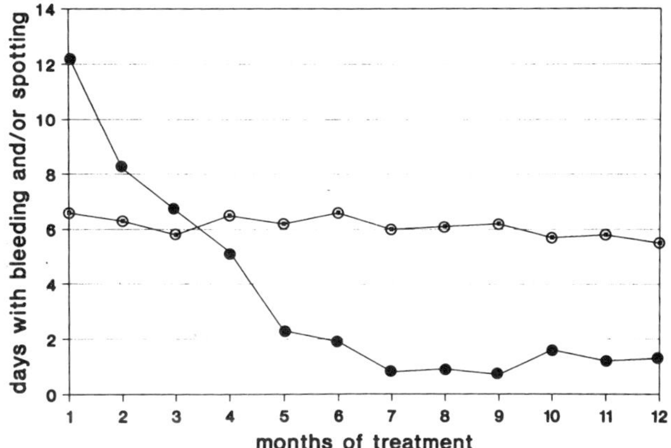

Fig 18–10.—The mean number of days with bleeding and/or spotting each month in perimenopausal women during estrogen-progestogen treatment. For explanation, see legend to Figure 18–9. (Courtesy of Andersson K, Mattsson L-Å, Rybo G, et al: *Obstet Gynecol* 79:963-967, 1992.)

women became amenorrheic after 12 months (Fig 18–10). In the IUD group, endometrial biopsy specimens taken after 12 months of treatment showed no endometrial proliferation or atypia in any specimen, and 16 samples showed a pronounced progestogen effect with decidua-like stroma. There were no IUD-related side effects, such as expulsion, pelvic inflammatory disease, or pain.

Conclusion.—Intrauterine release of levonorgestrel, in combination with oral E2 valerate, prevents endometrial proliferation and reduces uterine bleeding. These results are promising and should be confirmed in large-scale studies. This new approach to continuous combined hormone replacement therapy provides a well-tolerated alternative in perimenopausal women.

▶ The only purpose of adding a progestin to postmenopausal estrogen replacement therapy is to reduce the increased risk of adenocarcinoma of the endometrium developing in association with administration of unopposed estrogen. Administering the progestin systemically is associated with adverse effects on mood and adverse alterations in the lipid profile. Administering small amounts of the progestin locally in the endometrial cavity should keep the endometrium atrophic; it also avoids or minimizes the adverse effects of systemic progestins. This levonorgestrel-releasing IUD has an effective duration of action of 7 years and induces amenorrhea in the majority of women. This promising opportunity for an acceptable method of hormone replacement is deserving of more study.—D.R. Mishell, Jr., M.D.

19 Infertility

Prevalence of Out-of-Phase Endometrial Biopsy Specimens
Peters AJ, Lloyd RP, Coulam CB (Methodist Hosp of Indiana, Inc, Indianapolis)
Am J Obstet Gynecol 166:1738–1746, 1992 19–1

Purpose.—The prevalence of out-of-phase endometrial biopsy specimens in fertile and infertile women and women with recurrent pregnancy loss was studied in relation to 4 reference points for expected ovulation.

Methods.—A total of 485 women underwent endometrial biopsy 7–10 days after documented ovulation-based ultrasonographic evidence for follicle collapse was found. Of these 485 women, 340 were infertile, 115 had experienced recurrent pregnancy loss, and 30 were fertile. Histological dating of biopsy specimens was compared with 4 reference points, including last menstrual period (LMP), next menstrual period, luteinizing hormone (LH) surge testing, and ultrasonographic documentation of ovulation. Histological dating also was compared with midluteal phase serum progesterone concentrations.

Results.—The prevalence of out-of-phase endometrial biopsy specimens was 42% when LMP was used, 26% with next menstrual period, 21% with LH testing, and 4% with ultrasonographic documentation of ovulation. For all 3 groups of women, there were significantly fewer out-of-phase biopsy specimens when ultrasonography was used as reference point for histologic dating than the LMP, next menstrual period, or LH testing. Furthermore, when ultrasonographic documentation was used as reference point, the prevalence of out-of-phase endometrial biopsy did not differ significantly among infertile women (3%), those with recurrent spontaneous abortion (5%), and fertile women (10%). In infertile women, the prevalence of out-of-phase biopsy specimens was 4% in women with an explained cause of fertility and 3% in women with unexplained cause when ultrasonographic documentation was used as reference point. In infertile women, serum progesterone concentrations with out-of-phase biopsy specimens were similar to those with in-phase biopsy specimens.

Conclusion.—The prevalence of out-of-phase endometrial biopsy specimens varies markedly as a result of the point of reference used to date the endometrial biopsy specimens. Histological endometrial dating can be accurately determined by ultrasonographic monitoring.

▶ The diagnosis of luteal insufficiency very frequently is made among infertile women, because the conclusion that the endometrial histology is out of phase is usually made when a single biopsy specimen is dated by subtracting 14 days from the onset of the next menses. As this study and a previous study by Shoupe et al. (1) have shown, this method of dating usually yields an erroneous diagnosis compared with accurate dating by ultrasonographic determination of the time of ovulation. Because it originally was stated that the diagnosis would not be made unless the defect occurred in at least 2 cycles, the actual incidence of luteal deficiency in infertile couples is even lower than that reported in this study, in which only 1 biopsy specimen was obtained in a single cycle. In this study, the incidence of luteal insufficiency (as diagnosed by a single accurately dated biopsy specimen) was lower in infertile women than in fertile controls. Furthermore, when accurate dating criteria are used, no one has demonstrated that luteal deficiency is an actual cause of infertility. Treatment of this disorder by progesterone, human chorionic gonadotropin, or clomiphene citrate has never been shown to yield higher pregnancy rates than treatment with placebo. The necessity for performing luteal phase biopsies during the diagnostic evaluation of the infertile couple has not been demonstrated.—D.R. Mishell, Jr., M.D.

Reference

1. Shoupe D, et al: *Obstet Gynecol* 72:88, 1989.

Error in Histologic Dating of Secretory Endothelium: Variance Component Analysis

Gibson M, Lee KR, Badger GJ, Korson R, Byrn F, Trainer TD (Univ of Vermont, Burlington)

Fertil Steril 56:242–247, 1991 19–2

Introduction.—Histological dating of secretory endometrium is the cornerstone of clinical evaluation of the luteal phase. The extent and sources of imprecision in endometrial histological dating were investigated.

Methods.—Duplicate endometrial biopsy specimens were obtained on the same occasion from 25 women who were undergoing routine evaluation for infertility. Each of the 50 slides was examined by 5 evaluators on 2 separate occasions and assigned endometrial dates based on criteria of Noyes et al. None of the evaluators had previous formal teaching or consulting relationships concerning dating endometrial biopsy specimens. Estimates of intrauterine, intraevaluator, and interevaluator variability were determined using variance component analysis.

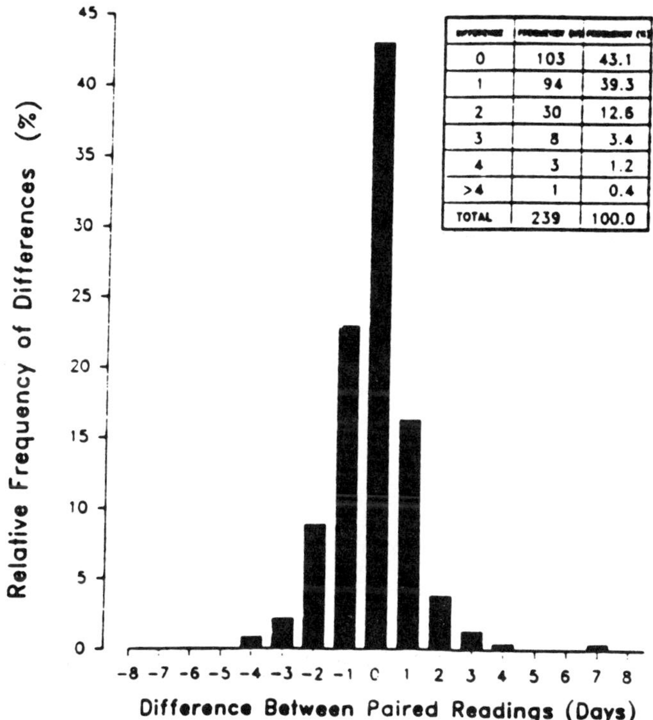

Fig 19–1.—Frequency distribution of differences between the dates assigned to endometrial biopsy specimens on the first and second readings as performed by 5 evaluators reading 50 slides. *Inset table* shows these data numerically. (Courtesy of Gibson M, Lee KR, Badger GJ, et al: *Fertil Steril* 56:242–247, 1991.)

Results.—Duplicate readings of the same slide by the same evaluator were in agreement in 43.1% of instances and were within 1 day of each other in another 39.3% (Fig 19–1), whereas only 5% were discordant by 3 days or more. Assignment of histological days between readers were in agreement in 25% of readings, within 1 day of each other in 62%, and within 2 days in 78%; the other 22% of readings were discordant by more than 2 days (Fig 19–2). The mean histological dates for the 2 biopsy specimens obtained at the same time agreed within 1 day in 56% of the subjects and within 2 days in 95%. Variance component analysis indicated that interevaluator inconsistencies accounted for 65% of the observed variability, intraevaluator differences for 27%, and intrauterine inconsistencies for 8%.

Conclusion.—These data show an overall variance of 2.58 associated with a single endometrial dating by a single reader. Assuming that the error is normal about the true histological date, 12% of biopsy specimens will be mistakenly identified as lagging by 2 days or longer. The overall error from intraevaluator, interevaluator, and intrauterine differ-

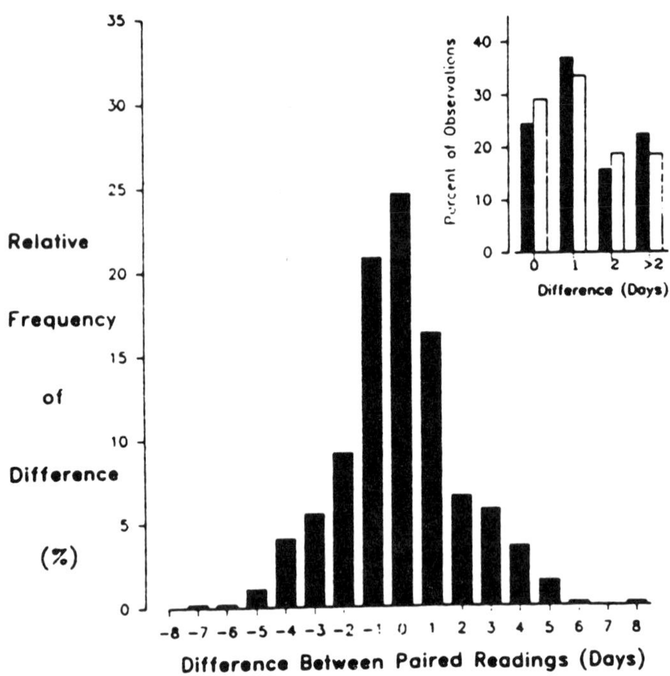

Fig 19–2.—Frequency distribution of all pair-wise differences between the 5 readers on the first reading of 50 slides (evaluable $n = 467$). Frequency difference in this study (*filled bars*) is compared with that reported by Noyes and Haman (*Fertil Steril* 4:504, 1953) (*open bars*) in the *inset.* (Courtesy of Gibson M, Lee KR, Badger GJ, et al: *Fertil Steril* 56:242–247, 1991.)

ences has the potential to result in a substantial false positive rate in the diagnosis of luteal phase defect.

▶ It has never been established whether the luteal phase defect, as diagnosed by out-of-phase endometrial dating, is a true cause of infertility. As shown by this and other studies, luteal insufficiency is greatly overdiagnosed because of the subjective means to estimate dating of the endometrium based on morphometric imprecise criteria established more than 40 years ago. The inter- and intraobserver variation in dating, as well as the lack of precision in determining the true date of ovulation, contribute to the overestimation of the diagnosis. Fortunately, administration of progesterone is harmless and, combined with timed intercourse and increased duration of attempts to conceive, fertility rates will increase. Whether progesterone is superior to placebo has never been determined in randomized prospective trials.—D.R. Mishell, Jr., M.D.

A Clinical Comparison of Sonographic Hydrotubation and Hysterosalpingography

Mitri FF, Andronikou AD, Perpinyal S, Hofmeyr GJ, Sonnendecker EWW

(Coronation and Johannesburg Hospitals, Univ of the Witwatersrand Med School, Johannesburg, South Africa)
Br J Obstet Gynaecol 98:1031–1036, 1991 19–3

Background.—The value of hysterosalpingography (HSG) in infertile women undergoing laparoscopy is limited to demonstrating intrauterine and intratubal abnormalities. In addition, HSG is time consuming, labor intensive, and associated with the risk of reaction to contrast media. The value of using vaginal sonographic hydrotubation instead was investigated.

Methods.—Sixty women undergoing routine infertility testing agreed to participate in the prospective, blind, comparison study of HSG and sonographic hydrotubation. Within the 4 weeks before or after HSG, sonographic hydrotubation was done. The uterus and tubes were identified using a 5-MHz vaginal ultrasound probe, and 10–20 mL of normal saline were injected into the uterine cavity through an endocervical catheter. The main outcome measures were the shape of the uterus and its cavity, the flow of saline through the tubes, the presence of hydrosalpinges before and after saline injection, and the presence of free fluid in the pouch of Douglas.

Results.—Sonographic and HSG uterine assessment findings were comparable in 82% of the women. Tubal findings were comparable in 72%. Twelve percent of the women had bipolar tubal disease on sonography and cornual block on HSG, with sonographic diagnosis confirmed at laparoscopy. Sonographic hydrotubation enabled a more certain diagnosis of septate uterus in 3 cases.

Conclusion.—Sonographic hydrotubation is a simple office procedure that should be used in the initial evaluation of the uterine cavity and fallopian tubes. The use of this technique will decrease the need for HSG and, in some cases, laparoscopy.

▶ Hysterosalpingography is a procedure that is a useful aid in the diagnosis of the cause of infertility. However, HSG is a cause of discomfort and is costly to perform. The technique of sonographic hydrotubation should cause less discomfort and should be less expensive than HSG. However, the main advantage appears to be the ability to diagnose the presence of both proximal and distal disease. With the use of HSG, it is only possible to detect the presence of proximal disease, because the dye does not fill the oviduct. In this study, all 7 (12%) women had bipolar disease diagnosed by sonographic hydrotubation—not by HSG. Once the diagnosis of bipolar disease is made, the women should be advised to have in vitro fertilization, and diagnostic laparoscopy need not be performed. The use of sonographic hydrotubation may shorten the time and expense of the infertility evaluation for some women.—D.R. Mishell, Jr., M.D.

Hysterosalpingography With Color Doppler Ultrasonography

Peters AJ, Coulam CB (Methodist Hosp of Indiana Inc, Indianapolis)

Am J Obstet Gynecol 164:1530–1534, 1991 19–4

Objective.—Color Doppler flow ultrasonography and hysterosalpingography were carried out in 129 infertile women, 85 of whom also had x-ray hysterosalpingography or chromopertubation, or both. Fifty-eight of the 85 underwent pelviscopic examination with chromopertubation.

Methods.—The ultrasonographic study was carried out by instilling 5–50 mL of saline transcervically into the endometrial cavity. Flow into and out of the fallopian tubes was monitored by using an ATL Ultramark 9-color Doppler unit. Doppler scans were made transabdominally or transvaginally. Tubal occlusion was diagnosed when no fluid passed through the fallopian tubes or when no fluid was seen entering the peritoneal cavity.

Findings.—Ultrasonography-hysterosalpingography indicated bilateral tubal patency in 66% of subjects, unilateral patency in 16%, and bilateral tubal occlusion in 18%. Comparison with x-ray hysterosalpingography or chromopertubation, or both, indicated agreement in 81% of cases. Ultrasonography-hysterosalpingography was falsely negative in 19% of cases and falsely positive in 6%. The corresponding figures for x-ray hysterosalpingography, compared with chromopertubation, were 45% and 18%.

Conclusion.—If chromopertubation is accepted as the standard for diagnosing tubal occlusion, the findings at ultrasonography-hysterosalpingography are at least as accurate as the findings at x-ray hysterosalpingography in demonstrating tubal occlusion. The method does not require anesthesia, administration of antimicrobials or contrast dye, and radiation exposure is avoided. It is an office procedure and is relatively inexpensive.

▶ These additional studies comparing ultrasonographic hysterosalpingography with x-ray hysterosalpingography demonstrate that the newer technique is as accurate as the older technique and has the advantage of avoiding the use of contrast dye and radiation exposure, as well as being less costly. The study by Schlief and Deichert (1) indicates it is unnecessary to use the expensive color Doppler ultrasonographic system instead of the more widely available office ultrasound unit with a vaginal probe.—D.R. Mishell, Jr., M.D.

Reference

1. Schlief R, Deichert U: *Radiology* 178:213, 1991.

Salpingitis Isthmica Nodosa in Female Infertility and Tubal Diseases

Skibsted L, Sperling L, Hansen U, Hertz J (Gentofte Hosp, Copenhagen)

Hum Reprod 6:828–831, 1991 19–5

Background.—Salpingitis isthmica nodosa (SIN) is a condition of nodular thickening of the proximal fallopian tube that is characterized by small diverticula in an irregularly hypertrophied myosalpinx. The occurrence, distribution, and frequency of SIN were evaluated in Danish women who underwent salpingectomy because of tubal pregnancy or salpingitis. In addition, correlations between SIN and infertility, pregnancies, outcome of pregnancies, births, pelvic inflammatory disease (PID), and salpingitis were investigated.

Methods.—Sections from the isthmus of 223 Fallopian tubes obtained from 193 patients were analyzed by the same pathologist. The results were compared among patients with SIN and those without SIN.

Findings.—A total of 24 women had SIN; only 1 had SIN in both tubes. The disease was located in the isthmus only in 72% of the patients, and in both the isthmus and the ampulla in 28%; SIN was never found in the ampulla alone. The median patient age was 32.5 years in women with SIN and 30.9 years in women without SIN. The incidence of SIN was 12.3% (19/155) in women with tubal pregnancies and 19.4% (12/62) in infertile women. Of the 15 women who had both SIN and tubal pregnancy, 40% had more than 1 tubal pregnancy. The women with SIN had a greater risk of 2 or more tubal pregnancies than the women without SIN (17.3%). Primary infertility was more common in the SIN group. The frequency of births before salpingectomy did not differ significantly among women with or without SIN. After SIN was diagnosed, no children were born to the SIN women; however, this did not differ significantly from the women without SIN. Although the women with SIN had histological signs of salpingitis more often than women without SIN, SIN complicated with salpingitis did not influence the number of children or tubal pregnancies.

Conclusion.—Salpingectomized women have reduced fertility. Although women with SIN can give birth to as many children as women without SIN, the women with SIN have a greater risk of 2 or more tubal pregnancies. The frequency of salpingitis is increased in women with SIN and tubal pregnancy.

▶ The etiology of SIN has not been completely clarified. Some believe the condition occurs after tubal infection, and others believe that it occurs in the absence of salpingitis, in a manner similar to the development of adenomyosis. Its etiology most likely is not congenital, because SIN is not found in the oviducts of children and is rarely found in the second decade of life. A causal relationship between SIN and infertility has not been established, because both entities increase with age and because SIN has been demonstrated in nearly 10% of the oviducts removed at the time of postpartum sterilizations.

In this study, 11 of the 24 women with SIN had previously given birth compared with 100 of 169 women without SIN, an insignificant difference.—D.R. Mishell, Jr., M.D.

Adenosine Triphosphate in Semen and Other Sperm Characteristics: Their Relevance for Fertility Prediction in Men With Normal Sperm Concentration

Rowe PJ, for the World Health Organization Task Force on the Prevention and Management of Infertility (World Health Organization, Geneva)

Fertil Steril 57:877–881, 1992 19–6

Purpose.—The relevance of conventional sperm characteristics, including concentration, motility, morphology, and adenosine triphosphate (ATP) content in predicting the occurrence of pregnancy in infertile couples was evaluated prospectively.

Subjects.—During 400 days of follow-up, 306 couples were studied; all had the following characteristics: infertility of at least 12 months' duration, anatomically normal female ovulating regularly, sperm concentration $> 20 \times 10^6$ mL, valid semen data, and ATP available before conception.

Outcome.—Ninety-six (31.4%) pregnancies occurred, for a cumulative life table pregnancy rate (PR) of 11.9%, 24.2%, 29.4%, and 32.7% at 3, 6, 9, and 12 months, respectively. The duration of infertility was an important predictor of PR, with a conception rate of 41.1% in couples with less than 3 years of infertility compared with 28.2% in couples with longer duration. None of the semen characteristics nor the ATP content were significant predictors of PR (Fig 19–3).

Conclusion.—In couples in which the female partner is normal and the male partner has a sperm concentration $> 20 \times 10^6$ mL, none of the conventional sperm characteristics and ATP concentrations can predict the occurrence of pregnancy.

► According to this study, if the female partner of an infertile couple is ovulatory without evidence of tubal obstruction and her male partner has a sperm concentration of more than 20 million sperm per mL, the chances of pregnancy occurring within the next 12 months did not vary according to other characteristics of the semen analysis, including ATP content. Therefore, it does not appear beneficial to routinely measure the ATP concentration of the semen of the male partner in the infertile couple whose sperm concentration is normal. Data were not given regarding the outcome of pregnancy in couples in whom the semen analysis had a normal sperm concentration but an abnormally low percentage of mobile sperm or morphologically abnormal sperm. This information could be useful for counseling and treating infertile couples.—D.R. Mishell, Jr., M.D.

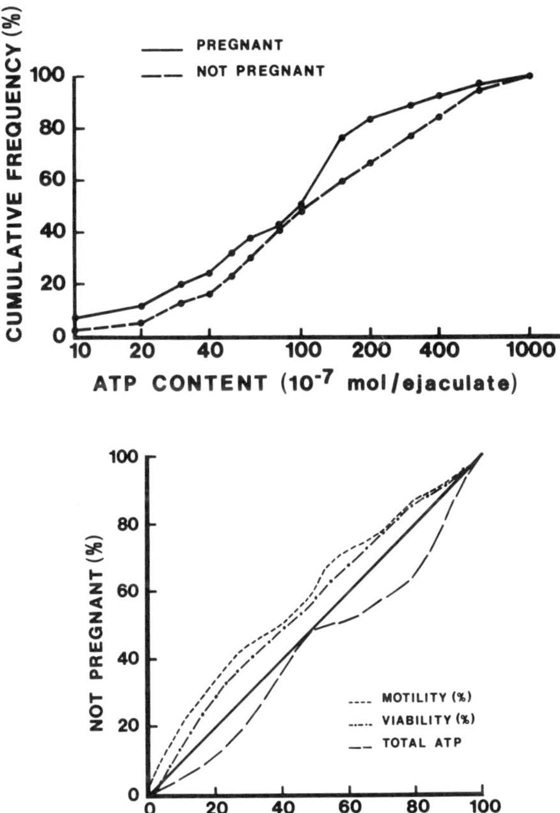

Fig 19–3.—Top, cumulative frequency distribution for total ATP (10^{-7} mol/ejaculate) among couples who did (*solid line*) or did not (*dotted line*) attain pregnancy. **Bottom,** receiver-operating-characteristic curves of the proportion of spermatozoa with progressive motility, proportion of viable spermatozoa, and total ATP among couples who did or did not attain pregnancy. (Courtesy of Rowe P, for World Health Organization Task Force on the Prevention and Management of Infertility: *Fertil Steril* 57:877–881, 1992.)

Ejaculatory Duct Obstruction in Subfertile Males: Analysis of 87 Patients

Pryor JP, Hendry WF (Inst of Urology, London)
Fertil Steril 56:725–730, 1991 19–7

Introduction.—Ejaculatory duct obstruction is considered to be a rare condition. The diagnosis may be suspected clinically from seminal analysis. The finding of a small volume of acid semen that does not contain fructose in a patient in whom the vasa are palpable is virtually pathognomic. However, the clinical picture may be complicated by the obstruction being unilateral, partial, or functional, and the diagnosis can only be

Number of Patients Successfully Treated/Number With Adequate Follow-up in the Various Groups

Group	Patency	Reservoirs	Pregnancies produced
Congenital			
Müllerian (n = 17)	10/12		5
Wolffian (n = 19)	1/6	1/3	1
Traumatic (n = 15)	2/6	4/4	1
Postinfective (n = 19)	4/6	1/4	2
Tuberculous (n = 8)			1
Megavesicles (n = 8)	1/1	1/1	
Neoplastic (n = 1)			
Total (n = 87)	18/31	7/12	10

(Courtesy of Pryor JP, Hendry NF: *Fertil Steril* 56:725-730, 1991.)

confirmed by vasography. Data from a 15-year clinical study were reviewed.

Methods.—Ejaculatory duct obstruction was found in 87 men who underwent scrotal exploration and concomitant vasography while under general anesthesia. Obstructing cystic congenital lesions in the region of the verumontanum were treated by incision of the verumontanum with the optical urethrotome. Ductal obstruction was treated by resection of the verumontanum. Coexisting epididymal obstruction was treated by epididymovasostomies when indicated.

Results.—Of the 87 patients, 67 had azoospermia, 17 had very severe oligozoospermia, 1 had oligozoospermia, and 2 had normal sperm concentrations. A small volume ejaculate with acid pH and low or absent fructose content was found in 65 (89%) of the 75 men for whom this information was available. In 17 men, vasography revealed single midline Müllerian duct cysts, 1-2 cm in diameter. Endoscopic incision of the cyst improved the seminal quality in 10 of 12 men with adequate follow-up data, and 5 female partners subsequently became pregnant. In 19 men with Wolffian malformations, surgery generally was unsuccessful, because patency was restored in only 1 of them. In 15 men, there were traumatic obstructions from previous operations, and 19 had a history of previous genital, urinary, or tuberculous infection. Patency was restored in 4 patients with previous infections, and 1 partner subsequently became pregnant. In all, patency was restored in 25 of 43 men with adequate follow-up, and 10 partners became pregnant (table). Treatment was primarily surgical in 31 men, of whom 18 achieved patency and 6 produced pregnancies in their partners. Reservoirs were inserted in 12 men, spermatozoa were obtained in 7, and 2 of them produced pregnancies.

Conclusion.—Ejaculatory duct obstruction in subfertile men is not as rare as was previously thought. Surgical intervention may restore fertility in some patients. Routine vasography is recommended to avoid overlooking this diagnosis.

▶ Although ejaculatory duct obstruction is a rare condition, if the male partner of an infertile couple has azoospermia or severe oligozoospermia, the clinician should perform the appropriate diagnostic studies to determine whether this condition is present. If so, it is one of the few causes of azoospermia that can be treated successfully.—D.R. Mishell, Jr., M.D.

Cervical Mucus Score and in Vitro Sperm Mucus Interaction in Spontaneous and Clomiphene Citrate Cycles

Randall JM, Templeton A (Univ of Aberdeen, Scotland)

Fertil Steril 56:465–468, 1991 19–8

Introduction.—Clomiphene citrate (CC) is frequently used to induce ovulation, including empiric use in patients with unexplained infertility; however, this indication has been questioned. The drug has been reported to have adverse effects on cervical mucus and sperm penetration, although not all studies agree.

Methods.—The cervical mucus score and in vitro sperm mucus interaction during spontaneous ovulatory cycles and CC cycles were studied retrospectively in 22 women with infertility of at least 3 years' duration and ovulatory midluteal progesterone level less than 30 nmol/L for at least 2 cycles. The mean patient age was 30.4 years, and the mean duration of infertility was 4.4 years. Each woman initially was studied during a spontaneous cycle and then in a cycle stimulated by CC, 150 mg, given on days 5–9. Cervical mucus was assessed as to amount, spinnbarkeit, ferning, and viscosity. Sperm-mucus penetration was assessed by a standardized Kremer test.

Results.—The mean cervical mucus score was 9.3 during the spontaneous cycle and 5.6 during the CC cycle. All of the cervical mucus score parameters were significantly reduced, despite the finding of a significantly increased mean serum estradiol level in the CC cycles. The mean sperm penetration scores were 11.4 in the spontaneous cycle and 3.9 in the CC cycle.

Conclusion.—Cervical mucus score and sperm-mucus penetration test score are reduced significantly in CC-stimulated compared with spontaneous ovulatory cycles. The components of the cervical mucus score are all relatively reduced. The empirical use of CC in infertile patients should be reassessed.

▶ Although this study shows that a high dose of clomiphene citrate, 150 mg/day given for 5 days, impairs cervical mucus amount and function when administered from days 5 to 9 of ovulatory cycles, it does not indicate that clomiphene citrate causes impaired sperm transport in the preovulatory mucus of women with anovulatory cycles treated with clomiphene citrate. Hammond et al. (1) showed that the monthly fecundability rate in women without infertility factors other than anovulation who ovulated with clomiphene citrate did not cause infertility in these women. Furthermore, Frisch et al. (the 1991 YEAR BOOK OF OBSTETRICS AND GYNECOLOGY, p 175) showed that women with unexplained infertility treated with clomiphene citrate at a dose of 100 mg/day for days 2–6 had a significant increase in their pregnancy rate. The dose of clomiphene citrate used in this study was too high, and it was given too late in the ovulatory cycle.—D.R. Mishell, Jr., M.D.

Reference

1. Hammond MG, et al: *Obstet Gynecol* 62:196, 1983.

Slow Release Intrauterine Insemination Versus the Bolus Technique in the Treatment of Women With Cervical Mucus Hostility

Muharib NS, Gadir AA, Shaw RW (Sabah Hosp, Kuwait Univ Health Sciences Center, Kuwait; The Royal Free Hosp and School of Medicine, London)

Hum Reprod 7:227–229, 1992 19–9

Background.—Intrauterine insemination of low sperm numbers in a slow release pattern may be more physiological if sperm motility is adequate. An attempt was made to simulate the natural cervical reservoir using an external, slow-release auto-syringe to inject small numbers of prepared motile spermatozoa in a continuous slow release pattern into the uterine cavity in patients with cervical mucus hostility.

Methods.—Thirty-eight infertile women, 24–36 years of age, were studied. Primary or secondary infertility caused by cervical mucus hostility was diagnosed by repeated negative postcoital tests (PCT) 8–12 hours after sexual intercourse, with good cervical mucus biophysical features and positive crossed hostility tests using Penetrak bovine mucus. Treatment assignment was random. Eighteen women began treatment with slow release intrauterine insemination and 20 began treatment with the bolus technique. They were then crossed over in subsequent alternating cycles.

Results.—In the follow-up period, no one had symptoms or signs of pelvic inflammatory disease. The total leukocyte and erythrocyte sedimentation rate values were not significantly changed after both types of treatment. None of the cervical swabs had significant bacterial growth. All insemination cycles were ovulatory. Eighty-five percent of the cycles had a spontaneous luteinizing hormone surge; human chorionic gonadotropin was given in 15%. Thirteen pregnancies occurred, 9 after slow-release intrauterine insemination and 4 after the bolus method. The cumulative pregnancy rates after these 2 treatments were 63.1% and 22%, respectively. The total number of spermatozoa inseminated during the first treatment was 9×10^6/cycle; in the second treatment, it was 31.5×10^6.

Conclusion.—The pregnancy rates were 3 times higher after slow release intrauterine insemination than after the bolus technique in these patients with cervical mucus hostility. Pregnancy rates may be improved using this method with a small number of prepared spermatozoa compared with the bolus technique.

▶ Although the technique of a 3-hour steady slow infusion of spermatozoa into the uterine cavity appears to be less convenient than a rapid insemination of sperm, the results of this study indicate that the inconvenience is certainly worthwhile in regard to pregnancy success. Other studies using the slow infusion technique are necessary before it can be recommended to replace rapid insemination; however, the intravenous similarity to what occurs with normal sexual intercourse appears to be a physiological rationale for the slow infusion.—D.R. Mishell, Jr., M.D.

Therapeutic Donor Insemination: A Prospective Randomized Trial of Fresh Versus Frozen Sperm

Subak LL, Adamson GD, Boltz NL (Stanford Univ, Stanford, California; Fertility Physicians of Northern California, Palo Alto, Calif)

Am J Obstet Gynecol 166:1597–1606, 1992 19–10

Background.—Under the new guidelines for therapeutic donor insemination issued by the American Fertility Society in February 1988, only sperm from donors who are seronegative for HIV 6 months after sperm donation and freezing would be used. The efficacy of fresh and frozen sperm in therapeutic donor insemination was compared in a prospective, randomized clinical trial.

Study Design.—Fifty-seven women underwent 72 courses of treatment, for a maximum of 6 therapeutic donor insemination (3 cycles with fresh and 3 cycles with frozen sperm). Each woman served as her own control and received a single, timed insemination of either fresh or frozen sperm from the same donor.

Outcome.—Overall, 30 conceptions occurred during 198 insemination cycles, for a fecundity of 15.2%. Of these, 83% occurred within three insemination cycles. Fecundity was significantly higher for fresh than for frozen sperm cycles (20.6% vs. 9.4%). Fecundity was significantly higher in fresh than in frozen (20.3% vs. 7.8%) cervical cap insemination cycles, but it was similar for fresh and frozen (21.2% vs. 15.8%) intrauterine insemination. The estimated cumulative pregnancy rates at 3 months were significantly greater for fresh than for frozen insemination cycles (48% vs. 22%) and for cervical cap insemination with fresh rather than frozen sperm (55% vs. 23%). Survival analysis with fixed covariates showed that fresh sperm correlated positively with pregnancy.

Conclusion.—Cycle fecundity is significantly greater with fresh sperm in women undergoing cervical cap insemination or intrauterine insemination cycles and cervical cap insemination only cycles. Although the percentage of couples conceiving would eventually be similar for fresh and frozen sperm, the use of frozen sperm requires up to double the time to conceive because the pregnancy rate is less. These findings have implications in the management of patients undergoing therapeutic donor inseminations with frozen sperm.

▶ Although the use of frozen or fresh sperm was randomized in this study, the technique of inseminating the sperm, either by cervical cap or intrauterine insemination, unfortunately was not randomized. Because it is now recommended that only frozen sperm be used from donors to determine that they have not been infected with HIV at the time of sperm donation, it would appear best to perform intrauterine insemination instead of using of the cervical cap. In this study, after 3 cycles there was no significant difference in pregnancy rates when frozen and fresh sperm were inseminated into the endometrial cavity after washing.—D.R. Mishell, Jr., M.D.

A Prospective Trial of Intrauterine Insemination of Motile Spermatozoa Versus Timed Intercourse

Kirby CA, Warnes GM, Flaherty SP, Matthews CD, Godfrey BM (Univ of Adelaide, Australia; The Queen Elizabeth Hosp, Woodville, South Australia)
Fertil Steril 56:102–107, 1991 19–11

Background.—Intrauterine insemination (IUI) as a treatment for male subfertility remains controversial. Promoted by the initial success with luteinizing hormone (LH)-timed IUI using motile sperm, a 5-year trial

TABLE 1.—Outcome of LH-Timed Intercourse and IUI Cycles With Respect to Infertility Category

	Timed intercourse			IUI		
Category	No. of couples	No. of cycles	No. of pregnancies	No. of cycles	No. of pregnancies	Logrank test
Mucus hostility	24	52	4 (7.8)*	58	7 (12.1)	$P > 0.05$
Unexplained	73	123	3 (2.4)	145	6 (4.1)	$P > 0.05$
Moderate semen defect	110	177	8 (4.5)	218	14 (6.4)	$P > 0.05$
Severe semen defect	78	154	2 (1.3)	179	10 (5.6)	$P < 0.05$
Overall	285	505	17 (3.4)	600	37 (6.2)	$P = 0.05$

* Values in parentheses are percents.
(Courtesy of Kirby CA, Warnes GM, Flaherty SP, et al: *Fertil Steril* 56:102–107, 1991.)

TABLE 2.—Effect of Number of Cycles of Treatment on the PR for Timed Intercourse and IUI in All Patient Categories Combined

	Timed intercourse		IUI	
Cycle no.	No. of cycles	No. of pregnancies	No. of cycles	No. of pregnancies
1	226	9 (4.0)*	266	27 (10.2)
2	125	5 (4.0)	141	7 (5.0)
3	79	2 (2.5)	98	2 (2.0)
4	49	1 (2.0)	56	1 (1.8)
5	19	0 (0.0)	27	0 (0)
6	7	0 (0.0)	12	0 (0)

* Values in parentheses are percents.
(Courtesy of Kirby CA, Warnes GM, Flaherty SP, et al: *Fertil Steril* 56:102–107, 1991.)

was conducted to extend the use of IUI to a larger group of male factor patients and to couples with cervical mucus hostility or unexplained infertility.

Study Design.—A prospective, randomized sequential trial was conducted to compare the efficacy of IUI with LH-timed intercourse. Cycles of IUI were alternated with LH-timed intercourse cycles. A modified swim-up procedure and discontinuous Percoll gradients were used to recover motile sperm, and inseminations were timed for 40 hours after the start of the endogenous LH increase. A total of 285 couples, including 73 with unexplained infertility, 24 with cervical mucus hostility, 110 with moderate semen defect, and 78 with severe semen defect, underwent 600 IUI cycles and 505 LH-timed intercourse cycles.

Outcome.—Overall, IUI was significantly more effective than LH-timed intercourse, with a pregnancy rate (PR) of 6.2% vs. 3.4% per cycle. However, the marked improvement was found only in the severe semen defect group, where PR was 5.6% vs. 1.3%, respectively (Table 1), and only during the first cycle of treatment when compared with the subsequent IUI cycles and the initial LH-timed cycle (Table 2). Overall, 74% of IUI pregnancies occurred in the first cycle, compared with 10.2% in LH-timed pregnancies.

Conclusion.—Intrauterine insemination is more effective than LH-timed intercourse in the treatment of severe male subfertility and only in the first cycle of treatment. However, given the low expectation of pregnancy, continued IUI is considered unrewarding, particularly if successful in vitro fertilization/gamete intrafallopian transfer (IVF/GIFT) programs are available.

▶ This prospective, randomized sequential trial provides evidence that IUI is more effective than LH-timed natural intercourse in couples whose male partner has a severe abnormality of the semen analysis, including abnormal motility or morphology in addition to sperm concentration. The pregnancy rate of 6% per cycle with IUI is not as high as that occurring with GIFT or IVF, but the success rate will probably increase if ovarian hyperstimulation is used in addition to IUI.—D.R. Mishell, Jr., M.D.

Clomiphene-Dexamethasone Treatment of Clomiphene-Resistant Women With and Without the Polycystic Ovary Syndrome

Singh KB, Dunnihoo DR, Mahajan DK, Bairnsfather LE (Louisiana State Univ, Shreveport)

J Reprod Med 37:215–218, 1992 19–12

Background.—The main treatment for patients with chronic anovulation resulting from hypothalamic-pituitary-ovarian dysfunction is clomiphene citrate, a nonsteroidal agent. The low pregnancy rates associated with the use of clomiphene have been a source of anxiety for many couples. The efficacy of a fairly simple protocol of clomiphene given simultaneously with dexamethasone in clomiphene-resistant women was assessed. The use of human chorionic gonadotropin (hCG) as an adjuvant was avoided.

Methods.—Forty clomiphene-resistant women with infertility and chronic anovulation from hypothalamic-pituitary-ovarian dysfunction were studied for approximately 5 years. A total of 45% met the criteria for the polycystic ovary (PCO) syndrome. The rest were thought to have idiopathic anovulation. All had been unsuccessfully treated with incremental clomiphene doses, 50–150 mg/day, with and without hCG. In the study protocol, clomiphene (50 mg/day) was given, beginning on day 5 of a spontaneous or progesterone-induced menstrual cycle. Dexamethasone, .5 mg, was taken orally every night, starting concurrently with clomiphene and continuing until conception or protocol discontinuation.

Results.—Ovulation was induced in 88.8% of the PCO group and in 90.9% of the non-PCO group. Overall, 52.8% of the women conceived. Probability of conception at 9 months of treatment was 87.5% in the PCO group and 46% in the non-PCO group. There were no major side effects or complications.

Conclusion.—In this series, a simple protocol of clomiphene and dexamethasone was successful. This treatment should be considered for clomiphene-resistant women with and without the PCO syndrome.

▶ Others have reported that dexamethasone treatment is beneficial for patients with PCO syndrome who fail to ovulate with clomiphene citrate—provided they have elevated levels of dehydroepiandrosterone sulfide. This study appears to indicate that dexamethasone is also beneficial for all women who are "clomiphene-resistant". Unfortunately, the authors did not define what the term "clomiphene-resistant" means, and they also did not include a placebo group as a control. Furthermore, the mean testosterone and dehydroepiandrosterone sulfate levels were not significantly different between the women with and without polycystic ovaries, which was a surprising finding. Despite these shortcomings, a trial of dexamethasone is certainly less expensive than human menopausal gonadotropin with or without a gonadotropin-releasing hormone analog, and it may be considered in the initial treatment of women with PCOS who fail to ovulate with clomiphene alone.—D.R. Mishell, Jr., M.D.

Combined Growth Hormone and Gonadotropin Treatment for Ovulation Induction in Patients With Non-Responsive Ovaries

Homburg R, West C, Ostergaard H, Jacobs HS (Middlesex Hosp, London; Novo-Nordisk A/S, Gentofte, Denmark)

Gynecol Endocrinol 5:33–36, 1991 19–13

Introduction.—The ovarian response to stimulation by human menopausal gonadotropin (hMG) can be markedly enhanced by coadministering growth hormone (GH). Therefore, this approach was tried in 4 women who exhibited no ovarian reponse to hMG alone.

Results.—A woman, aged 28 years, with idiopathic hypogonadotropic hypogonadism and undetectable serum gonadotropin had failed to respond to pulsatile luteinizing hormone-releasing hormone or to hMG alone. When GH was begun along with the same daily dose of hMG, the serum estradiol increased markedly within a week and ovulation occurred after human chorionic gonadotropin. A woman, aged 30 years, with autoimmune Addison's disease had a similar response to combined treatment with hMG and GH after failing to respond to hMG alone. The other 2 patients failed to respond to combined hormonal treatment.

Conclusion.—The combined administration of hMG and GH will initiate an ovarian response in some women who fail to respond to hMG alone. Those with clear evidence of primary ovarian failure, however, cannot be expected to respond to this treatment.

▶ Other investigators have reported in nonrandomized studies that treatment with gonadotropin-releasing hormone analogs combined with hMG successfully induces ovulation in women with polycystic ovarian syndrome (PCOS) who do not ovulate after treatment with hMG alone. This randomized study of women with PCOS who failed to ovulate with clomiphene indicates that it is not beneficial to treat all women with a combination of GnRH analogue and hMG, because this expensive regimen may be unnecessary. This combination therapy should be reserved for those women who fail to ovulate with hMG alone, because it requires greater amounts of hMG and a longer duration of therapy.—D.R. Mishell, Jr., M.D.

Low-Dose Gonadotropin Therapy for Induction of Ovulation in 100 Women With Polycystic Ovary Syndrome

Hamilton-Fairley D, Kiddy D, Watson H, Sagle M, Franks S (St Mary's Hosp Med School, London)

Hum Reprod 6:1095–1099, 1991 19–14

Background.—Women with anovulation caused by polycystic ovary syndrome (PCOS) are likely to have multiple follicles develop during gonadotrophin treatment. Therefore, their risk of multiple pregnancy is high. A low-dose regimen was assessed in these patients.

Methods.—One hundred women with clomiphene-resistant PCOS were treated. Low-dose gonadotrophin was injected intramuscularly every day. Eighty-three received human menopausal gonadtrophin, and 17 received follicle stimulating hormone. The initial doses were maintained for up to 14 days in the first cycle and up to 7 days in later cycles. The dose was increased from 1 to 1.5 ampoules per day if no response was seen on ultrasound. This dose was then maintained for another 7 days before increasing the dose by .5 ampoules a day. This stepwise increase was continued to a maximum of 3 ampoules per day; if no ovarian response occurred at this dose, the patient was considered unresponsive and treatment stopped. Once ovarian activity was seen ultrasonically, the same dose was continued until complete follicular maturation. Human chorionic gonadotropin, 5,000 IU, was administered for ovulation induction.

Results.—Ninety-five women ovulated at least once. A total of 72% of the 401 cycles induced were ovulatory, and 73% of these were uni-ovulatory. The overall 6-month cumulative conception rate was 55%. Only 2 multiple pregnancies occurred. The rate of early pregnancy loss was 32%, and the prevalence of complications was low. There were no cases of severe hyperstimulation, and less than 5% of the cycles were abandoned because multiple follicles developed. An increased baseline and/or mid-follicular luteinizing hormone level was associated with a poor response to treatment—anovulation, ovulation without conception, or early pregnancy loss. None of the women whose luteinizing hormone levels were persistently increased during ovulatory cycles had good pregnancy outcomes.

Conclusion.—Low-dose gonadotrophin treatment is a safe, effective way to induce ovulation. It is associated with a high incidence of single follicular development and a very low multiple pregnancy rate.

▶ Overall pregnancy rates after attempts at ovulation induction with hMG in women with polycystic ovaries who fail to ovulate with clomiphene citrate are not very high. The results of this regimen of administering to such women a low dose of hMG for a prolonged period of time are encouraging, with ovulation occurring in 95 of 100 women so treated; there is a cumulative pregnancy rate of 55% after 6 cycles of therapy. Although some centers have reported that the use of GnRH agonists enhances the success of hMG in these women, others have not been able to confirm these findings. Thus, the regimen reported here should be tried by other investigators to determine whether the good results reported by these investigators can be continued.—D.R. Mishell, Jr., M.D.

Transvaginal Ultrasound-Guided Follicular Aspiration in the Management of Anovulatory Infertility Associated With Polycystic Ovaries

Mio Y, Terado H, Toda T, Harada T, Tanikawa M, Terakawa N (Tottori Univ, Yonago, Japan)

Fertil Steril 56:1060–1065, 1991 19–15

Background.—Polycystic ovarian disease (PCOD) is associated with anovulation and hormonal abnormalities. Polycystic ovaries (PCO) without hormonal abnormalities have also been reported in patients with menstrual irregularity and an inability to conceive. Whether transvaginal ultrasound (US)-guided follicular aspiration can effectively induce ovulation and facilitate pregnancy in anovulatory women with PCO was determined.

Methods.—Eight patients with PCOD and 10 with PCO who failed to ovulate with medical therapies were studied. Most persistent follicles were punctured, their contents apsirated thoroughly during the midluteal phase. The ovarian stimulation regimen used in previous cycles was used in the cycles after aspiration. Evidence of ovulation and a subsequent pregnancy was monitored ultrasonically after aspiration. The responsiveness of pituitary gonadotropins to gonadotropin-releasing hormone was assessed.

Results.—Patients with PCOD had ovulation rates of 87.5% per individual and 52.6% per cycle. Those patients with PCO had rates of 100% per person and 63.3% per cycle. Half the patients with PCOD and half of those with PCO became pregnant after the aspiration. There was a significant decrease in basal and peak levels of serum luteinizing hormone after aspiration.

Conclusion.—Transvaginal US-guided follicular aspiration is a much less invasive and simpler technique for oocyte pick-up in an in vitro fertilization-embryo transfer program. This method therefore seems preferable for treating anovulatory patients with PCOD or with PCO with hormonal abnormalities. It is also helpful for clarifying the pathophysiology of anovulation such as PCOD and luteinized unruptured follicle.

► As mentioned in the discussion following Abstract 19–14, attempts to induce ovulation with hMG in women with PCOS who fail to ovulate when given clomiphene citrate are not highly successful. In attempts to replicate the success achieved decades ago with the surgical procedures of ovarian wedge resection, various investigators have destroyed portions of ovarian tissue by electrocautery or laser vaporization under laparoscopic visualization. Good success has been reported with these procedures, but this major surgical procedure requires general anesthesia and the use of an operating room facility. The minor operative procedure described in this study did not require either general anesthesia or use of an operating room, and the patients were able to be ambulatory and were discharged 30 minutes after the procedure was completed. Further studies of this innovative technique should be undertaken.—D.R. Mishell, Jr., M.D.

The Response of Patients With Polycystic Ovarian Disease to Human Menopausal Gonadotropin Therapy After Ovarian Electrocautery or a Luteinizing Hormone-Releasing Hormone Agonist

Gadir AA, Alnaser HMI, Mowafi RS, Shaw RW (Kuwait Univ Heart Science Ctr, Safat, Kuwait; The Royal Free Hosp, London)

Fertil Steril 57:309–313, 1992 19–16

Background.—Laparoscopic ovarian electrocautery and luteinizing hormone-releasing hormone agonists (LH-RH-a) are alternatives for inducing ovulation in women with polycystic ovarian syndrome (PCOS) who are unresponsive to simpler medications. The effect of laparoscopic ovarian electrocautery was compared to that of intranasal buserelin acetate medication on the response of patients with PCOS to human menopausal gonadotropin (hMG) medication.

Methods.—A group of 33 women with PCOS who had failed to conceive after 6 treatment cycles with hMG treatment was studied. By random assignment, 16 were treated with ovarian electrocautery followed by hMG on the third day after surgery (group 1). The 17 patients in group 2 began receiving buserelin acetate intranasal medication just after diagnostic laparoscopy, 800 μg/day, for 8 weeks. Eight weeks later, group 2 was given hMG medication for induction of ovulation in the same pattern as in group 1. Buserelin acetate medication was continued throughout the study. The treatment was offered for 6 cycles, unless pregnancy occurred.

Results.—The number of ovulatory cycles were 58 and 51, or 85.3% and 77.3%, in the respective groups. Group 1 patients needed fewer hMG ampules per cycle (with shorter induction time), and they had smaller leading follicles. However, the 2 groups had comparable midcycle serum luteinizing hormone and testosterone values. Women treated with LH-RH-a had more cycles with multiple dominant follicles and, accordingly, higher midcycle serum estradiol levels. Seven women in group 1 conceived, compared with 8 in group 2, for rates of 43.8% and 47.1%, respectively. The monthly fecundity rates per cycle were 12.1% and 15.7%, respectively. The 6-cycle cumulative pregnancy rates were 41.2% in group 1 and 49.9% in group 2. However, abortions occured in 4 women after LH-RH-a plus hMG medication, and only 1 occurred after electrocautery. The total multiple pregnancy rate was 20% in the entire series.

Conclusion.—Ovarian electrocautery performed during a planned diagnostic laparoscopy may be better than the more expensive LH-RH-a treatment for inducing ovulation in women with PCOS who do not conceive after gonadotropin treatment. In this series, the number of cycles with multiple dominant follicles, the luteal phase serum testosterone, and the miscarriage rate were lower after ovarian electrocautery.

▶ Patients with PCOS who fail to ovulate with clomiphene citrate are difficult to manage. Treatment with hMG, pure follicle-stimulating hormone, and pulsatile gonadotropin-releasing hormone (GnRH) is not very successful. Some groups have shown better results if the patients are pretreated with a GnRH agonist before receiving hMG, but the duration of therapy and the amount of hMG are both increased, thereby increasing the cost markedly. Partial surface destruction of the ovaries by laser or electrocautery frequently induces ovulation without the need for additional therapy. However, if ovulation does not occur, clomiphene citrate or hMG, as shown in this paper, is then usually successful.—D.R. Mishell, Jr., M.D.

The Effect of Short-Interval Laparoscopic Lysis of Adhesions on Pregnancy Rates Following Nd-YAG Laser Photocoagulation of Polycystic Ovaries

Gürgan T, Urman B, Aksu T, Yarali H, Develioglu O, Kisnisci HA (Univ of Hacettepe, Ankara, Turkey)

Obstet Gynecol 80:45–47, 1992 19–17

Background.—Laparoscopic ovarian electrocautery, laser vaporization, and laster photocoagulation of the ovaries have recently been advocated as alternative treatments in anovulatory patients with polycystic ovary disease who are resistant to clomiphene citrate-induced ovulation. The effect on pregnancy rates of short-interval second-look laparoscopy with lysis of adhesions in patients with polycystic ovary disease who had undergone laparoscopic Nd-YAG laser photocoagulation of the ovaries was determined.

Patients.—Forty anovulatory women with clomiphene citrate-resistant polycystic ovary disease, aged 21–31 years, underwent bilateral ovarian laparoscopic Nd-YAG laser photocoagulation. Twenty women were randomly assigned to second-look laparoscopy with lysis of adhesions within 3–4 weeks after initial laparoscopy, and 20 women were managed expectantly. At laparoscopy, all patients had normal-appearing pelvic organs and none had adhesions, but all ovaries had a polycystic appearance. The Nd-YAG laser photocoagulation consisted of the creation of 20–25 holes on the surface of each ovary, using a focused laser beam from a distance of 5–10 mm.

Results.—Nineteen patients assigned to second-look laparoscopy agreed to undergo the second-look procedure and 1 refused. There was no significant difference in the mean age and mean duration of infertility between the 2 groups. At second-look laparoscopy, 13 patients had minimal or mild adhesions, and in 12 of them, the adhesions were filmy, avascular, and localized to the periovarian site. The adhesions were easily lysed with sharp or blunt dissection, and significant bleeding did not occur. Thirteen parties (68%) in the second-look group and 15 observed patients (75%) ovulated spontaneously within 3 months after initial laparoscopic laser treatment. Nine women (47%) in the second-look group and 11 (55%) women in the observed group conceived during the 6-month follow-up period. All pregnancies were intrauterine and singleton gestations.

Conclusion.—Early laparoscopic lysis of adhesions after laparoscopic Nd-YAG laser photocoagulation of polycystic ovaries does not improve short-term conception rates.

▶ Selective partial ovarian destruction by means of electrocautery or laser increasingly is being used to induce ovulation in women with polycystic ovaries who fail to ovulate with clomiphene citrate therapy. The results of this study indicate that it is not cost effective or necessary to perform a second-look laparoscopy routinely in women who are so treated. If ovulation resumes but pregnancy does not occur within a year, then laparoscopic visualization may be worthwhile to determine whether periovarian adhesions are present.—D.R. Mishell, Jr., M.D.

Luteal Phase Support With hCG Does Not Improve Fecundity Rate in Human Menopausal Gonadotropin-Stimulated Cycles

Keenan JA, Moghissi KS (Wayne State Univ, Detroit)

Obstet Gynecol 79:983–987, 1992 19–18

Background.—It is generally accepted that a luteal phase deficiency may exist in human menopausal gonadotropin (hMG)-stimulated cycles. Luteal phase support with progesterone or human chorionic gonadotropin (hCG) is widely used to correct this deficiency and improve pregnancy rates.

Study Design.—The effects of luteal phase hCG administration on pregnancy rates during ovulation induction with hMG were studied in a randomized cross-over trial. In 67 infertile women, nontreatment cycles (no luteal phase support) were alternated with treatment cycles, in which patients received 2,500 IU of hCG on the third, sixth, and ninth days after the ovulatory dose of 10,000 IU of hCG (when serum estradiol > 400 pg/mL and 2 or more follicles with a mean diameter of at least 15 mm were present). Thirty-three women received luteal phase support during odd-numbered cycles (group A) and 34 during even-numbered cycles (group B).

Outcome.—There were 21 pregnancies, for an overall cycle fecundity of .14 and a total pregnancy rate of 31%. The mean number of cycles per patient was 2.2 for group A and 2.3 for group B. Of the 151 cycles of hMG therapy, 11 pregnancies occurred in 72 hCG-supported cycles, for a cycle fecundity of .15, compared with .13 for 79 unsupported cycles; the difference was not significant. The midluteal progesterone levels were significantly higher in supported than in unsupported cycles, but the mean peak estradiol levels did not differ significantly between supported and unsupported cycles.

Implications.—These findings do not support the routine use of luteal phase support with hCG in hMG-stimulated cycles.

▶ More well-designed studies such as this one are needed to determine the efficacy of many of the therapies used to treat the infertile couple. This study shows that, when hMG is used to stimulate ovulation in infertile women, it is not beneficial to administer additional injections of hCG during the luteal phase after the injection to induce ovulation is given. Avoiding the use of additional hCG will decrease the cost and inconvenience for the patient.—D.R. Mishell, Jr., M.D.

Fertility in Women With Late-Onset Adrenal Hyperplasia Due to 21-Hydroxylase Deficiency

Feldman S, Billaud L, Thalabard J-C, Raux-Demay M-C, Mowszowicz I, Kuttenn F, et al (Hôp Necker; Hôp Trousseau, Paris)

J Clin Endocrinol Metab 74:635–639, 1992 19–19

Background.—Few reports have addressed fertility in women with late-onset adrenal hyperplasia resulting from a partial enzyme defect. Fertility was assessed in 53 women with LAH resulting from partial 21-hydroxylase deficiency.

Patients.—The mean patient age was 24.6 years. Sixty-two percent of the patients came to attention for isolated hirsutism developing after normal puberty, and 17% were seen for sterility, which often was associated with menstrual disorders. None had any major signs of virilization. Seventy-one percent were treated for hirsutism, 24 with cyproterone acetate-containing antiandrogen therapy and 14 with hydrocortisone, 10 mg, given twice per day. Hydrocortisone was given to the 20 patients who wished to get pregnant.

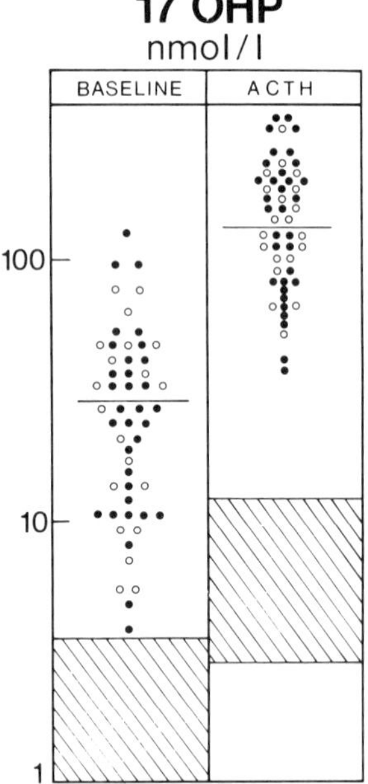

Fig 19–4.—Basal and adrenocorticotropic hormone (ACTH)-stimulated levels of 17-hydroxyprogesterone (17OHP) in 53 patients with late-onset adrenal hyperplasia who did (*open circles*) or did not (*filled circles*) achieve pregnancy. *Hatched areas* indicate normal ranges. (Courtesy of Feldman S, Billaud L, Thalabard J-C, et al: *J Clin Endocrinol Metab* 74:635–639, 1992.)

Findings.—The condition was diagnosed on the basis of plasma 17-hydroxyprogesterone (17OHP) level in excess of the normal value (Fig 19–4). All but 5 patients had high plasma androgen values; plasma testosterone, although often high, was normal in 15 patients (Fig 19–5). All patients had normal plasma dehydroepiandrosterone sulfate. There were 38 pregnancies in the women who wanted to get pregnant; 14 of 20 had ovulatory cycles as early as the first month of treatment with hydrocortisone only. That group had significant decreases in plasma androgen and 19 full-term pregnancies. Time to conception was less than 1 year in all cases.

Discussion.—Patients with late-onset adrenal hyperplasis are hypofertile, but they are much less so than women with the more severe 21-hydroxylase deficiency. Hydrocortisone treatment usually is quickly successful in women who wish to become pregnant; hydrocortisone usually is maintained at a dose of 20–30 mg when pregnancy occurs. Clomiphene citrate may be helpful if hydrocortisone fails.

▶ The signs and symptoms of late-onset adrenal hyperplasia, perhaps better named late-onset 21-hydroxylase deficiency, are similar to those of the polycystic ovarian syndrome; there usually is a more severe degree of hirsutism in the former condition. Late-onset adrenal hyperplasia is a genetically transmit-

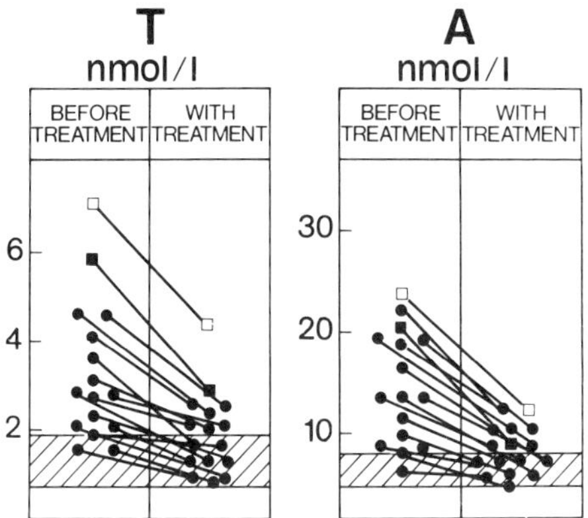

Fig 19–5.—Basal plasma testosterone (*T*) and androstenedione (*A*) levels before and after treatment in patients desiring pregnancy. *Hatched areas* indicate normal ranges. *Filled circles*, pregnancy after hydrocortisone treatment; *filled squares*, pregnancy after hydrocortisone and clomiphene citrate treatment; *open squares*, no pregnancy. (Courtesy of Feldman S, Billaud L, Thalabard J-C, et al: *J Clin Endocrinol Metab* 74:635–639, 1992.)

ted disorder that is more common in certain ethnic groups, such as Hispanics and Ashkenazi Jews, than it is in a diverse white population. As shown in this study, if women with this disorder are infertile, treatment with hydrocortisone yields very good pregnancy rates. These rates are comparable, if not better than, the use of clomiphene citrate in women with anovulation caused by the polycystic ovary syndrome.—D.R. Mishell, Jr., M.D.

Laparoscopic Distal Tuboplasty: Report of 87 Cases and a 4-Year Experience

Canis M, Manhes H, Mage G, Wattiez A, Pouly JL, Bruhat MA (Hôtel Dieu, Clermont-Ferrand, France)

Fertil Steril 56:616–621, 1991 19–20

Objective.—Although several authors have reported the value of laparoscopic distal tuboplasty in the treatment of tubal infertility, the procedure remains controversial. The fertility results after laparoscopic distal tuboplasty were evaluated, and these results were compared with those obtained previously with laser microsurgery.

Patients.—Between 1985 and 1989, 87 patients with a mean age of 29.1 years underwent laparoscopic surgery for distal tubal occlusion. Forty-two patients were treated for primary infertility and 45 for secondary infertility. The mean duration of infertility was 33 months. Tubal damage was evaluated at laparoscopy using a previously reported classification in which the disease severity is staged I, II, III, or IV, with IV being the worst.

Results.—Twenty-nine patients (33.3%) achieved intrauterine pregnancies (IUPs) and 6 (6.9%) had extrauterine pregnancies (EUPs). Twenty-

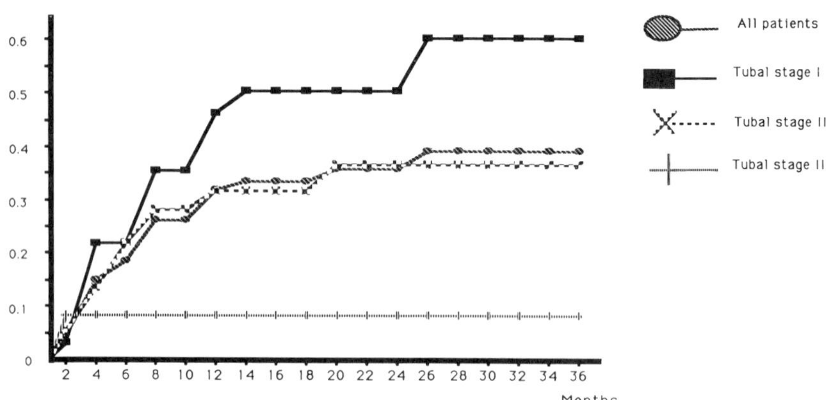

Fig 19–6.—Cumulative pregnancy rates. (Courtesy of Canis M, Manhes H, Mage G, et al: *Fertil Steril* 56:616–621, 1991.)

six of the 29 IUP occurred during the first year after laparoscopic surgery, and 93% of the pregnancies were obtained within 14 months (Fig 19–6). The monthly fecundity rate was 3.3% during the first postoperative year and only .6% during the following years. The overall monthly fecundity rate was 2.3%. None of the patients with stage IV disease became pregnant. The pregnancy rate (PR) was 5.6% for patients with stage II and IV tubal disease compared with 40.6% for patients with stage I and II disease. The difference was statistically significant. The EUP rates were 11.8% for stage I disease, 3.3% for stage II, 6.7% for stage III, and 10% for stage IV disease. A comparison of the PRs obtained after laparoscopic surgery with those obtained after laser microsurgical distal tuboplasty revealed no statistical difference in PRs between the 2 treatment modalities.

Conclusion.—Laparoscopic surgery represents a safe and effective alternative to laser microsurgery for the treatment of distal tubal occlusion.

▶ Although the use of laparoscopic salpingostomy was not prospectively compared with the microsurgical technique performed by laparotomy in this study, the retrospective comparison that was performed indicates that the pregnancy rates were comparable with the 2 techniques. It was recently reported by the Hopkins group (1) that the results with microsurgery were comparable to the treatments of tubal infertility by conventional surgery. It appears that the prognoses for fertility after salpingostomy by any operative technique are correlated more with the extent of disease than with the type of surgical procedure. Because laparoscopic salpingostomy results in less morbidity, length of hospitalization, and cost than performing the procedure by laparotomy, the former technique should become the procedure of choice to treat distal tubal disease when performed by experienced laparoscopic surgeons.—D.R. Mishell, Jr., M.D.

Reference

1. Hopkins MP, et al: *Fertil Steril* 54:984, 1991.

Buserelin Acetate Versus Expectant Management in the Treatment of Infertility Associated With Minimal or Mild Endometriosis: A Randomized Clinical Trial

Fedele L, Parazzini F, Radici E, Bocciolone L, Bianchi S, Bianchi C, Candiani GB (Università di Milano; Istituto di Ricerche Farmacologiche "Mario Negri"; Ospedali Civili Bergamo, Italy)

Am J Obstet Gynecol 166:1345–1350, 1992 19–21

Purpose.—Four hormonal regimens are available for treatment of pelvic endometriosis with infertility: danzol, progestins, gestrinone, and the gonadotropin-releasing hormone (GnRH) agonists. Their effectiveness in increasing conception rates in early endometriosis is largely unknown. This randomized clinical trial compared buserelin with expectant management for infertile women with stage I or II pelvic endometriosis.

Methods.—Seventy-one consecutive women with a laparoscopically confirmed diagnosis of minimal or mild endometriosis were studied.

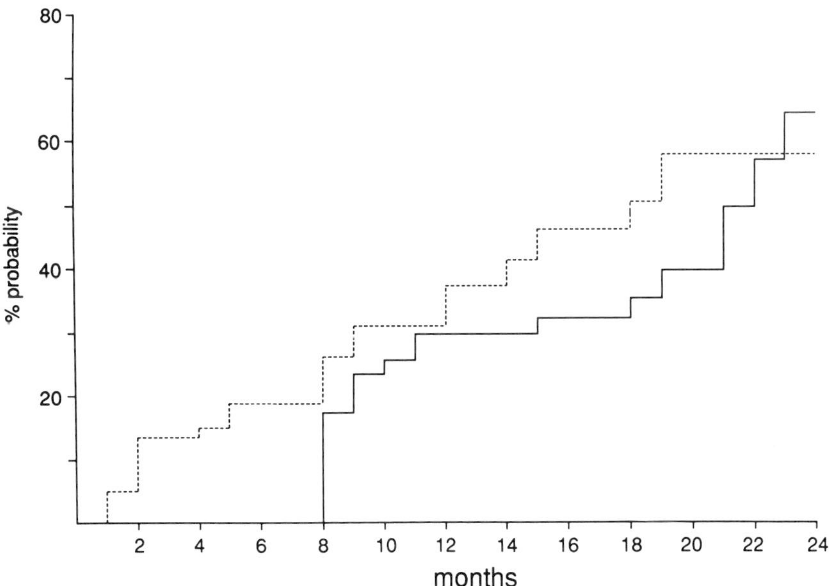

Fig 19–7.—Overall 24-month probability of becoming pregnant in 71 subjects with minimal or mild endometriosis according to treatment allocation, Milan, Italy, 1988 to 1990. *Solid line* indicates buserelin-treated group; *broken line* indicates expectant management group. χ^2_1 adjusted for stage = .69, P = .41 for 12-month analysis; χ^2_1 = .95, P = .33 for 24-month analysis. (Courtesy of Fedele L, Parazzini F, Radici E, et al: *Am J Obstet Gynecol* 166:1345–1350, 1992.)

The mean patient age was 32 years. The women were randomized to receive either intranasal buserelin, 400 μg 3 times per day for 6 months, or expectant management. The median follow-up was 17 months for the buserelin group and 18 months for the expectant management group.

Results.—Forty-three percent of the buserelin group and 39% of the no-treatment group received drugs to stimulate ovulation. There were 17 pregnancies in each group—of these 34, 13 occurred after treatment with clomiphene citrate and human chorionic gonadotropin. A mean of 4 cycles was induced in women who conceived after this treatment, with no significant differences between the 2 groups. The 12-month pregnancy rates were 30% in the buserelin group and 37% in the expectant management group; 24-month actuarial overall pregnancy rates were 61% in both (Fig 19–7).

Conclusion.—Intranasal buserelin does not appear to affect short-term reproductive outcome in women with minimal-to-mild endometriosis. This is the first known randomized study to compare treatment with a GnRH agonist with expectant management. The results are similar to those of the few previous studies of hormonal treatment that used the endpoint of reproductive outcome.

▶ No medical management of endometriosis with either progestins, danazol, or gonadotropin-releasing hormone agonists has been shown to improve the rates of conception in women with endometriosis compared with expectant management. Thus, it appears that minimal or moderate endometriosis without tubal adhesions is a result, not a cause, of infertility. The best way to maximally achieve pregnancy in such individuals is to offer them superovulation and intrauterine insemination or some form of assisted reproduction.—D.R. Mishell, Jr., M.D.

Menstrual Symptoms in Women With Pelvic Endometriosis

Mahmood TA, Templeton AA, Thomson L, Fraser C (Aberdeen Maternity Hosp, Aberdeen, Scotland)

Br J Obstet Gynaecol 98:558–563, 1991 19–22

Introduction.—Although endometriosis accounts for the second largest category of gynecological publications, the symptomatology of endometriosis is not clear. Many of the previous studies were retrospective and lacked suitable controls. A prospective, questionnaire-based study was conducted to examine menstrual symptoms in women with pelvic endometriosis.

Methods.—Of 1,250 questionnaires sent to women before planned admission, 1,200 (96%) were completed. The frequencies of dysmenorrhea, menorrhagia, menstrual regularity, premenstrual spotting, deep dyspareunia, and pelvic pain were evaluated in 598 women undergoing laparoscopic sterilization, 312 undergoing laparoscopy for infertility, 156

A Comparison of Menstrual Symptoms in Women With and Without Endometriosis
(n = 1,200)

Variables	Endometriosis (n = 201)		Pelvic adhesions (n = 278)		Normal pelvis (n = 721)		Significance with 2 df	
	n	(%)	n	(%)	n	(%)	χ^2	P
Dysmenorrhoea	137	(68)	140	(50)	358	(50)	24·48	<0·001
Present periods regular	154	(77)	206	(74)	632	(88)	9·92	<0·02
Menorrhagia	110	(55)	125	(45)	365	(51)	4·89	>0·05
Premenstrual spotting	56	(30)	79	(28)	190	(26)	2·28	>0·05
Deep dyspareunia	75	(37)	93	(33)	168	(23)	25·64	<0·001
Pain after intercourse	29	(14)	42	(15)	72	(10)	6·41	<0·05
Pelvic pain	118	(59)	165	(59)	346	(48)	17·95	<0·001

(Courtesy of Mahmood TA, Templeton AA, Thomson L, et al: *Br J Obstet Gynaecol* 98:558–563, 1991.)

undergoing laparoscopy for chronic pelvic pain, and 134 undergoing abdominal hysterectomy for dysfunctional uterine bleeding.

Results.—There were 201 (17%) women with endometriosis, most (73%) of whom had mild disease. The remaining patients had either postinfective pelvic adhesions (23%) or a normal pelvis (60%). Dysmenorrhea occurred more frequently in women with endometriosis than in women with normal pelvis or postinfective pelvic adhesions (table). Deep dyspareunia, pain after intercourse, and recurrent pain unrelated to menstruation or coitus occurred more often in women with endometriosis and those with postinfective pelvic adhesions than in women with a normal pelvis. Menorrhagia, menstrual irregularity, and premenstrual spotting were noted with equal frequency in all groups. In women with endometriosis, there was no relation between symptomatology and severity of the disease.

Conclusion.—Menstrual symptoms are not reliable indicators of disease in women with pelvic endometriosis. Dysmenorrhea is the most common symptom reported by women with endometriosis, but other menstrual symptoms are also common in women with postinfective pelvic adhesions and those with a normal pelvis.

▶ Other retrospective studies have suggested that women with endometriosis have a higher frequency of abnormal bleeding than those without this disease; therefore, endometriosis may be a cause of abnormal uterine bleeding. However, as shown in this nonrandomized, prospective study, women with endometriosis undergoing laparoscopy for a variety of reasons, including tubal sterilization, do not have a greater frequency of abnormal uterine bleeding than women without endometriosis. As expected, dysmenorrhea occurred significantly more frequently in women with endometriosis. Endometriosis does not appear to cause abnormal uterine bleeding, because it most likely does not cause infertility, unless the disease causes tubal pathology.—D.R. Miller, Jr., M.D.

A Prospective, Randomized Trial Comparing Two Different Intrauterine Insemination Regimens in Controlled Ovarian Hyperstimulation Cycles

Silverberg KM, Johnson JV, Olive DL, Burns WN, Schenken RS (Univ of Texas Health Science Ctr, San Antonio)

Fertil Steril 57:357–361, 1992 19–23

Background.—There are various methods for timing intrauterine insemination in natural cycles. The efficacy of a single intrauterine insemination done in the periovulatory period was compared with 1 done before and another done after ovulation.

Methods.—Thirty-one consecutive patients underwent 49 cycles of controlled ovarian hyperstimulation combined with intrauterine insemination. The initial dose was 150 IU of human menopausal gonadotropin given daily for 3 days. This dosage was increased by 75 when the serial estradiol levels increased by less than 50%. Human chorionic gonadotropin was given in a single, intramuscular dose of 10,000 IU when 2 follicles exceeded 16 mm in mean diameter and the serum estradiol levels were 400 pg/mL or more. Those patients randomly assigned to group 1 received hCG at midnight, followed by a single insemination in the periovulatory period 34 hours later. In group 2, 1 insemination was done before ovulation (18 hours after hCG), and the other was performed shortly thereafter (42 hours after hCG).

Results.—No patient in group 1 ovulated before insemination. All had ultrasonographic evidence of ovulation the day after insemination. Ovulation occurred after the first insemination (but before the second) in 22 of the 23 cycles in group 2 patients. Overall, significantly more clinical pregnancies occurred in group 2 cycles (cycle fecundity, 52.2%) than in group 1 cycles (cycle fecundity, 8.7%) (table).

Conclusion.—In this study, the 2 groups did not differ significantly in demographic characteristics, hMG requirements, or ovarian response to hMG stimulation. Every insemination done contained at least 1×10^6 motile spermatozoa, with a range of 1×10^6 to 124×10^6. The pregnancy rates were uncorrelated with sperm concentration. Using fresh or

Clinical Pregnancy Rate by Group

	Group I	Group II
No. of cycles	23	23
Clinical pregnancies	2	12
Cycle fecundity (%)	8.7[a]	52.2

[a] $P = .003$ vs. group II.

(Courtesy of Silverberg KM, Johnson JV, Olive DL, et al: *Fertil Steril* 57:357-361, 1992.)

cryopreserved sperm, 2 intrauterine inseminations timed as described are better than a single periovulatory intrauterine insemination in cycles of controlled ovarian hyperstimulation with hMG.

▶ Any technique that produces a cycle fecundity rate greater than 50% must be considered seriously. I wonder whether a slow infusion of sperm on 2 occasions will improve the changes of pregnancy success in couples with unexplained infertility even more.—D.R. Mishell, Jr., M.D.

Multiple Follicular Recruitment and Intrauterine Insemination Outcomes Compared by Age and Diagnosis

Horbay GLA, Cowell CA, Casper RF (Univ of Toronto, Toronto Hosp)

Hum Reprod 6:947–952, 1991 19–24

Background.—Intrauterine insemination (IUI) of washed semen has been used to treat infertility from various causes with varying results. The results of a large IUI plus a multiple follicular recruitment (MFR) program in a tertiary care facility were reported.

Methods.—A total of 190 couples, with a mean age of 33 years, completed 472 cycles of ovarian MFR with clomiphene citrate, human menopausal gonadotropin, and human chorionic gonadotropin and timed IUI in 1988 and 1989. The couples had been diagnosed as having pure male factor infertility, idiopathic infertility, ovulatory disorder, or other causes of infertility. Semen was prepared for IUI using wash and swim-up methods.

Results.—Pregnancy rates were greater in those younger than 36 years. The probability of conceiving after 3 treatment cycles was .402 overall—.481 for those younger than 36 years and .252 for those aged 36 years or older. The probability of conceiving for those with male factor was .469, and for those with idiopathic infertility, .411. An age effect was noted only in those with idiopathic infertility.

Conclusion.—Age appears to play a significant role in the ability to conceive after MFR plus IUI. However, pregnancy loss, multiple gestation, and spontaneous pregnancy in nontreatment cycles were unrelated to age. Life-table analyses suggest that patients 36 years of age or older will benefit from a maximum of only 3 MFR plus IUI treatment cycles. Those younger than 36 years may benefit from up to 4 to 6 cycles.

▶ Although this study was non-randomized, it contained a large number of infertile couples and confirmed the effectiveness of ovarian stimulation and washed intrauterine insemination for the treatment of not only unexplained infertility, but also male factor infertility. Interesting, but not unexpected conclusions are that pregnancy rates are greater for unexplained infertility in women younger than 36 years of age than in those who are older, and that there is continued effectiveness in treating these younger women for more than 3 cycles if they do not conceive. If conception fails to occur after these 6 cycles of treatment, in vitro fertilization or gamete intrafallopian transfer can be offered to these couples.—D.R. Mishell, Jr., M.D.

Effect of Controlled Ovarian Hyperstimulation on Pregnancy Rates After Intrauterine Insemination

DiMarzo SJ, Kennedy JF, Young PE, Hebert SA, Rosenberg DC, Villanueva B (Fertility Inst, San Diego)

Am J Obstet Gynecol 166:1607–1613, 1992 19–25

Background.—Use of intrauterine insemination for various forms of infertility has increased, despite the lack of adequately controlled studies demonstrating its efficacy. For patients with patent fallopian tubes, some clinicians recommend trying intrauterine insemination with controlled ovarian hyperstimulation for a few months before gamete intrafallopian transfer or in vitro fertilization is done. Pregnancy rates were reviewed in patients who had intrauterine insemination: those who had no ovarian stimulation, those who had clomiphene treatment, and those who had human menopausal gonadotropin (hMG) hyperstimulation.

Methods.—The analysis included 195 cycles with clomiphene stimulation, 79 with natural cycles only, and 53 with hMG stimulation. Couples often had 2 or more different treatments for 1 or more cycles as their workup progressed. Washed husband's sperm was always used for intrauterine insemination.

Results.—After 6 cycles, cumulative probability of pregnancy with no ovulation induction was 21%, with a monthly fecundability of 3.4% (Table 1). With clomiphene the pregnancy rate was 33%, and monthly fecundability was 6.1% (Table 2). With hMG, the pregnancy rate was 61% and the monthly fecundability was 13% (Table 3). Both pregnancy rates and monthly fecundability rates were significantly higher in the hMG group. This group had the highest pregnancy rate, although 38% of subjects had undergone an average of 5 insemination cycles with no induction of ovulation or administration of clomiphene before hMG was given. Of patients who became pregnant after hMG was given, 54% had had an average of 4 cycles in 1 or both of the other treatment groups. No significant differences were observed between the other 2 groups. The 3 groups showed no differences in ages of the women, the number of insemination cycles per treatment program, the number of motile sperm per insemination cycle, and the number of inseminations per treatment cycle.

Conclusion.—Compared with no ovulation or clomiphene, hMG stimulation results in a significantly higher pregnancy rate and monthly fecundability after intrauterine insemination. The differences are not attributable to differences in patient populations. Intrauterine insemination should continue to be offered for various causes of infertility, and

TABLE 1.—Cumulative Probability of Pregnancy After Intrauterine Insemination With No Ovulation Induction (Life-Table Analysis)

Cycle No.	*Observed at start of cycle*	*No. of pregnancies*	*No. lost to follow-up*	*Person months of follow-up*	*Probability of pregnancy/cycle*	*Probability of no pregnancy in cycle*	*Cumulative probability of pregnancy*
1	79	2	2	77	0.026	0.974	0.026
2	46	0	2	44	0	1	0.026
3	27	3	4	23	0.13	0.87	0.153
4	17	1	2	15	0.067	0.933	0.21
5	9	0	0	9	0	1	0.21
6	6	0	0	6	0	1	0.21
7	2	0	1	1	0	1	0.21
8	0	0	0	0	0	1	0.21

(Courtesy of DiMarzo SJ, Kennedy JF, Young PE, et al: *Am J Obstet Gynecol* 166:1607–1613, 1992.)

hMG stimulation should be considered sooner, particularly for patients who have failed 4–6 cycles with clomiphene.

▶ Although this study has the deficiency that it was retrospective, it is unlikely that a prospective, randomized study comparing these 3 methods of

TABLE 2.—Cumulative Probability of Pregnancy After Intrauterine Insemination With Clomiphene Administration (Life-Table Analysis)

Cycle No.	*Observed at start of cycle*	*No. of pregnancies*	*No. lost to follow-up*	*Person months of follow-up*	*Probability of pregnancy/cycle*	*Probability of no pregnancy in cycle*	*Cumulative probability of pregnancy*
1	195	12	14	181	0.066	0.934	0.066
2	127	8	4	123	0.065	0.935	0.127
3	81	8	4	77	0.104	0.896	0.218
4	49	0	2	47	0	1	0.218
5	34	1	3	31	0.032	0.968	0.243
6	19	2	1	18	0.111	0.889	0.327
7	12	0	1	11	0	1	0.327
8	7	0	0	7	0	1	0.327
9	6	0	0	6	0	1	0.327
10	4	0	0	4	0	1	0.327
11	3	0	0	3	0	1	0.327
12	2	0	0	2	0	1	0.327
13	1	0	0	1	0	1	0.327
14	0	0	0	0	0	1	0.327

(Courtesy of DiMarzo SJ, Kennedy JF, Young PE, et al: *Am J Obstet Gynecol* 166:1607–1613, 1992.)

treatment of couples with unexplained infertility ever will be performed. Superovulation combined with intrauterine insemination has been shown in several studies to yield higher pregnancy rates than intrauterine insemination alone. It appears that the use of the more complicated and expensive method of superovulation with human menopausal gonadotropin (hMG) is

TABLE 3.—Cumulative Probability of Pregnancy After Intrauterine Insemination With hMG Stimulation

Cycle No.	Observed at start of cycle	No. of pregnancies	No. lost to follow-up	Person months of follow-up	Probability of pregnancy/cycle	Probability of no pregnancy in cycle	Cumulative probability of pregnancy
1	53	6	3	50	0.12	0.88	0.12
2	27	4	1	26	0.154	0.846	0.256
3	13	1	0	13	0.077	0.923	0.313
4	7	1	0	7	0.143	0.857	0.411
5	3	1	0	3	0.233	0.667	0.607
6	1	0	0	1	0	1	0.607
7	0	0	0	0	0	1	0.607

(Courtesy of DiMarzo SJ, Kennedy JF, Young PE, et al: *Am J Obstet Gynecol* 166:1607–1613, 1992.)

superior to the use of clomiphene. Nevertheless, the monthly fecundability rate with clomiphene was double that of the group without ovarian stimulation. Therefore, if the clinician does not have the sonography equipment and laboratory aids necessary to monitor hMG, clomiphene plus intrauterine insemination can be used for a few cycles before referral for hMG or assisted reproductive techniques.—D.R. Mishell, Jr., M.D.

A Prospective Controlled Study of In-Vitro Fertilization, Gamete Intra-Fallopian Transfer and Intrauterine Insemination Combined With Superovulation

Mills MS, Eddowes HA, Cahill DJ, Fahy UM, Abuzeid MIM, McDermott A, Hull MGR (Bristol Maternity Hosp, Bristol, England)
Hum Reprod 7:490–494, 1992 19–26

Background.—The many comparative studies of in vitro fertilization (IVF), gamete intrafallopian transfer (GIFT), and intrauterine insemination (IUI) combined with superovulation have lacked sufficient controls. These 3 treatments were studied prospectively in matched groups of couples undergoing a single treatment cycle.

Methods.—In the 151 couples studied, the women were younger than 40 years of age and had normal ovulatory cycles and normal uteri, and the men had favorable sperm function. Treatments were chosen as appropriate for their condition—IVF for those with tubal disease and GIFT or IUI for nontubal causes. However, to overcome bias from the lack of randomization, all patients had favorable fertilization in a previous cycle of IVF.

Results.—Age, duration of infertility, peak serum estradiol concentration, and the number of follicles recruited were similar in the 3 groups. Those patients with tubal infertility had a higher fertilization rate those with unexplained infertility, who had a higher rate than those with endometriosis. Because of limited ovarian stimulation, the IUI group had lower estradiol levels and fewer follicles. With GIFT, pregnancy rate was 40% and birth rate 32%; with IVF, the figures were 28% and 23%. The pregnancy rate with IUI was 20%. These differences were not significant, but the implantation rate was 21% per egg transferred by GIFT and 11% per embryo transferred by IVF.

Conclusion.—Because of its better implantation rate, GIFT probably offers a significant advantage over IVF. In this study, no significant difference in pregnancy rate is noted. Intrauterine insemination with superovulation has about half the success rate of GIFT.

► Although this study was prospective, it was not randomized, and patients with tubal disease who had the highest fertilization rate were treated by in vitro fertilization only. Furthermore, superovulation in the IUI group was done with clomiphene as well as with human menopausal gonadotropin. It is important to realize that the pregnancy rates with the 3 different methods of treatment, although ranging from 20% to 40% in a single cycle, were not significantly different. Because superovulation and IUI are much less expensive and invasive than GIFT or IVF, unless tubal disease from salpingitis or endometriosis is present, the former therapy should be tried initially for a few cycles.—D.R. Mishell, Jr., M.D.

The ESHRE Multicentre Trial on the Treatment of Unexplained Infertility: A Preliminary Report

Crosignani PG, Walters DE, Soliani A (Univ of Milan; Cambridge Research Station, England)

Hum Reprod 6:953–958, 1991 19–27

Background.—Of an estimated 16% of couples classified as infertile, there is no obvious cause in 10% to 20% of cases. A multicenter study of the treatment of unexplained infertility explored the efficacy of superovulation alone and in combination with intrauterine insemination (IUI), intraperitoneal insemination (IPI), gamete intra-Fallopian transfer (GIFT), or in vitro fertilization (IVF).

Methods.—Nineteen European fertility centers participated in the controlled, randomized trial. Each was invited to use 2 of the 5 treatments being studied. Individual patients were randomly assigned to a treatment. The patients enrolled in the study had had more than 36 months of infertility and were required to be younger than 38 years of age. The patients also had normal fallopian tubes and evidence of spontaneous ovulation. Another criterion for study entry was that the male partner have normal fertility.

Results.—By the end of the trial, 444 patients had undergone a total of 649 cycles. Statistical analysis suggested that the pregnancy rate obtained from superovulation alone was inferior to that resulting from superovulation combined with a method of assisted conception. The pregnancy rate from each assisted procreation method was much better than various estimates of the spontaneous rates cited in the literature and estimates of the upper limit of the pregnancy rate implied by the pretreatment period of infertility.

Conclusion.—The use of one of the methods of assisted conception in this study enhanced the pregnancy rate beyond that expected from superovulation alone, but there was no evidence that one individual invasive methods was superior. All of the pregnancy rates obtained well exceeded various estimates of spontaneous rates.

▶ More large, prospective, randomized multicenter trials such as this one need to be performed in the field of infertility to provide valuable information as to how the infertile couple can best be managed. The main finding from this trial is that the use of some method of improved sperm selection and assisted sperm migration combined with superovulation significantly enhances the prospect of success compared with using superovulation and natural intercourse in couples with unexplained infertility. Because pregnancy rates were similar with the less invasive and less costly procedure of intrauterine or intraperitoneal insemination than with GIFT and IVF, the former procedure should be used initially for 3–6 months.—D.R. Mishell, Jr., M.D.

A Comparison of Intrauterine Insemination, Intraperitoneal Insemination, and Natural Intercourse in Superovulated Women

Evans J, Wells C, Gregory L, Walker S (Univ Hosp of Wales, Cardiff, England)

Fertil Steril 56:1183–1187, 1991 19–28

Background.—A simple, safe treatment is needed for couples with unexplained infertility, oligospermia, and asthenospermia, cervical mucus hostility, or antisperm antibodies. The results of intrauterine insemination (IU), intraperitoneal (IP) insemination, and natural intercourse in women receiving comparable ovarian stimulation were compared.

Methods.—Twenty-two couples with unexplained infertility, 22 with oligospermia or asthenospermia, and 12 with antisperm antibodies were recruited. Ovarian stimulation consisted of clomiphene citrate, 100 mg, on days 5 to 9, continuing with human menopausal gonadotropin, 150 IU, on days 6, 8, and 10. For continued treatment in that cycle, a maximum of 4 follicles of greater than 12 mm was allowed. At least 1 had to be greater than 16 mm. Those responding appropriately received human chorionic gonadotropin, 10,000 IU, to stimulate maturity of the oocyte and corpus luteum emergence. Insemination was done approximately 42 hours later. Initially, couples were assigned randomly to 1 of the 3 treat-

Overall PRS Per Cycle Relating to Type of Treatment in First and Second Part of the Study

Type of Treatment	No. of Cycles	No. of Pregnancies	% Pregnancy/ Cycle
Natural	63 (90)	2‡ (2)§	3.1 (2.2)
IUI	56 (77)	2‡ (2)¶	3.5 (2.5)
DIPI‖	84 (130)	10‡ (16)§,¶	11.9 (12.3)

Values not in parentheses relate to first part of the study only.

Values in parentheses relate to total numbers from the first and second part of the study.

‡ Statistical significance detected when pregnancies after IP insemination compared with those after natural intercourse and IUI in first part of study ($P < .05$).

§ Statistical significance detected when pregnancies in natural cycles are compared with those after IP insemination in the total numbers from the first and second part of the study ($P < .01$).

¶ Statistical significance detected when pregnancies after IUI are compared with those after IP insemination in the total numbers from the first and second part of the study ($P < .05$).

‖ Intraperitoneal insemination abbreviated to DIPI in table.

(Courtesy of Evans J, Wells C, Gregory L, et al: *Fertil Steril* 56:1183–1187, 1991.)

ments being studied. They progressed to the next treatment so that they had 4 cycles of each treatment in rotation.

Results.—Fourteen women became pregnant, for an overall rate of 25%. Seven of these aborted spontaneously. The pregnancy rate (PR) per cycle was significantly higher in cycles in which IP insemination was used compared with the other 2 methods (table). The PR was higher in the group with unexplained infertility, regardless of the method used. The highest PR occurred during the cycles in which patients with unexplained infertility underwent IP insemination, the rate being 17.5%.

Conclusion.—Pregnancy rates were significantly higher after IP than after IUI and natural intercourse after superovulation in this series. Pregnancy rates also were higher in those with unexplained infertility compared with those with semen factors. Intraperitoneal insemination combined with superovulation appears to be a simple, inexpensive, safe alternative to gamete intrafallopian transfer.

► After ovarian hyperstimulation of the woman with unexplained infertility, IP of washed sperm is being used by several European centers instead of the technique of IUI, which is used widely in the United States. In contrast to the results of the large multicenter study reported in the previous abstract, which showed no difference in success rates with the 2 techniques, the result of this randomized trial in one center indicates that IP resulted in higher pregnancy rates than did IUI or natural intercourse. Obviously, more randomized studies are needed to resolve the different results. Until then, if clinicians are not having good success with IUI of washed sperm, they should consider inseminating the washed sperm into the cul-de-sac through the vagina wall by a technique similar to culdocentesis.—D.R. Mishell, Jr., M.D.

Results of IVF From a Prospective Multicentre Study

Haan G, Bernardus RE, Hollanders JMG, Leerentveld RAL, Prak FM, Naaktgeboren N (Univ of Limburg, Maastricht; Free Univ Hosp, Amsterdam; St Radboud Univ Hosp, Nijmegen; Acad Hosp Dijkzigt, Rotterdam; St Elisabeth Hosp, Tilburg, The Netherlands, et al)

Hum Reprod 6:805–810, 1991 19–29

Introduction.—As part of a cost-effectiveness study of in vitro fertilization (IVF) in the Netherlands, the data on clinical results obtained during a predetermined 2-year period were analyzed. Data from all regular IVF treatments performed at 5 major IVF centers were prospectively collected in a uniform way.

Methods.—During the 2-year method, a total of 3,093 IVF treatments were performed at the 5 treatment centers, of which 2,466 were continued to follicle aspiration and 2,089 to embryo transfer. The clinical pregnancy rate was 20% per embryo transfer and 13.5% per started cycle. Of these clinical pregnancies, 93 ended in abortion or ectopic pregnancy;

84 ongoing pregnancies were multiple, including 14 triplets and 2 quadruplets. The rate of multiple pregnancy per ongoing pregnancy was significantly related to the number of embryos transferred.

Results.—Univariate analysis revealed huge differences in results. These differences were classified and analyzed according to patient characteristics and treatment center. Analysis of the patient characteristics revealed that tubal pathology was present in 90% of all cycles, and that the tubal factor was the sole indication in almost 75% of patients. Significantly better results were obtained in the tubal group as compared with all other categories. However, when tubal factor was associated with other factors such as male infertility, older age, or one ovary present, the favorable prognosis disappeared.

Conclusion.—When the data were analyzed according to treatment center, the average ongoing pregnancy per started IVF treatment was almost 3 times higher in the center with the best results compared with the center with the worst results. However, the differences in results at the different treatment centers could not be fully explained. Multivariate analysis confirmed that the differences in results were mainly caused by patient characteristics, the treatment episode, and the treating hospital.

▶ In this prospective multicenter study, the data were accumulated by individuals without a vested interest in the individual programs; the results of the weekly surveys of the centers involved are probably more valid than the data obtained from retrospective self-reporting to the United States IVF registry (1). Thus, the article contains much useful data regarding pregnancy success that can be presented when counseling couples contemplating the use of IVF. Even though the clinical pregnancy rate for embryo transfer was 20% in this series, the ongoing pregnancy rate per IVF treatment initiated was only half that figure, or 10%. Because couples undergoing IVF wish to have a baby—not just become pregnant—they should be counseled accordingly.—D.R. Mishell, Jr., M.D.

Reference

1. Hartz SC: *Fertil Steril* 55:14, 1991.

Expectations of Assisted Conception for Infertility

Hull MGR, Eddowes HA, Fahy U, Abuzeid MI, Mills MS, Cahill DJ, Fleming CF, Wardle PG, Ford WCL, McDermott A (BUPA Hosp, Bristol, England)

BMJ 304:1465–1469, 1992 19–30

Purpose.—Reliable prognostic data for couples undergoing in vitro fertilization and related techniques of assisted conception have been lacking. Analysis of 4 years of practice was done to provide reliable prognostic information to couples seeking assisted conception.

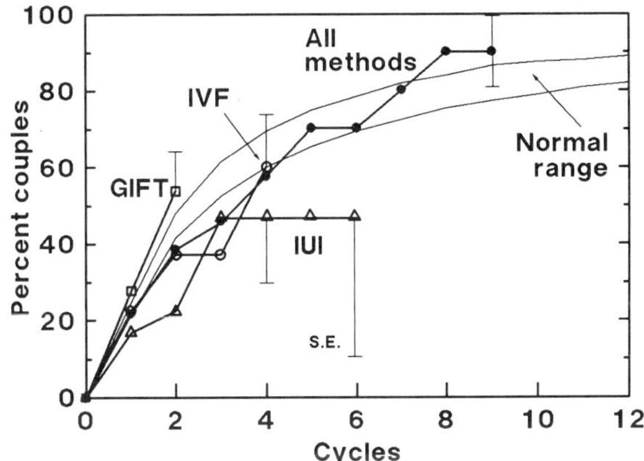

Fig 19–10.—Cumulative successful birth rates in women younger than 40 years and men with normal sperm. Some first pregnancies miscarried. Normal reference population is shown by *two curves*, the *upper* for parous women and the *lower* for nulligravid women (uncorrected for perinatal mortality). (Courtesy of Hull MGR, Eddowes HA, Fahy U, et al: *BMJ* 304:1465–1469, 1992.)

Methods.—The subjects were 804 couples who were offered treatment for various causes of subfertility, including tubal damage, endometriosis for more than 2 years, and sperm dysfunction. The median age of the women was 34 years; the median duration of subfertility was 5 years. A total of 1,280 cycles were completed; 950 in vitro fertilization cycles, 144 gamete intrafallopian transfers, and 186 superovulation and intrauterine inseminations. Pregnancy and birth rates per cycle, and cumulative pregnancy and take-home baby rates per couple were measured.

Findings.—Regardless of the cause of infertility, the results of in vitro fertilization improved steadily in women younger than 40 years of age and in men with normal sperm. The pregnancy rate per cycle was 30% in 1990 to 1991, and the birth rate per cycle was 29% in 1990. For gamete intrafallopian transfer, the pregnancy rate was 36% and the birth rate was 26%; for intrauterine insemination, the figures were 18% and 16%, respectively. After 4 cycles of in vitro fertilization and gamete intrafallopian transfer, the pregnancy rate was 78%. For women younger than 40 years of age and men with normal sperm, the cumulative pregnancy rate with all methods was 82%, and the take-home baby rate was 70% after 6 cycles (Fig 19–10). Miscarriage rates were 45% in women older than 40 years. 9% in those younger than 40 years. There was a 27% rate of multiple births, all in women younger than 40 years.

Conclusion.—Women older than 40 years of age and men with sperm dysfunction appear to have a decreased chance of success with assisted conception for infertility. Superovulation and intrauterine insemination, although not as successful as other methods, may be cost-effective choices in women younger than 40 years.

▶ The data provided in this study are of great use when counseling infertile couples about the probability of taking home a baby after using various methods of assisted reproductive therapy. Women older than 40 years and men with semen abnormalities should be informed about their relatively poor prognosis, and women younger than 40 years whose husbands have normal semen should be counseled that several cycles of therapy will be likely before conception occurs.—D.R. Mishell, Jr., M.D.

In Vitro Fertilization in Unstimulated Cycles: The University of Southern California Experience

Paulson RJ, Macaso TM, Sauer MV, Lobo RA, Francis MM (Univ of Southern California, California Med Ctr, Los Angeles)

Fertil Steril 57:290–293, 1992 19–31

Background.—Successful pregnancies occurring after in vitro fertilization (IVF) in unstimulated cycles triggered with human chorionic gonadotropin (hCG) have been reported. One center's experience with IVF in unstimulated cycles was presented.

Methods.—From 1988 to 1990, 46 women with partners who did not have a male factor began 101 cycles of unsimulated IVF. The patients ranged in age from 28 to 39 years. Fourteen of these women had had previous cycles of ovarian stimulation for IVF; 7 had had a poor response. Ovulation was triggered with hCG, 10,000 IU, administered intramuscularly at approximately midnight, when follicle maturity was considered adequate. Follicle aspirations were done 34–36 hours after hCG was given. All visible follicles were aspirated using transvaginal ultrasound guidance. A group of stimulated IVF cycles from the same center was used for comparison.

Results.—Twenty-three of the 101 cycles were canceled before oocyte retrieval. The remaining 78 aspirations yielded 127 oocytes, or which 91,

Comparison of Pregnancy Rates and Embryo Implantation Rates in Unstimulated and Stimulated IVF Cycles

Type of IVF cycle	No. of aspirations	Clinical pregnancies	Ongoing pregnancies	No.of embryos transferred	Clinical implantations*	Ongoing implantations*
Unstimulated	78	11 (14)†	9 (12)	82	11 (13)	9 (11)
Stimulated	178	49 (28)	35 (20)	730	66 (9)	47 (6.9)

* Per embryo implantation rate; clinical-intrauterine sac; ongoing-cardiac motion 8 weeks after embryo transfer.
† Values in parentheses are percentages.
(Courtesy of Paulson RJ, Sauer MV, et al: *Fertil Steril* 57:290–293, 1992.)

or 72%, were fertilized. All 66 occytes from the dominant follicles fertilized. In the unstimulated IVF group, 78 follicle aspirations resulted in 11 clinical pregnancies. Nine of these were ongoing. Therefore, the clinical pregnancy rate (PR) was 14% per aspiration, and the ongoing PR was 12% per aspiration. In the stimulated comparison group, 178 aspirations resulted in 49 clinical pregnancies, 35 of which were ongoing. The 2 PRs were 28% and 20% per aspiration, respectively. Thirteen percent of the 82 embryos transferred in the unstimulated group produced clinical implantations, with 11% ongoing. Nine percent of 730 transferred embyos implanted in the stimulated group; 6.4% were ongoing (table).

Conclusion.—In patients younger than 40 years of age with partners without male factor, unstimulated IVF can achieve PRs in the range of, but generally lower than, those attained in stimulated cycles. Despite the lower PRs, the individual per embryo implantation rates apparently are higher in unstimulated cycles.

▶ The unstimulated approach to in vitro fertilization has several advantages. First, it is more convenient, because human menopausal gonadotropin (hMG) does not have to be given daily for several days. Second, it is less expensive because hMG does not have to be purchased and less monitoring is required. Third, the incidence of multiple pregnancy is less than that associated with stimulated cycles, thereby resulting in a lower rate of preterm birth. These advantages appear to override the slightly lower pregnancy rate per treatment cycle.—D.R. Mishell, Jr., M.D.

Gamete Intrafallopian Transfer by Hysteroscopy as an Alternative Treatment for Infertility

Possati G, Pareschi A, Seracchioli R, Maccolini A, Melega C, Flamigni C (Univ of Bologna, Italy)

Fertil Steril 56:496–499, 1991 19–32

Objective.—The efficacy and safety of hysteroscopic cannulation of the fallopian tubes for gamete intrafallopian transfer (GIFT) were studied.

Procedure.—Twenty-six women, aged 21–41 years, were treated during a 6-month period. The causes of infertility were terminal tubal damage, male factors, unexplained factors, and endometriosis. Those patients with uterine tubal ostia unsuitable for gamete transfer or cervical incontinence were excluded.

All procedures were performed without hospitalization and general anesthesia. Ovulation was induced, and oocyte retrieval was performed by transvaginal ultrasonically guided puncture. Gamete transfer was performed under CO_2 hysteroscopic visualization using a flexible catheter put through the operating channel. The swim-up method was used to retrieve motile sperm.

Outcome.—The mean number of oocytes retrieved per cycle was 4.8. The mean number of mature oocytes transferred per hysteroscopic GIFT was 3.7, using only 1 tube for hysteroscopic GIFT. There were 7 clinical pregnancies, for a pregnancy rate of 25.9% per cycle. Two pregnancies were aborted during the first weeks of pregnancy, but no patient had ectopic pregnancy. The procedure was well accepted, and patients reported only low distress.

Conclusion.—Hysteroscopic GIFT is a safe and effective noninvasive alternative for treatment of infertility.

▶ The major disadvantage of GIFT (as now performed) is the necessity of general anesthesia and laparoscopy. The technique of aspirating oocytes by needles placed using transvaginally ultrasonic guidance is well established. The technique of cannulating the oviduct with a flexible catheter placed through the endometrial cavity under hysteroscopic visualization is only being performed in a few centers. However, if the results of this study can be repeated elsewhere, the technique will markedly reduce the cost and increase the safety of performing GIFT, because laparoscopy and general anesthesia can be avoided.—D.R. Mishell, Jr., M.D.

Transvaginal Peritoneal Oocyte and Sperm Transfer for the Treatment of Nontubal Infertility

Tan S-L, Balen A, Pampiglione J, Mills C, Steer C, Campbell S (Hallam Med Centre; Middlesex Hosp, London)

Fertil Steril 57:850–853, 1992 19–33

Introduction.—Peritoneal oocyte and sperm transfer (POST) has been tried as a means to simplify and reduce the cost of treatment for infertility. The feasibility and results of transvaginal POST were assessed prospectively.

Methods.—The subjects were 18 patients with unexplained infertility who had failed donor insemination or had oligoasthenozoospermia. Each had no more than 2 cycles of ovarian stimulation, with oocyte recovery performed transvaginally with ultrasonic guidance. After repeated aspiration of the fluid remaining in the pouch of Douglas, an embroyo transfer catheter was loaded with sperm using swim-up technique and as many as 4 oocytes. After the catheter was threaded through the needle, the sperm and oocytes were injected into the pouch under ultrasonic visualization.

Results.—One cycle of POST was conducted in 16 patients, and 2 cycles were done in 2 patients. The results were 5 clinical pregnancies, for a rate of 25%, and 4 live births, for a rate of 20%. When 1-9 oocytes were collected, the pregnancy rate was 20%; when 10 or more oocytes were collected, the pregnancy rate was 40%.

Conclusion.—The POST technique should be considered for patients with nontubal infertility. Measures should be taken to ensure adequate sperm concentration and number of oocytes placed in the pouch of Douglas, and to minimize bleeding at the time of oocyte aspiration. Transvaginal POST will be most useful as an adjunct procedure if superovulation, superovulation and intrauterine insemination, or direct intraperitoneal insemination are used and more than 4 large preovulatory follicles are generated.

▶ Transvaginal peritoneal oocyte and sperm transfer can be used as an alternative to superovulation and either intrauterine or intraperitoneal insemination, as well as gamete intrafallopian transfer in infertile women without tubal pathology. Whether its success rate is similar, less than, or greater than these other techniques of assisted reproduction needs to be determined by prospective comparative studies.—D.R. Mishell, Jr., M.D.

20 Contraception

Clinical Study of the Lactational Amenorrhoea Method for Family Planning

Pérez A, Labbok MH, Queenan JT (Pontificia Universidad Católica de Chile; Georgetown Univ, Washington, DC)

Lancet 339:968–970, 1992 20–1

Background.—In 1988, the Bellagio Consensus Conference proposed guidelines that became the basis for a family planning method called the lactational amenorrhea method (LAM). A woman who is fully or nearly fully breast-feeding her infant and who remains amenorrheic during the first 6 months post partum is protected from pregnancy during that time. The efficacy of LAM as a family planning method was studied prospectively in the context of a breast-feeding support program.

Subjects.—A total of 422 middle-class women from an urban community were offered LAM between 7 and 10 days post partum; 97% completed the 6-month study. The mean age of the women was 27.1 years, and the mean parity was 2.

Results.—The cumulative 6-month life-table pregnancy rate among women who used LAM as their only family planning method was .45%; only 1 woman became pregnant in month 6 (table). More than half (54.2%) of the women used LAM as their family method planning during the first 6 months post partum. Only 9% of exclusive breast-feeders restarted menses by 3 months, and 19% restarted at 6 months.

Life-Table Analysis of LAM Efficacy

Month	No of pregnancies	WM	WMAC	R × 100	P × 100
1	0	384	384	0·00	0·00
2	0	327	711	0·00	0·00
3	0	272	983	0·00	0·00
4	0	243	1226	0·00	0·00
5	0	224	1450	0·00	0·00
6	1	221	1671	0·45	0·45

Abbreviations: WM, number of women using LAM; WMAC, cumulative women-months of use; *R* × 100, monthly risk of conception; *P* × 100, cumulative risk of conception.

(Courtesy of Pérez A, Labbok MH, Queenan JT: *Lancet* 339:968–970, 1992.)

Conclusion.—The lactational amenorrhea method appears to be a highly effective family planning method for breast-feeding women. It is also highly accepted and can safely serve as an introductory method for breast-feeding women.

▶ The Bellagio Consensus Conference concluded that full lactation with frequent nursing episodes and no supplemental feedings is a very effective form of contraception during the first 6 months post partum—as long as the mother remains amenorrheic. This clinical study confirms the conclusions of the conference. Unfortunately, it requires a great deal of motivation for women exclusively to breast-feed their babies for 6 months. Therefore, when supplemental feeding is introduced, another method of contraception should be initiated.—D.R. Mishell, Jr., M.D.

Barrier Methods of Contraception and Cervical Intraepithelial Neoplasia

Coker AL, Hulka BS, McCann MF, Walton LA (Univ of South Carolina, Columbia; Univ of North Carolina, Chapel Hill)

Contraception 45:1–10, 1992 20–2

Background.—Most case-control studies of the topic suggest that barrier methods of contraception decrease the risk of cervical intraepithelial neoplasia (CIN). Not all studies have controlled for confounding variables, however, and the protective effect has not always been consistent. A case-controlled study of CIN II or III was evaluated to examine further the association between preinvasive cervical cancer and barrier methods of contraception.

Methods.—The study included 103 patients with confirmed CIN II or III that was newly diagnosed during a 14-month period. Only patients aged 18–45 years were included. The controls were 258 family practice patients with normal cytological findings on Papanicolaou smear. Women in both groups were interviewed as to their risk factors for CIN, including the use of barrier contraception.

Findings.—The women with CIN were younger, less educated, and of lower socioeconomic status (SES); they were also more likely to be divorced, to have ever been pregnant, to have had sex with more than 2 partners, to have had a sexually transmitted disease, and to smoke. Controlling for age, education, and number of partners, there was no increased risk of CIN for women who began having sex before age 18 years; there was no risk associated with use of an intrauterine device or oral contraceptives.

Barrier methods had been used by 24.3% of subjects and 58.2% of controls, for a crude odds ratio of .2. After adjustment for confounders, the odds ratio was .5, with no difference for level II and III CIN. There was a duration effect for increasing years of barrier method use, but there was no recency or latency effect. The adjusted odds ratio for diaphragm use was .3, and that for condom use was .5; the adjusted odds ratio for spermicide use was 1.3, suggesting no reduced risk. The odds ratio was .3 in the high SES, .5 in the middle SES, and .2 in the low SES.

Conclusion.—Barrier methods of contraception appear to reduce risk of preinvasive cervical neoplasia. Use of a condom or diaphragm reduces risk of CIN II/III, but use of spermicide alone does not. Barrier methods may help to decrease the risk of cervical neoplasia as well as unwanted pregnancy and sexually transmitted disease.

▶ Because CIN is thought to be causally related to infection with human papillomavirus that is sexually transmitted, one would expect that the use of barrier techniques that reduce the chance of transmission of this virus from the male to the female sexual partner would result in a decreased risk of CIN. Thus, the results of this study are those to be expected, and they agree with the results of most other epidemiological studies of different design. Women should be counseled that the use of condoms or diaphragms should reduce the risk of CIN developing with the problems of treatment, follow-up, and potential for invasive cancer developing.—D.R. Mishell, Jr., M.D.

Age-Specific Differences in the Relationship Between Oral Contraceptive Use and Breast Cancer

Wingo PA, Lee NC, Ory HW, Beral V, Peterson HB, Rhodes P (Ctrs for Disease Control, Atlanta; Radcliffe Infirmary, Oxford, England)

Obstet Gynecol 78:161–170, 1991 20–3

Background.—Almost all research on the use of oral contraceptives (OCs) and the aggregate risk of breast cancer indicates that the 2 are not associated in women aged 20–54 years. However, there are age-specific differences in the breast cancer–parity relationship and in other breast cancer risk factors. The Centers for Disease Control therefore reassessed data from the Cancer and Steroid Hormone Study to determine whether use of OCs has different effects on the risk of breast cancer at different ages of diagnosis.

Methods.—This population-based, case-control study was done in 8 geographic locations in the United States from 1980–1982. The cases were 4,711 women, aged 20–54 years, who had histologically confirmed breast cancer. The controls were 4,676 women matched to the geographic-age distribution of the cases.

Results.—Age-specific breast cancer incidence risks are seen in the table. The relationship between the risk of breast cancer risk and use of OCs appeared to vary by age at diagnosis. Those women aged 20–34 years at diagnosis or interview who had ever used OCs had a slightly higher risk of breast cancer than did same-aged women who had never used OCs. The odds ratio in the former group was 1.4. No trends of in-

Hypothetical Annual Age-Specific Breast Cancer Incidence Rates in United States Women Aged 20–54 in 1982

Age	OC Use History	Percent OC Use+	RR* (95% CI)	Incidence Per 100,000 Women per Year	Rate Difference Per 100,000 Women
20-34	Never	24.0	Ref	8.5	
	Ever	76.0	1.4 (1.0-2.1)	11.9	3.4
	All Women	100.0		11.1	
35-44	Never	28.6	Ref	74.8	
	Ever	71.4	1.1 (0.9-1.3)	82.2	7.4
	All Women	100.0		80.1	
45-54	Never	53.1	Ref	177.5	
	Ever	46.9	0.9 (0.8-1.0)	159.8	-17.7
	All Women	100.0		169.2	

* The age-specific estimates of percentages of never and ever use of oral contraceptives for controls younger than 45 years of age at interview in the Cancer and Steroid Hormone Study data were weighted to estimates from the 1982 National Survey of Family Growth. The estimates for older controls were not weighted.

† The age-specific relative risk estimates are from Table 3 (original article).

The breast cancer incidence data are annual age- and sex-specific rates from SEER (Surveillance Epidemiology and End Results [Program]) for 1978-1981. The estimates of the annual incidence of breast cancer by OC use are calculated using percent OC use, relative risk, and the age- and sex-specific SEER rates.

(Courtesy of Wingo PA, Lee NC, Ory HW, et al: *Obstet Gynecol* 78:161–170, 1991.)

creasing or decreasing risk could be found among those women with any measure of OC use. There was no association between OC use and breast cancer in women aged 35–44 years. Women aged 45–54 years who used OCs had a slightly reduced risk of breast cancer, with an odds ratio of .9. In this group, the risk estimates decreased significantly with increasing time since first and last use.

Conclusion.—The finding that younger women have a slightly higher risk of breast cancer with use of OCs is compatible with findings from other research. Fewer studies have reported a reduced risk estimate for the oldest age group. These data do not suggest that changes in prescription or use of OCs are necessary.

▶ The incidence of breast cancer steadily increases with increasing age, and the occurrence of this disease is uncommon among women younger than 35 years of age. Therefore, the findings of this study indicate that the use of high-dose OCs has a net effect of reducing the risk of breast cancer among women younger than 55 years. The slight reduction in the risk of breast cancer in women aged 45–54 years would result in a lower absolute number of cases of breast cancer than the consequences of the greater increased risk among women younger than 35 years. Studies need to be undertaken to determine the effect of OC use on the risk of breast cancer in women older than 55 years when the incidence of the disease is even higher.—D.R. Mishell, Jr., M.D.

Clinical and Metabolic Considerations of Long-Term Oral Contraceptive Use

Godsland IF, Crook D, Wynn V (Wynn Inst for Metabolic Research, London)
Am J Obstet Gynecol 166:1955–1963, 1992 20–4

Introduction.—With the availability of lower dose formulations of oral contraceptives, there is support for their use for longer periods and in older women. Data from a cross-sectional study were used to analyze the effects of duration of contraceptive use, age of the user, and risk of cardiovascular disease.

Duration of Use.—In women taking a common combination oral contraceptive (150 μg of levonorgestrel plus 30 μg of ethinyl estradiol), glucose tolerance deteriorated progressively for up to 3 years. No increase was seen in the area under the oral glucose tolerance test (OGTT) glucose concentration profile with up to 12 years of oral contraceptive use, unlike in other studies. Similarly, no progression was seen in the OGTT insulin area, fasting serum triglyceride levels, and low-density lipoprotein (LDL) and high-density lipoprotein subfraction 2 (HDL_2) cholesterol.

Age.—Linear regression equations for age derived with various factors showed a marked interaction with regard to an oral contraceptive-induced increased in fasting serum triglyceride levels, which increased with age in oral contraceptive users. There was less of an effect of age in oral contraceptive users with LDL cholesterol, and there was no difference in regard to HDL_2 cholesterol. Age had less of an effect on glucose tolerance in oral contraceptive users, but there was no difference in OGTT insulin response.

Previous Use.—The only differences between those who had and had not previously used oral contraceptives were in OGTT insulin response and HDL_2 cholesterol, and these differences became nonsignificant after adjustment for other factors.

Conclusion.—After 2 years of continuous oral contraceptive use, no apparent progression was found in the metabolic risk markers for cardiovascular disease. Older women using oral contraceptives appear to have increased triglyceride concentrations, but there is no potentially adverse interaction between age and duration of use. Also, no effect of previous oral contraceptive use was found. Oral contraceptive use may be extended in patients older than 35 years of age, but these women should have regular health checks and measurement of serum lipid levels.

▶ In 1991, the product labeling of all oral contraceptives was changed to state that the benefits of administering oral contraceptives to women older than 35 years may outweigh the risks. This study provides information indicating that neither increasing age nor increasing duration of use of oral contraceptives beyond 2 years causes progression of the changes in glucose or lipid metabolism produced by this strongly progestogenic agent. These data provide reassurance that continuation of low-dose oral contraceptive use after age 35 years will not worsen the health of healthy, nonsmoking women.—D.R. Mishell, Jr., M.D.

Oral Contraceptives and Non-Contraceptive Oestrogens in the Risk of Gallstone Disease Requiring Surgery

La Vecchia C, Negri E, D'Avanzo B, Parazzini F, Gentile A, Franceschi S (Istituto di Ricerche Farmacologiche "Mario Negri," Milan, Italy)

J Epidemiol Community Health 46:234–236, 1992 20–5

Introduction.—Research suggests that gallstone incidence may be related to female hormones. The frequency of this disease makes it a public health issue. The relationship between oral contraceptives, noncontraceptive estrogens, and risks of gallstone disease requiring surgery was studied.

Patients.—The hospital-based, case-control study included 235 women with gallstones requiring surgery and 538 controls admitted for acute diseases other than digestive or hormonal diseases or conditions that might affect the use of female hormone preparations. The median age of case patients was 54 years. All had a discharge diagnosis of cholelithiasis or "cholecystitis"; in no cases did the original diagnosis date back more than 1 year, and all case patients had undergone cholecystectomy.

Findings.—Seventeen percent of women with gallstones requiring surgery and 15% of controls had ever used oral contraceptives, for an age-adjusted relative risk of .8. There was no direct association with duration of use. Eight percent of case patients and 5% of control patients had ever used estrogen replacement therapy, for a relative risk of 1.7. This risk was also unrelated to duration of use, and none of the estimates were significant.

Conclusion.—Oral contraceptives and other estrogens appear to play no important role in the etiology of gallbladder disease. This confirms the results of previous studies.

▶ Although high-steroid–dose oral contraceptive formulations accelerated the development of symptomatic gallbladder disease, the overall risk was not increased with long-term use. This study indicates that both the lower-dose–steroid oral contraceptive formulations as well as estrogen replacement therapy have no appreciable effect on the development of gallbladder disease severe enough to require surgery.—D.R. Mishell, Jr., M.D.

Functional Ovarian Cysts in Relation to the Use of Monophasic and Triphasic Oral Contraceptives

Holt VL, Daling JR, McKnight B, Moore D, Stergachis A, Weiss NS (Fred Hutchinson Cancer Research Ctr, Seattle; Univ of Washington, Seattle; Ctr for Health Studies, Seattle)

Obstet Gynecol 79:529–533, 1992 20–6

Background.—Previous research suggests that the use of monophasic combination oral contraceptives is associated with a markedly reduced risk of functional cysts, whereas the use of progestin-only oral contraceptives is associated with an increased risk. However, past studies have had problems with internal and external validity. The effect of monophasic or triphasic OCs that are currently in use on the risk of functional ovarian cyst development was studied.

Methods.—The patients were all enrollees in a group health cooperative who had received either an inpatient primary diagnosis of functional ovarian cyst in 1988 or 1989, or an outpatient primary diagnosis of functional ovarian cyst from March 1988 through August 1989 at 1 of 5 primary care clinics. A total of 67 women had an inpatient diagnosis, and 39 had an outpatient diagnosis. The patients ranged in age from 15 to 39 years. The control subjects also were enrollees, chosen randomly and matched to the cases for age, primary care clinic, and enrollment date. There were 255 controls.

Findings.—A medical record review showed that 16% of the cases and 19% of the controls were currently using monophasic oral contraceptives. A total of 11% of the patients and 9% of controls were using triphasic oral contraceptives. Compared with women who did not use hormonal contraception, the relative risks of a diagnosed functional ovarian cyst among current oral contraceptive users were .8 for monophasic users and 1.3 for triphasic users.

Conclusion.—In contrast to previous research, it is suggested that current low-dose monophasic oral contraceptive use does not greatly reduce a woman's risk of functional ovarian cyst formation. The current findings also do not support recent speculation that current triphasic oral contraceptive use substantially increases the risk of functional ovarian cysts.

▶ This retrospective study indicates that the low-dose oral contraceptives in use today do not decrease the risk of functional ovarian cysts, as was demonstrated in earlier studies with the higher dose oral contraceptive formulations. However, a major difference between the studies is that the earlier studies investigated the risk in women who had ovarian cysts requiring hospitalization, whereas this study included all women (both inpatients and outpatients) with ovarian cysts larger than 2 cm. A reassuring finding is that there was no relationship between ovarian cyst development and women using multiphasic formulations, as was suggested by a small case series that was widely publicized.—D.R. Mishell, Jr., M.D.

Oral Contraceptive Type and Functional Ovarian Cysts

Lanes SF, Birmann B, Walker AM, Singer S (Epidemiology Resources Inc, Newton, Mass; Harvard School of Public Health, Boston; Maine Health Information Ctr, Augusta)

Am J Obstet Gynecol 166:956–961, 1992 20–7

Introduction.—The first study investigating the risk of functional ovarian cysts among women using multiphasic oral contraceptives compared with other types of oral contraceptives and nonuse of oral contraceptives was reviewed.

Study Design.—Using the automated files of Maine Medicaid, a cohort of 7,462 women (aged 15–44 years) who were prescribed an oral contraceptive from January 1, 1987, to December 31, 1988, was studied. Oral contraceptives were grouped as multiphasic pills, low-dose monophasic pills (≤ 35 μg estrogen), high-dose monophasic pills (> 35 μg estrogen), and progestin-only pills. The cases were defined as women with a principal diagnosis of a functional ovarian cyst > 20 mm in diameter that was diagnosed by pelvic ultrasound and required hospitalization or outpatient surgery.

Findings.—There were 32 women with functional ovarian cysts, and the incidence rate was greatest when no oral contraceptive was prescribed (Table 1). When compared with periods with no oral contraceptive prescribed, the incidence rate of functional ovarian cysts was reduced by 76% with high-dose monophasic pills, by 48% with low-dose monophasic pills, and by 9% with multiphasic pills (Table 2). When compared with women prescribed multiphasic pills, the rate of func-

TABLE 1.—Incidence Rates of Functional Ovarian Cysts by Oral Contraceptive Category

	No. of cases	*Person months*	*Rate (× 10,000)*
No prescription	19	42,738.0	4.4
Recent prescription	2	8,872.8	2.3
Active prescription	11	44,053.2	2.5
Progestin-only	0	219.6	0.0
Multiphasic	5	13,196.4	3.8
≤35 μg estrogen	5	22,251.6	2.2
>35 μg estrogen	1	8,385.6	1.2

(Courtesy of Lanes SF, Birmann B, Walker AM, et al: *Am J Obstet Gynecol* 166:956–961, 1992.)

TABLE 2.—Rate Ratio Estimates for Functional Ovarian Cysts Comparing Each Oral Contraceptive Category With No Oral Contraception

	*Rate ratio**	*95% Confidence interval*
No prescription	1.00	Reference category
Active prescription:		
Multiphasic	0.91	0.30-2.31
≤35 μg estrogen	0.52	0.17-1.33
>35 μg estrogen	0.24	0.01-1.34

* Rate ratios standardized to age distribution of index (i.e., "exposed") category.

(Courtesy of Lanes SF, Birmann B, Walker AM, et al: *Am J Obstet Gynecol* 166:956–961, 1992.)

tional ovarian cysts was 40% lower with low-dose monophasic pills and 67% lower with high-dose monophasic pills. The incidence of cysts across these oral contraceptives decreased progressively with increasing ovarian suppression. The overall incidence of cysts decreased with increasing duration of use.

Conclusion.—The preventive effect of oral contraceptives against functional ovarian cysts appears to be greater for monophasic pills, particularly with high-dose pills, than for the newer multiphasic pills.

▶ Unlike the study in Abstract 20–6, in this investigation, the rate of functional ovarian cysts diagnosed by pelvic ultrasound and requiring hospitalization or outpatient surgery was studied in the same cohort both when the women received and did not receive oral contraceptives. In contrast to the first study, the results of this study concluded that the lower dose monophasic oral contraceptives also reduce the formation of ovarian cysts. These diverse findings may be the result of differences in study design. Both studies failed to confirm the erroneous, but widely accepted, belief that multiphasic oral contraceptives increase the risk of formation of ovarian cysts.—D.R. Mishell, Jr., M.D.

Oral Contraceptive Use May Protect Against Low Bone Mass

Kleerekoper M, Brienza RS, Schultz LR, Johnson CC, Henry Ford Hosp Osteoporosis Cooperative Research Group (Henry Ford Hosp, Detroit)

Arch Intern Med 151:1971–1976, 1991 20–8

Objective.—A cross-sectional epidemiological review was undertaken to identify risk factors for low bone mineral density (BMD) in a series of 2,297 women, 75% of whom were postmenopausal. Bone mineral density was measured in the forearm using single-photon abosorptiometry, and in the lumbar spine by dual-photon absorptiometry.

Relationship of Duration of OC Use and Bone Density

Duration of OC Use, y	N	Odds Ratio	95% Confidence Interval
0*	1577	. . .	. . .
<2	170	0.52	0.27-1.00
2-<4	143	0.24	0.09-0.65
4-<6	93	0.37	0.14-1.03
6-<8	50	0.35	0.08-1.43
8-<10	34	0.25	0.03-1.85
10+	111	0.23	0.07-0.73

* All intervals compared with unexposed group. Women with 6 months or less OC use were classified with the never-used group ($n = 3$). Duration of use was unknown for 77 women.

(Courtesy of Kleerekoper M, Brienza RS, Schultz LR, et al: *Arch Intern Med* 151:1971-1976, 1991.)

Subjects.—Forty-eight percent of the premenopausal women and 25% of the postmenopausal group reported using oral contraceptives (OCs). The average time of OC use was 4.7 years. Older women tended to report OC use less often.

Observations.—Women reporting use of OCs were significantly less likely than others to have low BMD estimates, and they were significantly more likely to have high measurements. The proportion of women with a history of OC use increased the values of BMD, and women using OCs for 10 years or longer exhibited the greatest protective effect (table). In logistic regression analysis, both OC use and the duration of use correlated positively with BMD.

Implications.—Women who have used OCs exhibit some degree of protection against low bone mineral density. This study is large, and the effects of premenopausal OC exposure were assessed in a group of predominantly postmenopausal women. The protective effect of OC use apparently persists in the postmenopausal years.

▶ This large multicenter study provides evidence that the hyperestrogen state produced by OC use increases bone mass premenopausally and reduces the risk of osteoporosis developing postmenopausally. Because only 15% of American women take estrogen replacement postmenopausally and 25% of white and oriental postmenopausal women who are not taking estrogen have fractures develop as a result of osteoporosis, this effect on bone is another substantial noncontraceptive benefit of oral contraception use.—D.R. Mishell, Jr., M.D.

Is Oral Contraceptive Use Still Associated With an Increased Risk of Fatal Myocardial Infarction? Report of a Case-Control Study

Thorogood M, Mann J, Murphy M, Vessey M (Univ of Oxford, Oxford, England; Univ of Otago, Dunedin, New Zealand)

Br J Obstet Gynaecol 98:1245–1253, 1991 20–9

Background.—During the 1960s and 1970s, several studies showed an increased risk of myocardial infarction in women taking oral contraceptives. However, many changes have taken place in oral contraceptives since then, including changes in formulation and a decline in use by women older than 30 years of age. Whether there has been any change in this risk was determined in a case-control study of fatal myocardial infarction.

Methods.—The subjects were 161 British women younger than 40 years of age who died of myocardial infarction from 1986 to 1988. For each subject, 2 living controls, matched for age and marital status, were selected from the same general practice lists as the subject. The 2 groups were compared for oral contraceptive use, which was assigned to 1 of 3 categories: current use, meaning use in the month before death; previous use, meaning use in the preceding 10 years but not in the last month; and nonuse, meaning no use within the last 10 years.

Results.—The risk factors considered were diabetes, hyperlipidemia, hypertension, angina, or previous myocardial infarction. At least 1 of these occurred in 34% of the subjects and 3% of the controls; the estimated relative risk of myocardial infarction with at least 1 risk factor present was 7.6. The relative risk of myocardial infarction with current cigarette smoking was 19.3%. The subjects were somewhat more likely to take oral contraceptives, but not significantly so. The relative risk associated with current use compared with nonuse was 1.1; allowing for the effects of surgical sterilization and risk factors, the relative risk was 1.9. With previous use, the relative risk also was 1.9. However, when calculated for current and previous risk and adjusting for other risk factors, the relative risk decreased to 1.1. Subjects were more than 3 times as likely to use formulations containing 50 μg of estrogen, although this difference was nonsignificant. The relative risk associated with use of these preparations was 4.2. The duration of contraceptive use or the time since last contraceptive use appeared to have no effect on risk.

Discussion.—After adjusting for other risk factors for fatal myocardial infarction—including medical risk factors and surgical sterilization—the relative risk associated with current and previous use of oral contraceptives is estimated to be 1.9. Much of this effect may be attributable to smoking. If there has been any increase in risk, it may be solely with older combined preparations containing 50 μg of estrogen.

▶ The finding of this study is in agreement with the study performed in New England by Rosenberg et al., which reported that use of the current low-dose oral contraceptives is not associated with a significantly increased risk of myocardial infarction (1). As was found in the New England study, the majority of myocardial infarctions that occurred in oral contraceptive users were in those women who also smoked. Now, 3 studies have shown that the use of currently marketed oral contraceptives in nonsmoking women is not associated with an increased risk of myocardial infarction.—D.R. Mishell, Jr., M.D.

Reference

1. Rosenberg L, et al: *Am J Epidemiol* 131:1009, 1990.

Risk Factors for Fatal Venous Thromboembolism in Young Women: A Case-Control Study

Thorogood M, Mann J, Murphy M, Vessey M (Univ of Oxford, England; Univ of Otago, Dunedin, New Zealand)

Int J Epidemiol 21:48–52, 1992 20–10

Background.—Epidemiological studies have shown that the magnitude of the risk of venous thromboembolism associated with the use of oral contraceptives (OCs) correlates with the estrogen dose in the OC preparation. Because estrogen doses in OC formulations have been reduced in recent years, the statistics on fatal venous thromboembolism in young women were updated.

Methods.—All deaths that occurred in England and Wales among female patients (age, 16–39 years) between January 1986 and December 1988 for which the underlying cause of death was coded as pulmonary embolism (PE) or venous thromboembolism were included in the analysis. For each subject, 2 living controls matched for age and marital status were randomly selected from the records of a general practice. Sixty case patients and 115 controls met the criteria for inclusion in this analysis.

Results.—The cause of death was listed as PE without mention of venous thrombosis in 14 women and as venous thrombosis in the other 46. Five women (8%) had a history of previous deep venous thrombosis and 4 (7%) had a history of superficial venous thrombosis. Four cases (7%) and 1 control (1%) had a history of previous PE. The estimated odds ratio (OR) of fatal venous thrombosis associated with a history of previous venous thrombosis was 4. The estimated OR of fatal venous thromboembolism associated with recent surgery or an accident within 3 months was 11.1. None of the differences between cases and controls in the use of OCs was significant. The overall estimated OR associated with current use of an OC was 1.6. After controlling for the presence of other conditions, the estimated OR increased to 2.1.

Conclusion.—Surgery or an accident increase the risk of venous thrombosis. The estimated OR of venous thromboembolism associated with the current use of OCs in this study was considerably less than 3, and it did not reach statistical significance. This risk was considerably smaller than that reported in earlier studies.

▶ It has been established that the risk of pulmonary embolism associated with OC use is directly related to the dose of estrogen in the formulation. In the 1960s and 1970s, when the formulations contained estrogen in an amount of 50 μg or more, there was a markedly increased hepatic syntheses of the globulins involved in the clotting process. Therefore, the risk of both venous and arterial thrombosis developing and their fatal consequences of pulmonary embolism and myocardial infarction were significantly increased. Now that nearly all OC users ingest formulations with less than 50 μg of estrogen, the risk of fatal pulmonary embolism, as well as myocardial infarction, is not significantly increased.—D.R. Mishell, Jr., M.D.

Desogestrel and Gestodene in Oral Contraceptives: 12 Months' Assessment of Carbohydrate and Lipoprotein Metabolism

Petersen KR, Skouby SO, Pedersen RG (Diabetes Ctr, Copenhagen)

Obstet Gynecol 78:666–672, 1991 20–11

Objective.—A group of 34 healthy women was evaluated to determine whether a low-dose combination of desogestrel and gestodene (both third-generation progestogens) with ethinyl estradiol reduces the effects of oral contraceptives on carbohydrate and lipoprotein metabolism.

Treatment.—Fifteen women received 20 μg of ethinyl estradiol plus 150 μg of desogestrel, whereas the other 19 women received 30 μg of ethinyl estradiol combined with 75 μg of gestodene. Both regimens were given cyclically for 21 days, followed by 7 drug-free days, for 12 consecutive cycles.

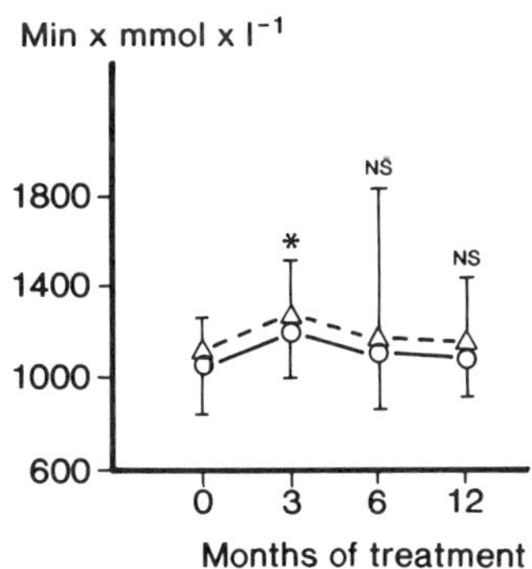

Fig 20–1.—Area under the glucose concentration curves during a 180-minute oral glucose tolerance test with 75 g of glucose. *Triangles* = ethinyl estradiol plus desogestrel; *circles* = ethinyl estradiol plus gestodene; *asterisk* indicates pretreatment vs. 3 months, $P < .05$; *NS* = not significant. (Courtesy of Petersen KR, Skouby SO, Pedersen RG: *Obstet Gynecol* 78:666–672, 1991.)

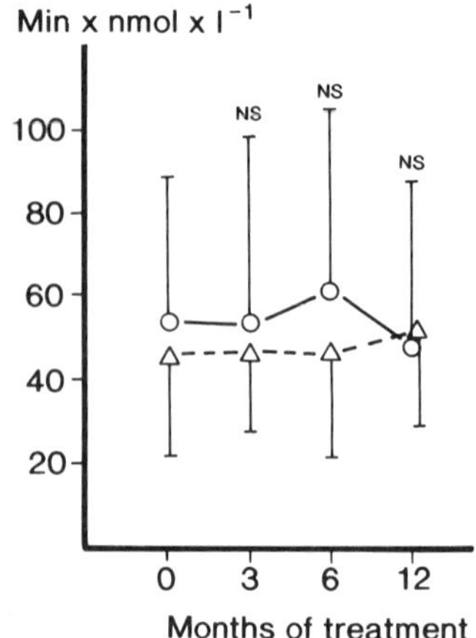

Fig 20–2.—Area under the insulin concentration curves during a 180-minute oral glucose tolerance test with 75 g of glucose. *Triangles* = ethinyl estradiol plus desogestrel; *circles* = ethinyl estradiol plus gestodene; *NS* = not significant. (Courtesy of Petersen KR, Skouby SO, Pedersen RG: *Obstet Gynecol* 78:666–672, 1991.)

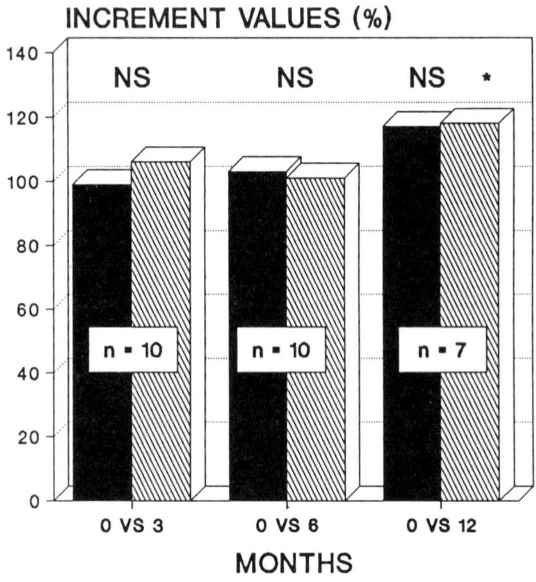

Fig 20–3.—Incremental values (in percent of pretreatment levels) of fasting plasma levels of high-density lipoprotein$_3$ cholesterol. *Asterisk* indicates pretreatment vs. 12 months, $P < .05$; *NS* = not significant. (Courtesy of Petersen KR, Skouby SO, Pedersen RG: *Obstet Gynecol* 78:666–672, 1991.)

Observations.—Both groups had a transient increase in the area under the glucose concentration curve (Fig 20–1) and no change in the area under the insulin curve (Fig 20–2). The plasma high-density lipoprotein (HDL) cholesterol levels increased in women given desogestrel, whereas total cholesterol remained unchanged. Both very-low-density lipoprotein cholesterol and triglycerides increased significantly. Similar changes occurred in gestodene-treated women. The HDL cholesterol increased for the first 6 months in gestodene-treated women. The increase in HDL_3 cholesterol at 12 months was significant only in women given gestodene (Fig 20–3).

Summary.—No marked changes in carbohydrate metabolism were associated with monophasic combinations of ethinyl estradiol with desogestrel or gestodene. Also, no persistent adverse effects on lipid levels were noted.

▶ Although neither of these oral contraception formulations are currently available in the U.S., they have been marketed in Europe for several years and soon will become available in the U.S. It is reassuring that neither of these formulations produces adverse changes in carbohydrates or lipid metabolism. Clinicians should also realize that some of the currently available low-dose ethanol estradiol norethindrone formulations also produce no adverse changes in carbohydrate or lipid metabolism. Trials comparing the effects of low-dose combination norethindrone formulations with gestodene and desogestrel formulations should be undertaken to see whether the newly developed "third-generation" progestins have less adverse metabolic effects than formulations with low doses of norethindrone.—D.R. Mishell, Jr., M.D.

Are Oral Contraceptive-Associated Liver Cell Adenomas Premalignant?

Tao L-C (Toronto Gen Hosp, Toronto)

Acta Cytol 36:338–344, 1992 20–12

Background.—A convincing relationship exists between the use of oral contraceptives and the development of liver cell adenoma; however, a relationship between contraceptive use and hepatocellular carcinoma remains speculative.

Series.—Transabdominal fine-needle aspiration biopsy was carried out in 1,670 patients seen in 1977–1990 with a liver mass or masses on imaging. Ninety-nine biopsy specimens were reported as "hepatocellular carcinoma," and 9 others as "consistent with liver cell adenoma." Three of the patients with carcinoma were known to have used oral contraception for 10–12 years. All those with liver cell adenoma had used oral contraceptives for 5–10 years.

Findings.—The mean duration of oral contraceptive use in those patients with liver cell adenoma was 7½ years. Two patients had foci of liver cell dysplasia develop within their adenomas after the prolonged and continuous use of oral contraceptives. The three oral contraceptive users with hepatocellular carcinoma had used contraception for a mean of 11 years.

Discussion.—Some patients using oral contraception for a prolonged period appear to have liver cell adenoma, dysplasia, and hepatocellular carcinoma develop sequentially. Only the transition to liver cell adenoma is reversible; this seems not to be a premalignant lesion. Liver cell dysplasia within an adenoma is, in contrast, irreversible. Liver cell adenomas should be resected, especially in women who have used oral contraception for longer than 8 years.

▶ The hypothesis suggested in the authors' discussion is speculative but cannot be dismissed. Even though epidemiological studies have suggested that oral contraceptive use is not associated with an increased risk of liver cancer, clinicians should routinely palpate the liver edge in women who have used oral contraceptives for 5 or more years. If an adenoma is found, use of oral contraceptive should be discontinued, and if spontaneous regression does not occur, surgical resection should be strongly considered.—D.R. Mishell, Jr., M.D.

Prolonged Intrauterine Contraception: A Seven-Year Randomized Study of the Levonorgestrel 20 mcg/day (LNg 20) and the Copper T380 Ag IUDS

Sivin I, Stern J, Coutinho E, Mattos CER, El Mahgoub S, Diaz S, Pavez M, Alvarez F, Brache V, Thevenin F, Diaz J, Faundes A, Diaz MM, McCarthy T, Mishell DR Jr, Shoupe D (Ctr for Biomedical Research, New York; Universidade Federal de Bahia, Salvador, Brazil; Ain Shams Univ, Cairo; Instituto Chileno de Medicina Reproductiva, Santiago, Chile; PROFAMILIA, Santo Domingo, et al)

Contraception 44:473–480, 1991 20–13

Background.—Theoretically, very long-acting methods of contraception are economical and desirable. A 7-year study of medicated intrauterine devices (IUDs) releasing copper or levonorgesterel was reported.

Methods and Results.—Five clinics participated in the 7-year randomized study. Two other clinics participated in a 5-year study. A levonorgestrel-releasing IUD (LNg20) was compared with the Copper T 380Ag IUD (TCu 380Ag). There were no pregnancies in either group in years 6 and 7. The cumulative pregnancy rates were 1.1 per 100 at 7 years for the steroid-releasing IUD and 1.4 per 100 for the copper-releasing IUD. Cumulative pelvic inflammatory disease rates did not differ significantly between groups and they were less than 4% for devices after 7 years of use. Infection rates seemed lowest in the sixth and seventh years of the study. The main contributor to differences in cumulative continuation rates between groups was termination attributable to amenorrhea. At the

Seven-Year Gross Cumulative Rates Per 100

Item	Rates: All Clinics LNg 20 Rate S.E.	All Clinics TCu Rate S.E.	Clinics with Seven-Year LNg IUD LNg 20 Rate	Clinics with Seven-Year LNg IUD TCu Rate	No. of Events All Clinics LNg 20	No. of Events All Clinics TCu 380Ag
Pregnancy	1.1±0.5	1.4±0.4	0.5	1.0	6	10
Expulsion	11.7±1.2*	8.4±1.0	11.7*	8.3	99	74
Amenorrhea	24.6±2.0***	1.1±0.6	21.9***	1.0	150	5
Other Menstrual/Pain	20.4±1.9**	30.0±1.9	18.2**	28.0	133	210
PID/Endometritis	3.6±0.8	3.6±0.8	3.6	3.4	24	24
Other Medical	23.3±2.2	20.4±1.9	22.6	19.4	121	116
Planning Pregnancy	29.4±2.0	33.8±2.1	29.5	33.5	169	195
Other Personal	15.5±2.0	14.2±1.7	15.6	12.2	71	72
End of Study[A]	15.6±2.2	4.1±1.2	3.6	4.4	47	14
Continuation	23.1±1.4*	27.2±1.5	24.9	29.4		
N., Enrolled			897	896	1125	1121
N.,Entered Month 84			172	189	172	211
Woman-Years			2831	3085	3371	3758
Users with <7 yrs			0	0	5	16
Percent LFU					11.5	16.2

A, includes women who stopped use before month 82; not counted as a relevant termination.
Abbreviation: LFU, Lost to Follow-Up
*P < .05, **P < .01, ***P < .001
(Courtesy of Sivin I, Stern J, Coutinho E, et al: *Contraception* 44:473–480, 1991.)

5 clinics carrying the study to 7 years, the cumulative continuation rates were 24.9 and 29.4 per 100 for the LNg20 and TCu 380Ag devices, respectively. Women using either method for 5–7 years had marked-to-mild increases in hemoglobin compared with admission levels (table).

Conclusion.—Approximately one fourth of the original cohort continued to use the device randomly allocated to them 7 years after study entry. With the average annual continuation rate of 80 per 100 for each device, these IUDs proved highly acceptable and effective for 7 years.

▶ The TCu 380A has been marketed in the United States for 4 years and has similar event rates to the TCu 380Ag. This device recently was approved by the United States Food and Drug Administration for 8 years' use, because the cumulative pregnancy rate at this time is only slightly higher than 1%. It previously was speculated that deposits that build up on the body of the IUD with increasing duration of use could harbor microorganisms and possibly increase the risk of infection. Therefore, it is reassuring to find that the rates of pelvic infection in these women actually diminished with length of time of use. The levonorgestrel-releasing IUD marketed recently in Finland and, in contrast to the progestin-releasing IUD, which has to be replaced annually, is also effective for 7 years. There are no immediate plans to market this device in the United States.—D.R. Mishell, Jr., M.D.

Two-Year Comparative Trial of the Gyne T* 380 Slimline and Gyne T* 380 Intrauterine Copper Devices

Sivin I, Diaz S, Pavez M, Alvarez F, Brache V, Diaz J, Odlind V, Olsson S-E, Stern J (Ctr for Biomed Research, New York; Inst Chileno de Medicina Reproductiva, Santiago, Chile; PROFAMILIA, Santo Domingo; Ctr de Pesquisas e Controle das Doencas, Materno-Infantis de Campinas, Sao Paulo, Brazil; Univ of Uppsala, Uppsala, Sweden)

Contraception 44:481–487, 1991 20–14

Introduction.—A variant of the collared Copper T* 380-intrauterine contraceptive was designed to facilitate insertion. To determine whether the design changes might alter the effectiveness or complication rate of the device, the new Gyne T* 380 Slimline was compared with the standard Gyne T* 380 in a randomized clinical trial. The 2-year follow-up results were reviewed.

Methods.—At 5 clinics, 700 women were randomized to receive the Gyne T* 380 Slimline and 300 received the standard Gyne T* device. Pregnancy, expulsion, medical removals, and continuation were assessed and compared.

Results.—The cumulative 2-year pregnancy rate for the Gyne T* 380 Slimline was .3 per 100, which was not significantly different from that of 1.5 for the standard model. After 2 years, the rates of removal for bleeding and pain were similar for the 2 models (11.6–13.7 per 100). Removal rates for other medical reasons were also almost identical for the variants (6.3–7 per 100). Expulsion of the Slimline model occurred at a rate of 7.1 per 100, which was higher than that of 3.2 per 100 for the Standard Gyne T*.

After 2 years, removals for planned pregnancy were 7–10 per 100. Based on life-table calculations, 35 per 100 women conceived within 1 month of removal, 65.8 after 3 months, and 86.3 after 1 year. At 2 years, the continuation rates were 64.7 per 100 for the Slimline and 68.9 for the Standard model; the average continuation rates were greater than 80 per 100 for both variants. Women younger than 30 years had lower continuation rates.

Conclusion.—Based on 2 years of experience, the gyne T* 380 Slimline provides the same protection against pregnancy with similar performance in other aspects as the standard Copper T* 380.

▶ The Slimline model of the Copper T* 380 has the copper bands on the horizontal arm extended to the tip rather than placed more medially over the plastic, as occurs with the standard model. The change in design allows greater ease of placement of the Slimline model into the inserter tube, and it provides a slightly smaller width of the device at the time of insertion into the uterine cavity than occurs with the standard model. The Slimline Copper T* 380 is not available in the United States, but it is marketed in Canada. This study shows no significant difference in any IUD event rate, indicating that clinicians can use either of these devices where both are available.—D.R. Mishell, Jr., M.D.

Intrauterine Devices and Pelvic Inflammatory Disease: An International Perspective

Farley TMM, Rosenberg MJ, Rowe PJ, Chen J-H, Meirik O (World Health Organization, Geneva; Health Decisions Inc, Chapel Hill, NC)

Lancet 339:785–788, 1992 20–15

Introduction.—There is worldwide concern about the possible association between the use of intrauterine devices (IUDs) and the occurrence of pelvic inflammatory disease (PID). Sexual behavior, smoking, and other factors may also be important causes of PID. The World Health Organization's clinical trials of IUDs were examined to elucidate the incidence and patterns of PID risk associated with IUD use.

Methods.—Data were drawn from 12 randomized studies comparing 2 or more IUDs and from 1 nonrandomized study of a single type of IUD. The analysis included 22,908 IUD insertions and 51,399 woman-years of follow-up from across the world. The criteria for the diagnosis of PID included temperature of at least 38°C, tenderness and guarding of the lower abdomen, and a pelvic examination showing tenderness on cervical motion, adnexal tenderness, or palpable adnexal mass.

Findings.—A total of 81 women had PID, corresponding to a rate of 1.58/1,000 woman-years. Risk was highest immediately after insertion; later, it became lower, but it was constant as long as 8 years after insertion (Fig 20–4). Closer examination of the early risk showed that the immediate postinsertion risk was high for as long as 20 days, decreasing

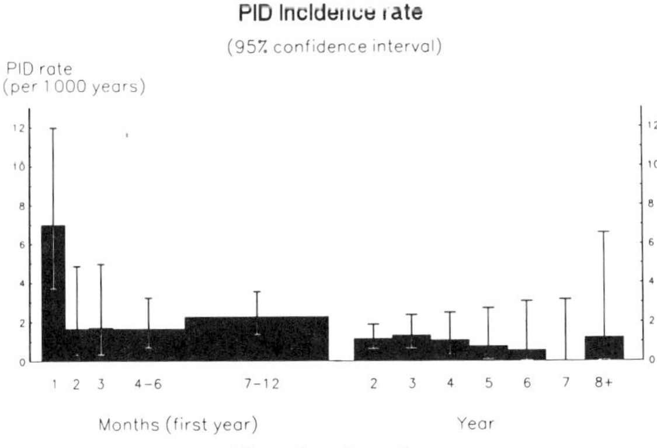

Fig 20–4.—Incidence of pelvic inflammatory disease by time since insertion. The incidence rate was estimated by the number of cases of PID and the years of exposure in each time interval. The 95% confidence intervals were calculated from the Poisson distribution. (Courtesy of Farley TMM, Rosenberg MJ, Rowe PJ, et al: *Lancet* 339:785–788, 1992.)

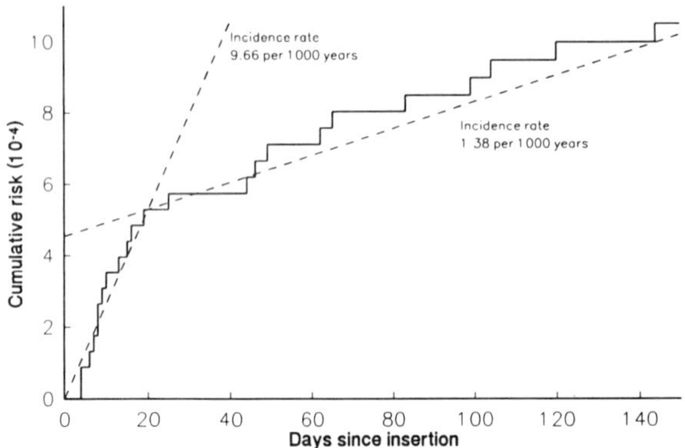

Fig 20–5.—The cumulative risk of PID by time since insertion. *Stepped lines* represent the Kaplan-Meier estimate of the cumulative hazard function. *Straight lines* are fitted from rates in Table 1 of the original article, with the optimum point of intersection estimated by eye from this plot. (Courtesy of Farley TMM, Rosenberg MJ, Rowe PJ, et al: *Lancet* 339:785–788, 1992.)

thereafter (Fig 20–5); this was the case in all regions. After 1980, the rate of PID was less than half what it had been in earlier years. The highest rate of PID was found in Africa; there were no cases among 4,301 Chinese women. Older women had less than half the risk of women aged 15–24 years at the time of insertion, who had the highest risk. The type of IUD had no significant effect on risk.

Conclusion.—In women who use an IUD, the risk of pelvic inflammatory disease is greatest during the first 20 days after insertion. Thereafter, risk is uniform and low for as long as 8 years of use. There is an inverse relationship between PID risk and age and the number of live births; this association varies according to region but not by type of IUD. The long-term use of an IUD does not appear to increase risk of PID.

▶ This study confirms data from another study indicating that IUDs do not cause PID, but that the PID in the IUD user is caused by sexually transmitted pathogenic bacteria. If these bacteria are in the cervical canal at the time of IUD insertion, then the risk of PID developing is increased, thereby resulting in the increased risk of PID found in this study in the first 3 weeks after IUD insertion. Because PID rates are constant in IUD users after the insertional risk is no longer present, development of PID more than 3 weeks after insertion of the IUD is caused by the sexual transmission of pathogenic bacteria. Insertion of IUDs should be as infrequent as possible to diminish the postinsertional risk of the transmission of bacteria. The United States Food and Drug Administration recently has lengthened the effective duration of use of the Copper T380A from 6 to 8 years. Thus, this device does not need to be replaced until 8 years after insertion.—D.R. Mishell, Jr., M.D.

Ultrasonically Guided Retrieval of Occult IUD in Early Pregnancy
Sviggum O, Skjeldestad FE, Tuveng JM (Univ Hosp, Trondheim, Norway)
Acta Obstet Gynecol Scand 70:355–357, 1991 20–16

Introduction.—The risk of spontaneous abortion in pregnancy associated with an intrauterine contraceptive device (IUD) in situ is approximately 50%. Removing the IUD during the first trimester reduces the abortion rate to approximately 15% to 25%. Although it is generally agreed that the IUD should be removed as soon as pregnancy is confirmed, there is no agreement on the proper method for removing an IUD when the string is not visible. In 9 women, an occult IUD was retrieved in early pregnancy under ultrasonographic guidance.

Technique.—Removal of an occult IUD is performed in the ultrasound laboratory by using a convex MHz probe. The cervix is cleansed with an antiseptic solution, and the anterior lip of the cervix is grasped with a uterine fenaculum. The forceps is introduced through the cervical canal under ultrasound guidance without cervical dilatation. The IUD is grasped and removed slowly. The procedure can be performed on an outpatient basis without analgesia or anesthesia.

Results.—During a 17-month period, removal of an occult IUD was successful in 8 of 9 women with an intrauterine first-trimester pregnancy. Two attempts were made in 1 woman, but removal failed because the IUD was located between the gestational sac and the posterior wall of the uterine fundus. She then elected to terminate her pregnancy by legal abortion. Another woman had a spontaneous abortion 1 week after removal of her IUD. Six women had uneventful pregnancies and gave birth spontaneously at term. One woman underwent cesarean section in the 35th week of gestation because of fetal growth retardation.

Conclusion.—The removal of an occult IUD in pregnancy under ultrasound guidance is a useful procedure.

▶ Before the refinement of pelvic ultrasonography, when a woman became pregnant with an IUD in place and wished to continue the pregnancy, it was recommended that the IUD be removed if the tailstrings were still visible; however, it was suggested that intrauterine manipulation to remove the IUD not be performed when the tail strings were not seen, because there was danger that the gestational sac could be entered causing abortion. Because the rate of spontaneous abortion is markedly lessened if the IUD can be removed, clinicians should now attempt to perform this procedure with the use of ultrasonography—even if the tail string is no longer visible. This series is the latest and largest to demonstrate the efficacy of this procedure.—D.R. Mishell, Jr., M.D.

Effect of Norplant® Implants on Liver, Lipid and Carbohydrate Metabolism

Singh K, Viegas OAC, Loke DFM, Ratnam SS (Natl Univ Hosp, Singapore)
Contraception 45:141–153, 1992 20–17

Introduction.—The Norplant® system is a relatively new, progestogen-only subdermal contraceptive. Progestogens are known to alter lipid and carbohydrate metabolism, and they may predispose to cardiovascular disease. The metabolic effects of the Norplant® system were studied in a population of Southeast Asian women.

Findings.—One hundred Singaporean women who had chosen the Norplant system for contraception were studied. The mean bilirubin level increased by 58% in the first year, decreased by 4.5% in the second year, and increased further in the third year. By the end of 5 years, it was 50% above the preinsertion mean. Total proteins and globulins decreased in the first 3 years but increased to preinsertion means in the next 2 years. Albumin and alkaline phosphatase were unchanged. Despite these changes, all levels stayed within the local limits of normal.

Total triglycerides decreased significantly in the first 3 years and then increased in the next 2 years; at the end of 5 years, they were still significantly lower than the preinsertion mean. Total cholesterol level decreased significantly in the first year, then increased steadily thereafter; at the end of 5 years, it remained below its preinsertion mean. The low-density lipoprotein cholesterol level showed a similar pattern but reached its preinsertion mean at the end of 3 years. The high-density lipoprotein (HDL) cholesterol level increased in the first year, decreased for the next 2 years, and increased to reach its preinsertion mean in the fifth year.

The ratio of the HDL to total cholesterol-HDL cholesterol increased in the first year, decreased during the next 2 years, and remained stable in the fourth year; in the fifth year, it increased to nearly its preinsertion values. The ratio of low-density lipoprotein to HDL cholesterol was significantly below its preinsertion value after 5 years. No change was seen on oral glucose tolerance testing.

Conclusion.—Use of the Norplant® implant contraceptive system does not appear to be associated with liver dysfunction or increased cardiovascular risk. If anything, it may protect against cardiovascular complications. This system seems ready for increased use as a reversible and long-term contraceptive.

▶ The Norplant® method of contraception, which currently is used by more than 100,000 American women, contains no estrogen and, therefore, unlike combination oral contraceptives, might be expected to have an adverse effect on serum lipids and glucose metabolism. However, with Norplant®, only a small amount of steroid is released into the circulation at a steady rate and the subdermal route avoids the first pass effect of orally ingested steroids on the liver. For these reasons, there is only a minimal effect of this method of contraception on hepatic lipid metabolism. Thus, this method of contraception should not be associated with the acceleration of atherosclerosis.—D.R. Mishell, Jr., M.D.

Rates and Outcomes of Planned Pregnancy After Use of Norplant Capsules, Norplant II Rods, or Levonorgestrel-Releasing or Copper TCu 380Ag Intrauterine Contraceptive Devices

Sivin I, Stern J, Diaz S, Pavéz M, Alvarez F, Brache V, Mishell DR Jr, Lacarra M, McCarthy T, Holma P, Darney P, Klaisle C, Olsson S-E, Odlind V (Population Council, New York; Instituto Chileno de Medicina Reproductiva, Santiago, Chile; PROFAMILIA, Santo Domingo, Dominican Republic; Univ of Southern California, Los Angeles; Natl Univ of Singapore; et al)

Am J Obstet Gynecol 166:1208–1213, 1992 20–18

Objectives.—Preservation of reproductive potential with the use of contraception is essential. Pregnancy rates and factors affecting fertility after the removal of very-long-acting contraceptive systems were reported. A copper T (TCu 380Ag) intrauterine device (IUD), a levonorgestrel-releasing IUD, the subdermal levonorgestrel (Norplant) capsule system, and the subdermal Norplant II rod implant system were evaluated.

Methods.—Of 2,748 women enrolled in a multicenter, prospective trial of these 4 long-acting contraceptive systems, 372 requested removal for a planned pregnancy. Removal was requested by 10% to 12% of the implant users and by 17% to 20% of the IUD users.

Results.—The 12-month life-table rate of pregnancy after the contraceptive device had been removed was 82% for the 372 women, ranging from 77% to 84% by individual contraceptive method. The combined 24-month pregnancy rate was 89% and ranged from 87% to 925 depending on which contraceptive regimen was used. Thus, conception rates 1 and 2 years after cessation were within normal limits. Pregnancy rates in the first 3 months after removal differed considerably between methods. Whereas 58% of former Norplant II rod users conceived within 3 months after removal, only 34% of former levonorgestrel-releasing IUD users conceived within 3 months after discontinuation. Forty-three percent of former copper T IUD users and 37% of former Norplant capsule users became pregnant within 3 months. No correlation was found between pregancy rate and former contraceptive regimen, duration of contraceptive use, or parity. In contrast, family planning intention and age were strongly associated with pregnancy rates.

Conclusion.—The use of any of the 4 very-long-acting contraceptive regimens does not appear to adversely affect fertility after removal.

▶ In contrast to male or female sterilization, which should be considered nonreversible methods of preventing pregnancy, the long-acting contraceptive methods investigated in this study do not affect the rate of resumption of fertility on their discontinuation. Norplant and the Copper T 3380 IUD are the most effective reversible methods of contraception available for American women. The former has an effective duration of 5 years and the latter 8 years. Because the user has to return to the health care facility for discontinuation, continuation rates are very high (in contrast to oral contraceptives, which can be discontinued easily without return visits).—D.R. Mishell, Jr., M.D.

Depot-Medroxyprogesterone Acetate (DMPA) and Risk of Invasive Squamous Cell Cervical Cancer

Thomas DB and Ray RM for the WHO Collaborative Study of Neoplasia and Steroid Contraceptives (Univ of Nairobi, Kenya; Hosp General de Mexico, Mexico City; Chiang May Univ, Chiang May, Thailand; Chulalongkorn Univ, Bangkok; Mahidol Univ, Bangkok; et al)

Contraception 45:299–312, 1992 20–19

Objective.—A hospital-based, case-control study was undertaken in Thailand, Mexico, and Kenya to determine whether the long-acting progestational contraceptive depot medroxyprogesterone acetate (DMPA) alters the risk of cervical cancer. Data were acquired from 2,009 women with invasive squamous-cell cervical cancer and 9,583 control women matched with the patients for age and place of residence.

Findings.—Depot medroxyprogesterone acetate was used by 16.8% of the women with cancer and 14.8% of the control women. Risk factors included more than 1 sex partner, early age of first intercourse, and sexually transmitted disease. A history of induced abortion and alcohol use also were risk factors. The use of DMPA at any time carried a relative risk of 1.11 — of borderline statistical significance. Higher risk was associated with smoking, anal/genital warts, and the presence of antibody against herpes simplex virus 2. A number of factors relating to the husband's sexual behavior correlated with the risk of invasive cervical cancer. The duration of use of DMPA and the time since the first or last use did not relate to the risk of cancer developing. Any increase in risk in women who had used DMPA was limited to those having a single sex partner.

Conclusion.—Use of DMPA appears not to be a risk factor for invasive cervical carcinoma. Like all sexually active women, those using DMPA should have regular Pap smears.

▶ A single 150-mg intramuscular injection of DMPA every 3 months is an extremely effective method of contraception. This method has been used by millions of women since its introduction in 1960, and it is approved as a contraceptive in more than 80 countries, including Great Britain. Currently, this method of contraception has not been approved by the United States Food and Drug Administration (FDA) because animal studies indicated that it may increase the risk of breast and endometrial cancer.

This paper is 1 of several large studies conducted by the World Health Organization (WHO) to determine the carcinogenic risk of DMPA in humans. This paper shows that DMPA has no effect on cervical cancer, which was one of the previous concerns of the FDA. Other WHO studies have shown no increase in breast cancer or ovarian cancer, and a significant reduction in the risk of endometrial cancer associated with the contraceptive use of DMPA. After receiving the WHO data, a Food and Drug Administration advisory committee unanimously recommended that DMPA be approved for contraceptive use in the United States. Hopefully, the Food and Drug Administration will agree with these recommendations and allow American women access to this effective, reversible, safe, and inexpensive method of contraception.—D.R. Mishell, Jr., M.D.

Practical Experience in the UK With an Oestrogen/Progestogen Contraceptive Vaginal Ring

Kirkman RJE, Bounds W, Colliver D, Jackson R, Barden E (Univ of Manchester; University College, London; Organon Labs, Cambridge; Warnford Hosp, South Warwickshire; Edinburgh, UK)

Br J Fam Plann 18:12–15, 1992 20–20

Introduction.—Four centers in the United Kingdom in an international trial evaluating the Organon combined contraceptive vaginal ring (CCVR). The ring is a 2-compartment system providing a steady release of 120 μg of 3-keto-desogestrel and 15 μg of ethinyl estradiol daily. Twenty-one of 41 women entering the trial completed 9 cycles.

Results.—A single pregnancy occurred, the only 1 reported to date in the entire European multicenter study. This subject had a history of previous combined pill failures. Three women complained of spontaneous expulsion of the ring. There was no increase in nonspecific vaginosis or *Candida* infection. A majority of users reported that their partners felt the ring during coitus, but only 9% of partners objected. The participants found the ring easy to insert.

Conclusion.—The CCVR provides an acceptable alternative to the combined contraceptive pill for women who have difficulty remembering to take the pill and those who experience nausea or breakthrough bleeding.

▶ Clinical trials with various forms of contraceptive vaginal rings that deliver effective contraceptive doses of steroids into the circulation by absorption through the vaginal epithelium have been ongoing for more than 25 years. This effective form of reversible steroid contraception avoids the necessity of remembering to ingest a pill every day, avoids the first pass hepatic effect of oral contraceptives, and provides nearly constant circulating levels of steroids while the ring is in the vagina. For these reasons, this new method of steroid contraception may be preferred by a certain segment of women needing contraception who have problems with the currently available effective reversible methods. It is encouraging that phase 3 trials of this particular contraceptive ring are yielding good results. The addition of another effective choice of contraception for women may increase the overall use of effective contraceptives and decrease the disturbingly high rate of unwanted pregnancies.—D.R. Mishell, Jr., M.D.

21 Abortion

Luteal Phase Defect in Habitual Abortion: Progesterone in Saliva
Tulppala M, Wahlström T, Björses U-M, Ylikorkala O, Stenman U-H (Univ Central Hosp of Helsinki)
Fertil Steril 56:41–44, 1991 21–1

Introduction.—A luteal phase defect (LPD) is 1 of the established causes of habitual abortion. Recent studies have used serial salivary progesterone (P) measurement in monitoring corpus luteum function. The applicability of serial salivary P measurement in the diagnosis of LPD in patients with habitual abortion has not been examined. The occurrence of LPD in habitual abortion was reevaluated, and the value of salivary P assay in its diagnosis was determined.

Patients.—Among 46 women with a mean age of 34.2 years and 3–8 consecutive miscarriages, 30 were studied during 2 menstrual cycles and 16 were studied during 3 menstrual cycles. Twenty-seven patients were primary aborters and 19 were secondary aborters. Twelve healthy age-matched women without a history of abortion served as controls. The diagnosis of LPD required that endometrial retardation be present during at least 2 consecutive cycles. Three blood samples for serum P measurement were collected between 1 and 12 days after the luteal hormone (LH) surge. In addition, 18 patients and 12 controls collected daily saliva samples themselves throughout the entire cycle.

Results.—Eight patients (17.4%), 5 primary aborters and 3 secondary aborters, exhibited a delay in endometrial maturation of more than 2 days during 2 consecutive cycles. In the remaining 38 patients (82.6%), endometrial maturation corresponded to the actual cycle day. Salivary P showed a distinct ovulatory increase, but the difference between patients, either with or without LPD, and health controls was not significant statistically. The serum P levels were also similar in these 3 groups. The average salivary P concentration was .5% of that in serum.

Conclusion.—In patients with habitual abortion, an endometrial maturation defect may be a factor in 17.4% of cases. However, this defect cannot be detected by the serial measurement of salivary P.

▶ Controversy exists regarding the optimal method to diagnose luteal deficiency and whether such deficiency truly is a cause of infertility. This study suggests, but does not prove, that luteal deficiency may be a cause of recurrent abortion. The diagnosis needs to be made by accurately timed endometrial biopsies rather than by serial serum or salivary progesterone levels, and it needs to show retardation of endometrial maturation in at least 2 cycles. Whether treating such women with exogenous progesterone rather than placebo results in higher successful pregnancies in a subsequent conception has not been shown.—D.R. Mishell, Jr., M.D.

Risk Factors for Spontaneous Abortion: A Case-Control Study in France

Coste J, Job-Spira J, Fernandez H (INSERM U.292, Hôpital de Bicêtre, Le Kremlin-Bicêtre; INSERM U. 187, Maternité Antoine Béclère, Clamart, France)

Hum Reprod 6:1332–1337, 1991 21–2

Introduction.—Spontaneous abortions are associated with chromosomal abnormalities, uterine/cervical causes, previous spontaneous abortion, and maternal age. The role of other previous reproductive events, exogenous, and psychological factors remains controversial.

Methods.—Women who had spontaneous abortions were compared with those who delivered to evaluate the role of several risk factors for spontaneous abortion. The 2 groups of 279 women each were compared for sociodemographic characteristics, reproductive history, and conditions of conception.

Results.—Increasing maternal age was associated with an increased risk of spontaneous abortion: the odds ratio (OR) for spontaneous abortion was .90 for women younger than 25 years compared with 2.98 for women aged 40 years or older. The risk of spontaneous abortion was not associated with employment or marital status, cigarette smoking, a prior sexually transmitted disease with or without a history of salpingitis, positive *Chlamydia trachomatis* serology, multiparity, previous ectopic pregnancy, or previous induced abortion. It also was not associated with previous use of combined contraceptive pill or intrauterine devices. Similarly, neither regularity of the mentrual cycle, apparent luteal phase deficiency, nor delayed ovulation was associated with increased risk of spontaneous abortions. However, 2 or more previous spontaneous abortions significantly increased the risk of spontaneous abortion. The presence of a psychological problem, whether or not related to pregnancy or infertility, was associated with a threefold increased risk.

Conclusion.—Maternal age and 2 or more previous spontaneous abortions appeared to independently increase the risk for spontaneous abortion in these women. These data also suggest that psychological problems at the time of conception increase the risk of spontaneous abortion, although investigational bias may account for this finding.

► Although this study shows that a history of 1 previous spontaneous abortion did not significantly increase the risk of abortion in a subsequent pregnancy, 2 previous abortions increased this risk 2.7 times. Therefore, when a woman has had 2 spontaneous first trimester abortions without a live birth, a diagnostic evaluation should be initiated. Because second trimester abortions are more likely the result of maternal rather than fetal causes and can therefore frequently be found with a hysterogram, we initiate a diagnostic evaluation after one second trimester loss if no live birth has occurred. Prospective parents also should be counseled that increasing maternal age not only increases the risk of infertility, it also increases the risk of abortion if they *do* conceive.—D.R. Mishell, Jr., M.D.

Methods for Detecting Lupus Anticoagulants and Their Relation to Thrombosis and Miscarriage in Patients With Systemic Lupus Erythematosus

Ferro D, Saliola M, Quintarelli C, Valesini G, Basili S, Grandilli AM, Bonavita MS, Violi F (Univ of Rome "La Sapienza")

J Clin Pathol 45:332–338, 1992 21–3

Objective.—The accuracy of 4 coagulation tests in detecting past thrombotic events was examined in 53 consecutive patients with systemic lupus erythematosus. Twenty-four patients had had venous and arterial thrombosis or miscarriage in the past 10 years.

Methods.—The tests compared included the activated partial thromboplastin time (aPTT), the dilute Russell's viper venom time (dRVVT), the kaolin clotting time, and the dilute aPTT. In addition, titers of anticardiolipin antibodies were determined in the patients and in 20 healthy subjects.

Findings.—The dilute aPTT was prolonged in 79% of the patients with a history of thrombosis or miscarriage, and 50% of them had an abnormal dRVVT. The kaolin clotting time was prolonged in 46% of the patients, and the aPTT was prolonged in 21% of the patients. Four patients with a negative history had a prolonged dilute aPTT, and 2 each had an abnormal dRVVT and kaolin clotting time. Nine of these subjects had high titers of anticardiolipin antibody. The dilute aPTT was the most sensitive correlate of a history of thrombosis or miscarriage. It also was more specific, although not significantly so. The only tests significantly associated with anticardiolipin antibody titers were the dilute aPTT and dRVVT.

Conclusion.—The dilute aPTT is a sensitive test for past thrombotic events in patients with systemic lupus erythematosus. It is a simple and inexpensive test, which in conjunction with a highly specific test (e.g., the dRVVT), could help identify patients at high risk of thrombosis.

▶ There is an association between the presence of lupus anticoagulant activity and recurrent pregnancy loss in patients with and without systemic lupus. Several different methods have been used to detect the presence of the lupus anticoagulant, which prolongs the clotting time in vitro but shortens it in vivo, thereby increasing the risk of thrombosis in the placental vessels leading to embryonic or fetal death. This comparative study indicates that, of the 4 tests used to detect this activity, the dilute aPTT has the best correlation with the presence of thrombotic activity and therefore should be the recommended screening test in women who have a history of recurrent pregnancy loss.—D.R. Mishell, Jr., M.D.

Intravenous Immunoglobulin Treatment of Women With Multiple Miscarriages

Christiansen OB, Mathiesen O, Lauritsen JG, Grunnet N (Aalborg Hosp, Aalborg, Denmark)

Hum Reprod 7:718–722, 1992 21–4

Background.—Immunotherapy has been reported for women who have had recurrent miscarriage. Studies of leukocyte immunization have given conflicting results. The results of intravenous immunoglobulin therapy in 11 patients with recurrent miscarriage who were at high risk of another miscarriage were reviewed.

Patients.—The 11 women (median age, 30 years) had had a total of 60 miscarriages. They had had 2 intrauterine fetal deaths and had delivered 5 live born infants, 2 of whom died perinatally. Previous leukocyte immunization was unsuccessful in 6 cases, and heparin/aspirin therapy had failed in 3. In most cases, intravenous immunoglobulin was begun before ultrasound could reveal fetal echoes or heart action, preferably in week 5. Planned minimum doses were 15 g in week 5, followed by weekly doses of 10 g until week 10 and twice weekly 10-g doses thereafter. This dosage was to be individualized according to clinical and paraclinical signs. Complement factors were measured both in the patients and in a random group of 33 women with normal early pregnancy.

Results.—Healthy infants were delivered by 9 women. All had full Apgar scores after 5 minutes and no congenital defects. Development has been normal up to 13 months of follow-up. The only side effect was a transient skin rash in 2 patients. No patient had a positive HIV, hepatitis B, or serum alanine-aminotransferase test develop. In most cases, more than the minimum planned dose of intravenous immunoglobulin was given. The patients had a significantly increased median level of complement C3 neodeterminants compared with controls.

Conclusion.—Intravenous immunoglobulin therapy appears more promising than leukocyte immunization for the treatment of recurrent miscarriage. Women who are negative for cardiolipin antibodies can also benefit from this treatment, and women with recurrent miscarriage may have increased complement turnover.

▶ Women with recurrent abortion who have no anatomical abnormality have been treated with a variety of agents in an attempt to have a live birth. These agents include progesterone, antibiotics, aspirin, glucocorticoids, heparin, and infusion of leukocytes from the husband. Success rates of approximately 80% have been reported with each of these therapies, and this paper reports a similar success rate with intravenous immunoglobulins. The problem with all these reports is the lack of a placebo control group. There is a lack of consistent studies demonstrating that any of these agents is more effective than placebo. Until significantly better success with the agent (rather than placebo) is consistently demonstrated, therapy with any of these agents must be regarded as experimental. Because both leukocyte and immunoglobulin infusion have the possibility of long-term serious harmful effects, patients should be suitably informed about the current status of these experimental and costly therapies before considering their use.—D.R. Mishell, Jr., M.D.

Serum β-Human Chorionic Gonadotropin, Estradiol and Progesterone as Early Predictors of Pathologic Pregnancy

Buyalos RP, Glassman LM, Rifka SM, Falk Rj, Macarthy PO, Tyson VJ, DiMattina M (Georgetown Univ Hosp and Columbia Hosp for Women, Washington, DC)

J Reprod Med 37:261–266, 1992 21–5

Background.—Some endocrine markers have been evaluated as markers of pregnancy outcome, but most are unreliable in early differentiation of normal vs. abnormal pregnancy. The efficacy of serum β-human chorionic gonadotropin (hCG), estradiol (E_2), and progesterone in detecting abnormal pregnancy was evaluated.

Methods.—The subjects were 126 infertile women who had a serum β-hCG level greater than 5 mIU/mL between 15 and 25 days after ovulation. After enrollment, patients underwent serial pelvic ultrasound examinations 3 times a week until an intrauterine gestational sac or evidence of pathologic pregnancy was seen, or until symptoms of miscarriage or ectopic pregnancy developed. No patient was studied more than 5 weeks postovulation. Hormonal assays of serum β-hCG, E_2, and progesterone were done every 48 or 72 hours.

Results. A total of 348 evaluations were done in 110 patients. Ovulation was induced in 40% of the cycles studied; the hormonal levels in these women were not significantly different than they were in those who did not undergo induction of ovulation. Sixty-seven percent of the women had viable pregnancies; 93% of these had at least a 66% increase in β-hCG in 48 hours or a 120% increase in 72 hours. In 87% of the patients with normal pregnancy outcomes, E_2 increased, plateaued, or decreased by less than 15% at 48 hours or by less than 20% at 72 hours. A total of 91% of the patients who had at least 2 consecutive serum progesterone measured showed an increase, plateau, or decrease of less than 25% in 48 hours or less than 33% in 72 hours.

Seventy-eight percent of the abnormal pregnancies had an abnormal β-hCG profile before confirmation; 63% had an abnormal E_2 profile and

Sensitivity, Specificity, Predictive Value, and Test Efficiency of β-Human Chorionic Gonadotropin, Estradiol, and Progesterone in the Detection of Pathologic Pregnancies in Early Gestation

Hormone	Sensitivity %	Specificity %	Predictive value of positive test (%)	Predictive value of negative test (%)	Efficiency of test (%)
β–Human chorionic gonadotropin	78	93	84	89	88
Estradiol	63	87	74	77	76
Progesterone	47	91	83	61	70
β–Human chorionic gonadotropin + estradiol	58	98	95	78	82
β–Human chorionic gonadotropin + progesterone	38	100	100	63	70
Progesterone + estradiol	41	97	92	65	70
β–Human chorionic gonadotropin + estradiol + progesterone	34	100	100	62	68

(Courtesy of Buyalos RP, Glassman LM, Rifka SM, et al: *J Reprod Med* 37:261–266, 1992.)

47% had an abnormal progesterone profile. The efficiency of the hormonal assays for detecting pathologic pregnancy before the fifth week after ovulation was between 68% and 88% (table).

Conclusion.—In sum, β-hCG continues to be the most efficient test for the early detection of pathologic pregnancy. Although specificity is not enhanced by the addition of E_2 or progesterone measurement, they do significantly decrease sensitivity and efficiency compared with β-hCG alone.

▶ This study confirms that the most useful early predictor of an abnormal pregnancy is serial measurement of serum β-hCG levels. Before 6–7 weeks' gestation (when ultrasonography should detect intrauterine fetal heart activity), a normal pregnancy measurement of β-hCG twice weekly at 3-day intervals should show a doubling of the levels. In high-risk pregnancies (infertility or recurrent abortions), I measure β-hCG on Monday and Thursday beginning 4 weeks after the onset of the last menses. A doubling of levels in this time indicates that approximately 90% of the pregnancies will be normal. If the levels do not double in this time interval, approximately 75% of the pregnancies will be abnormal.—D.R. Mishell, Jr., M.D.

Effectiveness of Prednisolone/Aspirin Therapy for Recurrent Aborters With Antiphospholipid Antibody

Hasegawa I, Takakuwa K, Goto S, Yamada K, Sekizuka N, Kanazawa K, Tanaka K (Niigata Univ, Niigata, Japan; Akita Red Cross Hosp, Akita-City, Japan)

Hum Reprod 7:203–207, 1992 21–6

Introduction.—In recurrent aborters with antiphospholipid antibody, the outcome of new pregnancies is very poor. Successful term pregnancy has been reported in women receiving prednisolone/low-dose aspirin (PSL/ASP) therapy; however, these reports have not compared their outcome with natural outcome, or mentioned the effect of the therapy on

Pregnancy Success Rate in Prednisolone/Low-Dose Aspirin (PSL/ASP)-Treated Cases and Untreated Cases

	PSL/ASP-treated	Untreated	*P*-value
No. of patients	17	12	
Age (years)	30.2 ± 4.4	29.8 ± 3.0	NS
No. of fetal losses	3.3 ± 1.3	3.3 ± 1.7	NS
APA titre	60.2 ± 32.6	57.8 ± 22.3	NS
Success rate	13/17 (76.5%)	1/12 (8.3%)	$P < 0.01$

Abbreviation: NS, not significant.
(Courtesy of Hasegawa I, Takakuwa K, Goto S, et al: *Hum Reprod* 7:203-207, 1992.)

antiphospholipid antibody. Pregnancy outcome was compared in recurrent aborters treated with PSL/ASP and in untreated controls.

Methods.—The study included 29 women with at least 2 recurrent spontaneous abortions. Seventeen received PSL/ASP therapy and the other 12, at their own request, received no therapy. Subsequent care was the same in both groups. The treatment group received PSL, 40 mg/day, for at least 4 weeks. The dosage was reduced when the antiphospholipid antibody titer decreased, and aspirin administration continued at a dosage of 81 mg/day. Treatment began as soon as pregnancy was diagnosed.

Findings.—All patients were positive for anticardiolipin and antiphosphatidylserine antibodies; lupus anticoagulant activity occurred in 5 treated and 3 untreated patients. Only 1 of 12 untreated women had a successful pregnancy outcome. In this group, there were 6 spontaneous abortions in the first trimester and 5 cases of severe fetal growth retardation in the middle trimester. Live infants were born to 13 of the 17 treated women, although 4 of them had fetal growth retardation (table). The treatment group had significantly decreased fetal growth retardation compared with previous untreated pregnancies. The anticardiolipin and antiphosphatidylserine titers decreased in this group after 4 weeks, significantly so by 8 weeks; the reduction of the antiphosphatidylserine titer was especially pronounced. Lupus anticoagulant activities also returned to normal within 8 weeks.

Conclusion.—When begun early in gestation, PSL/ASP therapy appears to be effective for the achievement of successful pregnancy in women with a history of recurrent spontaneous abortion. The treatment also prevents fetal growth retardation. Antiphosphatidylserine titer may be a good clinical marker for evaluating the effects of therapy.

▶ There are many reports that a higher percentage of women with recurrent abortion have elevated levels of antiphospholipid antibodies—as well as lupus anticoagulant activity—than do controls. However, there is no conclusive evidence that these antibodies are a cause of the abortion, or that reducing these levels by corticosteroid therapy increases the chances of a successful pregnancy oucome. Although several reports (similar to this one) have indicated that corticosteroid therapy is associated with an approximately 80% rate of successful pregnancy, there are no prospective randomized, double-blinded, placebo-controlled studies to prove that administration of corticosteroids and aspirin increases the chance of pregnancy success. This study was not prospective, not randomized, and not placebo controlled. Therefore, such therapy must still be regarded as investigational.—D.R. Mishell, Jr., M.D.

Mifepristone or Vacuum Aspiration in Termination of Early Pregnancy

Legarth J, Schnack Peen UB, Michelsen JW (Herlev Univ Hosp, Herlev, Denmark)
Eur J Obstet Gynecol Reprod Biol 41:91–96, 1991 21–7

Purpose.—This trial was designed to compare the efficacy and safety of RU 486, which is marketed as Mifepristone, and traditional vacuum aspiration for the termination of early pregnancy.

Patients.—Fifty healthy women with unwanted pregnancies of less than 43 days made up the study group. Twenty-five women were randomized to 600 mg of Mifepristone taken in 3 divided oral doses at home, and 25 women were allocated to dilatation and vacuum aspiration under general anesthesia at the hospital. After vacuum aspiration, each woman was given 1 mL of methylergometrine intravenously. Women allocated to Mifepristone with serum βhCG levels less than 25 IU/L or greater than 20,000 IU/L were excluded from the study and were rescheduled for vacuum evacuation. All women underwent a vaginal examination 1 week after treatment to verify that the abortion was complete.

Results.—Two women who underwent evacuation were excluded from analysis. One did not return for evaluation, and the other had an emergency laparotomy because of perforation of the uterus during the evacuation. Three women treated by evacuation had pelvic inflammatory disease develop after the procedure, which required antibiotic therapy. None of the women required repeat evacuation. Six women allocated to Mifepristone had an incomplete abortion and subsequently underwent evacuation. Five women with Mifepristone abortions and 12 with evacuation abortions reported that treatment had been painless, but the difference statistically was not significant. Bleeding in women who had uncomplicated Mifepristone abortions lasted longer than it did in women who underwent uncomplicated evacuation. The decrease in hemoglobin between the initial visit to the follow-up visit 1 week later was negligible in both groups, and the difference between the 2 groups was insignificant. However, the decrease in βhCG was significantly greater for evacuation than it was for Mifepristone. The decrease in βhCG between complicated and uncomplicated Mifepristone abortions also differed significantly. The mean number of days spent in bed was 1.1 days for uncomplicated evacuation and .2 days for Mifepristone. The mean duration of sick leave was 2.1 days for uncomplicated evacuation and 1.2 days for uncomplicated Mifepristone. The first menstrual period after uncomplicated abortion occurred significantly earlier after evacuation than it did after Mifepristone. Four patients in the Mifepristone group who previously had an abortion by vacuum evacuation preferred the drug treatment.

Conclusion.—Mifepristone is a simple, safe, and highly acceptable alternative method to vacuum aspiration for termination of early pregnancy. The reported complications compare favorably with the complications of vacuum aspiration.

▶ The drug RU 486 (Mifepristone) is now being routinely given in combination with a prostaglandin to increase its rate of success; thus, another study needs to be done to compare the use of these 2 agents with vacuum aspiration. If general medical therapy is preferable to surgical therapy and the effectiveness of the 2 treatments is similar, the complications of surgical therapy, such as the uterine perforation requiring laparotomy that was reported in this series, usually are more severe.—D.R. Mishell, Jr., M.D.

The Prevalence of Antiphospholipid Antibodies in Women With Recurrent Spontaneous Abortion, Women With Successful Pregnancies, and Women Who Have Never Been Pregnant

Parke AL, Wilson D, Maier D (Univ of Connecticut School of Medicine, Farmington)

Arthritis Rheum 34:1231–1235, 1991 21–8

Background.—In patients not fulfilling the criteria for connective tissue diseases, antibodies to negatively charged phospholipids are associated with a predisposition to arterial and venous thrombosis, recurrent fetal wastages, and thrombocytopenia. A prospective study was designed to determine the true prevalence of antiphospholipid antibodies in patients with recurrent spontaneous abortion (RSA) compared with those who had successful pregnancy outcomes and those who had never been pregnant.

Methods.—A total of 233 women were studied. Eighty-one had RSA, 88 had successful pregnancies, and 64 had no pregnancies. Recurrent spontaneous abortion was defined as 3 or more fetal losses.

Results.—Antiphospholipid antibodies were found in 16% of women with RSA, in 7% with successful pregnancies, and in 3% with no pregnancies. Only the biologically false positive test for syphilis (VDRL) reached statistical significance when the women with RSA were compared with the 2 control groups. The prevalence of IgG anticardiolipin was significantly different only when the 2 pregnancy groups were compared. Differences in the results of the lupus anticoagulant test and the IgM anticardiolipin antibodies (aCL) test were not significant, suggesting that the current tests for antiphospholipid antibodies, the VDRL and IgG aCL tests, seem to be more specific for fetal wastage. Of the 13 women with RSA who were found to have antiphospholipid antibodies, 2 had 3 positive results and 4 had 2 positive results. Therefore, 46% of the patients with antiphospholipid antibodies had 2 or more positive results. The presence of both a positive VDRL and an IgG aCL carried a relative risk for recurrent spontaneous abortion of 4.29. Only patients with systemic lupus erythematosus and women with RSA had significantly increased IgG aCL levels (Fig 21–1).

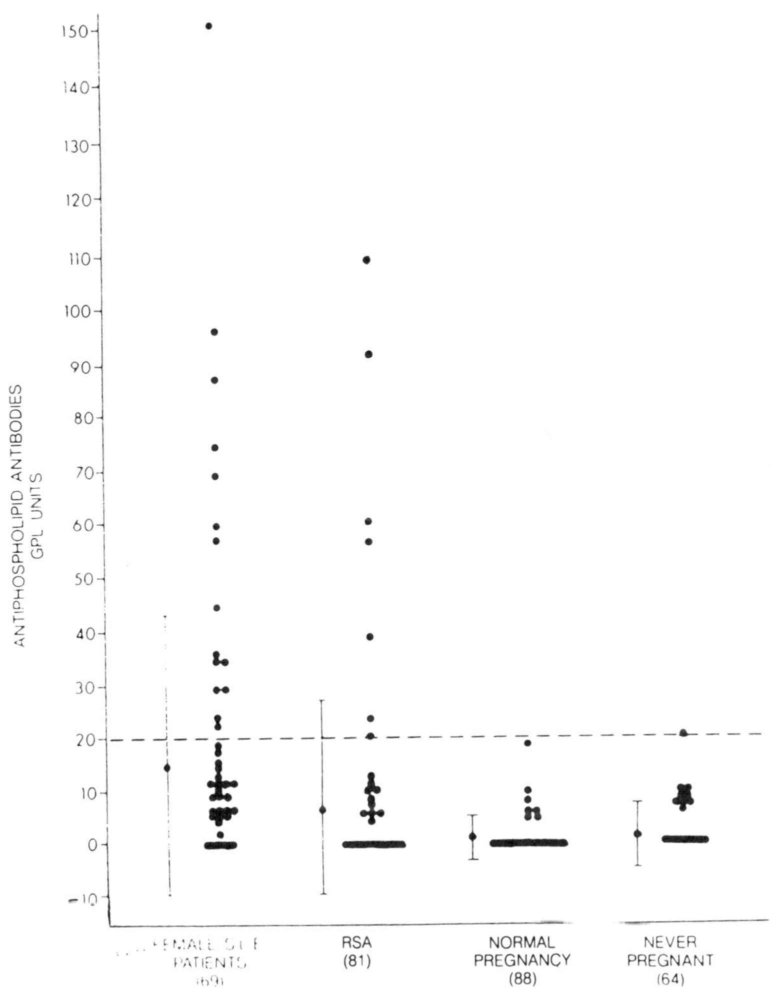

Fig 21–1.—Anticardiolipin antibodies in women with systemic lupus erythematosus *(SLE)*, women with *RSA* (3 or more fetal losses), women with successful pregnancies, and women who have never been pregnant (*n* values shown in parentheses). The values are given in IgG phospholipid *(GPL)* units. *Bars* show the mean ± 2 SD; the *broken line* marks the cutoff point for normal results (5 SD from the normal mean). (Courtesy of Parke AL, Wilson D, Maier D: *Arthritis Rheum* 34:1231–1235, 1991.)

Conclusion.—A biologically false positive test for syphilis is more specific for predicting fetal wastage than the test for lupus anticoagulant. The lupus anticoagulant test used in this study, the dilute tissue thromboplastin time, is not one of the most sensitive tests for lupus anticoagulant detection.

▶ There is no doubt that there is an increased prevalence of antiphospholipid antibodies among a group of women with RSA compared with controls who have had term pregnancies. To best detect these antibodies, one should screen women with recurrent abortion for the presence of both anticardiolipin antibodies by enzyme-linked immunosorbent assay, as well as lupus anticoagulant activity by a sensitive activated partial thromboplastin time. The latter technique was not used in this study. The real question, which remains unanswered, is whether treatment with steroids, aspirin, or anticoagulant therapy, in individuals who have these antibodies or lupus anticoagulant activity improves pregnancy outcome. No randomized prospective study has addressed this issue.—D.R. Mishell, Jr., M.D.

22 Ectopic Pregnancy

Risk Factors in Ectopic Pregnancy: Results of a Population-Based Case-Control Study

Nordenskjöld F, Ahlgren M (Univ Hosp, Lund, Sweden)

Acta Obstet Gynecol Scand 70:575–579, 1991 22–1

Background.—The rate of ectopic pregnancy (EP) has been increasing, possibly because of the increased rate of pelvic inflammatory disease, the increased use of intrauterine devices (IUDs), and improved early detection, among other reasons. A population-based, case-control study was conducted to assess the risk factors for ectopic pregnancy.

Methods.—A total of 119 women with EP and 357 age-matched controls with intrauterine pregnancy were studied. Each woman with EP was matched to 1 control with delivery, 1 with spontaneous abortion, and 1 with induced abortion. The risk factors evaluated included previous delivery, spontaneous abortion, induced abortion, and EP; history of salpingitis, appendectomy, gynecological surgery, or infertility; use of an IUD; and sterilization.

Findings.—Subjects had a significantly higher incidence of previous EP. They were also more likely to have had a previous spontaneous abortion, but this could have been a random effect. Twenty of the subjects had their EP despite having an IUD being in place at their last menstrual period. Compared with controls, the observed/expected ratio for IUD in situ was 4.36. At least 1 risk factor was present in 76.5% of the subjects, including pregnancy despite IUD use. The observed/expected ratio compared with controls with intrauterine pregnancy was thus 3.18 which was highly significant.

Conclusion.—A population-based, case-control study confirms the previously reported association between EP and a history of previous EP, history of salpingitis, history of infertility, history of fallopian tube operations, and pregnancy despite IUD use. Appendectomy may also be a risk factor, but other gynecological operations are not. An ectopic pregnancy rate of 2.4% of all identified pregnancies, which is one of the highest reported in the literature, was found.

▶ In this study performed in 1982–1983 in Sweden, 1 in every 40 identified pregnancies (including deliveries and spontaneous and induced abortions) was ectopic, an extremely high ratio. However, in the past year at Women's Hospital, LAC + USC Medical Center in Los Angeles, there were approximately 400 ectopic pregnancies and 16,000 deliveries, for a similar ratio. The annual ectopic pregnancy rate in this study was 1.8 per 1,000 women of reproductive age, which is similar to the 1987 rate of 1.5 per 1,000 women in the United States. During the past 30 years, the incidence of ectopic pregnancy has been steadily increasing in the United States as well as in Europe; therefore, it is important for clinicians to be aware of the risk factors for this potentially fatal pregnancy problem.—D.R. Mishell, Jr., M.D.

Controlled Ovarian Hyperstimulation as a Risk Factor for Ectopic Pregnancy

Fernandez H, Coste J, Job-Spira N (Hôpital A Béclère, Clamart, France; Hôpital de Bicêtre, Kremlin Bicêtre, France)

Obstet Gynecol 78:656–659, 1991 22–2

Introduction.—As part of a case-control study of ectopic pregnancy, the potential association between controlled ovarian hyperstimulation for ovulation induction and ectopic pregnancy was investigated. The risk of ectopic pregnancy with in vitro fertilization (IVF) was also examined.

Patients.—The index patients were 279 women with ectopic pregnancy confirmed at laparoscopy or laparotomy. The first woman who delivered in the same center after the operation on the index patient became a control. Only those women who planned to complete the pregnancy and who had no history of ectopic pregnancy were analyzed. The final study population consisted of 135 case patients and 244 controls. Sociodemographic characteristics, history of infertility, and history of cigarette smoking were similar in cases and controls. Because only 8.9% of case patients and 1.6% of controls used controlled ovarian hyperstimulation to become pregnant, the results of all forms of ovulation induction therapy were combined as 1 risk factor for the analysis of controlled ovarian hyperstimulation.

Results.—Ovulation induction alone was associated with an increased risk of ectopic pregnancy. The association remained valid after adjustment for the higher number of case patients using ovulation induction to become pregnant. Conversely, the risk of ectopic pregnancy was not further increased for IVF, but the number of women conceiving after IVF was small.

Conclusion.—The high rate of ectopic pregnancy in women treated with controlled ovarian hyperstimulation is likely to result from the hormone therapy, rather than from an underlying tubal disease or male factor.

▶ Because the incidence of tubal disease was similar in the 2 groups of ovarian hyperstimulated women, the increased risk of ectopic pregnancy after ovarian hyperstimulation is most likely the result of hormonal factors; probably hyperestrogenism—but possibly the high endogenous progestin levels—could inhibit the rate of tubal transport. In any event, clinicians should be aware of the increased risk of ectopic pregnancy associated with use of clomiphene citrate or hMG, and they should monitor patients who conceive after such treatment by ultrasonography to detect and treat ectopic pregnancy before tubal rupture occurs.—D.R. Mishell, Jr., M.D.

The Use of a Pretherapeutic, Predictive Score to Determine Inclusion Criteria for the Non-Surgical Treatment of Ectopic Pregnancy

Fernandez H, Lelaidier C, Thouvenez V, Frydman R (Hôpital Antoine Béclère, Clamart, France)

Hum Reprod 6:995–998, 1991 22–3

Introduction.—Nonsurgical management of ectopic pregnancy (EP) has recently become an alternative to surgery; however, there are no criteria to determine whether a surgical or a nonsurgical approach is indicated. In this study, the value of a pretherapeutic score was tested to define the indications for nonsurgical and surgical management of EP.

Patients.—Of 343 patients admitted with EP during a 5-year period, 61 (18%) were treated by a nonsurgical approach. Of the 61 patients, 16 were suitable for expectant management, 6 had a diagnosis of interstitial pregnancy and were treated with a local or systemic procedure, and 39 were treated with a dual local and systemic approach. Six criteria with a scale of 1 - 3 were used to arrive at a total score: gestational age, human chorionic gonadotropin (hCG) level, progesterone level, abdominal pain, hemoperitoneum volume, and hematosalpinx diameter (Table 1). The latter 2 measurements were obtained by laparoscopy or sonography. Three scores, 10, 11, and 12, were studied to define a threshold beyond which surgical treatment would be more preferable. Success was defined

TABLE 1.—Score for Nonsurgical Treatment

	1	2	3
Gestational age (weeks of amenorrhoea)	> 8	7–8	≤ 6
HCG level (mIU/ml)	< 1000	1000–5000	> 5000
Progesterone level (ng/ml)	< 5	5–10	> 10
Abdominal pain	Absent	Induced	Spontaneous
Haematosalpinx (cm)	< 1	1–3	> 3
Haemoperitoneum (ml)	0	1–100	> 100

(Courtesy of Fernandez H, Lelaidier C, Thouvenez V, et al: *Hum Reprod* 6:995–998, 1991.)

TABLE 2.—Results of Nonsurgical Treatment According to Initial hCG Level

HCG level (mIU/ml)	≤ 5000	> 5000
Success	38	8
Failure	5	10
Total	43	18

$P < .001$.
Sensitivity, 83%; specificity, 76%; positive predictive value, 88%; negative predictive value, 55%.
(Courtesy of Fernandez H, Lelaidier C, Thouvenez V, et al: *Hum Reprod* 6:995–998, 1991.)

as a complete resolution of EP confirmed by regression of the hCG level below 10 mIU/mL.

Results.—Nonsurgical treatment was successful in 46 patients (75%). When the threshold value for the score was fixed at 10 or 12, the success rate was significantly different; however, for a score of 11, the results were not significant. When the initial hCG level was below 5,000 mIU/mL, the success rate was 88% and the difference was significant (Table 2). The success rates were 75% with abstention, 66% with systemic methotrexate, and 77% with ultrasound puncture. Thus, the success rate was similar with no significant difference between the treatments used.

Conclusion.—A score of 12 or less permits nonsurgical management of EP with a success rate of 82%. A score greater than 12 is an indication that laparoscopic surgery may be more suitable. The use of different nonsurgical approaches does not affect the success rate.

▶ Whether it is safe and effective to use a nonsurgical method to treat early unruptured ectopic pregnancy has not yet been established. One can argue that a 20% failure rate is unacceptable, especially if the diagnosis is made without the use of laparoscopy, because many of the treatment "successes" may not have had an ectopic gestation, and the true failure rate is even higher. If laparoscopy is used to make the diagnosis, little appears to be gained by not surgically removing the unruptured ectopic pregnancy, because subsequent intrauterine pregnancy rates have not been shown to be higher with nonsurgical than surgical treatment.—D.R. Mishell, Jr., M.D.

Improved Sensitivity and Specificity of a Single Measurement of Serum Progesterone Over Serial Quantitative Beta-Human Chorionic

Gonadotrophin in Screening for Ectopic Pregnancy

Stovall TG, Ling FW, Andersen RN, Buster JE (Univ of Tennessee, Memphis)

Hum Reprod 7:723–725, 1992 22–4

Background.—The standard method for diagnosing ectopic pregnancy (EP) includes serial management of β-human chorionic gonadotropin (hCG) titers spaced by 48 hours. Several reports have shown that serum progesterone (PG) levels in EP are significantly lower than those in normal intrauterine (IU) pregnancy. Whether a single serum PG measurement is more effective than serial serum hCG determinations in screening for EP was determined.

Methods.—During a 6-month period, 1,120 patients entering an emergency room of a regional medical center with a positive urinary pregnancy test and who were in the first trimester of pregnancy according to their last menstrual period were screened for EP. Patients with serum PG levels of less than 25 ng/mL and those who did not have an increase of 66% or more in serial hCG measurements taken 48 hours apart were considered to have potentially abnormal pregnancies. Patients with serum PG levels of 25 ng/mL or greater or a 66% or greater increase in 2 serial hCG measurements were considered to have normal IU pregnancies.

Results.—Of 1,120 patients screened, 116 (10.4%) had laparoscopically documented EPs, 755 (67.4%) had IU pregnancies confirmed by US, and 249 (22.2%) had abnormal IU pregnancies including complete, incomplete, and missed abortions. Of 116 EPs, 113 (97.4%) had a serum PG level of less than 25 ng/mL, whereas 516 (68.3%) of viable IU pregnancies had serum PG levels of 25 ng/mL or greater. Of 1,120 patients, 402 (35.9%) had both a serum PG and 2 hCG measurements, and their data were included for analysis using receiver operating characteristic (ROC) curves. Setting a cut-off of 25 ng/mL, a single serum PG measurement was significantly more sensitive than 2 serial hCG measurements in screening for abnormal pregnancy, but the specificity decreased below that of serial hCG titers. However, when serial hCG determinations were added in the analysis, only 1 additional EP was identified.

Conclusion.—A single serum PG measurement should be added to serial hCG determinations as a standard diagnostic screening test for EP. Those patients with serum PG levels of 25 ng/mL or greater will have a 97% chance of a viable IU pregnancy, whereas those with PG levels of less than 25 ng/mL should undergo serial hCG testing and US scanning to determine the viability of the pregnancy.

▶ All patients coming to an emergency room during the first trimester of pregnancy with complaints of lower abdominal pain and/or abnormal uterine bleeding should be suspected of having an EP. If a rapid method to measure PG were available, all women with a progesterone level less than 25 μg/mL would then undergo further diagnostic evaluation, including vaginal probe pelvic ultrasonography and, if necessary, other diagnostic procedures in an attempt to establish a diagnosis of EP before the development of tubal rupture.—D.R. Mishell, Jr., M.D.

Ectopic Pregnancy: Evaluation With Endovaginal Color Flow Imaging

Pellerito JS, Taylor KJW, Quedens-Case C, Hammers LW, Scoutt LM, Ramos IM, Meyer WR (Yale Univ, New Haven, Conn)

Radiology 183:407–411, 1992 22–5

Introduction.—The vascular features of ectopic pregnancy are well demonstrated by color flow imaging. Endovaginal sonography alone was compared with endovaginal scanning plus color Doppler in the detection of ectopic pregnancy.

Methods.—A total of 155 women were referred for evaluation of suspected ectopic pregnancy. After scanning the uterus for evidence of intrauterine pregnancy, color Doppler was done if there was an abnormal intrauterine saclike structure or if the sac's appearance did not match the patient's serum human chorionic gonadotropin (hCG) level. The adnexa also were examined.

Results.—Ectopic pregnancy was confirmed surgically in 42% of the patients. When an ectopic fetus or extrauterine gestational sac was seen, the diagnosis was made with endovaginal sonography alone. Color flow imaging was used to make the diagnosis if an ectopic fetus or sac was seen or placental flow was noted in an adnexal mass that was separate from the ovary and uterus. The sensitivities were 54% for endovaginal sonography and 95% for endovaginal color flow imaging. Ectopic pregnancy could be ruled out by the finding of intrauterine gestation, failure to visualize an adnexal mass, or absence of extrauterine placental flow on color flow imaging. Specificity was 98% for both techniques. The negative predictive values were 75% for endovaginal sonography and 97% for endovaginal color flow imaging; the positive predictive value was 95% for both. Both methods failed to diagnose 2 cases of ectopic pregnancy.

Conclusion.—Color Doppler flow imaging is useful in detecting ectopic pregnancy. It is more sensitive than endovaginal scanning alone, helps differentiate ectopic pregnancies from the ovaries, and permits localization of placental flow for Doppler examination.

Diagnostic Efficacy of Endovaginal Color Doppler Flow Imaging in an Ectopic Pregnancy Screening Program

Emerson DS, Cartier MS, Altieri LA, Felker RE, Smith WC, Stovall TG, Gray LA (Univ of Tennessee, Memphis)

Radiology 183:413–420, 1992 22–6

Objective.—Although diagnosis of ectopic pregnancy (EP) has improved, considerable morbidity and mortality may result, mainly from delayed diagnosis. This may be addressed by an outpatient EP screening program. The addition of endovaginal color Doppler flow imaging with pulsed Doppler ultrasound (US) to an endovaginal sonography (EVS) screening protocol was assessed to determine whether Doppler could improve the sensitivity and specificity of screening.

Methods.—The study sample comprised 304 high-risk patients who underwent EVS within 48 hours of study enrollment. From this, they were assigned to diagnostic categories of viable intrauterine pregnancy (IUP), failed IUP, EP, or indeterminate. The same examiners then performed endovaginal color and pulsed Doppler US. Relative sensitivities and specificities were determined by comparing the results of EVS and EVS with color and pulsed Doppler US.

Results.—Final clinical diagnosis was EP in 12% of patients, failed IUP in 39%, and viable IUP in 48%. Diagnosis predicted clinical outcome in 62% of the cases with EVS alone vs. 82% with color and pulsed Doppler US. Sensitivities for the new protocol were 87% for EP, 59% for failed IUP, and 99% for IUP. The new protocol added diagnostic information in 54% of cases in the indeterminate category. For individual diagnoses, specificities ranged from 97% to 100%. The new protocol identified 55% of EPs, 48% of failed IUPs, and 93% of viable IUPs that initially were classified as indeterminate.

Conclusion.—Use of endovaginal color and pulsed Doppler US increases the diagnostic ability of EVS in a screening program for EP. Pelvic Doppler US appears to be more sensitive with EVS than with the transabdominal approach. The greatest benefit is in decreasing the percentage of indeterminate sonographic diagnoses. The increased sensitivity relies greatly on how early in gestation the study is performed.

▶ These 2 studies (Abstracts 22–5 and 22–6) indicate that the use of endovaginal color Doppler imaging greatly improves the ability to diagnose extrauterine pregnancies compared with ordinary EVS. Although the US machines that have the ability to perform color flow imaging are expensive, if the clinician suspects that an ectopic pregnancy exists and the diagnosis cannot be confirmed by routine endovaginal sonography, use of color Doppler imaging may avoid the need to perform a diagnostic laparoscopy, which is even more costly.—D.R. Mishell, Jr., M.D.

Multifactorial Analysis of Fertility After Conservative Laparoscopic Treatment of Ectopic Pregnancy in a Series of 223 Patients

Pouly JL, Canis M, Chapron C, Wattiez A, Manhes H, Bruhat M-A (Centre Hospitalier Universitaire, Clermont-Ferrand, France)

Fertil Steril 56:453–460, 1991 22–7

Objective.—A retrospective study of 223 patients undergoing laparoscopic treatment for ectopic pregnancy (EP) attempted to determine how to select patients with the worst outlook, in whom removal of the tube is preferable to removing only the EP. The women were followed for a mean of 6.4 years.

Findings.—Sixty-seven percent of the women had normal intrauterine pregnancies during follow-up, but 27 (12%) had recurrent EP. All but 6 of 39 recurrences were in the ipsilateral tube. Age did not influence future fertility. Nulliparous women had lower rates of intrauterine pregnancy and were more often infertile than those who were parous. Parity was a factor only when a past history of infertility was taken into account. The characteristics of the EP itself did not affect future fertility, but ipsilateral periadnexal adhesions made the outlook substantially worse. The state of the other tube also was important in fertility prognosis. A history of IUD use or previous abdominopelvic surgery did not compromise the outlook. In contrast, a history of infertility caused by tubal disease or peritubal adhesions or history of salpingitis was an adverse prognostic factor.

Implications.—Laparoscopic treatment for EP may protect later fertility. A scoring system was developed from the present findings, according to which conservative laparoscopy is indicated for a score of 0 to 3; salpingectomy for a score of 4; and salpingectomy with contralateral sterilization and in vitro fertilization for a score of 5 or higher. These recommendations are based on risk estimates for EP recurring.

▶ When it is technically possible to treat EP at the time of diagnostic laparoscopy, conservative treatment by salpingostomy or salpingotomy is nearly always performed. This study indicates that the overall rates of subsequent intrauterine pregnancy after this procedure are high—75% at 8 years. However, the various factors shown in the table reduce the chances of future intrauterine pregnancy and increase the risk of subsequent EPs and infertility. The authors suggest that, when several of these factors are present, it is better to remove the affected tube than to conserve it to reduce the risk of subsequent EP.—D.R. Mishell, Jr., M.D.

Low-Dose Oral Mehtotrexate as Second-Line Therapy for Persistent Trophoblast After Conservative Treatment of Ectopic Pregnancy

Bengtsson G, Bryman I, Thorburn J, Lindblom B (Univ of Göteborg, Göteborg, Sweden; Karolinska Inst, Stockholm)

Obstet Gynecol 79:589–591, 1992 22–8

Background.—Probably because of the trend toward more conservative surgery, persistent trophoblast after ectopic pregnancy has become more common in recent years. A second operation is generally done in these cases. An uncontrolled case series of the effects of orally adminis-

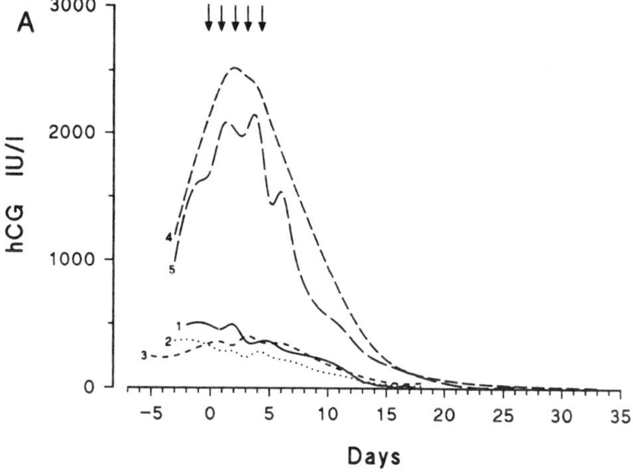

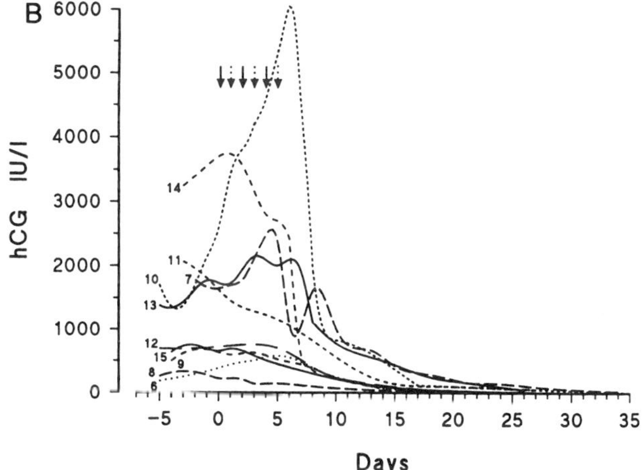

Fig 22–1.—The effect of methotrexate treatment (*solid arrows*) on serum human chorionic gonadotropin (hCG) levels. Day 0 = start of treatment. **A,** cases 1–5. **B,** cases 6–15, who also received citrovorum factor (*dotted arrows*). Note the variation in time from initiation of treatment until hCG started to decline. In several cases, hCG decreased after discontinuation of therapy and not during treatment. (Courtesy of Bengtsson G, Bryman I, Thorburn J, et al: *Obstet Gynecol* 79:589–591, 1992.)

tered methotrexate were evaluated in an uncontrolled case series of women with persistent trophoblast.

Methods.—Of 218 women who were treated for ectopic pregnancy, 15 with evidence of persistent trophoblast after conservative laparoscopic surgery were treated with orally administered methotrexate. In the first 5 patients, treatment consisted of 10–20 mg of methotrexate given daily for 4 or 5 days. The other 10 patients received citrovorum factor and methotrexate, 15 mg, on alternate days for 6 days, 3 days for each.

Results.—The serum human chorionic gonadotropin (hCG) levels were stable or continued to increase during treatment. They then decreased gradually, becoming normal at a mean of 24 days in all patients but 1 (Fig 22–1). This patient had a sharp increase in hCG during treatment and was managed with laparoscopic salpingectomy. No patient had any changes in blood and kidney function tests. During treatment, 4 patients had slight nausea; in the week after treatment, 4 had mild or severe stomatitis, 2 had mild hair loss, and 2 had urticaria. The side effects resolved within 3 weeks; those women who received citrovorum factor had no untoward effects.

Conclusion.—For those patients who have persistent trophoblast after surgery for ectopic pregnancy, orally administered methotrexate seems to be an effective and well-tolerated alternative to a second operation. Citrovorum factor prevents side effects. The timing of this treatment depends on the patient's hCG pattern after her initial operation.

▶ Most studies indicate that approximately 5% of women with ectopic pregnancy treated by conservative surgery, either salpingostomy or salpingotomy, will have evidence of persistent trophoblast activity by measurement of serial hCG levels that plateau or increase. These authors used a fairly large amount of methotrexate to treat the women studied, and side effects were common. Others have found that a similar degree of success can be obtained with a single dose of methotrexate without the use of citrovorum. The single regimen also has fewer side effects than the 3- or 4-day treatment schedule described in this paper.—D.R. Mishell, Jr., M.D.

Outpatient Laparoscopic Management of Ectopic Pregnancy With a Local Methotrexate Injection

Wolf GC, Witt BR (Univ of New Mexico, Albuquerque; Tulane Univ, New Orleans)

J Reprod Med 36:489–492, 1991 22–9

Background.—Ectopic pregnancy usually is treated with salpingostomy, and it often is performed via the laparoscope. Medical therapy using systemic methotrexate avoids the postoperative adhesions that can result from surgery, but it may be associated with undesired side effects. Data were reported on 9 cases of ectopic pregnancy treated with a laparoscopically directed injection of methotrexate.

Methods.—The women all had tubal ectopic gestations with no evidence of tubal rupture or active tubal bleeding. Methotrexate (15 mg) was injected directly into the gestational mass through the tubal wall. Three separate puncture sites were used to disperse the drug. A 15-cm, 25-gauge spinal needle was introduced under laparoscopic guidance and left in place for approximately 1 minute. The women were checked for serum levels of β-human chorionic gonadotropin (β-hCG) until the level was 5 mIU/mL or less.

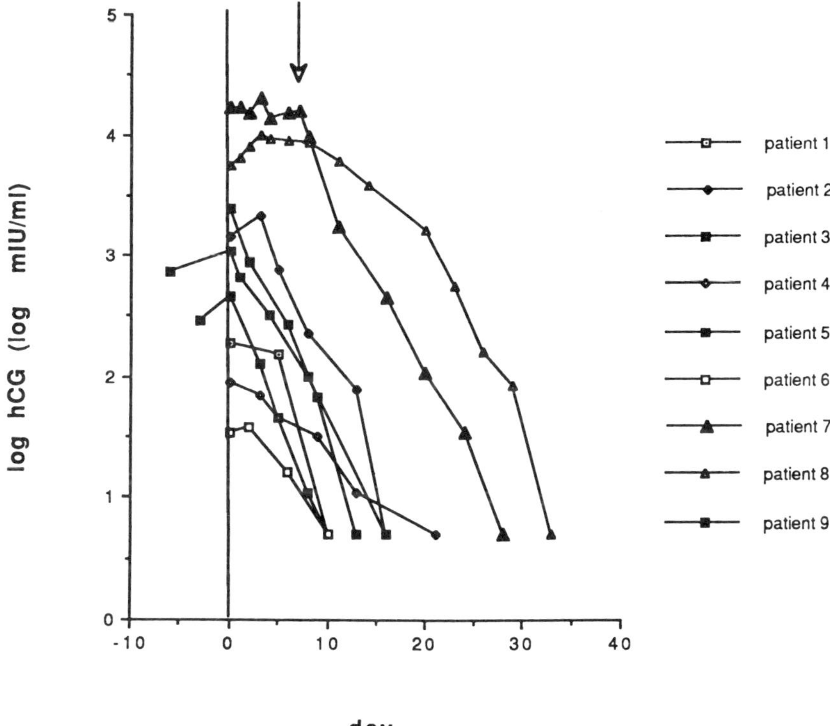

Fig 22–2.—Log of β-human chorionic gonadotropin levels in each patient over course of treatment. Vertical line at 0 days represents time of methotrexate injection in each patient. *Arrow* represents when laparotomy was performed in a patient aged 25 years, 8 days after initial laparoscopy. (Courtesy of Wolf GC, Witt BR: *J Reprod Med* 36:489–492, 1991.)

Results.—All patients underwent the procedure with no complications, and 8 of the 9 had a resolution of their symptoms. One woman required a salpingectomy 8 days later when her pelvic pain continued and the level of β-hCG did not show a downward trend. The levels of β-hCG decreased to undetectable levels in the remaining patients (Fig 22–2). The average time for a resolution of the level of β-hCG among responding patients was 16.5 days.

Conclusion.—Outpatient treatment of ectopic pregnancy is potentially hazardous, but all these women underwent laparoscopy so the risk of rupture could be assessed. Patients with initially high levels of β-hCG are less likely to respond to medical therapy. For a successful outcome, the use of a 25-gauge needle, a concentrated solution of methotrexate, and multiple injection sites is recommended.

Transvaginal Intratubal Methotrexate Treatment of Ectopic Pregnancy

Tulandi T, Falcone T, Atri M, Khalife S, Bret P (McGill Univ, Montreal)

Fertil Steril 58:98–100, 1992 22–10

Objective.—The value of intratubal methotrexate (MTX) as a treatment for tubal ectopic pregnancy (EP) was examined in 40 women aged 24–42 years who had early, unruptured tubal gestations diagnosed by transvaginal ultrasonography. The women were asymptomatic, but they had increasing serum levels of beta-human chorionic gonadotropin (*β*-hCG) at the time of treatment.

Management.—The patients received diazepam and fentanyl before the tubal contents were partially aspirated. A dose of 1 mg of MTX per kg was then instilled into the gestational sac or hematosalpinx using a 19-gauge needle. Transvaginal ultrasonography was repeated twice a week until tubal dilatation resolved.

Results.—The mean gestational age at the time of teatment was 6 ½ weeks. Twelve patients (30%) failed to respond to MTX treatment, 11 of whom underwent surgery. Two patients had tubal rupture after administration of MTX, despite decreasing levels of serum hCG. Another patient had surgery for abdominal pain and was found to have a dilated tube filled with clot. Four of 11 women who wished to conceive did so, but 2 of them had a recurrent EP on the treated side.

Conclusion.—Intratubal administration of MTX was an effective treatment for tubal EP in 70% of these patients. Rupture may occur even if the serum *β*-hCG is low and decreasing.

▶ There would be advantages in terms of cost and safety if EP could be treated by an outpatient transvaginal procedure instead of by laparoscopy or laparotomy. Several small series have reported limited success with intratubal injection of MTX, such as the results reported in Abstract 22–9, as well as with prostaglandins or potassium chloride when administered under direct vision at the time of laparoscopy. The series in this abstract indicates that the success rate is only about 70% if MTX is injected into the oviduct transvaginally. Furthermore, approximately 15% of the failures had subsequent tubal rupture, despite the fact that *β*-hCG levels had decreased. Further refinements to each of these therapeutic approaches need to be undertaken before they can be recommended for patients with EP.—D.R. Mishell, Jr., M.D.

23 Premenstrual Syndrome

Spontaneous Anovulation Causing Disappearance of Cyclical Symptoms in Women With the Premenstrual Syndrome

Hammarbäck S, Ekholm U-B, Bäckström T (Univ of Umeå, Sweden; Univ of Uppsala, Sweden)

Acta Endocrinol 125:132–137, 1991 23–1

Background.—Ovulation and the formation of corpus luteum seem to play an important role in the development of premenstrual syndrome. Previous studies have shown that the physical and emotional changes typical of the syndrome disappear when ovulation is disturbed. The symptom scores of ovulatory and anovulatory menstrual cycles were compared in the same patient.

Methods.—A group of 124 consecutive patients who had premenstrual symptoms rated their symptoms on a daily basis for at least 2 menstrual cycles, and they gave weekly blood samples for estradiol and progesterone radioimmunoassays. Eight of these patients had 1 ovulatory cycle with premenstrual syndrome and 1 spontaneously occurring anovulatory menstrual cycle. These cycles were observed to determine whether the patients experienced a significant worsening of their symptoms before menstruation.

Results.—The mean ovulatory cycles were 27 days, and the mean anovulatory cycles were 25 days. All anovulatory cycles were followed by menstrual bleeding. During the ovulatory cycles, all the women had cyclical symptoms that worsened significantly before menstruation (Fig 23–1). In the anovulatory cycles, the cyclical symptoms disappeared, resulting in relief of premenstrual syndrome.

Conclusion.—Menstrual bleeding alone, or its anticpation, does not seem to provoke the negative symptoms of premenstrual syndrome. This supports the finding that hysterectomized but still ovulating women have persistent cyclical changes. Symptom-provoking factors appear to be produced in the corpus luteum after ovulation.

▶ This study adds some evidence to the belief that premenstrual syndrome is associated with the levels of decreasing sex steroid that occur in ovulatory menstrual cycles during which conception does not take place. Both premenstrual syndrome and dysmenorrhea occur much less frequently in anovula-

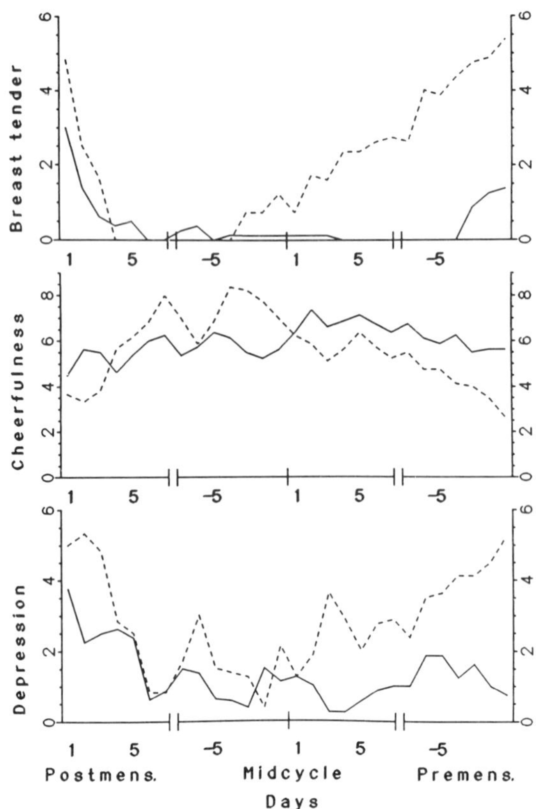

Fig 23–1.—The mean ratings of symptom scores for the group as a whole in standardized 28-day ovulatory (*dashed lines*) and anovulatory (*solid lines*) menstrual cycles. The data are centered around the day of ovulation or midcycle and the first day of menstrual bleeding in ± 7-day periods. (Courtesy of Hammarbäck S, Ekholm U-B, Bäckstroöm T: *Acta Endocrinol* 125:132–137, 1991.)

tory than in ovulatory cycles. For this reason, low-dose combined oral contraceptives that inhibit ovulation are useful initial therapy for both these problems.—D.R. Mishell, Jr., M.D.

The Epidemiology of Premenstrual Symptoms in a Population-Based Sample of 2650 Urban Women: Attributable Risk and Risk Factors

Ramcharan S, Love EJ, Fick GH, Goldfien A (Univ of Calgary, Calgary, Alta; Calgary Gen Hosp, Alta; Univ of California, San Francisco)

J Clin Epidemiol 45:377–392, 1992 23–2

Purpose.—Although the premenstrual syndrome (PMS) has received much attention, it remains a poorly defined clinical entity of unknown etiology. Problems in the definition and diagnosis of PMS have contributed to conflicting prevalence rates. Because there is a need to obtain a reliable measure of the prevalence of severe PMS symptoms, the characteristics of women who are more likely to experience severe PMS were identified using a large representative cross-sectional sample as the data base.

Patients.—The population sample consisted of 6,232 women of all reproductive statuses, including naturally cycling women aged 20–49 years. To avoid the bias of small or selected samples and subjective expectation, the women were identified through random sampling of all urban households in a defined area. The women were predominantly Caucasian and English speaking. Only those who could complete a self-administered questionnaire were included in the study. Symptoms experienced in the past 24 hours were measured using the Moos' Menstrual Distress Questionnaire (MDQ), which contains 47 symptom items pertaining to 8 major symptom categories. The MDQ made no reference to the cycle phase that was determined from follow-up interviews in a subgroup of 2,650 naturally cycling women.

Results.—The prevalence of distressing symptoms characteristic of PMS was not higher in the premenstrual phase than it was in other phases of the menstrual cycle. Only the prevalence of symptoms related to water retention was higher among those who were in the premenstrual phase, but high scores on this scale also peaked—almost to the same degree in the menstrual phase. High negative affect scores showed a positive relationship with increasing duration of reported stressful life experiences during the past year. The proportion of women with high negative affect scores among those reporting no stressful life changes was quite small, and no relationship to cycle phase could be detected. However, among women reporting stressful life changes during the past year, the prevalence of high negative affect scores in the premenstrual phase was more than double that in the mid-cycle. The relationship between PMS risk factors and high negative affect scores was not related to high water retention scores. The actual risk of affective symptoms attributable to the premenstrual state was 1%.

Conclusion.—Severe premenstrual symptoms appear to reflect a discrete mood disorder affecting women aged 25–35 years who are vulnerable to stress.

▶ This well-designed, population-based study avoids the biases of selection and information found in most other studies of PMS. It appears that PMS is a discreet disorder affecting, at most, about 5% of women in their lifetime. It does not appear to be the extreme manifestation of a physiological gradient of psychological distress that, to some degree, affects all women in the premenstrual phase of ovulatory cycles. These data should provide reassurance to women in their 30s who do not have PMS that they are unlikely to have this problem develop.—D.R. Mishell, Jr., M.D.

Oral Magnesium Successfully Relieves Premenstrual Mood Changes

Facchinetti F, Borella P, Sances G, Fioroni L, Nappi RE, Genazzani AR (Univ of Modena, Modena; Univ of Pavia, Pavia, Italy)

Obstet Gynecol 78:177–181, 1991 23–3

Objective.—Because reduced magnesium levels have been described in women with premenstrual syndrome (PMS), an oral magnesium preparation (pyrrolidone carboxylic acid) was evaluated in 32 women (mean age, 32.5 years) with confirmed PMS for 3–18 years who had symptoms that often affected social relationships and work.

Methods.—Premenstrual syndrome was diagnosed using the Moos Menstrual Distress Questionnaire. After a 2-month baseline period, the women were assigned to receive magnesium or placebo for 2 cycles. The daily dose of magnesium ion was 360 mg. Magnesium levels were measured by atomic absorption spectrophotometry.

Findings.—Treatment did not influence pain scores significantly, but it did significantly affect both questionnaire scores and "negative affect." Magnesium levels increased in lymphocytes and polymorphs, but they did not increase significantly in red cells or plasma.

Conclusion.—An oral magnesium supplement can effectively relieve the mood-related symptoms of PMS. The treatment appears to be safe and well tolerated.

▶ The use of magnesium in the luteal phase of the menstrual cycle appears to be well tolerated, without complications, and effective at improving some of the mood-related symptoms of PMS. A trial of magnesium supplementation may be warranted in some women with premenstrual adverse mood changes and depression.—D.R. Mishell, Jr., M.D.

Fluoxetine in the Treatment of Late Luteal Phase Dysphoric Disorder

Stone AB, Pearlstein TB, Brown WA (Univ of Massachusetts Med School, Worcester; Brown Univ School of Medicine, Providence, RI; VA Med Ctr, Providence, RI)

J Clin Psychiatry 52:290–293, 1991 23–4

Background.—Late luteal-phase dysphoric disorder (LLPDD), according to the *Diagnostic and Statistical Manual of Mental Disorders, Third Edition, Revised,* has many associations with major depression; however, placebo-controlled trials of antidepressant therapy are lacking. Nortriptyline has proved effective in open trials of women with LLPDD, and clomipramine and fluoxetine has been proved effective in those with a diagnosis of PMS.

Study Design.—A double-blind, randomized, placebo-controlled trial of fluoxetine was carried out in 20 women who met the criteria for

Premenstrual Symptom Increase Before and After Treatment in the Fluoxetine Group (N = 10) in Each Late Luteal Phase Dysphoric Disorder Symptom Category

DSM-III-R Category	Premenstrual Symptom Increase (%) Before	After	p[a]
Affective lability	146.7	41.2	< .0020
Irritability	142.1	25.9	< .0020
Anxiety	105.3	14.6	< .0005
Depression	150.3	15.9	< .0003
Anhedonia	163.0	24.2	< .0005
Fatigue	155.7	45.9	< .0075
Difficulty concentrating	107.1	16.5	< .0045
Increased appetite	149.4	61.4	< .0210
Hypersomnia	133.9	42.9	< .0160
Physical symptoms	123.9	66.5	< .0105

[a]P value determined by 1-tailed matched-pairs *t*-test.
(Courtesy of Stone AB, Pearlstein TB, Brown WA: *J Clin Psychiatry* 52:290–293, 1991.)

LLPDD after a single-blind trial of placebo. The dose of fluoxetine was 20 mg daily. Medication was taken each morning for 2 complete cycles.

Findings.—Nine of 10 women receiving fluoxetine responded, with 5 no longer meeting the criteria for LLPDD in the final treatment cycle. Final Global Assessment Scale scores showed a significant difference between the fluoxetine and placebo groups (table). Side effects from fluoxetine usually were resolved by the final cycle. Seven of 8 women who failed to respond to placebo elected to receive fluoxetine openly, and 6 of them responded.

Conclusion.—Fluoxetine appears to be an effective and safe treatment for women with diagnosed LLPDD. Whether fluoxetine exerts a general antidepressant effect or specifically inhibits the reuptake of serotonin needs to be learned.

▶ This double-blind, randomized, placebo controlled trial of the antidepressant fluoxetine indicates that it effectively relieves some of the symptoms of the premenstrual syndrome. Nevertheless, the sample size of the study was small, and larger studies are needed to confirm these results.—D.R. Mishell, Jr., M.D.

The Response of American Women to the Threat of AIDS and Other Sexually Transmitted Diseases

Campbell AA, Baldwin W (Natl Inst of Child Health and Human Development, Bethesda, Md)

J Acquir Immune Defic Syndr 4:1133–1140, 1991 23–5

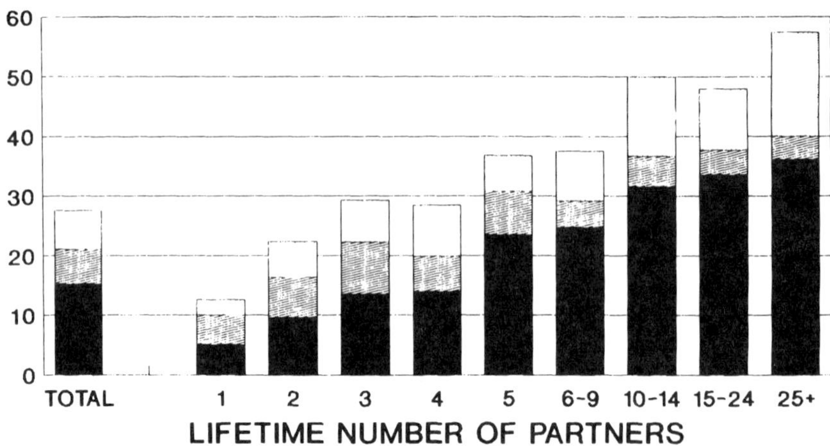

Fig 23–2.—Percentage of women reporting behavior change and/or condom use to prevent STDs, by number of partners. *Black bars* indicate behavior change; *hatched bars*, condom use; *white bars*, both. (Courtesy of Campbell AA, Baldwin W: *J Acquir Immune Defic Syndr* 4:1133–1140, 1991.)

Background.—The number of AIDS cases among women is increasing more rapidly than that among men. Several questions were included on the National Survey of Family Growth in 1988 to determine what precautions American women are taking to protect themselves from AIDS and other sexually transmitted diseases (STDs).

Methods.—Personal interviews were conducted with 8,450 women, aged 15 to 44 years, in the first half of 1988. The questions were designed to elicit whether a woman changed her sexual behavior to avoid acquiring STDs. Data included whether a woman has stopped having sexual intercourse, has stopped having other types of sexual relations, has sex less often, has or stopped having sex with more than one man, men she didn't know well, bisexual men, or men who used intravenous drugs.

Findings.—The most common change was limiting sexual relations to 1 man, which was reported by 13%. Nearly the same proportion said they used condoms. The least frequently reported change was stopping other types of sexual relations, reported by 1%. More than one fourth of the respondents said they changed their behavior or that their partners used condoms. Behavioral change was more common than condom use. The greatest precaution was taken by 6%, who said they changed their behavior *and* used condoms. Another 6% reported condom use only, and 15% reported behavioral change only. The 1% of women who thought they had a "very strong chance" of getting AIDS reported the highest proportion changing sexual behavior (54%) and the highest proportion whose partners used condoms (30%). These proportions dropped off as the perceived risk of AIDS decreased. The number of lifetime partners was strongly related to efforts to prevent infection (Fig 23–2).

Conclusion.—Large numbers of American women say they are responding to the rising danger of AIDS and other STDs. However, many women report doing nothing to protect themselves against infection, despite the fact that they engage in sexual and contraceptive behavior that puts them at high risk.

▶ Concern about acquiring sexually transmitted disease, not only AIDS but also genital herpes, genital warts, chlamydia, and gonorrhea, is gradually changing the sexual practices of American women. This survey was taken 4 years ago, so it will be interesting to observe whether the next nationwide survey shows that the trend of changing sexual activity, including less sexual partners, is continuing. Fear of contracting disease is changing the sexual life-style introduced by the sexual revolution of the 1970s.—D.R. Mishell, Jr., M.D.

24 Breast Diseases

The Role of the Gynecologist in the Diagnosis and Management of Breast Disease

Buytaert Ph, Coppens M (Antwerp Univ, Antwerp, Belgium)

Eur J Obstet Gynecol Reprod Biol 43:215–218, 1992 24–1

Background.—Breast cancer accounts for nearly 30% of all malignancies in women and is the leading cause of death in women between the ages of 40 and 50 years. Women with breast complaints frequently will consult a gynecologist rather than a specialist or their general practitioner. The need for the gynecologist to have the latest and most accurate information concerning breast problems was emphasized.

Breast Examination and the Gynecologist.—The search for early breast cancer must be aggressive. Gynecologists should have a thorough knowledge of the role exogenous estrogens play in mammary carcinogenesis. In women taking hormonal replacement, breast examination and mammographic screening are important during follow-up. Gynecologists must also acquire expertise of the surgical modalities and be broadly informed in the areas of the radiology, chemotherapy, and hormonal therapy. In this way, the gynecologist can become an equal discussion partner in the multidisciplinary approach required in the treatment of breast cancer. The gynecologist also should become actively involved in breast cancer screening.

Conclusion.—Postgraduate teaching in breast disease must become an important part of the basic training program for all resident gynecologists/obstetricians. In some countries, 2 groups of gynecologists have formed: the generalist and the breast specialist. The generalist, however, still has an important task to fulfill in screening, early detection, and management of breast cancer. Patients needing surgery can be referred to the breast specialist.

▶ This urgent message from Belgium can equally be applied to the United States. Although only a few American gynecologists are prepared to perform major breast surgery, which is common in parts of Europe and South America, they should be prepared to evaluate breast complaints, establish a definitive diagnosis, treat benign breast disease, coordinate the multidisciplinary care of women with breast cancer, and provide counseling and follow-up for all breast problems.—W.H. Hindle, M.D.

Causes of Breast Cancer Malpractice Litigation: A 20-Year Civil Court Review

Kern KA (Hartford Hosp, Hartford, Conn)

Arch Surg 127:542–547, 1992 24–2

Background.—The failure of a physician to diagnose breast cancer is the second most common medicolegal allegation filed against physicians and is the single greatest source of liability costs in settling malpractice suits. All cases tried in the United States federal and state civil court system during a 20-year period were reviewed. The aim was to produce a risk management educational tool for physicians by determining where and why failures occur.

Method.—Medical information was extracted from the court records of United States civil court trials involving malpractice with the diagnosis of breast cancer. During 1971 to 1990, the 45 cases from 31 states all involved delayed diagnosis. Six of the verdicts favored the defendants, 18 favored the plaintiffs, and the decision was unknown in 19 cases. Medical information was extracted from court records.

Findings.—The patients had a mean age of 40 years. Eighty-two percent of the patients found a painless breast mass by self-examination, but there also were other presenting signs. Fifty-one percent of the patients had no workup beyond visual observation and physical examination alone. Of 20 mammograms performed, 80% were read as normal. Workup results, largely mammography showing no evidence of malignancy, lead to a mean delay in diagnosis of 15 months. Of 12 patients with known death or metastases, 83% initially were seen with an isolated mass, and 17% involved asymmetric nodularity. General surgeons accounted for 42% of the liability payments and were responsible for the largest compensation awards in terms of total dollars paid and total dollars paid per case. Obstetricians and gynecologists were responsible for the second highest compensation payments, followed by family practitioners, internists, and radiologists.

Conclusion.—To avoid misdiagnosis or delayed diagnosis, physicians must be aware of the real potential for young or pregnant women to have breast cancer develop. Aggressive cytological investigation also is warranted to evaluate asymmetric nodularity. Reliance on mammogram findings in women younger than 30 may lead to misdiagnosis caused by a high false negative rate in this age group. The patients who were seen with a mass seemed to have a worse prognosis in terms of reported deaths or metastases. A study of the factors that contribute to delayed diagnosis of breast cancer may help improve the diagnostic abilities of all physicians who manage breast disease.

▶ Court records reveal the tip of the iceberg in malpractice litigation. This review validates the axiom that a persistent, palpable, dominant breast mass must be diagnosed definitively. From a medicolegal standpoint, this is particularly true for young and for pregnant women. Documentation in the medical record and liberal use of consultations are the best defensive measures to prevent adverse medicolegal judgments. With a persistent, palpable, dominant breast mass, delay in diagnosis should be assiduously avoided, and a "normal" or "negative" mammogram never should be relied upon to rule out cancer.—W.H. Hindle, M.D.

Breast Cancer—Biology and Malpractice

Plotkin D, Blankenberg F (Mem Cancer Research Found of Southern California, Inc, Los Angeles; Stanford Univ, Palo Alto, Calif)

Am J Clin Oncol 14:254–266, 1991 24–3

Background.—Strictly defined, curing breast cancer means eliminating the hazard of death from this disease. However, in the medical community, 5-year survival is often inaccurately equated with cure. Statements that invasive breast cancer is incurable are in conflict with reports of improved survival rates. The biology of invasive breast cancer was discussed with the goal of establishing more realistic expectations in everyday practice.

Discussion.—Available evidence indicates that curing invasive breast cancer is not possible with current treatment methods. The primary tumor can be controlled effectively, unless it is advanced locally at presentation. Death from metastatic disease can sometimes be postponed, but it is never avoidable, unless a competing fatal disease intervenes. Statements about early diagnosis of breast cancer can seriously mislead the medical and legal communities, as well as the public at large. Although numerous studies have suggested that screening results in improved survival rates, they do not claim true curability, and lead time and selection bias are limitations of such studies. The public at large may greet such "breakthroughs" with enthusiasm, and when treatment failures occur, patients may conclude that they are the result of a physician's negligence. Thus, the stage is set for a distressingly high volume of medical malpractice actions.

Conclusion.—The incidence of breast cancer has been increasing for more than 50 years, and an increase in mortality from the disease may also be starting. When treatment expectations are high and there is no improvement or a worsening in mortality, malpractice suits can occur.

▶ The natural history of breast cancer is poorly understood (1). Breast cancer is an insidious and protracted disease. Although life can be prolonged by treatment of palpable cancer, "cure" may not be possible. Current data strongly suggest that small nonpalpable cancers detected by screening mammography and treated appropriately can be "eradicated." However, because breast cancer is known to recur 20–30 years after initial diagnosis and treatment, long-term follow-up will be necessary to confirm this hopeful outcome. Lacking confirmed data on the etiology and final treatment outcomes of breast cancer makes obtaining informed consent difficult. If not clearly communicated, it can lead to unrealistic expectations by the patient and her family. Physicians should be cautious about prognosis.—W.H. Hindle, M.D.

Reference

1. Mittra I, MacRae KD: *Eur J Cancer* 27:1574, 1991.

Drug Treatments for Mastalgia: 17 Years Experience in the Cardiff Mastalgia Clinic

Gateley CA, Miers M, Mansel RE, Hughes LE (Univ of Wales College of Medicine, Heath Park)

J R Soc Med 85:12–15, 1992 24–4

Background.—The severity of mastalgia can affect quality of life and require drug treatment. Placebo-controlled studies show a placebo response in approximately 19% of patients. Only treatments tested in controlled studies should be recommended. The overall results of 3 placebo-proven agents used in mastalgia treatment were reviewed.

Methods.—The Cardiff Mastalgia Clinic is a dedicated mastalgia clinic that was established in 1973. Three hundred twenty-four patients with cyclical mastalgia and 90 with noncyclical mastalgia received a therapeutic trial of drug treatment. The drugs used were danazol, bromocriptine, and evening primrose oil.

Findings.—Overall, 92% with cyclical mastalgia and 64% with noncyclical mastalgia has a clinically useful response to treatment. Danazol was the most effective (Figs 24–1 and 24–2). Bromocriptine and evening primrose oil had equivalent efficacies. Patients treated with evening primrose oil complained of fewer side effects than did those receiving danazol or bromocriptine.

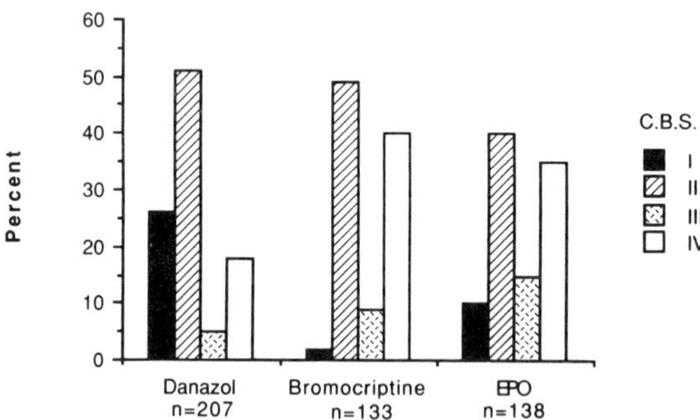

Fig 24–1.—The overall response of patients with cyclical mastalgia to drug treatment (*EPO* , evening primrose oil). (Courtesy of Gateley CA, Miers M, Mansel RE, et el: *J R Soc Med* 85:12–15, 1992.)

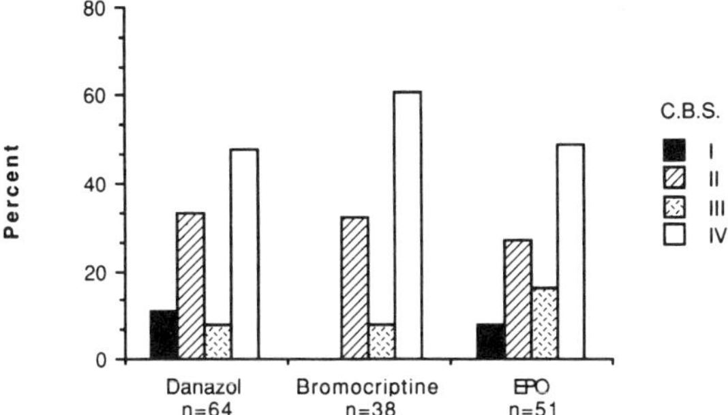

Fig 24–2.—The overall response of patients with noncyclical mastalgia to drug treatment. (*EPO*, evening primrose oil.) (Courtesy of Gateley CA, Miers M, Mansel RE, et al: *J R Soc Med* 85:12-15, 1991.)

Conclusion.—Mastalgia can be treated successfully. All responses to mastalgia treatment should be compared with the placebo response obtained in 19% of patients.

▶ The Cardiff Mastalgia Clinic continues to be a leading source of clinical information on the treatment of mastalgia. After complete evaluation, most women seen with mastalgia respond to reassurance that there is no evidence of breast cancer, and they do not require pharmacological treatment. For those women who do require therapy, danazol is the only United States Food and Drug Administration–approved medication. Evening primrose oil seems to be a regional product confined to the United Kingdom. Any hormone manipulation that suppresses the luteinizing hormone surge and ovulation is effective in the treatment of cyclic mastalgia. Noncyclic mastalgia always responds at a lesser rate. Both cyclic and noncyclic mastalgia tend to recur after therapy is completed.—W.H. Hindle, M.D.

The Natural History of Macroscopic Cysts in the Breast
Sterns EE (Queen's Univ; Kingston Gen Hosp, Kingston, Ont)
Surg Gynecol Obstet 174:36–40, 1992 24–5

Background.—Although cystic masses of the breast are common and cause significant patient anxiety, little is known about the relationship between these cysts and carcinoma. To explore the natural history of macrocystic changes, 4,207 patients were reviewed during a 14-year period to determine the age at which most cysts were discovered, the frequency of multiple cysts, and any association with carcinoma of the breast.

Methods.—Patients were examined either for screening or because of a problem of the breast. Macroscopic cysts were defined as clinically apparent lesions that resolved after percutaneous fluid aspiration.

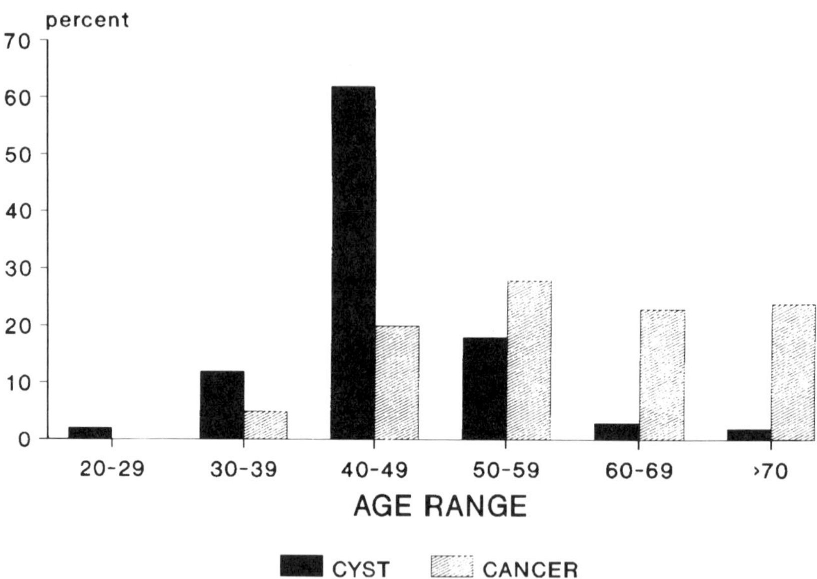

Fig 24–3.—Age of first occurrence of cysts (*solid columns*) and carcinoma (*cross-hatched columns*) of the breast is illustrated. (Courtesy of Sterns EE: *Surg Gynecol Obstet* 174:36–40, 1992.)

Results.—From 1976 to 1990, 767 biopsies were performed in 737 patients. A total of 286 patients had single or multiple aspiration-proved cysts on 561 occasions. Seventy-three percent of diagnosed cysts were single, the remainder were multiple. A previous study showed that cysts lined with flattened cells are usually single whereas apocrine-lined cysts are more likely to be multiple. In this study, lumps were discovered by patients in 83% of the cases. Often, sudden appearance of lumps, associated with slight discomfort occurred. The mean patient age at diagnosis of the first cyst was 48 years, and 62% were diagnosed when the women were between 40 and 50 years of age. Only 5% of cysts occurred in women older than 60 years of age. See Figure 24–3 for age of first occurrence of cysts and carcinoma.

Sixty percent of the patients experienced no recurrences, 36% experienced 2–5 recurrences, and 4% experienced more than 5 recurrences. The mean interval between aspirations of recurrent cysts was 17 months. Recurrences rarely occurred at the same site as previous aspirations. Three of the 286 patients with cysts subsequently had carcinoma of the breast. These women had cysts diagnosed at ages 36, 48, and 53 years; malignancies were diagnosed 3–5 years later.

Conclusion.—Macroscopic cysts appear common in premenopausal and perimenopausal women, usually occurring slightly with few or no recurrences. The development of carcinoma of the breast seems unrelated to cysts.

▶ Palpable breast cysts usually occur during a woman's reproductive years. Fine-needle aspiration (FNA) is diagnostic and usually is therapeutic if all the cyst fluid is drained. Cytology of cyst fluid rarely is rewarding, because the incidence of intracystic carcinoma is approximately 1:1000. When there is a suggestion of an intracystic lesion, pneumocystography can be helpful. Both the decreased Na:K ratio of cyst fluid and an apocrine cell lining may be associated with an increased risk of breast cancer. In this series, it is of clinical interest that a subsequent cyst developed in 40% of patients after the initial FNA; however, the "recurrent" cyst usually was at another site in the breast.—W.H. Hindle, M.D.

Complementary Roles of Mammography and Physical Examination in Palpable Cyst Aspirations

Angeid-Backman E, Ikeda DM, Andersson I, Linell F (Univ of Michigan Hosps, Ann Arbor; Malmö Gen Hosp, Malmö, Sweden)

Breast Dis 5:1–9, 1992 24–6

Diagnosis.—Breast cysts, which are common both before and near menopause, may appear as nodules on mammography. To differentiate cystic from solid lesions in the case of a palpable mass, some radiologists will use fine needle aspiration (FNA). In 3 cases, the correlation of mammographic and physical findings after FNA prevented misdiagnosis of palpable breast masses.

Conclusion.—Carcinomas and cysts can be difficult to distinguish by palpation or mammography. The palpable mass caused by simple cysts usually resolves after FNA. These 3 cases illustrate the need for follow-up physical examination after aspiration of fluid from palpable breast masses. The findings of mammography, cytology, physical examination, and pneumocystography may need to be correlated for an accurate diagnosis of breast lesions.

▶ During the initial evaluation of a palpable breast mass, FNA will identify a cyst immediately. Complete removal of the fluid often is therapeutic. However, it is essential to palpate for a residual mass after cyst aspiration. If a mass is present, FNA for cytology can be performed. The area should be reevaluated after 1 month and again 2 months later to be certain that the cyst does not reform, and that no associated mass is palpable. With a persistent palpable mass, if FNA cytology does not establish a definitive diagnosis, then open surgical biopsy should be performed.—W.H. Hindle, M.D.

Benign Papillary Neoplasms of the Breast: Mammographic Findings

Cardenosa G, Eklund GW (St Francis Med Ctr, Peoria; Univ of Illinois, Peoria)

Radiology 181:751–755, 1991 24–7

Background.—It has been suggested that patients with multiple peripheral papillomas are at increased risk for breast cancer; however, this proposal is controversial. Clinical, mammographic, and ductographic findings in 77 patients with histologically proved benign papillary neoplasms of the breast were studied retrospectively.

Methods.—Patients were classified as having solitary or multiple papillomas. Multiple papilloma cases were further subclassified as being central or peripheral.

Findings.—Sixty-six percent (51) of the patients had solitary papillomas. Thirty-seven of these 51 patients were symptomatic; 36 had spontaneous nipple discharge, and 1 had a palpable mass. Of the 35 women undergoing ductography, 32 had positive results. Biopsy was prompted in the 14 asymptomatic patients, by subareolar mammographic abnormalities in 10, and by peripheral mammographic abnormalities in 4. Fourteen patients had multiple peripheral papillomas. One also had bilateral central solitary papillomas. Eleven of these women were not symptomatic, and 2 were seen with palpable abnormalities. Another had spontaneous bilateral discharge. Mammography showed microcalcifications in 5 and clustering nodules in 2. Six of the 14 women with multiple peripheral papillomas had associated atypical ductal hyperplasia. Some also had lobular carcinoma in situ and radial scars. All 12 women with multiple central papillomas were seen with spontaneous nipple discharge and had positive ductograms.

Conclusion.—The risk for breast cancer may increase progressively in patients with benign papillary neoplasms according to the number and location of the lesions, the lowest risk occurring in those with solitary papillomas. The risk may also be higher in patients with multiple central papillomas than in those with multiple peripheral papillomas.

▶ Papillomas (benign papillary neoplasms) are the most common cause of watery, serous, and bloody, spontaneous, single-duct nipple discharge. Mammography is now detecting subareolar lesions (papillomas) without associated nipple discharge. The etiology of papillary carcinoma is unknown, although the theory of malignant transformation of multiple papillomas is attractive. All papillary neoplasms must be excised: even with optimum ductography, benign papillomas can not be confidently differentiated from the malignant papillary carcinomas, other than by histological diagnosis.—W.H. Hindle, M.D.

A Prospective Study of Benign Breast Disease and the Risk of Breast Cancer

London SJ, Connolly JL, Schnitt SJ, Colditz GA (Univ of Southern Calif, Los Angeles; Harvard Med School, Boston)

JAMA 267:941–944, 1992 24–8

Introduction.—Although it has long been known that benign breast disease is associated with an increased risk of breast cancer, the pathological abnormalities associated with risk have not been codified. The relationship between proliferative benign breast disease with and without atypical hyperplasia and the subsequent risk of breast cancer were assessed.

Methods.—A case-control study was nested within a prospective cohort study, the Nurses' Health study, which includes 121,700 registered nurses. All cases had breast cancer and had undergone a previous biopsy for benign disease. Controls had a benign breast biopsy specimen but no cancer, and they were matched by year of biopsy and year of birth. There were 121 cases and 488 controls. Slides from the benign biopsy specimen were reviewed blindly by 2 breast pathologists.

Results.—The relative risk for breast cancer, relative to women with no proliferative disease, was 1.6 for proliferative disease without atypia and 3.7 for proliferative disease with atypia. The association with atypia was stronger in premenopausal women than in postmenopausal women.

Conclusion.—A significant association between proliferative disease with atypia and increased breast cancer risk was confirmed. This association is strongest in premenopausal women. Therefore, it is suggested that these women be encouraged to undergo frequent screening for breast cancer. Research into the progression of atypical hyperplasia to breast cancer may be important in breast cancer prevention.

▶ This confirms the landmark work of Dupont and Page (1) and suggests that there is a progressive continuum of proliferative breast disease, with the potential of transformation to in situ carcinoma and, ultimately, invasive cancer. These are histological diagnoses. Clinically, most noncancerous proliferative breast lesions are asymptomatic and have no associated characteristic findings by palpation or mammography.—W.H. Hindle, M.D.

Reference

1. Dupont WD, Page DL: N *Engl J Med* 312:146, 1985.

Suggested Readings

Krieger N, Hiatt RA: Risk of breast cancer after benign breast diseases. *Am J Epidemiol* 135:619–631, 1992.

▶ With an average of 16 years of follow-up after a biopsy specimen showing histological benign breast disease was obtained, 2,731 women were evaluated and were found to have a cohort's age-adjusted rate of breast cancer 1.8 times that of the general population (confidence interval, 1.6–2.2). The greatest rate ratios were for intraductal papilloma (3.9), adenosis (2.5), and fibrocystic changes (1.5). The ratios increased with age at the time of biopsy and decreased with increasing cancer-free interval after biopsy; there was no difference after 10–15 years.—W.H. Hindle, M.D.

McDivitt RW, Stevens JA, Lee NC, et al: Histologic types of benign breast disease and the risk for breast cancer. *Cancer* 69:1408–1414, 1992.

▶ This population-based study of 433 women with newly diagnosed breast cancer and a control group with a history of benign breast disease by biopsy, calculated the odds ratio (relative risk of breast cancer) for specific histological diagnoses. In agreement with other studies (Dupont WD, Page DL: *N Engl J Med* 312:146, 1985; Carter CL, Corle DK, Micossi MS, et al: *Am J Epidemiol* 128:467, 1988), benign breast disease correlated with a slightly increased odds ratio; epithelial hyperplasia without atypia was somewhat more increased; and atypical hyperplasia increased significantly. Fibroadenoma was an independent risk factor (odds ratio, 1.7; confidence limits, 1.1–2.5), which is similar to Carter's findings but is at variance with those of Dupont.—W.H. Hindle, M.D.

The Clinical and Histologic Criteria That Predict Metastases From Cystosarcoma Phyllodes

Hawkins RE, Schofield JB, Fisher C, Wiltshaw E, McKinna JA (Royal Marsden Hosp, London)

Cancer 69:141–147, 1992 24–9

Background.—Cystosarcoma phyllodes is a rare breast tumor. The estimated incidence of malignant tumor is 25%, and the frequency of metastases is approximately 17%. The records of 33 patients with cystosarcoma phyllodes were retrospectively reviewed to evaluate the clinical and histological criteria that may predict the development of metastases.

Predictive Values of Clinical and Histological Features for the Development of Metastases

Characteristic	Predictive values: Positive	Predictive values: Negative	Statistical significance*
Age ≥ 50 yr	4/11 = 0.36	10/14 = 0.71	NS
Nulliparous	2/10 = 0.20	9/15 = 0.60	NS
Size ≥ 10 cm	5/6 = 0.83	16/19 = 0.84	0.01
Local recurrence	6/12 = 0.50	11/13 = 0.85	NS
Mitotic count (per 10 HPF)			
≥ 5	8/16 = 0.50	9/9 = 1.00	0.02
≥ 10	8/11 = 0.73	14/14 = 1.00	0.0003
Stromal overgrowth	8.10 = 0.80	15/15 = 1.00	0.00008
Severe nuclear pleomorphism	8/9 = 0.89	16/16 = 1.00	0.00002
Marked stromal cellularity	7/14 = 0.50	10/11 = 0.91	NS
Necrosis	5/7 = 0.71	15/18 = 0.83	0.03
Absence of cysts	6/19 = 0.32	4/6 = 0.67	NS
Infiltrating margins	6/8 = 0.75	15/16 = 0.94	0.003
Specialized stroma	4/5 = 0.80	16/20 = 0.80	0.05

Abbreviation: HPF, high-power field.
* P value calculated from 2-tailed Fisher exact test. NS indicates $P > .05$.
(Courtesy of Hawkins RE, Schofield JB, Fisher C, et al: *Cancer* 69:141–147, 1992.)

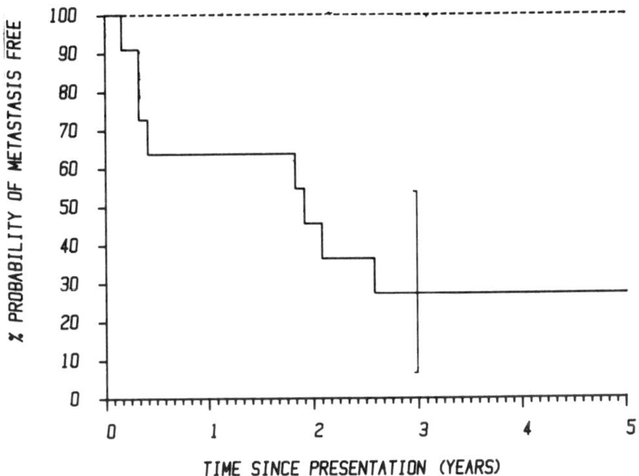

Fig 24–4.—Metastasis-free survival for patients with (n = 11; *solid line*) and without (n = 22, *broken line*) stromal overgrowth. The difference is significant ($P < .005$). The actuarial risk of metastasis for those with stromal overgrowth is 73% at 5 years. The *vertical bar* indicates the 95% confidence interval on metastasis-free survival at 3 years. (Courtesy of Hawkins RE, Schofield JB, Fisher C, et al: *Cancer* 69:141–147, 1992.)

Data Analysis.—Eight patients (24%) had metastases and 7 (21%) died of their disease. The median interval between the initial diagnosis and metastases was 14 months; between metastases and death, it was 10 months. The factors that were significantly associated with metastases included severe nuclear polymorphism, stromal overgrowth, high mitotic count (> 10 per high-power field), and infiltrating margins (table). Furthermore, 6 of 12 (50%) patients with locally recurrent disease had metastases. On the basis of this study and other series previously reported in the literature, stromal overgrowth was the most reliable predictor for the development of metastases. None of the patients without stromal overgrowth in the original tumor had metastases, for a negative predictive value of 100%. The actuarial risk of metastasis among patients with stromal overgrowth was 73% at 5 years (Fig 24–4).

Conclusion.—Stromal overgrowth appears to be the most reliable predictor of metastatic potential in cystosarcoma phyllodes. In addition, metastasis also is more likely if there is local recurrence among high-risk patients. Patients with primary tumors that contain areas of stromal overgrowth should be followed closely, because metastases occur within the first 5 years.

▶ This report demonstrates the importance of a precise histological diagnosis of the specific subclassification of these uncommon tumors. Excision with clear margins is appropriate for the benign tumors. The biological behavior of the histologically malignant tumors is variable, but those that do metastasize are almost invariably fatal in spite of all methods of treatment. The World

Health Organization recommends that the term "cystosarcoma phyllodes" no longer be used, and that these tumors be classified as phyllodes tumors: (1) benign; (2) borderline; or (3) malignant (Histological typing of breast tumors, in *International Histological Classification of Tumours,* ed 2. Geneva, World Health Organization, 1981).—W.H. Hindle, M.D.

Prognostic Factors in Cystosarcoma Phyllodes: A Clinicopathologic Study of 77 Patients

Cohn-Cedermark G, Rutqvist LE, Rosendahl I, Silfverswärd C (Karolinska Hosp, Stockholm)

Cancer 68:2017–2022, 1991 24–10

Objective.—Current available data on the prognostic significance of various clinical and histopathologic parameters of primary cystosarcoma phyllodes (CSP) of the breast are conflicting. The independent prognostic factors in CSP were identified in a retrospective study.

Methods.—Seventy-seven patients with primary CSP of the breast were studied. The median patient age was 50 years. Treatment included local excision in 24 patients, simple or radical mastectomy in 53, and adjuvant radiation therapy in 24. Median follow-up time was 8 years (range, .5–39). The prognostic significance of age, symptom duration, clinical tumor size, type of surgery, and various histopathologic parameters, including stromal cellularity, stromal cellular atypism, mitotic activity, atypical mitoses, stromal overgrowth, tumor contour, tumor necrosis, and heterologous stromal elements, were studied.

Results.—Distant metastases occurred in 16 (21%) patients, and all died of CSP. Local recurrence developed in 15 (20%) patients, and it occurred significantly more often in patients treated with local excision of the tumor (54%) than in those treated with simple or radical mastectomy (4%). Local recurrence, however, did not affect the risk of subsequent distant metastasis or overall survival. Other clinical parameters did not affect prognosis. When tested univariately, mitotic activity, stromal overgrowth, stromal cellular atypism, stromal component other than fibromyxoid tissue, tumor necrosis, and subjective classification of the pathologist yielded significant prognostic information. However, multivariate analysis showed that the only independent prognostic factors were tumor necrosis and the presence of stromal elements other than fibromyxoid tissue.

Conclusion.—These data and previously published reports are in conflict regarding prognostic factors in CSP. Additional studies are warranted to clarify these issues.

▶ This relatively large case series of phyllodes tumors (the current terminology that is replacing "cystosarcoma phyllodes") from Stockholm found tumor necrosis and heterologous stromal elements to be statistically significant histopathological prognostic factors. Rates of 21% for biologically malignant behavior and 20% for local recurrences are consistent with other published reports. Most local recurrences are thought to be caused by inadequate excision at the initial surgery. Confirmed clear surgical margins are essential for surgical success, although clinical outcome is not effected.—W.H. Hindle, M.D.

Suggested Reading

Grimes MM: Cystosarcoma phyllodes of the breast; Histologic features, flow cytometric analysis, and clinical correlations. *Mod Pathol* 5:232–239, 1992.

▶ The overall recurrence rate, which was about equivalently distributed between histologically benign, borderline, and malignant tumors, was 28% in this review of 187 cases of phyllodes tumors (the preferred histopathologic terminology, according to Page DL, Anderson TJ: *Diagnostic Histopathology of the Breast.* New York, Churchill Livingstone, 1987, p 341). Of those with available clinical follow-up, 8% had metastases develop. Wide local excision is recommended as initial treatment for phyllodes tumors.—W.H. Hindle, M.D.

Phylloides Tumor: Findings on Mammography, Sonography, and Aspiration Cytology in 10 Cases

Buchberger W, Strasser K, Heim K, Müller E, Schröcksnadel H (Univ of Innsbruck, Austria)

AJR 157:715–719, 1991 24–11

Introduction.—The phyllodes tumor accounts for only .3% to 1% of all breast neoplasms. The local recurrence rate of 16% to 28% after mastectomy or wide-wedge resection and 28% to 46% after simple enucleation of the tumor is probably a function of inadequate excision. Repeated relapses are common with occassional metastases through the vascular route. The clinical findings include a palpable mass, often of remarkably large size. Large tumors are usually correctly diagnosed by mammography because of their size and benign-looking appearance, but mammography cannot differentiate benign from malignant tumors.

Methods.—The sonographic appearance of the phyllodes tumor and the use of sonography and fine-needle aspiration (FNA) cytology in its diagnosis were reviewed. The findings on physical examination, mammography, sonography, and FNA cytology of 9 histologically benign and 1 malignant phyllodes tumor were correlated with the histological diagnosis of resected specimens.

Results.—Mammography missed 1 small tumor, but it showed a round or lobulated benign-appearing opacity in 9 patients. Sonography depicted all tumors as mostly solid masses, with intramural cysts in 6 cases. Neither mammography nor sonography reliably differentiated between benign and malignant phyllodes tumors. Fine-needle aspiration cytology accurately diagnosed benign tumors. The malignant tumor was correctly classified by FNA, but it could not be definitely differentiated from a carcinoma; 2 histologically benign phyllodes tumors were misdiagnosed as carcinomas by FNA cytology.

Conclusion.—Phyllodes tumor should be considered when there are mammographically benign-appearing breast masses and sonography demonstrates intramural cysts within a solid lesion. Although FNA cytology gives good results, it is not completely reliable, because the tumors are heterogeneous. Permanent sections are necessary for correct histological diagnosis.

▶ Phyllodes tumors are uncommon in clinical practice. Fortunately, the biologically malignant phyllodes are rare and usually are reported as approximately 20% of the histologically malignant phyllodes tumors. Evaluation of a palpable breast mass by the diagnostic triad of clinical breast examination, mammography, and FNA cytology can usually differentiate between histologically benign and malignant phyllodes tumors. For definitive histological diagnosis, multiple permanent sections are required. Treatment is by wide excision with clear surgical margins, if cosmetically feasible.—W.H. Hindle, M.D.

Fine Needle Aspiration of Breast Lesions in Women Aged 30 and Under

Maygarden SJ, McCall JB, Frable WJ (Virginia Commonwealth Univ, Richmond; Univ of North Carolina, Chapel Hill)

Acta Cytol 35:687–694, 1991 24–12

Background.—Fine needle aspiration (FNA) is primarily used to diagnose malignancy, but it also is helpful in confirming a clinically benign diagnosis. In young adult patients with breast masses, FNA is a quick and accurate method of identifying frank malignancy and cytologic atypia. In 48 patients aged 30 years and younger, a cytological diagnosis was made at the time of FNA, and histological follow-up material was available.

Methods.—Forty-three of the 48 women were between the ages of 20 and 30 years; 3 were pregnant. Aspirates were obtained by a cytopathologist using standard FNA techniques. All cytology and histology slides were reviewed independently.

Results.—Both the cytological and histological diagnoses were benign in 37 cases, including the 5 patients younger than 20 years. The most common benign lesions were fibroadenoma (20) and fibrocystic changes (14). In the 2 pregnant women in the benign cytology/histology group, histological material revealed fibroadenomas with lactational changes. Eight patients with atypical cytological diagnoses underwent excision; 4 lesions were benign and 4 malignant (table). Atypia in benign lesions resulted from epithelial proliferation in fibroadenomas and from fibrocystic changes and cellular stroma in a fibroadenoma-mimicking phyllodes tumor.

Summary of Pathologic Findings

Cytologic diagnoses (no. of cases)	Corresponding histologic diagnoses (no. of cases)
Benign cytology	
Fibroadenoma (13)	Fibroadenoma (11)
	Fibrocystic changes (2)
Benign duct cells (12)	Fibrocystic changes (7)
	Fibroadenoma (5)
Fibrocystic changes (4)	Fibrocystic changes (3)
	Fibroadenoma with lactational changes (1)
Benign stroma (2)	Fibroadenoma (1)
	Fibrocystic changes (1)
Sclerosing adenosis (2)	Sclerosing adenosis (1)
	Fibrocystic changes (1)
Reactive epithelium (1)	Fibroadenoma with lactational changes (1)
Myoepithelial cells (1)	Fibroadenoma (1)
Granular debris (1)	Fat necrosis (1)
Mastitis (1)	Mastitis (1)
Atypical cytology	
Atypical duct cells (1)	Fibrocystic changes (1)
Atypical duct cells, carcinoma not excluded (1)	Fibrocystic changes (1)
Fibroadenoma with atypia (1)	Fibroadenoma (1)
Fibroadenoma vs. cystosarcoma (2)	Juvenile fibroadenoma (1)
	Carcinoma, infiltrating duct (1)
Favor fibroadenoma, carcinoma not excluded (1)	Carcinoma, infiltrating duct (1)
Atypical duct cells, probable lactational changes (1)	Carcinoma, infiltrating duct (1)
Severely atypical duct cells, carcinoma not excluded (1)	Carcinoma, atypical medullary (1)
Malignant cytology	
Ductal carcinoma (3)	Carcinoma, infiltrating duct (3)

(Courtesy of Maygarden SJ, McCall JB, Frable WJ: *Acta Cytol* 35:687–694, 1991.)

Conclusion.—There may be a reluctance to perform a biopsy in a young woman with a breast mass because of the rarity of carcinoma in this age group. The use of FNA should identify those patients requiring a surgical biopsy. If FNA shows unequivocally malignant cells and the clinical impression is positive for carcinoma, then 1-step surgical therapy is possible.

▶ Fine-needle aspiration is a near ideal diagnostic technique for a persistent breast mass in a young patient. With an adequate cell sample, specific cytological diagnoses of benign and malignant neoplasms are possible. Why not do FNA first and reserve open surgical biopsy for those masses that remain undiagnosed by FNA?—W.H. Hindle, M.D.

Suggested Reading

Gupta RK, McHutchison AGR, Simpson JS, et al: Value of fine needle aspiration cytology of the breast, with an emphasis on the cytodiagnosis of colloid carcinoma. *Acta Cytol* 35:703-709, 1991.

▶ A review of 6,941 breast lesions evaluated by FNA cytology (FNAC) revealed a sensitivity of 100%, a specificity of 99%, a positive predictive value of 96%, and a negative predictive value of 100%. All suspicious and malignant FNAC results were confirmed by open biopsy histology. Benign FNAC results were followed for 1-5 years without clinical evidence of malignancy. The specific cytological criteria for colloid carcinoma diagnosis by FNAC (13 cases) are presented.—W.H. Hindle, M.D.

Fine Needle Aspiration of Benign and Malignant Breast Masses Associated With Pregnancy

Novotny DB, Maygarden SJ, Shermer RW, Frable WJ (Med College of Virginia, Richmond; Univ of North Carolina, Chapel Hill)

Acta Cytol 35:676–686, 1991 24–13

Background.—The reported incidence of cancer in pregnancy is approximately 1 in 1,000. The most frequently diagnosed cancers in pregnant women are those of the breast and cervix. Gestation and lactation make palpable breast masses difficult to detect, and the resulting delay in diagnosis means that pregnant women initially may be seen with relatively advanced disease. The results of fine-needle aspiration (FNA) biopsy of breast masses in 25 pregnant patients were evaluated.

Methods.—During a 7-year period, 25 (1.5%) of 1,612 FNAs performed at the study institution were from women with breast lesions associated with pregnancy. The charts of these women were reviewed for age, family and obstetric history, estimated gestational age (EGA) at the time of FNA, clinical presentation, biopsy confirmation, and follow-up data.

Results.—The mean patient age was 27 years; gestational age at the time of FNA ranged from 3 months to 3 months post partum or after breast-feeding. Twenty-two women had benign cytological diagnoses of galactocele, lactating adenoma, or fibroadenoma; none subsequently had carcinoma at a mean follow-up of 27 months. Infiltrating duct carcinoma found in 3 patients involved multiple axillary lymph nodes. In 1 of those cases, the carcinoma was advanced and the woman died within a year of diagnosis.

Conclusion.—Aspirates from breast masses in pregnant or lactating women may exhibit cellular atypia indicative of malignancy. The pregnancy-associated clinical and cytological findings described can aid in identifying those breast masses that do not require surgical biopsy.

▶ Pregnancy breast changes decrease the accuracy of clinical breast examination and mammography. However, if palpable dominant breast mass is discovered during pregnancy or lactation, the mass must be diagnosed definitively. Fine-needle aspiration can be performed during pregnancy and lactation without hesitation or delay. The cytological changes associated with pregnancy are well known. With an adequate cell sample, FNA will usually provide a specific cytological diagnosis of a persistent dominant breast mass.—W.H. Hindle, M.D.

Pneumothorax: A Complication of Fine Needle Aspiration of the Breast

Gateley CA, Maddox PR, Mansel RE (Univ Hosp of South Manchester, England; Univ of Wales, Cardiff)

BMJ 303:627–628, 1991 24–14

Introduction.—Fine-needle aspiration (FNA) cytology is a standard procedure in diagnosing breast lumps. Minor bruising was the complication most frequently described in 1 study. Iatrogenic pneumothorax is a recognized complication of needle-aspiration lung biopsy. It is also a rare but potential complication after fine-needle aspiration of the breast. Data were reviewed on 7 patients in whom pneumothorax developed after FNA of the breast.

Methods.—In most of these patients, the aspirations were performed at the periphery of the breast or in the axilla. At this location, the breast depth is minimal and the multiple passes at different angles required by the FNA technique increase the chance of breaching the pleura. In aspirating lumps at the periphery of the breast, the needle should be passed parallel to the chest wall rather than at right angles toward it.

Conclusion.—Although routine chest radiography is not indicated for this rare complication, patients should be informed that persistent chest pain is abnormal. Pneumothorax usually is amenable to observation or simple aspiration of the pneumothorax rather than to the more traumatic chest drainage.

▶ This documentation presents in the English language literature what has been known for years and what has occasionally been published elsewhere: pneumothorax is a complication of FNA. The technique of immobilizing a dominant breast mass over a rib should preclude this complication. The aspirator should mentally visualize the needle tip within the mass constantly during aspiration. Chest x-rays are indicated when there is suspicion of a pneumothorax. It is reassuring that conservative management is successful in treating this rare complication.—W.H. Hindle, M.D.

Mammographically Guided Fine-Needle Aspiration Biopsy of Nonpalpable Breast Lesions: Can It Replace Open Biopsy?

Layfield LJ, Parkinson B, Wong J, Giuliano AE, Bassett LW (Univ of California at Los Angeles Med Ctr; Jonsson Comprehensive Cancer Ctr, Los Angeles; Iris Cantor Ctr for Breast Imaging, Los Angeles)

Cancer 68:2007–2011, 1991 24–15

Introduction.—Fine-needle aspiration (FNA), although widely used as an initial biopsy procedure, has a small but significant false negative rate in the evaluation of palpable breast nodules. Less well documented is the value of FNA in the diagnosis of nonpalpable breast lesions. The accuracy of mammographically guided FNA for the evaluation of nonpalpable breast lesions in 71 patients was reported.

Methods.—Coordinates were obtained from 2 mammographic views of the lesions taken 30 degrees apart. Guided by these coordinates, the needle was inserted and 2 aspirates were taken from the lesion. Hookwire localization of the lesion was achieved after FNA, and an open biopsy of the area was performed. The cytological findings were correlated with the surgical pathological diagnoses.

Results.—Mammographically guided FNA correctly diagnosed benign disease in 36 of the 71 patients. Seven patients were shown to have ma-

TABLE 1.—Correlation Results Between Cytologic and Histological Diagnoses

	Total cases	Mass lesions	Calcifications
True-negatives	36	19	17
True-positives	7	7	0
False-negatives	3	1	2
False-positives	0	0	0
Insufficient, histologic condition malignant	4	2	2
Insufficient, histologic condition benign	15	7	8
Cytologic condition atypical, histologic condition benign	4	2	2
Cytologic condition atypical, histologic condition malignant	2	0	2

(Courtesy of Layfield LJ, Parkinson B, Wong J, et al: *Cancer* 68:2007–2011, 1991.)

TABLE 2.—Diagnostic Accuracy Rate (%) for FNA of Nonpalpable Lesions

	Total cases	Mass lesions	Calcifications
Sensitivity	78	88	0
Specificity	100	100	100
Predictive value of a positive test	100	100	—
Predictive value of a negative test	92	95	89

(Courtesy of Layfield LJ, Parkinson B, Wong J, et al: *Cancer* 68:2007-2011, 1991.)

lignancy on FNA and excisional biopsy, but 3 cancers were not detected in aspirates judged to be sufficient for diagnosis. There were no false positive FNA diagnoses (Table 1). Nineteen aspirates, 15 from patients with benign lesions and 4 from patients with adenocarcinoma, were insufficient for evaluation. For adequate specimens, FNA had a sensitivity of 78% and a diagnostic accuracy of 94%. The overall predictive value of a negative diagnosis was 92% (Table 2).

Conclusion.—The majority of open biopsies performed as a result of screening mammography of asymptomatic women will have negative results. Mammographically guided FNA has been proposed as a cost-effective alternative to open biopsy in nonpalpable breast disease, but FNA is not sufficiently sensitive for this purpose.

▶ With the expanding use of screening mammography, suspicious nonpalpable lesions are becoming the most common breast lesions requiring definitive diagnosis. Most of these lesions prove to be benign. Stereotactic FNA with an adequate cell sample permits cytological diagnosis of mass lesions, but it has a low diagnostic yield for clustered calcifications that are becoming the most common indication for needle-dirercted open biopsy. Definitive diagnosis by needle-core biopsy, directed either by ultrasound or mammography, is currently being evaluated by clinical investigation in many centers.—W.H. Hindle, M.D.

Nonpalpable Breast Lesions: Findings of Stereotaxic Needle-Core Biopsy and Fine-Needle Aspiration Cytology

Dowlatshahi K, Yaremko ML, Kluskens LF, Jokich PM (Rush-Presbyterian-St Luke's Med Ctr, Chicago)

Radiology 181:745–750, 1991 24–16

Background.—Although there have been advances in the technique of mammography, it still is hard to predict accurately the benign or malignant nature of mammographically detected breast lesions. The findings of stereotaxic needle-core biopsy and fine-needle aspiration cytology in cases of nonpalpable breast lesions were reviewed.

Methods.—Two hundred fifty mammographically detected nonpalpable lesions that were suspicious for malignancy were localized stereotaxically. These lesions were found in women undergoing routine screening mammography. In each case, fine-needle aspiration (FNA) cytological specimens and needle-core biopsy specimens were obtained before open biopsy.

Findings.—Seventy-six of the lesions (30%) were malignant; 83% of these were 1 cm long or smaller. Needle-core biopsy alone conclusively diagnosed 41% of these cancers. The FNA cytological study alone was diagnostic in 32%. There were no false positive results in either test. The same diagnosis was reached in 54% when the results of both tests were combined. When the 2 needle tests were applied to 125 mammographically defined low-suspicion lesions, 68% were found to be benign by either 1 or both needle tests. There was 1 lobular carcinoma in situ. Applying this algorithm, 34% of patients with abnormal mammograms, or one third of those recommended for open biopsy, could have avoided surgery.

Conclusion.—This and other studies suggest that stereotaxic needle biopsy of nonpalpable breast lesions can play an important role in the future diagnosis and management of breast cancer. It can reduce the number of unnecessary breast biopsies and the associated cost.

► With the increasing use of screening mammography, a large percentage of the estimated 500,000 breast biopsies performed in the United States in the past year were for mammographically suspicious nonpalpable lesions. Stereotaxic needle aspiration and biopsy have been performed effectively in European breast centers for some time. This technology is now being used in the United States. Each institution will have to use its own quality assurance and accuracy determinations for stereotaxic technology. Potentially, the number of open surgical biopsies could be decreased significantly. With current methods of therapy, small cancers—such as the malignant lesions found in this study, which were mostly less than 1 cm in diameter—have a very favorable prognosis. Also, the absence of false positives is encouraging.—W.H. Hindle, M.D.

Nonpalpable Breast Lesions: Stereotactic Automated Large-Core Biopsies

Parker SH, Lovin JD, Jobe WE, Burke BJ, Hopper KD, Yakes WF (Radiology Imaging Associates, Englewood, Colo; Fitzsimons Army Med Ctr, Aurora, Colo; Pennsylvania State Univ Hershey)

Radiology 180:403–407, 1991 24–17

Objective.—If needle-core biopsy of the breast could be made accurate and dependable, it probably could replace most surgical excision biopsies. Therefore, surgical excision biopsy of the breast was compared with automated stereotactic large-gauge, needle-core gun biopsy (exclusively using 14-gauge needles) in 102 patients with mammographically suspicious nonpalpable lesions.

Results.—The gun biopsy results and the surgical excision biopsy results agreed histologically in 98 cases (96%), including 22 of 23 carcinomas (96%). Two benign cases were missed by surgical biopsy but were correctly diagnosed by gun biopsy. Two cases (1 cancer) were missed by gun biopsy, but they correctly diagnosed by surgical biopsy.

Conclusion.—Stereotactic gun biopsy can be an acceptable alternative to surgical biopsy in women with mammographically suspicious lesions, particularly if a 14-gauge needle is used.

▶ Routine screening mammography has uncovered an expanded spectrum of breast disease, especially small lesions resulting in an increased number of needle localization breast biopsies. Most of these mammographically detected lesions prove to be benign. Automated stereotactic gun biopsy is a technique that has the potential to decrease the number of open surgical biopsies markedly. However, as with fine-needle aspiration cytology, unless a specific diagnosis is obtained, open surgical biopsy is still required for definitive diagnosis. Ultrasound with a hand-held linear array, 7.5-mHz head is an alternative technique for needle-core gun biopsy, which currently is being clinically investigated.—W.H. Hindle, M.D.

Screening Mammography: Reasons for Non-Compliance in a Family Medicine Teaching Unit

Abdeen N (Ottawa)

Can Fam Physician 37:2569–2573, 1991 24–18

Background.—Annual mammographic screening for older women has been recommended in Canada. Good compliance with screening would be expected in an urban setting where availability of screening is high, transport is easy, and the procedure is free of charge to the patient. The compliance rates and the reasons for noncompliance were investigated.

Methods.—All women aged 52–62 years who were attending a family medicine unit from October 1989 to January 1990 were asked to participate in the survey. A questionnaire was developed and tested on 20 of the 351 women attending the clinic. Ten of the remaining 331 women contacted refused to participate, and 145 either could not be reached after 5 attempts, had no telephone, or spoke neither English nor French. The response rate was 54.8%.

Findings.—Approximately half the women contacted had had screening mammography in the past 2 years. Few women said they had problems with transportation or time or reported anxiety sufficient to prevent them from going. Twenty-five percent to 36% said that radiation risk was a concern. A similar proportion cited concerns about pain or discomfort. A high percentage of women said they would go if their physician asked them to do so. The most common reason for not going was a lack of symptoms or signs of breast disease, which fostered the belief that everything was all right. The next most common response that they had no particular reason to go.

Conclusion.—To improve screening rates, primary care physicians need to educate women about screening mammography and identify their concerns. Considerable progress is still needed in realizing the full benefits of screening mammography. The primary care physician's role is important.

▶ The main reason given for noncompliance in this telephone survey was the absence of breast symptoms. Asymptomatic women are precisely those who should have periodic screening mammography. The mammographic detection of small breast cancers, which have an excellent prognosis when treated, is the only proven method of significantly reducing breast cancer mortality. If guidelines for screening mammography are recommended by their physicians, women will follow them.—W.H. Hindle, M.D.

Suggested Reading

Glockner SM, Hilton SVW, Holden MG, et al: Women's attitudes toward screening mammography. *Am J Prev Med* 8:69–77, 1992.

▶ The physician's recommendation was found to be the highest incentive for women to have screening mammography. The gynecologist's recommendation was particularly effective, and gynecologists as a group recommended mammography more often than did any other specialty. Cost was the most significant deterrent.—W.H. Hindle, M.D.

Self-Referred Mammography Patients: Analysis of Patients' Characteristics

Reynolds HE, Jackson VP (Indiana Univ, Indianapolis)

AJR 157:481–484, 1991 24–19

Background.—Some women refer themselves directly for mammographic screening, without the suggestion of their physicians. This group is in the minority, but it is highly motivated and growing. Mammography patients were surveyed to determine the ways in which self-referred mammography patients differ from physician-referred patients.

Survey.—The survey included 485 patients who underwent mammography during a 3-month period. The patients completed the 2-page questionnaire while waiting for their examination. The questionnaire addressed demographics, health-promoting practices, knowledge about cancer, motivation for mammography, and potential barriers to examination. The response rate was about 40%.

Results.—There were 437 physician-referred and 48 self-referred patients. Overall, the patients tended to be in their late 40s and white. The self-referred group was more likely to be married and to have a family income of greater than $30,000 per year. These women were also more likely to have a college education and to regard their own health as excellent or good. In both groups, approximately two thirds of patients performed other health promoting practices. Members of the self-referred group were more likely to have a friend who had breast cancer and to believe that cancer was curable. The self-referred group worried less about exposure to radiation and was more likely to indicate that $50 was a reasonable cost for the examination. Sixty-two percent of self-referred patients sought the examination for health promotion and disease prevention.

Conclusion.—The self-referred group is generally wealthier, better educated, and less worried about the associated cost and radiation dose. More education and moderate costs will probably cause more patients to refer themselves for screening mammography.

▶ Questionnaire surveys of self-referred patients vs. physician-referred patients having mammography revealed self-referred women to be more often older, white, of higher income status and higher education status, in good health, to believe cancer is curable, to have a friend with breast cancer, and to be less worried about radiation and mammography cost. However, the overall demographics for the 2 groups are quite similar.—W.H. Hindle, M.D.

Suggested Reading

Rickard MT, Lee W, Read JW, et al: Breast cancer diagnosis by screening mammography: Early results of the Central Sydney Area Health Service Breast X-ray Programme. *Med J Aust* 154:126–131, 1991.

▶ This preliminary report of 7,193 women older than 45 years of age who were screened in a mobile van by 2-view mammography during a period of 18 months found 7 cancers per 1,000 women and a biopsy-to-cancer ratio of 2:1. Sixty percent of the cancers were nonpalpable, and 19% had involved axillary nodes.—W.H. Hindle, M.D.

Why Do Some Women Get Regular Mammograms?

Rimer BK, Lerman C, Trock B, King E, Engstrom PF (Fox Chase Cancer Ctr, Philadelphia)

Am J Prev Med 7:69–74, 1991 24–20

Background.—Breast cancer is common, and mammography is a proven technique for diagnosing early, curable disease; however, most women do not have regular mammograms. To gather information for programs to foster adherence to routine mammographic screening, characteristics of women who had more than 1 mammogram were identified.

Methods.—The study was based on the framework of the Health Belief Model and social learning theory. The subjects were drawn from the membership of a large health maintenance organization. The investigators performed a random telephone survey of 910 women (age, 50–74 years) approximately half of whom were members of the HMO. The completion rate was 84% for HMO patients and 76% among control women.

Results.—Two thirds of the respondents had had mammograms, and approximately 60% had had 1 or 2 mammograms. The HMO patients were more likely to have had mammograms and to have had them in the past year. Most women who did not have mammograms said they were unnecessary, they were afraid of finding something, or they were too busy. According to logistic regression models, the most important variable was physician support. Cost was another consistent variable, with women willing to pay $75 to $100 being 1½ times more likely to have a mammogram than those willing to pay up to $50. Other important variables included visiting a physician at least annually—even when healthy, being a nonsmoker, and recognizing the increased risk of breast cancer in women older than 50 years of age.

▶ In this random telephone survey, women who had not had mammograms said that mammograms were not necessary, that they were afraid something would be found, and that they were too busy. Cost was another consistent variable. The most important positive variable was physician support.—W.H. Hindle, M.D.

Suggested Reading

Turner BJ, Schwartz JS, Amsel Z, et al: Breast cancer screening: effect of physician specialty, practice setting, year of medical school graduation, and sex. *Am J Prev Med* 8:78–85, 1992.

▶ Of the 3 specialties surveys (cardiopulmonary, general medicine, and obstetrics-gynecology), obstetrician-gynecologists reported higher performance levels in performing clinical breast examinations, ordering mammography, and following the American Cancer Society (ACS) mammography guidelines. Obstetrician-gynecologists reporting compliance in more than half of eligible patients reported rates of 90% for examination, 49% for mammography, and 28% for following ACS guidelines. We must do better. Practice setting, year of medical school graduation, and gender did not have major impact on this performance.—W.H. Hindle, M.D.

Breast Screening, Prognostic Factors and Survival: Results From the Swedish Two County Study

Duffy SW, Tabar L, Fagerberg G, Gad A, Gröntoft O, South MC, Day NE (MRC Biostatistics Unit, Cambridge, England; Central Hosp, Falun, Sweden;

Univ Hosp, Linköping, Sweden)
Br J Cancer 64:1133–1138, 1991 24–21

Background.—Mammographic screening for breast cancer allows earlier diagnosis of tumors and reduces the rate of larger tumors and metastases. Using the results of the Swedish 2-county trial of mammographic screening, researchers examined tumor size, nodal status, malignancy grade, and the relationship of these prognostic factors to screening and mortality reduction.

Methods.—The trial invited 66,741 women between the ages of 40 and 69 years to undergo regular mammographic screening. A control group of 48,678 women did not take part in the regular screening program. The follow-up for breast cancer mortality ended on December 31, 1990, with an average follow-up period since randomization of 11 years. Data obtained on 1,582 cases of breast cancer included tumor size, axillary lymph node involvement, and malignancy grade.

Results.—These 3 tumor characteristics—diameter of the primary cancer, nodal status, and malignancy grade—accounted for the favorable prognosis of screen-detected cancers. The women screened—compared with those who did not take part—had smaller tumors and an appreciably lower proportion of node positive cancers. As expected, screen-detected cancers had much better survival. Malignancy grade, as a measure of inherent malignant capacity, appears to evolve as a tumor grows. Independent of the length bias of screening, the proportion of cancers with poor malignancy grade is severalfold lower for cancers less than 15 mm in diameter than for cancers greater than 30 mm in diameter.

Conclusion.—If malignancy does evolve with tumor growth, then the benefit from screening comes not only from the smaller size at which cancers are detected, but also from a reduction in the degree of malignancy. Breast cancer mortality, especially in women older than 50 years of age can be substantially reduced by regular screening.

▶ This further analysis of the landmark Swedish 2-county screening mammography study (1–3) adds to the evidence that tumor size and nodal status correlate inversely with disease free survival. In addition, malignancy grade (4, 5) seems to be a measure of inherent malignant capacity and to increase with increasing cancer size. This principle may prove to be important for estimating prognosis and to further validate the benefits of screening mammography.

The original report (Fagerberg et al.) described the methodology of single view mammography every 33 months and demonstrated a 40% reduced mortality from breast cancer during a 10-year period by screening women older than 50 years of age. Two-view screening mammography at more frequent intervals might well have produced a greater reduction in mortality (6).—W.H. Hindle, M.D.

References

1. Fagerberg CJG, et al: *Acta Radiol* 24:465, 1985.
2. Tabar L, et al: *Lancet* i:829, 1985.
3. Tabar L, et al: *J Epidemiol Commun Health* 43:107, 1989.
4. Scarff RW, Torloni H: Histological typing of breast tumors, in *International Histological Classification of Tumors*, no. 2. Geneva, World Health Organization, 1968.
5. Bloom HJG, Richardson WW: *Br J Cancer* 11:359, 1957.
6. Tabar L, et al: *Br J Cancer* 55:547, 1987.

Usefulness of Mammography and Sonography in Women Less Than 35 Years of Age

Bassett LW, Ysrael M, Gold RH, Ysrael C (Univ of California, Los Angeles)
Radiology 180:831–835, 1991 24–22

Introduction.—The American Cancer Society recommends that asymptomatic women undergo baseline mammography between the ages of 35 and 39 years, and periodic mammography screening from age 40 years on. Although breast cancer develops in less than 5% of women younger than 35 years, some physicians order mammography screening for symptomatic and asymptomatic women in this younger age group. However, the usefulness of mammography in women younger than 35 years is controversial, because it is apparently less effective in the evaluation of the radiodense breasts of younger women than of the less radiodense breasts of older women. The usefulness of mammography in women younger than 35 years was evaluated.

Methods.—During an 8-year period, 1,016 women aged 17–34 years underwent mammography. The indications for mammography were palpable mass (44.7%), screening (23.3%), lumpiness (14.9%), tenderness (8%), nipple discharge (5%), and adenopathy (1.9%). The clinical records of 787 women with localized clinical findings were reviewed to determine the effect of the mammographic findings on their treatment.

Results.—Breast carcinomas were found at biopsy in 3 women with a palpable mass, 1 woman with a personal history of breast cancer, 1

Mammographic Results in 6 Women with Cancer

Indications	Number of Patients	Age (y)	Mammographic Results			Delay in Biopsy Because of Mammography
			Negative	Benign	Suspicious	
Palpable mass	3	30, 33, 33	0	3	0	2
Personal history	1	30	1	0	0	0
Localized tenderness	1	34	0	0	1	0
Unilateral discharge	1	27	1	0	0	1

(Courtesy of Bassett LW, Ysrael M, Gold RH, et al: *Radiology* 180:831–835, 1991.)

woman with localized breast tenderness, and in 1 woman with unilateral nipple discharge (table). Mammograms were interpreted as benign in all 3 women with a palpable mass, which led to a delay of biopsy in 2. Of the mammograms in the other 3 women with breast cancer, 2 were negative and 1 was suspicious. No breast cancers were detected on any of the screening mammograms. In 30% of the mammograms of this age group, the breast was mostly fatty with excellent mammograms. However, in 40%, more than two thirds of the breast was mammographically radiodense. Sonography performed in 389 women was useful in preventing unnecessary biopsy of cysts, but it was not useful in differentiating benign from malignant solid masses.

Conclusion.—A mammographic examination tailored to a specific area or problem may be useful in women younger than 35 years of age with persistent localized breast symptoms. However, a biopsy or fine-needle aspiration should always be performed if there is a persistent palpable solid breast mass, even when the mammographic findings are negative or benign.

▶ Except for individualized cases (such as when a patient is seen with a family history of early onset breast cancer in a first-degree relative) screening mammography is not indicated for women younger than 35 years of age because (1) the incidence of carcinoma is so low, and (2) the dense glandular breast tissue of young women makes mammographic interpretation significantly less accurate. However, diagnostic mammography has the same indications in this young age group as in older women.

At any age, a persistent dominant breast mass must be diagnosed. Fine-needle aspiration can specifically diagnose most palpable breast masses. Mammographic needle-directed surgical biopsy usually is required to specifically diagnose a nonpalpable persistent dominant breast mass. Open surgical biopsy with histological diagnosis by permanent sections is the definitive diagnostic procedure if previous breast-mass evaluation has not established a specific diagnosis.—W.H. Hindle, M.D.

The Prevalence of Carcinoma in Palpable vs Impalpable, Mammographically Detected Lesions

Bassett LW, Liu T-H, Giuliano AE, Gold RH (Univ of California at Los Angeles)

AJR 157:21–24, 1991 24–23

Introduction.—One of the barriers to breast cancer screening with mammography that has been cited is the excessive number of false positive mammograms leading to unnecessary investigations and surgical interventions.

Methods.—In a retrospective study, the biopsy results in palpable vs. impalpable (nonpalpable) mammographically detected lesions from the practice of an experienced breast surgeon working with experienced mammographers were compared.

Results.—In 1980–1989, 372 biopsies were performed in 346 women. Of 143 biopsy specimens of palpable abnormalities, 48 yielded a primary malignant lesion. Of the 48 biopsies, 16 were performed in patients with positive axillary lymph nodes, and 5 were performed in patients who had distant metastases at the time of biopsy. In 229 biopsies for impalpable, mammographically detected lesions, 72 yielded a primary breast carcinoma. None of these patients had distant metastases at the time of biopsy, but 11 of the biopsies were performed in patients with positive axillary nodes. The positive predictive values, the number of cancers detected divided by the number of biopsies recommended, were not significantly different for palpable vs. impalpable mammographically detected abnormalities. The mammographically detected cancers were smaller, more often noninvasive, less often associated with axillary metastases, and without distant metastases.

Conclusion.—The positive predictive values for detecting breast carcinoma were not significantly different for palpable lesions and impalpable, mammographically detected lesions. Therefore, screening mammograms did not result in a larger percentage of negative or benign biopsy specimens than did biopsy of palpable masses. The lesions detected by mammography were smaller and noninvasive with less likelihood of distant metastases. Stereotaxic mammography guided fine-needle aspiration cytology may reduce the need for excisional biopsies of impalpable mammographically detected abnormalities.

▶ Compliance with the accepted guidelines for screening mammography should shift the typical diagnosed breast cancer to a smaller size and stage. The median length (diameter) in this review was 2.8 cm for palpable cancers and 1.5 cm for nonpalpable cancers. The percentage of in situ cancers was 4% of the palpable cancers and 32% of the nonpalpable cancers. The latter theoretically are 100% curable. There is growing clinical evidence that only those cancers less than 1.5 cm have an increased overall survival with current methods of treatment. The goal of primary care providers for women should be to diagnose all breast cancers before they are palpable.—W.H. Hindle, M.D.

Suggested Reading

Bauer TL, Pandelidis SM, Rhoads JE Jr, et al: Mammographically detected carcinoma of the breast. *Surg Gynecol Obstet* 173:482–486, 1991

▶ In this series of 2,077 consecutive mammographically guided needle-localization biopsies performed in a community hospital, 13.8% of the specimens proved to be carcinoma. Compared with palpable cancers diagnosed in the same institution, the mammographically detected cancers were smaller, were more frequently without axillary lymph node involvement, and were found in younger women. In the final year of this ten-year review, 42.1% of the breast cancers found were nonpalpable and mammographically detected.—W.H. Hindle, M.D.

Seltzer MH: The significance of breast complaints as correlated with age and breast cancer. *Am Surg* 58:413–417, 1992

▶ This thoughtful article from St. Barnabas Medical Center reveals that, in their surgical practice, approximately 7% of the women referred for breast evaluation proved to have breast cancer. How best to evaluate and follow the others? Gynecologists and other primary care physicians for women can serve a valuable function of initially evaluating women with breast complaints and overseeing diagnostic procedures. Open surgical biopsy (recommended in 40% of the referred women) should be the final step when the diagnosis cannot be established by less costly and invasive procedures.—W.H. Hindle, M.D.

The Influence of Ethnicity, Socioeconomic Status, and Psychological Barriers on Use of Mammography

Stein JA, Fox SA, Murata PJ (Univ of California, Los Angeles)

J Health Soc Behav 32:101–113, 1991 24–24

Objective.—Ethnicity is recognized as influencing sociomedical attitudes and behaviors. The effects not only of ethnicity, but also of psychological barriers and socioeconomic status on the use of mammography were assessed.

Study Design.—The sample included 586 white, 227 black, and 150 Hispanic women. The mean age of the respondents was 52 years. The Hispanic women were poorer and less educated than the women in the other groups. Data were initially analyzed with the EQS covariance structure analysis program, which tests the plausibility of a hypothesized covariance structure by comparing it with an actual data set. Confirmatory factor analysis served to demonstrate whether various psychological measures could be combined in a meaningful way.

Findings.—Factors that correlated significantly with the use of mammography included socioeconomic status, fear of irradiation, embarrassment, pain, anxiety, and concern over the cost. Both white and black women expressed cost concerns, whereas black and Hispanic women feared pain. The association with socioeconomic status was most evident among Hispanic women. After controlling for socioeconomic status and ethnicity, psychological barriers—particularly concern over cost—remained significant predictors of the use of mammography.

Implications.—Concern over cost emerged as the main perceived barrier to mammography in this survey. Many women also were concerned about radiation exposure. If women are convinced of the efficacy and value of mammography, they might be more willing to pay for the examination.

▶ Knowing their proven value in decreasing the mortality from breast cancer, why aren't all eligible women having mammograms? This interview study adds to the evidence that cost and fear of radiation are major deterrents to women of all backgrounds. Socioeconomic status is an important consideration. Screening mammography programs should be adapted to the cultural, racial, and economic attitudes of the various targeted groups. If they are within the health care system, women will have mammograms when recommended by their physicians. More education about breast cancer and the value of screening mammography is needed directly to women and to health care professionals.—W.H. Hindle, M.D.

Breast Cancer Screening Behaviors and Attitudes in Three Racial/Ethnic Groups

Vernon SW, Vogel VG, Halabi S, Jackson GL, Lundy RO, Peters GN (Univ of Texas, Houston; MD Anderson Cancer Ctr, Houston; Kelsey-Seybold Clinic, Houston; William Beaumont Army Med Ctr, El Paso, Tex; Baylor Univ Med Ctr, Dallas)

Cancer 69:165–174, 1992 24–25

Background.—Racial and ethnic differences have been found in stage of breast cancer at diagnosis, suggesting that there may be differential exposure to breast cancer screening. Data from a large sample of women participating in a breast cancer screening program in Texas were analyzed to compare the attitudes and behaviors of whites, blacks, and Hispanics to screening.

Methods.—More than 64,000 women completed mammography in the program. Fifty-six percent completed a self-report questionnaire inquiring about the risk factors for breast cancer, health behaviors, and factors affecting cancer screening behaviors.

Findings.—Similar patterns of association between a number of demographic and risk factors and prior mammography and recent clinical

Reasons for Not Having Mammography in the Past by Race/Ethnicity for Participants in the Texas Breast Screening Project, 1987

	Racial/ethnic groups				
Reason	*Blacks*	*Hispanics*	*Whites*	**Chi-square**	***P* value**
Not ordered by physician	34.7 (479)	31.2 (871)	30.2 (13,565)	20.51	< 0.001
Cost	30.0 (497)	33.9 (957)	23.5 (13,330)	71.23	< 0.001
Location of facility	15.0 (427)	13.8 (797)	8.6 (12,229)	44.65	0.001
Transportation	6.3 (426)	3.6 (798)	2.4 (12,074)	78.32	< 0.001
Time off work	6.4 (475)	8.0 (803)	4.7 (12,130)	46.21	< 0.001

* Importance was rated on a 5-point continuum from very important to not important. Statistical tests were done comparing the categories as very important, more or less important (the middle 3 categories), and not important. *Numbers in parentheses* represent the number of women in each group who rated that factor. Only women who had not had mammography previously were included in this analysis.

(Courtesy of Vernon SW, Vogel VG, Halabi S, et al: *Cancer* 69:165–174, 1991.)

breast examination (CBE) were found across racial and ethnic groups. However, the magnitude of the associations varied somewhat according to race and ethnicity. Thirty-three percent of whites had previously undergone a mammogram, compared with 27% of blacks and 24% of Hispanics. Reasons for not having had previous mammography examinations were similar across groups. The 2 most important reasons were lack of physician referral and cost. However, Hispanics were less likely than blacks or whites to report previous breast cancer screening, including CBE, mammography, and self-examination (table).

Conclusion.—Women of different racial and ethnic backgrounds can successfully be recruited to participate in a community-based, patient-initiated breast screening program. However, such programs must be augmented with other intervention strategies to reach low-income women. Women with more years of education and higher family incomes were overrepresented in all 3 racial and ethnic groups studied.

▶ To be successful as public health measures, population-based screening mammography programs require modification for various ethnic, social, and economic groups. Ready access to health care should be available, and positive health behaviors should be encouraged. Out-of-pocket cost is a significant barrier for low-income women. Physician referral is the most affirmative factor for most women.—W.H. Hindle, M.D.

Suggested Reading

Thomas DB, Noonan EA, and the WHO Collaborative Study of Neoplasia and Steroid Contraceptives. Breast cancer and specific types of combined oral contraceptives. *Br J Cancer* 65:108–113, 1992

▶ Even with the statistical power of this WHO collaborative study, when the data is stratified for dose, duration, and type of estrogen and progestin, only epidemiologically weak associations can be documented. Evaluation is further compounded by the lack of analysis of the biological activity of the estrogens/progestins and the effect of the hormonal interactions. Considering the wide confidence levels, no clinically significant consistent changes in relative risk were identified.—W.H. Hindle, M.D.

Breast Cancer and Depot-Medroxyprogesterone Acetate: A Multinational Study

WHO Collaborative Study of Neoplasia and Steroid Contraceptives, Thomas DB, Noonan EA (Fred Hutchinson Cancer Research Ctr, Seattle)

Lancet 338:833–838, 1991 24–26

Introduction.—Depot-medroxyprogesterone acetate (DMPA), a long-acting injectable progestational contraceptive, appeared to enhance the risk of breast cancer in animal studies and in certain human studies. The WHO Collaborative Study of neoplasia and Steroid Contraceptives was initiated in 1979, in part to determine whether use of DMPA enhances the risk of breast cancer. The final results from the WHO Collaborative Study on DMPA and breast cancer were reported.

Methods.—A hospital-based, case-control study was conducted in 5 participating hospitals in Nairobi, Kenya, Mexico City, Mexico, Bangkok, Thailand (2 hospitals), and Chiang Mai, Thailand. A total of 869 women who were young enough to have used DMPA for contraception were matched with 11,890 women of similar age who had been admitted to the hospital for conditions unrelated to steroid contraceptive use. Interviews on previous use of steroid contraceptives and suspected risks for breast cancer revealed that 12.5% of case women and 12.2% of control women had used DMPA.

Findings.—The relative risk of breast cancer in women who had ever used DMPA was 1 in 21, with an increased risk during the first 4 years of exposure—mainly in women younger than 35 years. The increased risk observed during the first 4 years of use was not a result of selective surveillance for breast cancer. There was no increased risk with duration or in women who had started to use DMPA 5 years previously.

Conclusion.—The relative risk of breast cancer in this study was increased in women who first used DMPA within the 4 previous years, and it decreased with time since first exposure. The overall relative risk estimate in ever-users of DMPA was 1 in 21. Results from the WHO Collaborative Study and an earlier population-based case-control study in New Zealand suggest that women who have used DMPA for a long time and who initiated use many years previously are not at increased risk of breast cancer.

► The epidemiological low level of increased relative risk (weak association) for breast cancer in woman who had depot-medroxyprogesterone for contraception is within the 95% confidence levels (C1, .96–1.52) of chance. This is reassuring to physicians prescribing this method of contraception. Because of the indolent nature of breast cancer, further long-term follow-up data would be of keen interest, as would dose and duration effects. However, the statistical power of this collaborative study is impressive. Pharmacological doses of progesterone had no demonstrable adverse effect (or benefit) on the breast ductal epithelium.—W.H. Hindle, M.D.

Suggested Readings

Berkel H. Birdsell DC, Jenkins H: Breast augmentation: A risk factor for breast cancer? *N Engl J Med* 326:1649–1653, 1992.

► This and other studies (Deapen DM, Brody GS: *J Plast Reconstr Surg* 88:660, 1992; Silverstein MJ, et al: *Arch Surg* 123:681, 1988) reaffirm that silicone implants do not increase the relative risk of breast cancer. Probably because of the selection bias in this report, the relative risk for breast cancer was found to be decreased. At least this aspect of silicone breast implants is clear and well documented.—W.H. Hindle, M.D.

Dunn KW, Hall PN, Khoo CTK: Breast implant materials: Sense and safety. *Br J Plast* 45:315–321, 1992

▶ This detailed review from England (with 71 references) is potentially objective and free of US political and Food and Drug Administration influences. A causal relationship between "Human Adjuvant Disease" and silicone breast implants has not been established. There is no proof that breast augmentations/implants are carcinogenic in humans.—W.H. Hindle, M.D.

Polycystic Ovaries and the Risk of Breast Cancer

Gammon MD, Thompson WD (Columbia Univ; New York; Univ of Southern Maine)

Am J Epidemiol 134:818–824, 1991 24–27

Background.—A positive association between polycystic ovaries and postmenopausal breast cancer has been previously reported. Because of the etiological implications of this finding, an attempt was made to corroborate this relationship.

Methods.—Data from a case-control study conducted between 1980 and 1982 were analyzed. This multicenter, population-based study involved in-home interviews with 4,730 women with breast cancer and 4,688 control subjects, aged 20–54 years.

Findings.—For women with a self-reported history of polycystic ovaries that had been diagnosed by a physician, the age-adjusted odds ratio for breast cancer was .52. Many covariates were assessed. Age, age at first birth, history of infertility, number of spontaneous abortions before the first birth, and menopausal status confounded the association, but only slightly. After these covariates were adjusted for, the odds ratio decreased to .47.

Conclusion.—Because women with polycystic ovaries have abnormal levels of certain endogenous hormones, the low risk of breast cancer in this group may offer new insights into the hormonal effects on breast cancer. Research on the etiology of breast cancer may benefit from more precise hormonal characterization of patients to recognize those with high levels of testosterone and luteinizing hormone in relation to normal levels of estradiol or increased levels of estrone.

▶ This adds to the data suggesting an altered hormone milieu in women who have breast cancer. The low incidence of breast cancer in males is the most compelling endocrine evidence. However, numerous studies of the measurement of various hormones have failed to demonstrate a consistent characteristic endocrine pattern of patients with breast cancer.—W.H. Hindle, M.D.

Breast Biopsy Techniques and Adequacy of Margins

Ngai JH, Zelles GW, Rumore GJ, Sawicki JE, Godfrey RS (Kaiser Permanente Med Ctr, Oakland, Calif)
Arch Surg 126:1343–1347, 1991 24–28

Background.—The shift toward the use of breast-conserving surgery for cancer has changed the role of the initial biopsy. Two initial biopsy techniques—traditional excisional biopsy and lumpectomy—were compared to assess their efficacy as procedures for breast-conserving surgery.

Methods.—The medical records of women who had positive breast biopsy results for cancer in 1988 and 1989 at 1 center were reviewed retrospectively. Forty-seven women had a traditional excisional biopsy, and 44 had a lumpectomy.

Findings.—Lumpectomy required a mean 53 minutes to do, whereas traditional biopsy required 37 minutes. The margins were verified as clear by microscopic assessment in 73% of those undergoing lumpectomy and in 17% of those undergoing traditional biopsy. Patients having lumpectomy subsequently had more axillary dissections (31%) than those having traditional biopsy (4%). Fewer modified radical mastectectomies were done in the lumpectomy than the traditional biopsy group, 49% and 71%, respectively. Extensive intraductal components were correlated with positive margins in those undergoing lumpectomy.

Conclusion.—As the initial biopsy technique, lumpectomy provides adequate margins more often than traditional excisional biopsy. Lumpectomy may also reduce the number of subsequent procedures required for breast-conserving surgery.

▶ For the treatment of stage I and II breast cancers, there is growing opinion that a malignant breast mass should be completely excised along with 1 centimeter of surrounding tissue, a lumpectomy by National Surgical Adjuvant Breast Project (NSABP) guidelines (Margolese R, et al: *Surgery* 102:828, 1987). Verified clear surgical margins are critical. If the margins are clear, local tumor removal for breast conserving surgery has been performed. If the margins are not clear, reexcision is indicated, unless a modified radical mastectomy is going to be performed.—W.H. Hindle, M.D.

Selection Criteria for Successful Immediate Breast Reconstruction

Dowden RV (Cleveland Clin Foundation)
Plast Reconstr Surg 88:628–634, 1991 24–29

Background.—Some investigators have reported high failure rates associated with immediate breast reconstruction after mastectomy, possibly because of lack of "complete muscle coverage." The factors affecting outcome of immediate reconstruction after mastectomy were evaluated.

Technique.—During a 5-year period, 176 consecutive immediate breast reconstructions were performed, using regular implants in 40, temporary expanders in 77, and "permanent" expanders in 59. The pectoralis muscle and/or serratus anterior were used between the skin incision and the implant if necessary. There was no attempt to secure complete muscle/fascia coverage of the lower pole of the implant; all implants were covered only by subcutaneous tissue and skin at the lower pole. Suction drains were placed adjacent to the implants. All patients received systemic antibiotics.

Results.—There were 5 (2.8%) failures, including 1 elective and 4 forced by infection/extrusion. Failure occurred in 1 of 40 regular implants and 4 of 77 temporary expanders; none occurred among the permanent expanders. One implant loss occurred in a previously irradiated patient. None of the implant losses involved extrusion through the lower pole of the implant. Implant losses did not occur in 19 patients with bilateral reconstructions.

Conclusion.—Failure in immediate breast reconstruction after mastectomy is not related to the use of drains, bilaterality, or lack of complete muscle coverage, but rather, to implant type, prior radiation, and suboptimal patient selection. The primary factor determining success is careful patient selection, and the second is interposing muscle between the implant and incision.

▶ When modified radical mastectomy is indicated or chosen by the patient, information about immediate or delayed reconstruction should be given as part of obtaining informed consent. Although seemingly psychologically advantageous, immediate reconstruction requires prolonged time under anesthesia with close coordination of the oncologic surgeon and the plastic surgeon. Careful patient selection is essential for optimum outcome. This treatment option may not be readily available in many locations, particularly rural areas.—W.H. Hindle, M.D.

Ten-Year Results of Breast-Conserving Surgery and Definitive Irradiation for Intraductal Carcinoma (Ductal Carcinoma In Situ) of the Breast

Solin LJ, Recht A, Fourquet A, Kurtz J, Kuske R, McNeese M, McCormick B, Cross MA, Schultz DJ, Bornstein BA, Spitalier J-M, Vilcoq JR, Fowble BL, Harris JR, Goodman RL (Univ of Pennsylvania, Philadelphia; Harvard Med School, Boston; Institut Curie, Paris; Univ Hosp, Basel, Switzerland; Washington Univ, St Louis; et al)

Cancer 68:2337–2344, 1991 24–30

Objective.—The combination of breast-conserving surgery and definitive irradiation has proved as effective as mastectomy in selective patients with invasive breast cancer. However, the use of this approach for noninvasive intraductal carcinoma remains controversial.

Patients.—A total of 259 patients from 9 centers had 261 breasts treated during the period from 1967 to 1985. The mean age was 50 years.

Management.—All patients had grossly complete excision of the primary tumor and definitive breast irradiation. Thirty-nine patients had reexcision of a biopsy site, and 86 underwent axillary node staging—all with negative results. The median radiation dose to the whole breast, including a booster dose, was 6,000 cGy. Eleven patients received systemic treatment as well.

Results.—Only 3% of patients were dead of breast cancer at 10 years. The 10-year rate of local failure in the breast was 16%. Three patients had chest wall recurrences after receiving salvage treatment for breast failure. Six patients (2%) had metastatic disease develop. Eight (3%) of the patients treated initially for unilateral carcinoma later had cancer develop in the other breast.

Conclusion.—These findings emphasize the need to follow women for a prolonged period after radiotherapy for intraductal breast cancer.

▶ The appropriate treatment of ductal carcinoma in situ is a major controversy in breast cancer therapy. The treatment of each case should be individualized. Frequent life-long follow-up is mandatory. The patient should clearly understand all aspects of the therapeutic options and probably outcomes before she makes her personal choice and gives her informed consent.—W.H. Hindle, M.D.

Suggested Readings

Cataliotti L, Distante V, Ciatto S, et al: Intraductal breast cancer: Review of 183 consecutive cases. *Eur J Cancer,* 28A:917–920, 1992.

▶ This series showed a sensitivity of 61% for clinical examination, 74% for mammography, 70% for fine-needle aspiration, and 93% for clinical examination and mammography combined. The ductal carcinoma in situ (DCIS) was multifocal in 60%, multicentric in 22%, and contralateral in 7%. Local recurrence occurred in 10% of lumpectomies and 3% of mastectomies. The authors note the recent tendency at their hospital toward treating DCIS by lumpectomy (81%), with approximately 60% having postoperative radiation.—W.H. Hindle, M.D.

McCormick B, Rosen PP, Kinne D, et al: Duct carcinoma in situ of the breast: An analysis of local control after conservation surgery and radiotherapy. *Int J Radiat Oncol Biol Phys* 21:289–292, 1992.

▶ Fifty-four patients treated by lumpectomy and radiation therapy (median follow-up, 3 years) demonstrated a recurrence rate of 18%, with 22% projected at 6 years. Of those with recurrent carcinoma, 30% had close/involved margins in spite of 50% reexcisions compared with 4% involved margins after a reexcision rate of 20% for patients considered controlled. There were no metastases or death within the follow-up range of 2–13 years. The authors consider residual microcalcifications a contraindication to breast conservation.—W.H. Hindle, M.D.

Underutilization of Breast-Conserving Surgery and Radiation Therapy Among Women With Stage I or II Breast Cancer

Lazovich D, White E, Thomas DB, Moe RE (Fred Hutchinson Cancer Research Ctr, Seattle)

JAMA 266:3433–3438, 1991 24–31

Background.—In 1990, a consensus panel of the National Institutes of Health (NIH) concluded that breast conservation with axillary dissection followed by radiation therapy was preferable to mastectomy for the treatment of most women with stage I or II breast cancer. Time trends and factors associated with breast-conserving surgery (BCS) and delivery of postoperative radiation therapy among such women were identified.

Methods.—Data on 8,095 women given a diagnosis of stage I or II breast cancer between 1983 and 1989 and registered with a population-based cancer registry in the Seattle area were obtained.

Findings.—In 1985, the frequency of BCS peaked, then returned to pre-1985 levels for women with stage II breast cancer, with a more moderate decrease for those with stage I breast cancer. The likelihood of BCS decreased with increasing age with stage II disease and with residence outside the region's major urban center. It increased with level of education or median income. The proportion of women treated with irradiation after BCS decreased with age, was lower for women with stage II disease compared with those with stage I, and was lowest in counties without radiation therapy facilities (Fig 24–5).

Conclusion.—Although clinical research demonstrates that BCS with radiation therapy is as effective as modified radical mastectomy in women with stage I or II disease, BCS is not being performed on most

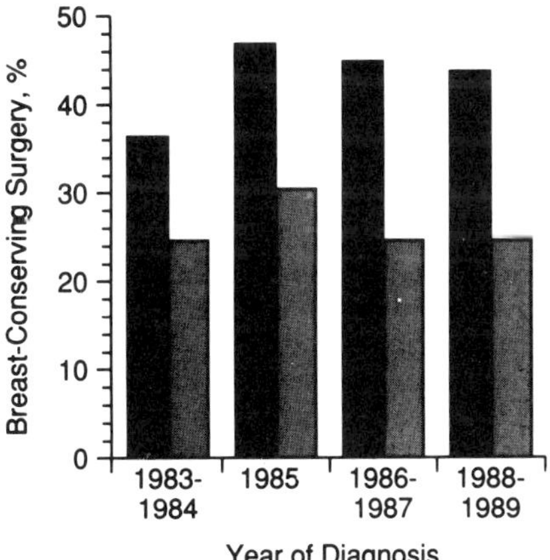

Fig 24–5.—Percentage of women with stage I (*solid bars*) or stage II (*shaded bars*) breast cancer who underwent breast-conserving surgery according to year of diagnosis. (Courtesy of Lazovich D, White E, Thomas DB, et al: *JAMA* 266:3433–3438, 1992.)

such women, as recommended as the preferred treatment by the National Institutes of Health.

▶ Behavior changes slowly, even with documented consistent medical data and a strong recommendation from a prestigious national panel of experts. The health care delivery system in the United States is largely a function of individual clinicians practicing in local hospitals. Changes in traditional practice come about slowly in such a decentralized system. However, women and their primary care physicians should be appropriately informed and should be aware of the treatment options available for stage I and II breast cancer. In most states, such counseling is a legal requirement; however, the giving of full current information and the obtaining of true informing consent before treatment is just good medical practice. Particularly with quality of life issues, only the patient herself can judge what is best for her.—W.H. Hindle, M.D.

Breast Conservation *Versus* Mastectomy: Is There a Difference in Psychological Adjustment or Quality of Life in the Year After Surgery?

Ganz PA, Schag CAC, Lee JJ, Polinsky ML, Tan S-J (Univ of California, Los Angeles)

Cancer 69:1729–1738, 1992 24–32

Introduction.—There still is little systematic information on the effect of surgery on psychological adjustment and quality of life in women with breast cancer. Despite an intuitive bias favoring segmental mastectomy (SM) (lumpectomy) and radiotherapy over modified radical mastectomy (MRM), several studies suggest there is no difference in psychological adjustment after these 2 treatments.

Methods.—The quality of life, performance status, and psychological adjustment were prospectively evaluated in 109 women treated for breast cancer during a 1-year period. Of these women, 52 were treated by SM and 57 were treated by MRM. The quality of life was estimated using the Global Adjustment to Illness Scale (GAIS).

Results.—The 2 operative groups did not differ significantly with respect to quality of life, mood disturbance, performance status, or global adjustment. Both groups improved significantly during the year of follow-up. Those patients who had MRM reported more problems with body image and dressing, but these did not seem to influence the reported quality of life.

Conclusion.—Limited surgery for breast cancer does not assure a better quality of life or better psychological adjustment compared with mastectomy. Women who have breast conservation treatment may actually require more intensive psychosocial intervention because of the added burden of radiotherapy.

▶ Psychological support should be offered to all women being treated for breast cancer. This and other studies indicate that body image and clothing are more problematic for women treated by modified radical mastectomy. However, radiation therapy used in breast conserving treatment is now identified as a significant psychosocial stress. Ideally, compassionate emotional support should be readily available for the patient with breast cancer, her family, and her companions.—W.H. Hindle, M.D.

Suggested Readings

Clark RM, McCulloch PB, Levine MN, et al: Randomized clinical trial to assess the effectiveness of breast irradiation following lumpectomy and axillary dissection for node-negative breast cancer. *J Natl Cancer Inst* 84:683–689, 1992.

▶ In this randomized series of 837 patients, less than 6% of the radiated group had local recurrence compared with 26% of the nonradiated group (Figure 2 of the original article). No survival advantage was noted up to 4 years. Age, tumor size, and nuclear grade were significant predictors of recurrence.—W.H. Hindle, M.D.

Janjan NA, Murray KJ, Conway P, et al: Prognosis for breast cancer surgery and radiation therapy compared with mastectomy alone. *Cancer* 69:2842–2848, 1992.

▶ A total of 558 patients treated by mastectomy and 201 treated by lumpectomy were evaluated with a median follow-up of 34 months. When corrected for axillary node status, lumpectomy showed more favorable results, but only in the node-negative patients. Selection or radiation control of microscopic cancer could account for the improved prognosis with lumpectomy.—W.H. Hindle, M.D.

Integration of Conservative Surgery, Radiotherapy, and Chemotherapy for the Treatment of Early-Stage, Node-Positive Breast Cancer: Sequencing, Timing, and Outcome

Recht A, Come SE, Gelman RS, Goldstein M, Tishler S, Gore SM, Abner AL, Vicini FA, Silver B, Connolly JL, Schnitt SJ, Coleman CN, Harris JR (Harvard Med School; Beth Israel Hosp; Harvard School of Public Health; Dana-Farber Cancer Inst; Harvard Community Health Plan, Boston)

J Clin Oncol 9:1662–1667, 1991 24–33

Background.—In patients with early stage breast cancer, the combination of breast-conserving surgery, radiotherapy, and adjuvant systemic therapy is being used more frequently. However, the optimal combination of these therapies remains to be established. Nine years of experience with such treatment were reviewed, focusing on the affect of treatment delay after surgery.

Patients and Treatment.—The patients were 295 women with breast cancer. The median age at diagnosis was 45 years, 200 patients being 50 years of age or younger. At surgery, all had positive axillary nodes. No gross residual disease was left in the breast or axilla postoperatively. All patients received breast irradiation (median dose, 66 Gy), and 86% had nodal irradiation. The patients also received at least 3 cycles of a cyclophosphamide, methotrexate, and fluorouracil-based regimen or a doxorubicin-containing regimen. The sequence of the various treatments was decided by consultation between the patients' oncologists and was not randomized. The median follow-up for all patients was 72 months.

Results.—In 99 patients who had radiotherapy before chemotherapy the actuarial 5-year breast failure rate was 4%. Failure rate was 8% in 54 patients who received some chemotherapy, followed by radiotherapy, then further chemotherapy, and it was 6% in 116 patients who received concurrent chemotherapy and radiotherapy. In 26 patients who had all chemotherapy before radiotherapy, the failure rate was 41%. Local failure within 4 years occurred in a crude incidence of 3%, 2%, 4%, and 15%, respectively. Two hundred fifty-two patients who received irradiation within 16 weeks after surgery had an actuarial 5-year local failure rate of 5% compared to 35% for 34 patients who received irradiation more than 16 weeks after surgery. Local failure within 4 years occurred in a crude incidence of 4% and 12%, respectively.

Conclusion.—In women with breast cancer, the likelihood of local failure is increased if radiotherapy is delayed. These results await confirmation by randomized, controlled studies, which will also improve the integration of the three therapies.

▶ This study of various sequence treatments of 295 women with early stage breast cancer and involved axillary nodes (median follow-up, 72 months) revealed failure rates of 41% with chemotherapy before radiation, 8% with mixed sequence, 6% with concurrent treatment, and 4% with radiation before chemotherapy. This suggests that indicated radiation therapy should not be delayed.—W.H. Hindle, M.D.

Relationship Among Outcome, Stage of Disease, and Histologic Grade for 22,616 Cases of Breast Cancer: The Basis for a Prognostic Index

Henson DE, Ries L, Freedman LS, Carriaga M (Natl Cancer Inst, Bethesda, Md; Georgetown Univ, Washington, DC)

Cancer 68:2142–2149, 1991 24–34

Background.—Histological grade can be used to estimate outcome independent of disease stage for cancers in most sites. However, the histological grading of breast cancer is not widely accepted. The association among the histological grade, stage, and outcome in patients enrolled in the Surveillance, Epidemiology, and End Results (SEER) program were reported.

Methods.—The survival rates for 22,616 patients listed in SEER were stratified on outcome according to the histological grade and disease stage. Two staging systems were used: a "local, regional, and distant"

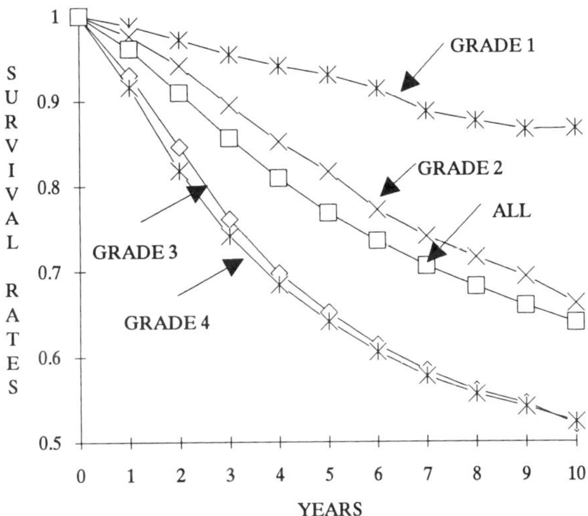

Fig 24–6.—Survival according to grade only. All stages combined. "Al" represents cases not graded. (Courtesy of Henson DE, Ries L, Freedman LS, et al: *Cancer* 68:2142–2149, 1991.)

and a modified American Joint Committee on Cancer system. Five- and ten-year relative survival rates were calculated (Fig 24–6).

Findings.—Patients classified as stage II, grade 1 had a survival rate comparable to patients classified as stage I, grade 3. Their survival was superior to those in stage I, grade 4. The 5-year survivals for those with stage I, grade 1 and for those with stage I, grade 2 were 99% and 98%, respectively. At 10 years, those in the former group had a 95% survival rate. Patients with histologic grade 1 tumors smaller than 2 cm and posi-

Distribution of Histological Grade by Tumor Size

Tumor diameter (cm)	Grade 1 (%)	Grade 2 (%)	Grade 3 (%)	Grade 4 (%)
< 0.5	26	41	27	6
0.5–0.9	24	46	25	4
1.0–1.9	12	45	37	5
2.0–2.9	7	40	47	6
3.0–3.9	4	35	52	8
4.0–4.9	4	33	57	6
> 5.0	3	26	62	9

Note: Based on analysis of 17,153 microscopically confirmed cases with known grade and tumor size. The rows add to 100%. All stages combined. Data from 1983 to 1987 only.

(Courtesy of Henson DE, Ries L, Freedman LS, et al: *Cancer* 68:2142–2149, 1991.)

tive axillary lymph nodes had a 99% 5-year survival rate. Histological grade increased as the size of tumor increased (table).

Conclusion.—These findings suggest that the staging system should be considered in linking histological grade with disease stage. When used in conjunction with disease stage, histological grade can improve the prediction of outcome. A prognostic index can be created for breast cancer using a combination of disease stage and histological grade. Only 3 grades appear to be needed for breast cancer.

▶ The search for a reliable prognostic index for patients with breast cancer continues. Histological grade seems to be useful. Nuclear grade, especially with in situ cancers, may prove to be valuable. However, the heterogeneity of breast cancer and the apparent histological and nuclear transformation of breast cancer as the tumor increases in size, have limited the clinical usefulness of these subjective evaluations. Inter- and intra-observer variability compounds the difficulty in applying such information to individual patients.—W.H. Hindle, M.D.

Paget's Disease of the Nipple

Dixon AR, Galea MH, Ellis IO, Elston CW, Blamey RW (City Hosp, Nottingham, England)

Br J Surg 78:722–723, 1991 24–35

Introduction.—Sir James Paget first recognized the relationship between chronic eczema of the nipple and underlying impalpable (nonpalpable) breast carcinoma in 1874. The origin of the large, clear intraepidermal Paget cells are thought to be derived from an underlying breast carcinoma, with migration upward to the epidermis along the mammary ducts. To determine the optimal surgical approach to this unusual malignancy, data were reviewed on 48 patients with Paget's disease of the nipple without palpable lumps.

Patients.—The median patient age at diagnosis was 62 years. All lesions were unilateral, with nipple discharge, crusting, bleeding or erythema of 1 month to 12 years' duration. All patients underwent nipple biopsy followed by a simple mastectomy with node biopsy in 37 patients. In 10 patients, conservative surgery was performed with excision of the nipple-areola complex and a cone of underlying breast tissue; 1 patient was treated with tamoxifen alone.

Results.—In situ ductal carcinoma (DCIS) was found in 96% of the operative specimens, with associated invasion in 8 patients (17%). The DCIS was predominantly large cell solid/comedo in type and was multifocal in 7 patients. There was local recurrence in 4 patients treated with cone excision by a median follow-up period of 56 months. Metastases developed in 2 of these patients. Of the 37 patients who underwent mastectomy, there were locoregional recurrences in 2 patients who had invasive foci at their first operation; at 8 years, both were disease-free.

Conclusion.—Mammography was not reliable in the diagnosis of Paget's disease. Of 34 patients with histological evidence of an underlying carcinoma 11 (32%) had a normal mammogram. Conservative surgery had a 40% recurrence rate. The high rate of invasive components found and the extensive DCIS of mastectomy specimens support the use of simple mastectomy for Paget's disease of the nipple.

▶ This unique clinical manifestation of underlying ductal carcinoma accounts for less than 2% of the breast cancers in most series. However, any moist or dry eczematoid lesion of the nipple must be evaluated to rule out this malignancy. Neither mammography nor ultrasound is diagnostic. Fine-needle aspiration cytology is helpful only if there is a palpable mass and is then significant only if malignant cells are identified. Open surgical nipple biopsy usually is required for diagnosis. The large are of tumor involvement within the breast usually makes breast conservation surgery cosmetically unacceptable.—W.H. Hindle, M.D.

Fear of Recurrence, Breast-Conserving Surgery, and the Trade-Off Hypothesis

Lasry J-CM, Margolese RG (Jewish Gen Hosp, Montreal)

Cancer 69:2111–2115, 1992 24–36

Introduction.—Although breast-conserving surgery presumably leads to a better body image, patients are expected to be more concerned about recurring cancer, because only a small part of the breast is excised.

Methods.—Fear of disease recurrence was compared in patients randomized into the National Surgical Adjuvant Breast Project trial who underwent total mastectomy, lumpectomy alone, or lumpectomy followed by radiotherapy. A "Fear of Recurrence" index included questions about the patient's own concern and her perception of her family's concern.

Results.—The type of treatment itself created no differences in fear of recurrence, but patients who had multiple operations were more fearful of recurrence and also had a worse body image, resembling those who underwent total mastectomy. Patients who had a radical operation did not fear recurrence less than those who had lumpectomy.

Conclusion.—The reputed trade-off between breast conservation and fear of cancer recurrence is not a reality. There seems to be little reason to raise this matter as a significant factor in selecting a surgical treatment for breast cancer.

▶ This adds to the increasing evidence that the treatment selected by the patient with stage I or II breast cancer is clearly her choice; there is little scientific evidence to tip the balance of probability toward survival or psychological advantage. Perception of adverse body image and clothing difficulties seem to be the 2 consistent psychological findings associated with modified radical mastectomy compared with breast conservation therapy. The individual woman's evaluation of her own quality of life appears to be the crucial factor in making her informed choice of breast cancer treatment.—W.H. Hindle, M.D.

Relative Effect of Steroid Hormone Receptors on the Prognosis of Patients With Operable Breast Cancer: A Univariate and Multivariate Analysis of 3089 Japanese Patients With Breast Cancer From the Study Group for the Japanese Breast Cancer Society on Hormone Receptors and Prognosis in Breast Cancer

Nomura Y, Miura S, Koyama H, Enomoto K, Kasumi F, Yamamoto H, Kimura M, Tominaga T, Iino H, Morimoto T, Tashiro H (Natl Kyushu Cancer Ctr, Fukuoka; Aichi Cancer Ctr, Nagoya, Japan; Osaka Adult Disease Ctr, Osaka, Japan; Keio Univ, Tokyo; Cancer Research Inst, Tokyo; et al)

Cancer 69:153–164, 1992 24–37

Background.—Estrogen (ER) and progesterone receptor (PgR) measurement is known to be useful in predicting responses to endocrine treatment in patients with advanced breast cancer. The correlation between ER and/or PgR in primary breast cancer with patient prognosis was investigated.

Methods.—Two hospitals participated in the study. Of 3,118 patients with operable breast cancer who were undergoing surgery between 1972 and 1982, 3,089 were evaluable. Fifty-six percent had ER-positive cancers, and 34% had PgR-positive cancers.

Findings.—The ER and PgR positivities decreased as tumor size increased, but they were independent on lymph node metastasis. No significant differences were found in relapse-free survival according to receptor status. In patients with 4 or more positive nodes, those with PgR-positive disease survived free of relapse for a longer time. Those with ER-positive disease survived significantly longer than those with ER-negative cancers. The greatest difference occurred in those with 4 or more positive nodes. The patients with ER-positive cancer had a significantly longer postrelapse survival (PRS) rate because of the different distribution of the major metastasis and the better responses to first-line and subsequent therapy. According to Cox's multivariate analysis, overall survival—but not PRS—was influenced by ER because of the longer PRS in ER-positive patients.

Conclusion.—Estrogen status appears to be the most important clinical factor predicting PRS. The ER-expressed hormone dependency in primary breast cancer appears to be retained at the time of the first recurrence and in the subsequent course, despite adjuvant and variable treatment. Information on hormone receptors in primary cancer can be used to predict recurrence status, response to endocrine therapy, PRS, and overall survival.

▶ Although the biological characteristics and incidence of ER-positive breast cancers in Japan are distinctly different from those reported in most western cultures, this detailed analysis of more than 3,000 surgically treated stage I, II, and III breast cancers confirms the more favorable prognosis of women, as a group, who have ER-positive cancers at the time of diagnosis. However, not even sophisticated multivariant analysis of all the known prognostic factors reliably predicts the outcome for an individual patient with breast cancer.—W.H. Hindle, M.D.

Optimal Mastectomy Timing

McGuire WL, Hilsenbeck S, Clark GM (Univ of Texas Health Science Ctr, San Antonio)

J Natl Cancer Inst 84:346–348, 1992 24–38

Background.—Based on results of a retrospective study of 249 cases, researchers at Guy's Hospital in London recommended in May 1991 that premenopausal patients with breast cancer have their surgery delayed until at least 12 days after their most recent menstrual period. Other studies, however, had not found an association between mastectomy timing and rates of recurrence and survival. The literature was reviewed to determine whether data support the existence of an optimal timing for mastectomy.

Discussion.—In September 1991, results similar to those noted at Guy's Hospital appeared in a study of 283 patients from Memorial Sloan-Kettering Cancer Center in New York. Women whose mastectomy was performed during days 7–14 of the menstrual cycle had a higher rate of recurrence. However, a review of the literature showed that each report of a significant result found a different prognostically favorable cycle window. The probability of finding a significant outcome by chance increases dramatically when multiple windows are tested on a single dataset to select the best one.

Conclusion.—Data on 675 patients with breast cancer from the San Antonio Tumor Bank were examined according to 14 possible pairs of 14-day windows. This simulation study showed that at least 1 ostensibly significant time period was found in 28 of 100 trials. There are insufficient data at this time to schedule surgery according to the menstrual period. A definite answer to the question must carefully define the day of the menstrual cycle by hormonal measurements and take into account the statistical problems discussed here.

▶ Most unfortunately, Dr. McGuire is no longer with us; however, his intense research continues to benefit women with breast cancer. The timing of mastectomy is controversial. Careful epidemiological and statistical analysis of the basic data is required. This carefully done article reveals no proof of an optimum time in the menstrual cycle for performing mastectomy.—W.H. Hindle, M.D.

Systemic Treatment of Early Breast Cancer by Hormonal, Cytotoxic, or Immune Therapy: 133 Randomised Trials Involving 31,000 Recurrences and 24,000 Deaths Among 75,000 Women

Early Breast Cancer Trialists' Collaborative Group (Oxford, England)

Lancet 339:71–85, 1992 24–39

Objective.—A worldwide collaborative effort was undertaken to analyze recurrences and deaths in randomized trials begun before 1985, that dealt with any aspect of systemic adjuvant treatment for early breast cancer. Data were available for 75,000 women, approximately 90% of those ever randomized into trials. Approximately one third of these women had died, and another 10% had had recurrences. There were nearly 30,000 women in trials of tamoxifen and 3,000 women in trials of ovarian ablation.

Tamoxifen.—Tamoxifen reduced recurrences by 25% and deaths by 17%. In addition, it reduced the risk of the development of contralateral breast cancer by 39%. Tamoxifen was of value in women 70 years of age and older. Recurrences were chiefly reduced in the first 4 years of follow-up.

Ovarian Ablation.—Women younger than 50 years of age who were managed by ovarian ablation had a 26% reduction in recurrences and a 25% decrease in mortality. Ablation at older ages was ineffective.

Polychemotherapy.—In 11,000 women participating in trials of polychemotherapy, recurrences were 28% less frequent and mortality decreased by 16%. As with tamoxifen, recurrences were avoided chiefly during the first years of follow-up, but mortality remained reduced after this time. Polychemotherapy was significantly more effective than single-agent chemotherapy. Treatment for 6 months was as effective as long-term treatment. In women aged 50–69 years, chemotherapy plus tamoxifen was more effective than chemotherapy alone. With combined chemo-endocrine therapy in middle-aged women, the absolute improvement in 10-year survival was about twice as great for node-positive as for node-negative patients.

Reprints available from EBCTCG Secretariat, ICRF/MRC Clinical Trial Service Unit, Nuffield Dept of Clinical Medicine, Radcliffe Infirmary, Oxford OX2 6HE, UK

▶ This collaborative report on adjuvant therapy should become a classic article because of the impressive statistical power (numbers) that validates the effectiveness of tamoxifen (Figure 3 in the original article) and ovarian ablation for women younger than 50 years of age (Figure 8 in the original article). Anyone involved with adjuvant therapy for breast cancer should read the original article in detail. Its conclusive data provide a rational basis for the treatment of women with breast cancer.—W.H. Hindle, M.D.

Suggested Reading

Cancer Research Campaign Breast Cancer Trials Group: The effect of adjuvant tamoxifen: The latest results from the Cancer Research Campaign Adjuvant Breast Trial. *Eur J Cancer* 28A:904–907, 1992.

▶ This collaborative randomized trial of 2,230 patients with stage I or II breast cancer demonstrated no benefit from perioperative cyclophosphamide therapy (treatment for 2 years with a median 7.8-year follow-up). In contrast, tamoxifen therapy demonstrated improved disease-free survival. The findings suggest that the benefit from tamoxifen was similar in patients with node-negative and node-positive tumors, in both premenopausal and postmenopausal women, and in all patients irrespective of tumor size. However, no overall survival benefit was demonstrated.—W.H. Hindle, M.D.

Effects of Tamoxifen on Cardiovascular Risk Factors in Postmenopausal Women

Love RR, Wiebe DA, Newcomb PA, Cameron L, Leventhal H, Jordan VC, Feyzi J, DeMets DL (Univ of Wisconsin Clinical Cancer Ctr, Madison)

Ann Intern Med 115:860–864, 1991 24–40

Background.—Tamoxifen citrate is now a front-line treatment for all stages of breast cancer. Investigators have also been considering tamoxifen as a chemosuppressive hormonal replacement therapy. However, the effects of tamoxifen treatment on the risk factors for cardiovascular

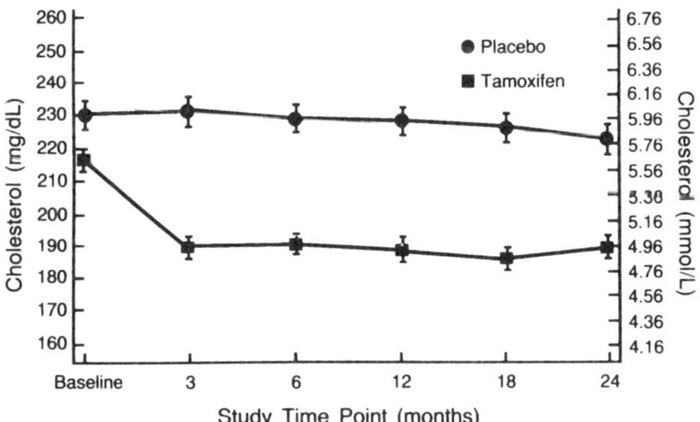

Fig 24–7.—The mean fasting levels of total cholesterol over time in patients receiving tamoxifen or plecebo. *Circle* = control patients; n = 70 at baseline and n = 70, 68, 67, 64, and 62 patients at 3, 6, 12, 18, and 24 months, respectively. *Square* = patients receiving tamoxifen; n = 70 at baseline and n = 66, 66, 65, 64, and 64 patients at 3, 6, 12, 18, and 24 months, respectively. *Bars* indicatc 95% Cls. Cholesterol levels decreased significantly at all time points in patients receiving tamoxifen. (Courtesy of Love RR, Wiebe DA, Newcomb PA, et al: *Ann Intern Med* 115:860–864, 1991.)

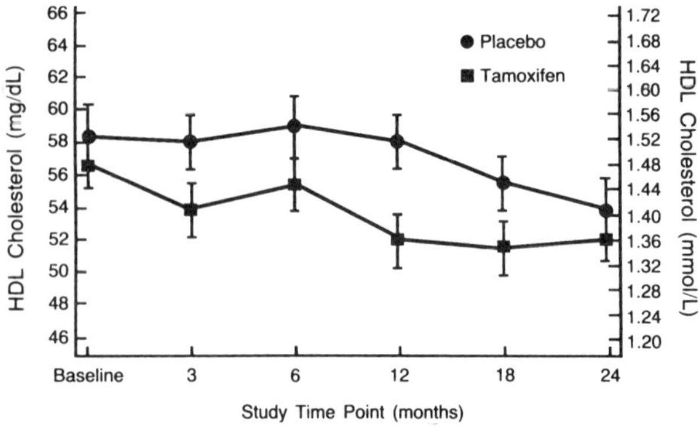

Fig 24–8.—The mean fasting levels of HDL cholesterol over time in patients receiving tamoxifen or plecebo. *Circle* = control patients; n = 70 at baseline and n = 70, 68, 67, 64, and 62 patients at 3, 6, 12, 18, and 24 months, respectively. *Square* = patients receiving tamoxifen; n = 70 at baseline and n = 66, 66, 65, 64, and 64 patients at 3, 6, 12, 18, and 24 months, respectively. *Bars* indicate 95% Cls. The difference between the 2 groups is only significant at 12 months. (Courtesy of Love RR, Wiebe DA, Newcomb PA, et al: *Ann Intern Med* 115:860–864, 1991.)

disease are very important in such contexts. The effects of tamoxifen on these risk factors in disease-free postmenopausal women were studied.

Methods.—One hundred and forty women were enrolled in the double-blind, placebo-controlled, randomized 2-year trial. The women were clinically postmenopausal with a diagnosis of axillary node-negative breast cancer and were disease-free by laboratory and clinical criteria.

Findings.—Women receiving tamoxifen, who were assessed every 3 or 6 months for 2 years, had a mean reduction of 12% in total cholesterol

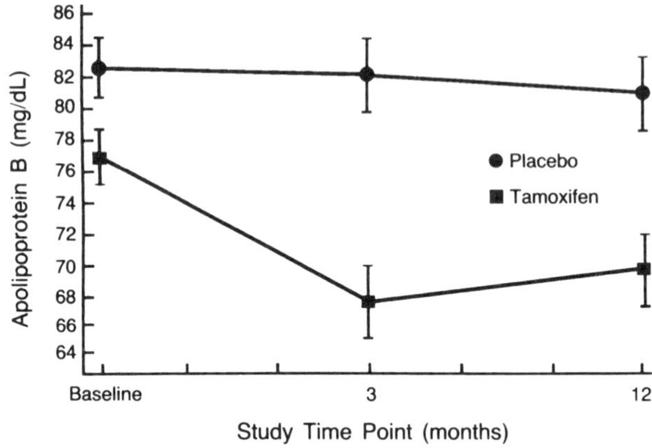

Fig 24–9.—The mean fasting levels of apolipoprotein B at 3 time intervals in patients receiving tamoxifen or placebo. *Circle* = control patients; n = 68 at baseline and n = 64 and 66 patients at 3 and 12 months, respectively. *Square* = patients receiving tamoxifen; n = 68 at baseline and n = 59 and 63 patients at 3 and 12 months, respectively. *Bars* indicate 95% Cls. Apolipoprotein B levels were significantly decreased at 3 and 12 months in patients receiving tamoxifen. (Courtesy of Love RR, Wiebe DA, Newcomb PA, et al: *Ann Intern Med* 115:860–864, 1991.)

levels. They also had a mean decrease of 20% in calculated low-density lipoprotein cholesterol levels. Those with higher baseline cholesterol levels had greater reductions with tamoxifen therapy. High-density lipoprotein cholesterol levels decreased in women treated with tamoxifen, but this decrease usually was nonsignificant. Apolipoprotein A-I levels increased significantly at the 2 time points at which it was measured. Apolipoprotein B levels were reduced significantly at these times in tamoxifen-treated patients. Tamoxifen therapy did not change plasma glucose levels, reported exercise and work activity, smoking, weight, or systolic and diastolic blood pressures (Figs 24–7, 24–8, and 24–9).

Conclusion.—Tamoxifen therapy produced generally favorable effects on the lipid and lipoprotein profile of postmenopausal women in this 2-year study. These effects may partly explain the decrease in adverse events and in mortality related to coronary heart disease in women receiving adjuvant tamoxifen treatment.

▶ The antiestrogenic actions of tamoxifen raised the concern that treated women might have adverse effects with resultant increased cardiovascular disease and osteoporosis. This short-term study is reassuring in that the lipoproteins were affected favorably. Other studies have shown favorable effects on osteoporis relative risk. Because tamoxifen therapy is long-term and probably will become life-long, these favorable metabolic effects are encouraging.—W.H. Hindle, M.D.

Suggested Reading

Love RR, Mazess RB, Barden HS, et al: Effects of tamoxifen on bone mineral density in postmenopausal women with breast cancer. *N Engl J Med* 326:852–856, 1992.

▶ There has been concern that tamoxifen (acting as an antiestrogen) might predispose to osteoporosis. This 2-year randomized, double-blind placebo study of 140 postmenopausal women with node-negative breast cancer found a .6% per year increase in the mean bone mineral density of the lumbar spine as measured by photon absorptiometry.—W.H. Hindle, M.D.

Lobular Carcinoma In Situ of the Breast: Clinical, Pathologic, and Mammographic Features

Beute BJ, Kalisher L, Hutter RVP (St Barnabas Med Ctr, Livingston, NJ)

AJR 157:257–265, 1991 24–41

Introduction.—Lobular carcinoma in situ (LCIS) is a rare lesion of the lobule of the breast that is difficult to diagnose by mammography. In an effort to identify the mammographic features or predictors of LCIS, 165 breasts diagnosed with LCIS were examined.

Findings.—Lobular carcinoma in situ was more common in younger women than other breast cancers. Multifocal disease was detected in the breast in 70% of cases. When both breasts were examined, bilateral foci were detected 50% of the time. In 37% of the breasts, simultaneous invasive cancers occured within the breast.

Mammography was normal in 44% of the LCIS breasts. In an N1 breast or in a breast with less than 25% of its parenchymal area occupied by fibroglandular density, LCIS was rare. Compared with an age-matched control group, LCIS breasts had more than 50% fibroglandular density and a significantly higher frequency of the DY pattern. In postmenopausal women, these 2 prognostic factors were nearly double the rate detected in the control group.

Conclusion.—In postmenopausal women, mammographically dense breasts are a marker for increased cancer risk. In the premenopausal age group, this marker is too nonspecific to be useful diagnostically. Mammography does not appear to be useful in the specific detection of LCIS.

► Lobular carcinoma in situ (LCIS) remains an enigma. Is it cancer? What is the optimum treatment? Neither mammography nor physical examination (clinical breast examination) is characteristic or clinically reliable for detecting LCIS. Fine-needle aspiration (FNA) cytology might show cancer cells, but it does not define invasion vs. in situ, and because there rarely is a mass, the lesion is often missed by FNA. In this series, LCIS was 70% multifocal, 50% bilateral, and 37% invasive carcinoma.—W.H. Hindle, M.D.

Suggested Readings

Bolla M, Chedin M, Colonna M, et al: Prognostic value of epidermal growth factor receptor in a series of 303 breast cancers. *Eur J Cancer* 28A:1052–1054, 1992.

► Measurements of epidermal growth factor receptors revealed 50.8% of the samples to be positive, inversely related to estrogen receptor expression, and with decreased expression correlated with tumor differentiation. However, in this group of patients, 70% of whom had adjuvant medical treatment, progesterone receptor assays were the strongest predictor of disease-free survival.—W.H. Hindle, M.D.

Brower ST, Schally AV, Redding TW, et al: Differential effects of LHRH and somatostatin analogs on human breast cancer. *J Surg Res* 52:6–14, 1992

► Direct action of LHRH and somatostatin analogues on the growth of human mammary tumor cells in vitro demonstrated the effects to be analogue specific and concentration dependent. Although such information does not translate directly into clinically useful applications for breast cancer in vivo, it does suggest endocrine actions and may be useful as a basis for clinical trials.—W.H. Hindle, M.D.

Cabanes PA, Salmon RJ, Vilcoq JR, et al: Value of axillary dissection in addition to lumpectomy and radiotherapy in early breast cancer. *Lancet* 339:1245–48, 1992.

► This prospective randomized series of 658 women with cancers less than 3 cm revealed increased survival and reduced visceral and supraclavicular metastases and less lymph node recurrence in the lumpectomy/axillary dissection group vs. the lumpectomy alone group. With a mean 54-month follow-up, survival related to age older than 35 years, absence of involved nodes, histological grading, and estrogen and progesterone receptor status. Whereas the authors were unable to conclude whether dissection itself or adjuvant treatments were responsible for the increased survival of the lumpectomy/axillary dissection group vs. the lumpectomy alone group, the Institut Curie now systematically uses the combined procedures in treating early breast cancers.—W.H. Hindle, M.D.

Improving Physicians' and Nurses' Clinical Breast Examination: A Randomized Controlled Trial

Campbell HS, Pilgrim CA, Fletcher SW, Morgan TM, Lin S (Univ of North Carolina at Wilmington; Bowman-Gray School of Medicine, Winston-Salem, NC)

Am J Prev Med 7:1–8, 1991 24–42

Introduction.—Clinical breast examination (CBE) is the major breast cancer screening method practiced, but health professional examination competence is not optimal. A randomized trial evaluated the changes in health professionals' lump detection accuracy and examination skills following a training program using lifelike silicone breast models.

Methods.—Thirty-two graduate nurses and 64 internal medicine residents participated in the randomized pretest, posttest design. The training emphasized systematic examination and development of tactile skills to detect lumps of varying sizes, degrees of hardness, and depth of placement in the silicone breast models. The experimental group of participants received instruction within 2 weeks of the pretest in lump discrimination and search techniques. All participants were pretested 4 months later.

Results.—Mean sensitivity increased in the experimental group but decreased in the control group. Specificity decreased in the experimental group and increased in the control group. The experimental group improved significantly in 5 of 6 techniques, whereas the control group improved in only one. The duration of the examination was an independent predictor of sensitivity. The medical records of women seen by a subset of the experimental and control groups during the 6 months after training showed no significant differences in the proportion of abnormal breast examinations reported or the number of mammograms ordered between the 2 groups.

Conclusion.—Health professionals who participated in a training program using silicone breast models to develop lump detection accuracy and tactile skills. The experimental group that received the training had increased sensitivity but decreased specificity; however, the training program improved the health professionals' clinical breast examination accuracy and skills.

▶ Physicians and nurses can increase their sensitivity of lump detection by training with silicone breast models with various lumps. However, when office records were reviewed, the specificity of clinical breast examination did not change significantly after the training.—W.H. Hindle, M.D.

Suggested Reading

Catania S, Zurrida S, Veronesi P, et al: Mondor's disease and breast cancer. *Cancer* 69:2267-2270, 1992.

▶ This series of 63 cases of Mondor's disease (thrombophlebitis of the subcutaneous veins of the anterior chest region) demonstrated multiple idiopathic etiologies and a 12.7% incidence of breast cancer. Thus, mammographic evaluation is essential to check for cancer associated with this otherwise benign disease.—W.H. Hindle, M.D.

Clark JA, Kent RB III: One-day hospitalization following modified radical mastectomy. *Am Surg* 58:239-242, 1992.

▶ The authors report a personal prospective study of 29 consecutive patients with breast cancer. Of these, 2 patients subsequently refused early discharge. Drains were removed in the office on day 5 after surgery. Seroma formation required aspiration at least once in 45%. There were no significant complications. An average 35% reduction in hospital cost was achieved.—W.H. Hindle, M.D.

Occult Breast Masses: Use of a Mammographic Localizing Grid for US Evaluation

Conway WF, Hayes CW, Brewer WH (Med College of Virginia, Richmond)
Radiology 181:143–146, 1991 24–43

Introduction.—Ultrasound (US) is a useful method for the characterization of mammographically detected, nonpalpable breast masses, but it may be difficult for the examiner to positively determine that the mass seen on the US scan is the same mass seen on the mammogram when there is more than 1 mass in the breast. Ultrasound demonstrates many areas of varying echogenicity, and some normal breast parenchyma may mimic solid masses. The use of a fenestrated mammographic compression grid to stabilize the breast and guide the US examination was described.

Technique.—Fifty mammographically distinct masses were identified in 47 patients scheduled to undergo needle localization. In 6 cases, the masses were localized in an area of the breast that contained other opacities which could have interfered with identification. Freehand US results were compared with a fenestrated mammographic compression guide to guide the US evaluation. Needle localization was performed while the breast was still in the grid.

Findings.—In five of 50 cases (10%), masses detected by freehand US and identified as the mammographically detected masses were found to represent different areas of the breast when US was used with the compression grid. There is a potential for misidentification of masses with freehand US.

Conclusions.—Because of the small number of patients studied, grid-directed US of the breast is not universally recommend, but the real potential for misidentification of masses with freehand US if identified. Grid-directed US is recommended when there are adjacent mammographic masses, when the mass is in dense tissue, when there is a significant size difference between the mammographic and US depiction of the mass.

▶ Grid-directed US of the breast revealed 10% more specific masses than freehand US when there were multiple masses, dense breasts, or mass size difference.—W.H. Hindle, M.D.

Suggested Reading

Crowe JP, Gordon NH, Hubay CA, et al: Estrogen receptor determination and long term survival of patients with carcinoma of the breast. *Br J Cancer* 64:1133–1138, 1991.

▶ Multivariant analysis of life-table estimates for 1,392 women with stage I–III breast cancer treated by modified radical mastectomy and grouped by estrogen receptor (ER) status revealed a 10% maximum difference for disease-free survival after 3 years, and a similar difference for overall survival at 3–10 years. The authors interpret their data to suggest that ER-positive tumors are less aggressive, and that ER assay is useful for predicting survival after recurrent cancer, with initially ER-positive cancers being more response to treatment.—W.H. Hindle, M.D.

Significance of Ipsilateral Breast Tumour Recurrence After Lumpectomy

Fisher B, Anderson S, Fisher ER, Redmond C, Wickerham DL, Wolmark N, Mamounas EP, Deutsch M, Margolese R (Natl Surgical Adjuvant Breast and Bowel Project Headquarters, Pittsburgh)

Lancet 338:327–331, 1991 24–44

Introduction.—The 8-year results of a prospective breast cancer treatment trial comparing total mastectomy, lumpectomy alone, and lumpectomy plus breast irradiation found no significant differences between the 3 treatment modalities in terms of distant-disease-free survival (DDFS) and survival (S). The 9-year follow-up data from that trial were used to examine the significance of ipsilateral breast tumor recurrence (IBTR) in relation to DDFS.

Methods.—All women had been treated for breast cancer between 1976 and 1984. Only those women with primary operable breast tumors of 4 cm or less were enrolled in the trial. Lumpectomy patients in whom IBTR developed were treated by total mastectomy, but they remained in the study group to which they were assigned. All patients were followed for disease-free survival (DFS), DDFS, and S, but only the relation between IBTR and DDFS was analyzed here. Although IBTR is the end of

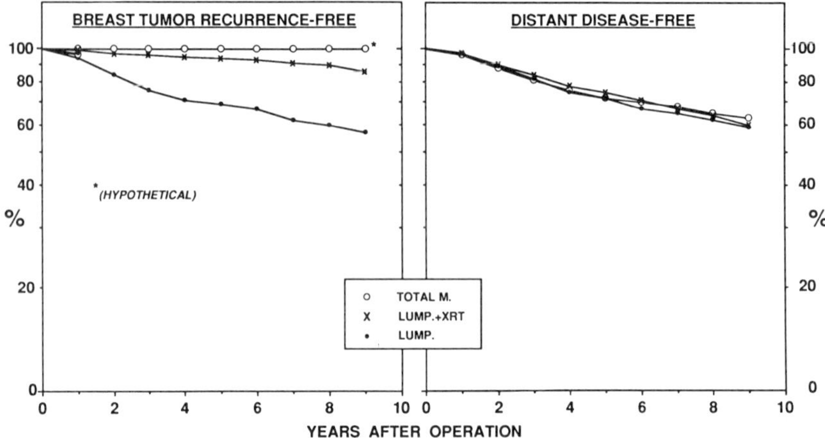

Fig 24–10.—Relation of IBTR to DDFS. (Courtesy of Fisher B, Anderson S, Fisher ER, et al: *Lancet* 338:327–331, 1991.)

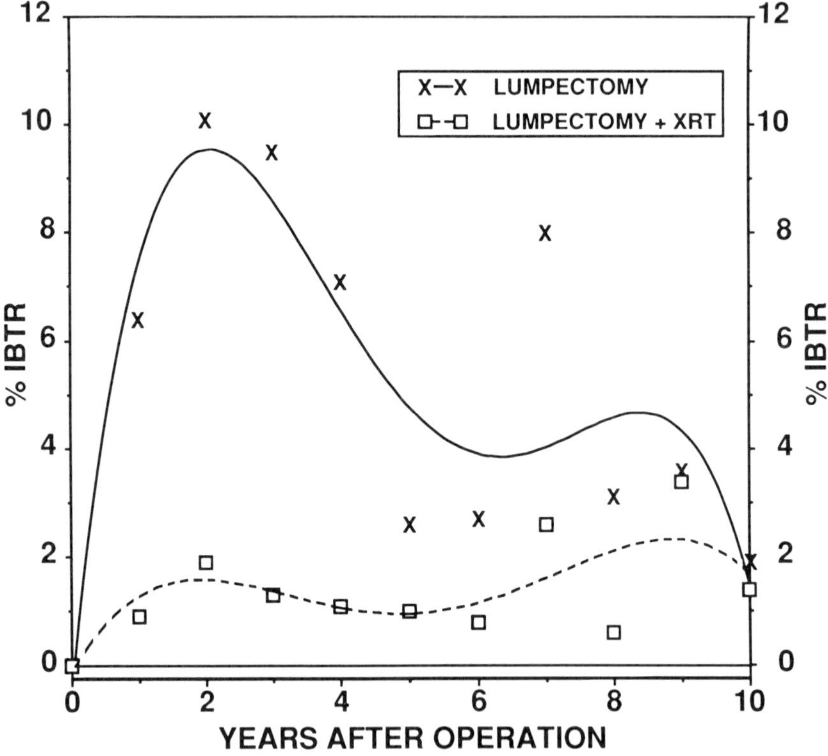

Fig 24–11.—Smoothed yearly hazard plots for IBTR. (Courtesy of Fisher B, Anderson S, Fisher ER, et al: *Lancet* 338:327–331, 1991.)

DFS, it was not considered an end-point because patients randomized to total mastectomy were not at risk for IBTR.

Results.—At 9 years, 88% of the lumpectomy-plus-irradiation patients and 57% of lumpectomy-alone patients were free of IBTR. Thus, post-operative breast irradiation significantly increased the probability of remaining IBTR-free after lumpectomy (Fig 24–10). Regression analysis of 8 fixed features present at surgery such as tumor size and tumor type revealed that only mode of treatment and tumor size were significant predictors of time to IBTR. At 9 years, DDFS was 63% for total mastectomy, 59% for lumpectomy, and 60% for lumpectomy plus irradiation. The differences were statistically not significant, and the probability of remaining free of distant disease was similar for the 3 treatments. However, the risk of distant disease was 3.41 times greater in patients with IBTR than in those without IBTR. Thus, IBTR is a highly significant predictor of distant disease. A comparison between women with early and late IBTR showed that earlier IBTR had less favorable DDFS. The average annual hazard rates for IBTR can be seen in Figure 24–11.

Discussion.—Although IBTR is a powerful independent predictor of distant disease, the occurrence of IBTR only shows that the patient was already at increased risk of distant disease when the primary tumor was removed. Although IBTR is a marker for risk of distant disease already present at operation, it is not a new risk factor for distant disease. Whereas mastectomy and irradiation after lumpectomy obscure this existing risk, lumpectomy alone enables this risk to manifest itself in an IBTR, thereby allowing timely additional systemic therapy at the time an IBTR is diagnosed and treated.

▶ This 9-year follow-up from the National Surgical Adjuvant Breast and Bowel Project B-06 confirms equal disease free survival for women treated by total mastectomy, lumpectomy, or lumpectomy plus radiation. Ipsilateral breast tumor recurrence (IBTR) was a significant predictor of distant disease. In women treated by lumpectomy alone, IBTR identified high-risk cancers and allowed timely adjuvant therapy.—W.H. Hindle, M.D.

Suggested Readings

Frierson HF Jr: Ploidy analysis and S-phase fraction determination by flow cytometry of invasive adenocarcinomas of the breast. *Am J Surg Pathol* 15:358–367, 1991.

▶ The clinical application of flow cytometry for the prognosis of breast cancer remains experimental, although some reports have been encouraging. This review of 56 publications covers 10,323 breast cancers. Ploidy usually correlates with histological type, S-phase fraction values, and tumor grade. The S-phase fraction values are associated with estrogen and progesterone receptor status, histological type, and tumor grade.—W.H. Hindle, M.D.

Gordon NH, Crowe JP, Brumberg DJ, et al: Socioeconomic factors and race in breast cancer recurrence and survival. *Am J Epidemiol* 135:609–618, 1992.

▶ In this study of 1,392 patients with breast cancer, multivariant analysis revealed that the number of involved lymph nodes, larger tumor diameter, lower socioeconomic status, and negative estrogen receptor status have an adverse correlation with disease-free survival. Age and obesity were not related.—W.H. Hindle, M.D.

Hillner BE, Smith TJ, Desch CE: Efficacy and cost-effectiveness of autologous bone marrow transplantation in metastatic breast cancer. *JAMA* 267:2055-2061, 1992.

▶ Decision analysis modeling revealed autologous bone marrow transplantation to give substantial survival benefit in patients with metastatic breast cancer; however, the cost may not be acceptable. Randomized clinical trials are urged.—W.H. Hindle, M.D.

Comparison of Breast Carcinomas Diagnosed in the 1980s With Those Diagnosed in the 1940s to 1960s

Joensuu H, Toikkanen S (Univ Central Hosp of Turku; Univ of Turku, Finland)
BMJ 303:155–158, 1991 24–45

Introduction.—According to available statistics, the incidence of breast cancer is increasing, whereas survival is improving. These trends may be the result of earlier detection, improved treatment, or less aggressive tumor behavior. To examine trends in these prognostic factors, a retrospective comparative cohort study was conducted of 439 patients with breast cancer diagnosed in 1945–1965 and 370 patients breast cancer diagnosed in 1980–1984 in Turku.

Results.—The age-adjusted incidence of breast cancer increased from about 31/100,000 person-years in 1953 to 62/100,000 in 1983 to 1987. Breast cancer mortality increased from 16.7 to 17.2/100,000 person-years during the same period. The survival of patients with stage II–IV disease improved, whereas the survival of those with stage I disease did not improve during this time period. The average age at diagnosis increased from approximately 56 years in 1945 to 63 years in 1980. The proportion of patients with TO-1 carcinomas increased from 13% to 41%, and the proportion with pNO carcinomas increased from 43% to 55%. In the 1980–1984 cohort, carcinomas were more likely to be well differentiated, have lower mitotic counts, have less nuclear polymorphism, have a more defined tumor margin, and have less tumor necrosis than in the earlier cohort. There was no difference in these variables between these 2 cohorts when tumors of the same size were compared.

Conclusion.—Improved breast cancer survival can be explained at least in part by early detection of increased numbers of small carcinomas with favorable histological characteristics.

▶ This comparison of 439 patients with breast cancer diagnosed between 1945 and 1965 and 370 patients with breast cancer diagnosed in 1980–1984 reveals an age-adjusted incidence increase from 31/100,000 (1953) to 62/100,000 (1983), slightly increased mortality, improved late stage survival, a 7-year increase in the average age at diagnosis

(1945–1980), 43% to 55% increased pNO cancers, and 13% to 41% increased TO-1 cancers. The authors ascribe the major improvements to early detection.—W.H. Hindle, M.D.

Breast Cancer Screening Among Relatives of Women With Breast Cancer

Kaplan KM, Weinberg GB, Small A, Herndon JL (Ctrs for Disease Control, Atlanta; Pennsylvania Dept of Health, Harrisburg, Pa)

Am J Public Health 81:1174–1179, 1991 24–46

Background.—Although breast cancer ranks second only to lung cancer as a cause of cancer mortality in women, national surveys show that screening measures are still underused. Screening behaviors were examined among women who have had at least 1 first-degree relative with diagnosed breast cancer and are considered to be at increased risk of breast cancer compared with women in the general population.

Methods.—Of 4,012 women with histologically confirmed breast cancer identified from hospital cancer registries, 1,862 were interviewed to identify their first-degree female relatives. A total of 3,860 eligible first-degree relatives were identified; of these, 2,539 were interviewed and asked to describe their breast cancer screening practices. Because 68 relatives had already had breast cancer, their data were excluded from this analysis.

Results.—Overall, 83% of the first-degree relatives reported having done breast self-examination (BSE), and 96% had had at least 1 breast examination done by a medical professional. Of 983 women 50 years of age or older, 49% had had at least 1 mammogram and 28% had had a mammogram within the previous 12 months. However, only 14% of these women reported having a mammogram annually. Of the women aged 50 years or older who reported that they had never had a mammogram, 92% said that a mammogram had never been recommended to them by a medical professional.

Conclusion.—The breast self-examination and mammography use of first-degree relatives of patients with breast cancer does not differ substantially from those of women in the general population. Although higher rates of professional breast examinations were reported among the high-risk women, enhanced efforts to educate medical professionals and encourage women to demand screening mammography are needed to reduce breast cancer mortality.

▶ In this interview survey of 2,471 first-degree relatives of patients with breast cancer, the use of BSE and mammography did not differ from the use by women in the general population. Seventy percent had annual clinical breast examinations. Only 14% of the women older than 50 years of age were having annual mammograms. We (physicians and patients) must do better.—W.H. Hindle, M.D.

Epidermal Growth Factor Receptor-Negative Tumors Are Predominantly Confined to the Subgroup of Estradiol Receptor-Positive Human Primary Breast Cancers

Koenders PG, Beex LVAM, Geurts-Moespot A, Heuvel JJTM, Kienhuis CBM, Benraad TJ (Univ Hosp of Nijmegen, The Netherlands)

Cancer Res 51:4544–4548, 1991 24–47

Background.—There have been various reports, using different preparation techniques and assays, on the prognostic significance of epidermal growth factor receptor (EGFR) content in human primary breast cancer. A ligand binding assay, standardized according to the recommendations of the European Organization for Research and Treatment of Cancer Receptor Study Group, was used to estimate the EGFR content in a series of tumors. The associations between EGFR and steroid hormone receptors also were reported.

Methods.—The multipoint assay was used in analysis of 725 stored human primary breast tumor biopsy samples. A lower cell membrane protein threshold of .2 mg of membrane protein per milliliter of assay buffer was established. This led to exclusion of 194 EGFR determinations because of insufficient assay membrane protein content and left 531 biopsy samples for analysis.

Results.—On Scatchard analysis, 57% of samples were EGFR positive; the median value was 40 fmol of membrane protein per mg. Seventy-two percent of samples were estrogen receptor (ER) positive, and 65% were progesterone receptor (PgR) positive. Forty-six percent of ER-positive and 85% of ER-negative specimens were EGFR positive. Forty-nine percent of PgR-positive and 72% of PgR-negative specimens were EGFR positive. The ER-positive samples had a mean EGFR level of 40 fmol/mg compared with 72 fmol/mg for ER-negative samples. The EGFR levels were also higher in PgR-positive samples than in PgR-negative samples: 41 vs. 70 fmol/mg. As steroid hormone receptor levels increased, EGFR positivity and levels decreased. Only ER was independently associated with EGFR.

Conclusion.—The EGFR assays should be standardized to ensure uniformity and comparability of data. This is vital in trying to assess the importance of EGFR in prognosis and tumor biology. Epidermal growth factor receptor appears to remain stable in stored cell membrane preparations. If the cell membrane protein level decreases below a certain point, measurement by ligand binding assay is likely to give a false negative outcome.

▶ The search continues for clinically useful prognostic indicators. This report shows a general inverse correlation between both EGFR positivity and EGFR levels and steroid hormone receptor levels.—W.H. Hindle, M.D.

Suggested Readings

Ma L, Fishell E, Wright B, et al: Case-control study of factors associated with failure to detect breast cancer by mammography. *J Natl Cancer Inst* 84:781–785, 1992.

▶ Extensive parenchymal density, lobular carcinoma, and small cancer size were found to be correlated significantly with false negative diagnostic mammograms.—W.H. Hindle, M.D.

McKinna JA, Davey JB, Walsh GA, et al: The early diagnosis of breast cancer: A twenty-year experience at the Royal Marsden Hospital. *Eur J Cancer* 28A: 911–916, 1992.

▶ More than 30,000 women with minimal breast symptoms were screened from 1968 to 1987. A total of 542 breast cancers were diagnosed. The breast cancer rates were 8.5:1000 for prevalence and 6.1:1000 for incidence. The stage was T_1 or less in 47% of the prevalence group and 70% of the interval screened group. The actuarial 10-year survivals after treatment are 73% for the prevalence group and 80% for the incident group.—W.H. Hindle, M.D.

Nattinger AB, Gottlieb MS, Veum J, et al: Geographic variation in the use of breast-conserving treatment for breast cancer. N *Engl J Med* 326:1102–1107, 1992.

▶ Medicare data (1986) on 36,982 women (aged 65–79 years) who were treated surgically for breast cancer revealed that only 12% had lumpectomies with a range of 3.5% to 21.2% in various states. Lumpectomies were performed most often in large urban teaching hospitals with on-site radiation therapy and geriatric services. When the data were adjusted for differences in hospital and patient characteristics, the geographic variations persisted.—W.H. Hindle, M.D.

Omne Pontén M, Holmberg L, Burns T, et al: Determinants of the psycho-social outcome after operation for breast cancer. Results of a prospective comparative interview study following mastectomy and breast conservation. *Eur J Cancer* 28A:1062–1067, 1992.

▶ This Swedish study of 99 women with stage I and II breast cancer shows that psychosocial adjustment remains a major clinical problem for women treated for breast cancer. In those treated by modified radical mastectomy, there were trends of increased depression, anxiety, sleep disturbance, and social adjustment compared with those treated by breast-conserving surgery. At 13 weeks after surgery, the differences were statistically significant for depression and social adjustment. Living with a spouse seemed to be psychologically protective. Employed women and those receiving radiation therapy showed poor adjustment after 4 months. However, the radiation therapy group showed a beneficial effect at 13 months. The breast conservation group showed a trend of sexual dysfunction at both 4 and 13 months.—W.H. Hindle, M.D.

Spontaneous and Induced Abortions and Risk of Breast Cancer

Parazzini F, La Vecchia C, Negri E (Istituto di Ricerche Farmacologiche "Mario Negri," Milan, Italy; Univ of Lausanne, Switzerland)

Int J Cancer 48:816–820, 1991 24–48

Introduction.—Whereas several epidemiological findings have suggested that a term pregnancy in early life is protective against breast cancer, the effect of an incomplete pregnancy is less clear. To further analyze the effect of an incomplete pregnancy on the risk of breast cancer, a case-control study of 2,394 patients with breast cancer and 2,218 controls was conducted in Milan.

Findings.—There was no consistent relationship between spontaneous or induced abortion and breast cancer. This lack of association was seen in all ages and states of parity. Those who had an abortion before their first full-term pregnancy had an increased risk of breast cancer that did not reach statistical significance.

Conclusion.—These results do not support the hypothesis that spontaneous or induced abortion significantly increases the risk of breast cancer.

▶ In this case-control study of 2,394 patients with breast cancer, no consistent relationship between spontaneous or induced abortion (either before or after full-term pregnancy) and subsequent breast cancer was identified.—W.H. Hindle, M.D.

Suggested Readings

Poen JC, Tran L, Juillard G, et al: Conservation therapy for invasive lobular carcinoma of the breast. *Cancer* 69:2789–2795, 1992.

▶ Sixty patients with stage I and II invasive lobular carcinoma treated by lumpectomy, axillary lumpectomy, axillary lymph node dissection, and radiation therapy (mean follow-up, 5.5 years) are reviewed. The 5-year actuarial disease-free survival was 84%, and the overall survival was 91%, which is comparable to results with ductal carcinoma in situ. There was a .6% per year rate of contralateral breast cancer. Long-term (10- to 15-year) results will be of interest.—W.H. Hindle, M.D.

Roisman I, Barak V, Robinson E, et al: Breast malignancies in adolescents in Israel (1967–1989). *Breast Dis* 5:149–168, 1992.

▶ This study of breast cancer in adolescents presents 7 cases in girls aged 14–17 years who were treated in hospitals in Israel during 1967–1989. There were 2 undifferentiated carcinomas, and 2 were malignant phyllodes tumors. Five patients died of their cancers. A review of 91 references and 33 clinical cases is presented.—W.H. Hindle, M.D.

Prognosis in $T_2N_0M_0$ Stage I Breast Carcinoma: A 20-Year Follow-Up Study

Rosen PP, Groshen S, Kinne DW (Mem Sloan-Kettering Cancer Ctr, New

York; Univ of Southern California, Los Angeles)
J Clin Oncol 9:1650–1661, 1991 24–49

Background.—Reports of long-term outcome in women with $T_1N_0M_0$ and $T_1N_1M_0$ breast cancer, including detailed analyses of pathologic prognostic factors, have been previously reported. Data on patients with $T_2N_0M_0$ breast carcinoma also were collected, and prognosis in 293 such patients who were treated during a 6-year period was determined.

Methods.—Data were drawn from review of pathology records for the years in question. The patients were treated by mastectomy and axillary dissection; the median follow-up was 19.8 years. Recurrence-free survival was estimated by the Kaplan-Meier method, and the estimated probability of cure was determined by the method of Brinkley and Haybittle.

Results.—The overall probability of surviving 20 years was 41.3%. Ten-year recurrence-free survival was 68.6%; this decreased to 63.2% at 20 years. The probability of cure estimate was 63%. Primary tumor size affected prognosis—those measuring 2.1-3cm carried a 33% chance of recurrence at 20 years compared with 44% for those measuring 3.1–5 cm. Recurrence at 20 years was 34% for women with invasive duct carcinoma and 42% for those with lobular carcinoma; however, those with medullary, mucinous, papillary, and other special types had a 25% chance of recurrence.

Twenty-nine patients had contralateral breast carcinoma, and 4 died of these tumors. Thus, they accounted for only 4.6% of breast carcinoma deaths. Nonmammary malignant neoplasm developed after the ipsilateral breast carcinoma in 32 patients; 69% of these lesions were fatal.

Conclusion.—Those patients with $T_2N_0M_0$ breast cancer may be stratified into recurrence risk groups depending on the size and histological type of their tumors. Investigators planning clinical trials of adjuvant therapy should bear these factors in mind. Part of the routine follow-up for patients with $T_2N_0M_0$ breast cancer should include measures for early detection of common nonmammary malignant neoplasms.

▶ This is the Memorial Sloan-Kettering Cancer Center experience with 293 patients and a median follow-up of 19.8 years. The overall 20-year survival was 41%, with a 63% rate of recurrence-free survival. Primary tumor size inversely affected prognosis. The recurrence rate at 20 years was 42% for invasive lobular carcinoma, 34% for invasive ductal carcinoma, and 25% for other types.—W.H. Hindle, M.D.

Contralateral Primary Tumors in Breast Cancer Patients in a Randomized Trial of Adjuvant Tamoxifen Therapy

Rutqvist LE, Cedermark B, Glas U, Mattsson A, Skoog L, Sommell A, Theve T, Wilking N, Askergren J, Hjalmar M-L, Rotstein S, Perbeck L, Ringborg U (Karolinska Hosp; Sodersjukhuset; Sabbatsberg Hosp; Danderyd Hosp; Huddinge Hosp, Stockholm)

J Natl Cancer Inst 83:1299–1306, 1991 24–50

Background.—Estrogens may promote the pathogenesis of breast cancer; therefore, prophylactic treatment with tamoxifen, an antiestrogen, may decrease breast cancer risk. A significant decrease in contralateral cancers in postmenopausal patients treated with adjuvant tamoxifen therapy was previously reported. These results were updated and included a group of patients randomized to 5 years of tamoxifen therapy.

Methods.—A total of 1,846 postmenopausal women with invasive breast cancer were randomized to receive tamoxifen, 40 mg/day, for 2 years postoperatively, or to receive no adjuvant endocrine therapy. After 2 years, disease-free patients in the tamoxifen group were randomized to either cease treatment or continue for an additional 3 years. The patients were followed for a median of 7 years.

Results.—There were 29 cases of contralateral breast cancer in the 931 patients who received tamoxifen compared with 47 cases in 915 control patients. The 10-year cumulative incidence was 5% in the tamoxifen group and 8% in the control group.

► This is the Swedish experience with 1,846 postmenopausal women in a randomized tamoxifen trial. The 10-year cumulative incidence of contralateral breast cancer was 5% in the tamoxifen group and 8% in the control group. Most of the benefit of tamoxifen therapy was seen in the first 2 years. However, risk reduction continued to 10 years after cessation of tamoxifen.—W.H. Hindle, M.D.

Obesity at Diagnosis of Breast Carcinoma Influences Duration of Disease-Free Survival

Senie RT, Rosen PP, Rhodes P, Lesser ML, Kinne DW (Ctr for Disease Control, Atlanta; Mem Sloan-Kettering Cancer Ctr, New York; North Shore Univ Hosp-Cornell Univ Med College, Manhasset, NY)

Ann Intern Med 116:26–32, 1992 24–51

Objective.—Prompted by previous reports of an association between excess body weight and breast cancer prognosis, disease-free survival was evaluated prospectively at 10 years in relation to obesity at the time of diagnosis among consecutively treated patients with primary breast cancer.

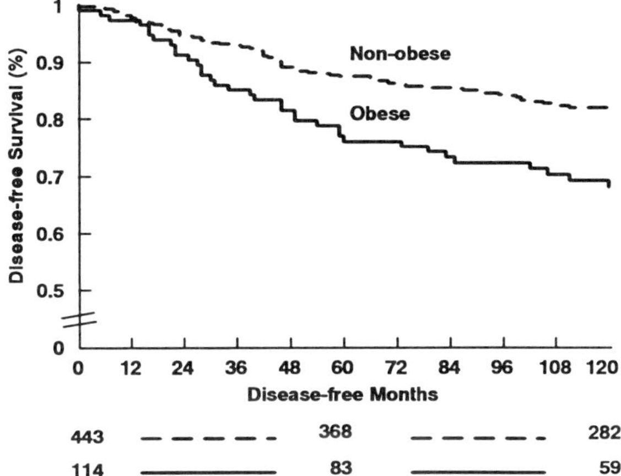

Fig 24–12.—Disease-free survival of 557 patients with breast cancer and negative nodes according to obesity at diagnosis. The number of patients at risk at time 0, at 5 years, and at 10 years is shown for each set of survival curves. Hazard ratio, 1.93 (95% confidence interval, 1.29-2.88; *P* = .001). (Courtesy of Senie RT, Rosen PP, Rhodes P, et al: *Ann Intern Med* 116:26–32, 1992.)

Patients.—A total of 923 women with primary breast cancer treated by mastectomy and axillary dissection were studied. The mean body weight was 143.5 pounds and, on average, the patients were 11.6% over optimal weight.

Findings.—The risk of recurrence was significantly greater among women who were obese with body weight 25% or more over the optimal weight for height at the time of primary breast cancer compared with nonobese patients (42% vs. 32%; hazard ratio, 1.45). Multivariate analyses showed that obesity remained a significant prognostic factor, even after controlling for measured tumor size, number of positive axillary lymph nodes, age at diagnosis, and adjuvant chemotherapy. Among the 557 patients free of lymph node metastases, 32% of obese patients had recurrent disease compared with 19% of nonobese women. The risk of recurrence was significantly increased in these patients with negative nodes (hazard ratio, 1.59) (Fig 24–12).

Conclusion.—Obesity at the time of diagnosis of primary breast cancer is a significant independent factor that effects prognosis, expecially among patients with negative lymph node metastases. These findings suggest that obesity may limit the reduction in breast cancer mortality attainable through detection at an early stage of disease. Because the prevalence of obesity increases with age, as it does for breast cancer, weight control may have a substantial effect on breast cancer survival.

▶ This report from the Centers for Disease Control and Memorial Sloan-Kettering Cancer Center demonstrated a risk of recurrence of 42% for obese women and 32% for nonobese women (hazard ratio, 1.45; CI, 1.13–1.86) in a group of 923 women treated by modified radical mastectomy for primary breast cancer and analyzed for 10-year disease-free survival. Among the 557 women without lymph node involvement, recurrent disease occurred in 32% of the obese women and 19% of the nonobese women (hazard ratio, 1.59; CI, 1.06–2.39) (Fig 24–12).—W.H. Hindle, M.D.

Suggested Readings

Singletary SE, McNeese MD, Hortobagyi; GN: Feasibility of breast-conservation surgery after induction chemotherapy for locally advanced breast carcinoma. *Cancer* 69:2849–2852, 1992.

▶ One hundred forty-three patients with stage IIB, IIIA, and IIIB breast cancer were treated with 3 cycles of multidrug chemotherapy before mastectomy. The diagnosis had been established by fine-needle aspiration or tissue core-needle biopsy. Twenty-three percent became eligible by criteria for lumpectomy, with mean decrease in tumor size from 5 cm to less than 1 cm. Of these, no residual cancer was found in 42%, and 45% had negative nodes. The overall survival and disease-free survival compared with traditional postoperative chemotherapy will be of keen clinical interest.—W.H. Hindle, M.D.

Tsangaris TN, Knox SM, Cheek JH: Tumor hormone receptor status and recurrences in premenopausal patients with node-negative breast carcinomas. *Cancer* 69:984–987, 1992.

▶ In this retrospective review of 147 premenopausal patients (mean follow-up, 85.4 months), estrogen/progesterone receptor status did not predict the disease-free survival or overall survival. Tumor size of less than 2 cm correlated with favorable prognosis in all groups. Furthermore, there were no recurrences of any cancers less than 1 cm.—W.H. Hindle, M.D.

Nonpalpable Invasive Breast Cancer

Wilhelm MC, Edge SB, Cole DD, deParedes E, Frierson HF Jr (Univ of Virginia Health Sciences Ctr, Charlottesville)

Ann Surg 213:600–605, 1991 24–52

Introduction.—Mammographic screening has yielded an increasing number of noninvasive and small invasive breast cancers that are not palpable. An 1980-1989 experience with impalpable lesions, in which a total of 1,464 women underwent biopsy of clinically occult, impalpable breast lesions, was reviewed. All lesions were excised using mammography-directed needle localization.

Findings.—Carcinoma was present in 18% of these women. Two thirds of the cancers were in situ lesions. Mammography demonstrated a mass in 63 of the 86 women with invasive cancer. Microcalcifications were present in 25 cases.

Treatment and Follow-Up.—Mastectomy was carried out in 71 patients with invasive breast cancer. Fourteen others had lumpectomy alone. The frequency of positive nodes increased with the size of the primary lesion, increasing to 32% in patients whose lesions were greater than 1 cm in diameter. In all, 23% of patients had positive nodes. Seven women had recurrences during a median follow-up of 44 months. Most patients with negative nodes did not receive adjuvant treatment.

Discussion.—Other studies also suggest a significant incidence of nodal metastases in patients with imalpable invasive breast cancers. Axillary dissection is appropriate in these cases; this is not minimal breast cancer.

▶ During a period of 10 years, 1,464 nonpalpable mammographic abnormalities were biopsied at the University of Virginia. Eighteen percent proved to be cancer; of these cancers, 67% were in situ. Of the invasive cancers, a mass was mammographically present in 73%; microcalcifications in 29%; and involved axillary lymph nodes in 23%. With a median follow-up of 44 months, the disease-free survival was 92% and the overall survival was 94%.—W.H. Hindle, M.D.

Suggested Reading

Uzan S, Denis C, Pomi V, et al: Double-blind trial of promegestone (R 5020) and lynestrenol in the treatment of benign breast disease. *Eur J Obstet Gynecol Reprod Biol* 43:219–227, 1991.

▶ This short-term study revealed an equivalent response to promegestone at .5 mg or 1 mg daily, and to lynestrenol at 10 mg daily, in 132 women (age, 19–50 years) with pronounced mastalgia and breast nodularity/tenderness. The improvement in symptoms was excellent/good in about 66%, and there was similar improvement by examination in about 51% to 59% with a clinical tolerance of therapy in 60% to 78%. Although this use of synthetic progestin is encouraging for the treatment of mastalgia, long-term prospective randomized studies with placebo control and crossover will be necessary.—W.H. Hindle, M.D.

Surgical Options in 424 Patients With Primary Breast Cancer Without Systemic Metastases

Wolberg WH (Univ of Wisconsin, Madison)

Arch Surg 126:817–820, 1991 24–53

Background.—Despite the appeal of conservation therapy of breast cancer, physicians who have offered it find that only 5% to 15% of their patients with primary breast cancer actually are managed in this way. Comprehensive management protocols for T1 and small T2 primary invasive breast cancers were developed at the University of Wisconsin in 1981.

Treatment Plan.—Conservation is considered for tumors less than 4 cm in size, although women with small breasts who have smaller tumors often require mastectomy. Node-positive patients and premenopausal node-negative women who are estrogen receptor-negative receive 4 cycles of doxorubicin-containing combination chemotherapy. Radiotherapy follows in patients having breast conservation and also in those with tumors of 5 cm or larger who have mastectomy.

Outcome.—Fifty-nine percent of 424 consecutive patients seen with invasive cancer but no systemic metastasis were considered suitable for conservation surgery. Most of the others had tumors that were too large. Of the 122 patients who elected conservation, 100 achieved it, representing about one fourth of all patients considered. Women aged 35-54 years elected conservation most frequently.

Discussion.—Nearly one fourth of women in this series with invasive, nonmetastatic breast cancer were managed by conservation. Women who elect conservation value their breasts more highly than those who choose mastectomy. The latter patients are concerned about the possible ineffectiveness of radiotherapy and about its side effects.

▶ Only about 25% of 424 consecutive patients with invasive, nonmetastatic breast cancer achieved breast conserving surgery in this University of Wisconsin experience. Approximately half of those considered suitable for local excision elected mastectomy, and intraoperative findings led to mastectomy in 20% of the women desiring breast conservation. Tumor size was the major indication for mastectomy in 41% of the cases.—W.H. Hindle, M.D.

Suggested Reading

Yoo, KY, Tajima K, Kuroishi T, et al: Independent protective effect of lactation against breast cancer: A case-control study in Japan. *Am J Epidemiol* 135:726-733, 1992.

▶ This hospital-based study comparing 521 women with breast cancer with controls, revealed a decreased odds ratio of .62 for breast cancer among parous women (CI, .37-1.04), suggesting a trend. This trend correlated with increasing the average months of lactation. With premenopausal women who had lactated for 7-9 months, the adjusted odds ratio was .39 (CI, .15-.97), epidemiologically suggesting lactation as an independent protective factor for Japanese women.—W.H. Hindle, M.D.

Subject Index

A

Abdomen
as hysterectomy route (*see* Hysterectomy, abdominal)
Abortion
habitual
antiphospholipid antibody-associated, prednisolone/aspirin therapy for, 511
antiphospholipid antibody prevalence and, 514
luteal phase defect in, 505
induced
breast cancer and, 596
ectopic pregnancy and, 517
recurrent (*see* habitual *above*)
spontaneous
(*See also* Miscarriage)
breast cancer and, 596
ectopic pregnancy and, 517
habitual (*see* Abortion, habitual *above*)
risk factors for, 506
Abscess
pelvic, ultrasound-guided transvaginal drainage of, 367
tubo-ovarian, percutaneous drainage of, 368
Acquired immunodeficiency syndrome (*see* AIDS)
ACTH (*see* Corticotropin)
Actinomycin D
in gestational trophoblastic tumors, 347
Acyclovir
for varicella pneumonia in pregnancy, 113
Adenocarcinoma
vagina, diethylstilbestrol-associated clear cell, risk factors for, 350
Adenomas
hepatocellular
danazol-induced, 407
oral contraceptives and, 493
Adenosarcoma
uterus, study of, 321
Adenosine
triphosphate in semen and fertility prediction, 440
Adhesions
laparoscopic lysis of, after laser photocoagulation of polycystic ovaries, pregnancy rates after, 453
Adnexal
cysts, simple, in postmenopausal women, 245
Adolescence
cancer during, early menopause in long-term survivors of, 410
height and weight in, and diethylstilbestrol-associated clear cell vaginal adenocarcinoma, 351
Adrenal
cells, fetal, regulation of corticotropin responsiveness in, 7
hyperplasia, late-onset, due to 21-hydroxylase deficiency, fertility after, 455
Adrenocorticotropin (*see* Corticotropin)
Age
abortion and, spontaneous, 506
body mass and endometrial cancer, 309
effect on follow-up after borderline Pap smear, 294
at first birth and borderline ovarian tumors, 346
gestational
amniotic fluid infection and preterm labor, 66
fetus large for, at term, sonographic diagnosis of, 173
obstetric performance and, 61
placental blood flow and combined ventricular output and, 25
oral contraceptives and breast cancer, 481
outcome of multiple follicular recruitment and intrauterine insemination and, 463
AIDS
(*See also* HIV)
threat, response of American women to, 533
Airway
epithelium, in vivo transfer of cystic fibrosis gene to, 240
Albumin
infusions in preeclampsia, 64
levels, effects of Norplant implants on, 500
Alcohol
use in pregnancy, two-year follow-up, 227
Alkaline
phosphatase levels, effects of Norplant implants on, 500
Allograft
renal, perinatal outcome in recipients of, 114
Alpha-fetoprotein (*see* α-Fetoprotein)
Alphaprodine
effect of sinusoidal fetal heart rate pattern in early labor, 146
Amenorrhea

method, lactational, for family planning, 479
in runners, and total body bone density, 387
Amniocentesis
/fetal blood sampling in prenatal diagnosis of cytomegalovirus infection, 125
in multiple gestation, 132
Amnioinfusion
prophylactic, for oligohydramnios in labor, 126
Amnionitis
after fetal intravascular transfusion for hemolytic disease, 121
Amniotic
cavity, microbial invasion of
amniotic fluid white cell count in diagnosis of, 109
in spontaneous rupture of membranes at term, 60
fluid
estriol, dehydroepiandrosterone sulphate and hCG levels in Down's syndrome, 138
infection, anaerobic coverage for, 57
infection and preterm labor, 66
white blood cell count, 109
Ampicillin
in intra-amniotic infection, 57
Anaerobic
coverage for intra-amniotic infection, 57
Analgesia
epidural
cesarean section for dystocia and, 182
in labor, computerized analysis of fetal heart rate after, 149
in labor, sufentanil addition to, and instrumental deliveries, 183
patient-controlled, demand-dose, 167
Androgen(s)
added to postmenopausal hormone replacement therapy, xxvii-xxviii
blockade vs. suppression in hirsutism, 396
Anemia
fetal, cordocentesis in prediction of, 131
Anesthesia
for cesarean section
in preeclampsia, 180
regional, ECG changes during, 169
Angioplasty
transluminal, in renovascular hypertension during pregnancy, 41
Angiotensin
converting enzyme inhibitors in pregnancy, fetal and neonatal effects of, 198
sensitivity, maternal, and fetal Doppler umbilical artery flow waveforms, 160
Anomalies
Ebstein's, and pregnancy outcome, 97
Anorectal
physiology, effect of hysterectomy on, 252
Anovulation
spontaneous, causing disappearance of cyclical symptoms in premenstrual syndrome, 529
Antenatal (*see* Prenatal)
Antibody
absorption test, fluorescent treponemal, for syphilis, 231
anticardiolipin (*see* Anticardiolipin, antibodies)
antiphospholipid (*see* Antiphospholipid, antibodies)
IgA, viral-specific, in early diagnosis of perinatal HIV infection, 229
mononclonal, FDC-6 measurement of fetal fibronectin in cervical and vaginal secretions, 38
status, maternal, and outcome of congenital cytomegalovirus infection, 119
Anticardiolipin
antibodies
fetal loss and, 53
during third trimester, 94
Anticoagulant
lupus (*see* Lupus, anticoagulant)
Anti-DNA
antibodies during third trimester pregnancy, 94
Antiepileptic drug
concentrations, plasma, during pregnancy, 55
Antigen
p24, for HIV replication during first weeks of life, 214
Antihepatitis
Be positive maternal mononuclear cells causing perinatal hepatitis B infection, 211
Antinuclear
antibodies during third trimester pregnancy, 94
Antiphospholipid
antibodies
in aborters, recurrent, prednisolone/aspirin therapy for, 511
prevalence of, 514
Antithyroglobulin

antibodies during third trimester pregnancy, 94
Antithyroid
microsomal antibodies during third trimester pregnancy, 94
Anuria
neonatal, after angiotensin converting enzyme inhibitors in pregnancy, 198
Apheresis
lipoprotein, for hypertrigylceridemia-induced pancreatitis during pregnancy, 79
Apolipoproteins
during endometriosis treatment with goserelin implant or danazol, 406
in postmenopausal women, tamoxifen effects on, 585
Appendectomy
ectopic pregnancy and, 517
Arrhythmia
in Ebstein's anomaly, and pregnancy outcome, 98
Artery(ies)
coronary, disease, and postmenopausal estrogen therapy, 423, 425
placental bed spiral, in hypertensive disorders of pregnancy, 104
umbilical (*see* Umbilical, artery)
Arthritis
rheumatoid, juvenile, and pregnancy, 95
Asphyxia
birth
endothelin-1 in fetal blood and, 6
outcome, phosphorus magnetic resonance spectroscopy in prediction of, 123
Aspiration
biopsy (*see* Biopsy, aspiration)
follicular, ultrasound-guided, for ovulation induction in polycystic ovary syndrome, 451
vacuum, in termination of early pregnancy, 512
Aspirin
controlled-release, effect on thromboxane A_2 and prostacyclin, 17
low-dose
in prevention of fetal growth retardation, 40
in prevention of pregnancy-induced hypertensive disease, 47
/prednisolone for recurrent aborters with antiphospholipid antibody, 511
Autoantibodies
during third trimester pregnancy complicated by hypertension or fetal growth retardation, 94
AZT
in HIV infection in pregnancy, 75

B

Bacterial
vaginosis (*see* Vaginosis, bacterial)
Bacteroides ureolyticus
infection, amniotic fluid, and preterm labor, 66
Balloon
mitral valvotomy, percutaneous, during pregnancy, 100
Barrier contraception (*see* Contraception, barrier)
Beta-blockade
in fetus, after labetalol in maternal hypertension, 17
Betamethasone
prenatal, respiratory disease in very low birth weight infant after, 219
Biology
of breast cancer, 539
Biopsy
aspiration, fine-needle
of breast cysts, palpable, 543
of breast lesions in women aged 30 and under, 550
of breast masses associated with pregnancy, 552
of breast, pneumothorax after, 553
in cystosarcoma phyllodes of breast, 549
mammographically guided, of nonpalpable breast lesions, 554
stereotactic, of nonpalpable breast lesions, 555
breast, techniques and adequacy of margins, 570
colposcopic-directed, of transformational zone, histologic differences between loop excision and, 303
endometrium, prevalence of out-of-phase specimens, 433
endomyocardial, in preeclampsia, 39
needle-core, stereotactic, of nonpalpable breast lesions, 555, 556
in Paget's disease of nipple, 578
Birth
asphyxia (*see* Asphyxia, birth)
first, age at, and borderline ovarian tumors, 346

preterm (*see* Delivery, preterm)
rate, cesarean, influence of hospital teaching status on, 175
-related events, effect on fetal metabolism (in sheep), 29
weight (*see* Weight, birth)
Blacks
breast cancer screening behaviors and attitudes of, 566
gonorrhea and syphilis trends in 1980s in, 358
infant mortality in, and college-educated parents, 33
pelvic inflammatory disease in, self-reported, 364
preterm delivery in, 65
Bladder
injury, iatrogenic, during gynecological surgery, early repair of, 255
neck suspension for stress incontinence
colpo-needle, 288
Pereyra, modified, outcome, 273
urethrovesical junction position and mobility after, 278
urodynamic evaluation and transvaginal ultrasound after, 276
Bleeding
(*See also* Hemorrhage)
breakthrough, with continuous therapy, treatment of, xxi-xxii
endometrial, after 8 years of continuous estrogen/progestogen therapy, 428
postmenopausal, from endometrial polyps due to tamoxifen, 314
uterine, dysfunctional
depot gonadotropin-releasing hormone agonist and cyclical hormone replacement therapy for, 402
presenting as menorrhagia, danazol and norethisterone in, 400
Blood
cell count, white, amniotic fluid, 109
cultures in fever evaluation in perioperative patients, 261
donations screened for HIV-1, evaluation by culture and DNA amplification of pooled cells, 77
fetal, endothelin-1 in, relation to asphyxia, 6
flow
placental, and combined ventricular output in fetus, 25
resistance, uteroplacental, in second trimester, Doppler studies of, 155
gases, fetal, related to computer analysis data of fetal heart rate patterns in small for gestation fetuses, 146
loss after ovarian cancer operations, 342
maternal
lipid peroxide/vitamin E imbalance in preeclampsia in, 48
prenatal diagnosis with fetal cells isolated by flow cytometry from, 199
pressure
in hyperthyroid pregnancy, 102
in preeclampsia, effect of albumin infusions on, 64
sampling, fetal, in prenatal diagnosis of cytomegalovirus infection, 125
transfusion (*see* Transfusion)
volume changes, fetal, acute response of umbilical artery pulsatility index to (in sheep), 141
Boari flap
in iatrogenic ureteral injury after gynecological surgery, 256
Body
fat distribution, central, and hormone replacement therapy, 414
mass, age, and endometrial cancer, 309
Bone
density, total body, in amenorrheic runners, 387
loss, postmenopausal, prevention of
estradiol and estradiol/testosterone implants in, 422
estradiol in, micronized 17β-, 420
mass and oral contraceptives, 487
mineral content in Turner syndrome, effect of estrogen replacement therapy on, 389
Bowel
complications after ovarian cancer operations, 342
Bradycardia
fetal, after intrauterine transfusion for fetal hemolytic disease, 121
paradoxical, after nitroprusside in preeclampsia, 90
Breakthrough bleeding
with continuous therapy, treatment of, xxi-xxii
Breast
biopsy
aspiration, fine-needle, pneumothorax after, 553
techniques and adequacy of margins, 570
cancer (*see* Cancer, breast)
carcinoma (*see* Carcinoma, breast)
-conserving surgery
for cancer, early-stage, node-positive, 575

for cancer, primary nonmetastatic, 601
for cancer, stage I or II, underutilization of, 573
for carcinoma, intraductal, 571
fear of recurrence and trade-off hypothesis, 579
vs. mastectomy, 574
cyst (*see* Cyst, breast)
cystosarcoma phyllodes of (*see* Cystosarcoma, phyllodes of breast)
disease
benign, and risk of breast cancer, 544
diagnosis and management, role of gynecologist in, 537
examination
clinical, physicians' and nurses', 587
self-, in relatives of breast cancer patients, 593
-feeding and HIV transmission, 218, 221
lesions
nonpalpable, biopsy of, fine-needle aspiration, 555
nonpalpable, biopsy of, fine-needle aspiration, mamographically guided, 554
nonpalpable, biopsy of, stereotactic needle-core, 555, 556
palpable and impalpable, mammographically detected, prevalence of carcinoma in, 563
in women aged 30 and under, fine-needle aspiration of, 550
masses
pregnancy associated, fine-needle aspiration of, 552
ultrasound of, mammographic grid-directed, 588
reconstruction, immediate, selection criteria for, 570
screening, prognostic factors, and survival, 560
tumor
benign papillary, mammography of, 543
ipsilateral, recurrence after lumpectomy, 589
ultrasound in women less than 35 years of age, 562
Breathing
movements, fetal, effect of glycemia on (in sheep), 12
Breathlessness
in pregnancy, and inspiratory effort, 13
Bromocriptine
in mastalgia, 540
Bupivacaine
/sufentanil epidural analgesia during labor, and instrumental deliveries, 183
Burch suspension
ultrasound and urodynamic evaluation after, 276
urethrovesical position and mobility after, 278
Buserelin
in infertility with endometriosis, 459
for ovulation induction in polycystic ovary syndrome, 452

C

CA-125
in postmenopausal palpable ovary syndrome, 330
Cachectin
decidua as source of, 26
Calcitonin
in prevention of postmenopausal bone loss, xxix
Calcitriol
in osteoporosis, postmenopausal, 418
Calcium
supplementation
in hormone replacement therapy, postmenopausal, xxviii-xxix
in hypertensive pregnancy, 35, 42
in osteoporosis prevention, postmenopausal, 416
in osteoporosis treatment, postmenopausal, 418
Cancer
(*See also* Carcinoma)
adolescent, early menopause in long-term survivors of, 410
breast
abortion and, 596
biology and malpractice, 539
contralateral, primary, after tamoxifen therapy, 598
early, hormonal, cytotoxic, or immune therapy in, 582
epidermal growth factor receptor content in, 594
estrogen-progesterone therapy and, xxxiii-xxxiv
fear of recurrence, breast-conserving surgery, and trade-off hypothesis, 579
hormone replacement therapy and, postmenopausal, xxx-xxxiv
invasive, nonpalpable, 600
medroxyprogesterone acetate and, depot-, 567

node-positive, early-stage, conservative surgery, radiotherapy, and chemotherapy for, 575
operable, effect of steroid hormone receptors on prognosis, 580
oral contraceptives and age, 481
polycystic ovarian syndrome and, 569
primary, nonmetastatic, surgical options in, 601
relationship among outcome, stage of disease, and histologic grade, 576
risk, and benign breast disease, 544
screening among relatives of women with breast cancer, 593
screening behaviors and attitudes, effect of race and ethnicity on, 566
stage I or II, underutilization of breast conservation and radiotherapy for, 573
tamoxifen in (*see* Tamoxifen, in breast cancer)
cervix
invasive, in pregnancy, maternal and fetal outcome after, 306
natural history, and dysplasia, 298
papillomavirus infection and, 296
smoking and, 305
squamous cell, invasive, and depot-medroxyprogesterone acetate, 502
endometrium
gonadotropin releasing-hormone analogue in, 320
in postmenopausal women, increased steroid production by ovarian stromal tissue in, 311
progestogen/estrogen replacement therapy and, 427
risk, and body mass at different ages, 309
risk, and depot-medroxyprogesterone acetate, 310
family syndrome, endometrial carcinoma in, 312
ovaries
familial, ultrasound screening for, 327
after hysterectomy, 324, 325
operations for, mortality and morbidity of, 341
oral contraceptives for protection against, 323
in postmenopausal women, asymptomatic, screening by transvaginal ultrasound, 326
survival in, long-term, 342
syndrome, correct, diagnosing, 328
taxol in, 344
after tubal sterilization, 324
Candidal
vaginitis (*see* Vaginitis, candidal)
Cannabinoid
metabolites in newborn, meconium analysis for, 203
Captopril
in pregnancy, fetal and neonatal effects of, 198
Carbohydrate
metabolism
desogestrel and gestodene in oral contraceptives and, 491
Norplant implants and, 500
Carbon
dioxide laser cervical excisional conization, thermal injury zones in, 302
monoxide intoxication in pregnancy, hyperbaric oxygen in, 27
Carcinoma
(*See also* Cancer)
adenocarcinoma, diethylstilbestrol-associated clear cell vaginal, risk factors for, 350
breast
diagnosed in 1980s compared with those diagnosed in 1940s to 1960s, 592
intraductal, breast-conserving surgery and irradiation for, 571
lobular in situ, features of, 585
macroscopic cysts and, 541
prevalence in palpable vs. impalpable mammographically detected lesions, 563
prognosis, and obesity, 598
stage I, $T_2N_0M_0$, prognosis in, 596
cervix
recurrence after radiotherapy, cervicovaginal cytology in detection of, 308
stage IB, ovarian metastases in, 332
endometrium
in cancer family syndrome, 312
early, surgical staging and survival rates in, 315
irradiation in, adjuvant, complications after, 318
noninvasive, recurrence in, 319
simultaneous ovarian carcinoma and, 344
squamous differentiation in, 317
ovaries
early, intraperitoneal chromic phosphate in, 340
early, surgery without adjuvant chemotherapy in, 338

simultaneous endometrial carcinoma and, 344
stage I, survival after definitive treatment, 339
uterus, papillary serous, 319
vagina, invasive, upper vaginectomy in, 349
vulva
epidemiology and pathogenesis of, 352
minimally invasive, surgical management, 353
Cardiac
(*See also* Heart)
hemodynamics, fetal, reproducibility of ultrasonic measurement of, 158
index in untreated preeclampsia, 89
output in hyperthyroid pregnancy, 102
Cardiovascular
benefit of estrogen, does progesterone subtract from? xxii-xxvii
disease and postmenopausal estrogen therapy, 423
risk factors in postmenopausal women, effects of tamoxifen on, 583
Catheter
-assisted endoluminal transcervical ultrasound of embryo, 201
Cefamandole
in pelvic inflammatory disease, 365
Cefixime
in gonorrhea, 369
Cefoxitin
in pelvic inflammatory disease, 370
Ceftriaxone
in gonorrhea, 369
Cell(s)
adrenal, fetal, regulation of corticotropin responsiveness in, 7
blood, white, amniotic fluid count, 109
fetal, isolated from maternal blood by flow cytometry, prenatal diagnosis with, 199
granulosa, ovarian, effect of immunoglobulins on in vitro growth of, 388
killer, natural, activity in pregnancy, effect on RU 486 on, 14
mononuclear, maternal antihepatitis Be positive, causing perinatal hepatitis B infection, 211
stem, fetal liver, in-utero transplantation into fetuses, 235
T cell etiology for postpartum thyroid dysfunction, 73
Cerebral palsy
in low birth weight infants, 214
MRI in, 212
Cerebrospinal
fluid shunts and pregnancy, 68
Cervix
cancer (*see* Cancer, cervix)
carcinoma (*see* Carcinoma, cervix)
cytology in detection of recurrent cervical carcinoma after radiotherapy, 308
dysplasia
minor, papillomavirus-associated, management of, 300
natural history of cervical cancer and, 298
in transformation zone, histological differences between colposcopic-directed biopsy and loop excision of, 303
excision
conization, thermal injury zones in, 302
loop electrosurgical (*see* Electrosurgical, loop excision)
infections, gonococcal and chlamydial, nonoxynol-9 in prevention of, 358
mucus
hostility, and slow release vs. bolus intrauterine insemination, 444
score in clomiphene cycles, 443
neoplasia, intraepithelial
barrier contraception and, 480
excision in, loop electrosurgical, 304
grade III, endocervical gland involvement by, 301
secretions, fetal fibronectin in, as predictor of preterm delivery, 36
smear test results, borderline, long-term follow-up, 294
transcervical ultrasound of embryo, endoluminal catheter-assisted, 201
Cesarean section
anesthesia in, regional, ECG changes during, 169
aspirin prevention in pregnancy-induced hypertension and, 47
birth rate, influence of hospital teaching status on, 175
dystocia and (*see* Dystocia)
hemorrhage in preterm infant and, intraventricular, 168
HIV transmission and, mother-to-child, 218
infant mortality risk in, 164
in preeclampsia, anesthesia in, 180
rate in post-term pregnancy with labor induction vs. serial antenatal monitoring, 34
Chemoprophylaxis

intrapartum, for group B streptococcus, 82
Chemotherapy
of breast cancer
early node-positive, 575
primary, nonmetastatic, 601
cisplatin in (*see* Cisplatin)
EMA/CO, in high-risk gestational trophoblastic tumors, 347
in ovarian tumors, borderline, 334
platinum-based, in stage I ovarian epithelial carcinoma, 339
polychemotherapy in early breast cancer, 582
Chlamydial
cervical infections, nonoxynol-9 in prevention of, 358
tests, rapid, comparison of three, 372
Cholesterol
fractions during endometriosis treatment with goserelin implant or danazol, 406
levels
after estrogen therapy, postmenopausal, 426
after Norplant implants, 500
after oral contraceptives, long-term, 483
after tamoxifen in postmenopausal women, 584
Chorionic
gonadotropin (*see* Gonadotropin, chorionic)
villus sampling
limb abnormalities and, 186
Medical Research Council European Trial of, 117
mosaicism diagnosis in, follow-up and pregnancy outcome after, 137
Christmas disease
obstetric and gynecological problems in, 84
Chromic phosphate
intraperitoneal, in early ovarian carcinoma, 340
Cigarette smoking (*see* Smoking)
Circulation
fetal-placental
thromboxane release and action in, effect on endothelin-1-induced vasoconstriction, 59
vasoconstrictor effects of thromboxane and endothelin in, attentuation by nitric oxide, 18
Circulatory
distress after nitroprusside in preeclampsia, 90
Cisplatin
addition to EMA/CO for gestational trophoblastic tumors, 348
in ovarian cancer, long-term survival after, 342
in ovarian tumors of low malignant potential, stage III, 307
in uterine sarcoma, 322
Citrovorum
/methotrexate for persistent trophoblast after surgery for ectopic pregnancy, 525
Clearview chlamydial EIA
vs. Surecell, 372
Cleft
lip, fetal surgery for, 236
Clindamycin
cream in bacterial vaginosis, 377
in intra-amniotic infection, 57
in labor, preterm, 45
in pelvic inflammatory disease, 365
gentamicin combined with, 370
Clomiphene
cycle, cervical mucus score and in vitro sperm interaction in, 443
-resistant women, clomiphene/dexamethasone in, 448
Clotting
time, kaolin, in detection of lupus anticoagulants, 507
Coagulopathies
congenital, and obstetric and gynecologic problems, 84
Cocaine
metabolites in newborn, meconium analysis for, 203
use during pregnancy
incidence in surburban setting, 223
limb deficiencies related to, physiatric management of, 185
two-year follow-up, 226
Colcher-Sussman x-ray pelvic measurement, 175
Collagen
implantation, para-urethral, for stress incontinence, 283
College
-educated parents, and infant mortality, 33
Colostrum
as route of HIV transmission from mother to child, 223
Colpo-needle suspension
for stress incontinence, 288
Colporrhaphy
anterior, 25-year experience, 284
Colposacropexy
for vaginal vault prolapse, 254
Colposcopy

-directed biopsy of transformational zone, histologic differences between loop excision and, 303
after hyperkeratosis on Pap smear, 294
Computed tomography
-guided drainage of tubo-ovarian abscesses, 368
pelvimetry vs. x-ray pelvimetry, 178
in puerperal febrile morbidity, 207
in tentorial subdural hemorrhage diagnosis, in newborn, 225
Computer
analysis of fetal heart rate
in labor, 144, 149
in small for gestation fetuses, related to fetal blood gases, 146
Conception
assisted, for infertility, expectations of, 472
Condoms
sexually transmitted diseases and, 360
use by American women, 534
Conization
cervical excisional, thermal injury zones in loop electrical vs. laser, 302
Contraception
barrier
cervical intraepithelial neoplasia and, 480
sexually transmitted diseases and, 360
intrauterine (*see* IUD)
Norplant system (*see* Norplant)
oral
bone mass and, 487
breast cancer and age, 481
desogestrel for, 491
gallstones and, 484
gestodene for, 491
liver cell adenomas and, 493
long-term, clinical and metabolic considerations of, 483
myocardial infarction and, 489
ovarian cancer and, 323
ovarian cysts and, functional, 485, 486
ovarian tumors and, borderline, 346
in perimenopausal women, xxxv
venous thromboembolism and, 490
sponge for, and sexually transmitted diseases, 361
vaginal ring for, estrogen/progestogen, 503
Contraction
uterine, role of platelet-activating factor binding sites in myometrium in, 9
Copper
IUD (*see* IUD, copper)
Cord
occlusion at birth, and fetal metabolism (in sheep), 29
Cordocentesis
in fetal hemolytic disease
prediction of fetal anemia, 131
treatment outcome after, 121
Coronary
disease and postmenopausal estrogen, 423, 425
Corticotropin
-releasing hormone level increase in preterm labor, 3, 191
responses to vasopressin during pregnancy (in baboon), 5
responsiveness in fetal adrenal cells, regulation of, 7
Cortisol
responses to vasopressin during pregnancy (in baboon), 5
Cost
differential between indomethacin and ritodrine in preterm labor, 44
of endometrial resection vs. abdominal hysterectomy in menorrhagia, 250
CT (*see* Computed tomography)
Culture
blood, in fever evaluation in perioperative patients, 261
for HIV replication during first weeks of life, 214
of pooled cells from screened blood donations for HIV-1, 77
Curette
Novak, vs. Pipelle endometrial sampling device, 313
Cyanosis
in Ebstein's anomaly, and pregnancy outcome, 97
Cyclophosphamide
/cisplatin in ovarian cancer, long-term survival after, 342
in gestational trophoblastic tumors, 347
Cyst
adnexal, simple, in postmenopausal women, 245
breast
macroscopic, natural history of, 541
palpable, aspirations, complementary roles of mammography and physical examination in, 543
ovaries
functional, and oral contraceptives, 485, 486
laparoscopic management of, 246
Cystic
fibrosis gene transfer to airway epithelium, in vivo, 240

kidney disease, prenatal diagnosis of, 190
polycystic ovaries (*see* Polycystic, ovarian syndrome)
Cystosarcoma
phyllodes of breast
mammography, sonography, and aspiration cytology in, 549
metastases from, prediction of, 546
prognostic factors in, 548
Cystoscopy
after urinary tract infections, recurrent, 267
Cytobrush
efficacy and safety during pregnancy, 293
Cytology
aspiration (*see* Biopsy, aspiration)
cervicovaginal, in detection of recurrent cervical carcinoma after radiotherapy, 308
Cytomegalovirus
infection
congenital, and maternal antibody status, 119
congenital, outcome of, 232
fetal, prenatal diagnosis of, 124
Cytometry
flow
DNA, in simultaneous carcinoma of endometrium and ovary, 344
in hydropic placentas, 346
prenatal diagnosis with fetal cells isolated from maternal blood by, 199
Cytophotometry
DNA, in ovarian tumors of borderline malignancy, 331
Cytotoxic
therapy in early breast cancer, 582

D

Danazol
in endometriosis
cholesterol fractions and apolipoproteins after, 406
vs. nafarelin, 403
-induced hepatocellular adenomas, 407
in mastalgia, 540
in menorrhagia, 400
Dating
histologic, of secretory endometrium, error in, 434
DDAVP
in labor in prevention of hemorrhage in Ehlers-Danlos syndrome patient, 108
Deafness
sensorineural, due to congenital cytomegalovirus infection, 232
Death (*see* Mortality)
Decidua
as source of cachectin-tumor necrosis factor, 26
Dehydroepiandrosterone
sulphate levels, amniotic fluid, in Down's syndrome, 138
Delivery
analgesia during, patient-controlled epidural, 167
cesarean (*see* Cesarean section)
forceps, long-term effects of, 163
instrumental, and epidural analgesia in labor, 183
mode, effect on neonatal outcome after immune thrombocytopenic purpura in pregnancy, 81
preterm
amniotic fluid white blood cell count in prediction of, 109
fetal fibronectin in cervicovaginal secretions as predictor of, 36
prevention, antenatal social support in, 51
risk factors associated with, and race, 65
vacuum, long-term effects of, 163
Deoxyribonucleic acid (*see* DNA)
Depressive symptoms
estrogen use in postmenopausal women and, 412
Desmopressin
in labor, in prevention of hemorrhage in Ehlers-Danlos syndrome patient, 108
Desogestrel
in oral contraceptives, 491
Dexamethasone
/clomiphene in clomiphene-resistant women, 448
in hirsutism, 397
Dextran-70
effect on respiratory function in severe gestational proteinuric hypertension, 80
Diabetes mellitus
during pregnancy, and shoulder dystocia, 127
prorenin and, 23
Diaphragm
sexually transmitted diseases and, 361
Diet

osteoporosis and, postmenopausal, xxix
Diethylstilbestrol
-associated clear cell vaginal adenocarcinoma, risk factors for, 350
Digoxin
in fetal supraventricular tachycardia and hydrops fetalis, 237
Dipyridamole
/aspirin in prevention of fetal growth retardation, 40
DNA
amplification of pooled cells from screened blood donations for HIV-1, 77
analysis in fragile X syndrome, 188
cytophotometry in ovarian tumors of borderline malignancy, 331
flow cytometry
in hydropic placentas, 346
in simultaneous carcinoma of ovary and endometrium, 344
hybridization, in situ, in herpes simplex infection of placenta, 128
in paraffin-embedded sections in linkage analysis in familial retinoblastoma, 187
Donor
insemination, therapeutic, 445
Doppler ultrasound (*see* Ultrasound, Doppler)
Down's syndrome
amniotic fluid estriol, dehydroepiandrosterone sulphate and hCG levels in, 138
Doxorubicin
in breast cancer, primary nonmetastatic, 601
Doxycycline
in pelvic inflammatory disease, 365
cefoxitin combined with, 370
Drainage
percutaneous, of tubo-ovarian abscesses, 368
ultrasound-guided transvaginal, of pelvic abscesses and fluid collections, 367
Drug(s)
antiepileptic, plasma concentrations during pregnancy, 55
polydrug/cocaine use in pregnancy, two-year follow-up, 226
screening of newborns by meconium analysis, 203
therapy for mastalgia, 540
Ductus arteriosus
effect of indomethacin for preterm labor on, 135
Dyskaryosis
high-grade, after borderline Pap smear, 294
Dysmenorrhea
endometriosis and, 461
Dysphoric
disorder, late luteal phase, fluoxetine in, 532
Dysplasia
cervical (*see* Cervix, dysplasia)
Dysplastic
nevi, vulvar, 351
Dystocia
cesarean section for
active management of labor and, 170
analgesia and, epidural, 182
birth weight and, 127

E

Ebstein's anomaly
pregnancy outcome and, 97
Echocardiography
M-mode, of maternal left ventricular dimension in fetal growth-retarded pregnancies, 122
Echography
prenatal, positive for obstructive uropathy, predictive value of, 238
Econazole
topical, in candidal vaginitis, 375
Ecotopic pregnancy (*see* Pregnancy, ectopic)
Education
college, of parents, and infant mortality, 33
Ehlers-Danlos syndrome
patient, DDAVP in labor for hemorrhage prevention in, 108
Ejaculatory
duct obstruction in subfertile males, 441
ELCAT
ultrasound of embryo, 201
Elderly
hormone replacement therapy in, xxix-xxx
pelvic muscle exercise for stress incontinence in, 279
Electrocardiographic
changes during cesarean section under regional anesthesia, 169
Electrocautery
effect on midline laparotomy wound infection (in rat), 259
ovarian, for ovulation induction in polycystic ovary syndrome, 452
Electrosurgical
loop excision

in cervical intraepithelial neoplasia, 304
histologic findings, difference between colposcopic-directed biopsy findings and, 303
thermal injury zones in, 302
EMA/CO
regimen in high-risk gestational trophoblastic tumors, 347
Embryo
ultrasound of, endoluminal catheter-assisted transcervical, 201
Employment
maternal, effects on family and preterm infants at age 3 months, 209
Enalapril
in pregnancy, fetal and neonatal effects of, 198
Endocervical
gland
atypia in Pap smears, 295
involvement by grade III cervical intraepithelial neoplasia, 301
Endometriosis
danazol in (*see* Danazol, in endometriosis)
goserelin implant in, effect on cholesterol fractions and apolipoproteins, 406
infertility with, buserelin for, 459
menstrual symptoms and, 460
nafarelin in, 403
Endometrium
biopsy specimens, out-of-phase, prevalence of, 433
cancer (*see* Cancer, endometrium)
carcinoma (*see* Carcinoma, endometrium)
histology and bleeding patterns after 8 years of continuous estrogen/progestogen therapy, 428
polyps, postmenopausal bleeding from, after tamoxifen therapy, 314
resection for menorrhagia, 398
vs. abdominal hysterectomy, 249
sampling device, Pipelle, vs. Novak curette, 313
secretory, error in histologic dating of, 434
Endomyocardial
ultrastructural findings in preeclampsia, 39
Endothelin-1
in fetal blood, relation to asphyxia, 6
in fetal-placental circulation, effect of nitric oxide on vasoconstrictor effects of, 18
-induced vasoconstriction, effect of thromboxane release and action on, 59
Enzyme
immunoassay
monitoring for salivary progesterone in return of postpartum fertility, 386
rapid, for chlamydial infections, comparison of three, 372
rapid, for streptococci, group B, in pregnancy, 52
inhibitors, angiotensin converting, in pregnancy, fetal and neonatal effects of, 198
Epidermal
growth factor receptor content in breast cancer, 594
Epidural
analgesia (*see* Analgesia, epidural)
Epilepsy
in pregnancy, and plasma antiepileptic drug concentrations, 55
Epithelium
(*See also* Intraepithelial)
airway, in vivo transfer of cystic fibrosis gene to, 240
Erythromycin
/penicillin, intrapartum, for group B streptococcus, 83
therapy in preterm premature rupture of membranes, 31
Escherichia coli
urinary tract infection, norfloxacin in, 291
Estradiol
implants in prevention of postmenopausal bone loss, 422
levels, effects on bone density after postmenopausal hormone replacement therapy, 422
receptor content of breast cancers related to epidermal growth factor receptor content, 594
serum, as early predictor of pathologic pregnancy, 509
17β-, micronized, in postmenopausal bone loss prevention, 420
Estriol
levels, amniotic fluid, in Down's syndrome, 138
Estrogen
in amenorrheic runners, 387
deficiency as cause of hot flushes, xxxvi
non-contraceptive, and gallstones, 484
/phenylpropanolamine for stress incontinence, in elderly, 279

/progestogen (*see* Progestogen, /estrogen)
receptor measurement in prognosis of operable breast cancer, 580
replacement therapy
postmenopausal (*see below*)
in Turner syndrome, 389
replacement therapy, postmenopausal (*See also* Hormone, replacement therapy, postmenopausal)
cardiovascular benefit of, does progesterone subtract from? xxii-xxvii
cardiovascular disease and, 423
depressive symptoms and, 412
effects on lipid values and coronary disease, 425
progesterone combined with (*see* Progesterone, /estrogen replacement therapy)
progestogen combined with (*see* Progestogen, /estrogen, replacement therapy)
psychological function after, 411
thrombosis and, venous, 426
Ethnicity
breast cancer screening and, 566
mammography use and, 565
Etidronate
in prevention of postmenopausal osteoporosis, xxix
Etoposide
in gestational trophoblastic tumors, 347
Examination
breast (*see* Breast, examination)
physical, of palpable breast cysts after aspiration, 543
Exercise
Kegel (*see* Kegel exercise)
osteoporosis and, postmenopausal, xxix, 416

F

Fallopian tube (*see* Tubal)
Family
planning, lactational amenorrhea method for, 479
of preterm infant, effect of maternal employment at 3 months on, 209
Fat
body, central distribution, and hormone replacement therapy, 414
FDC-6
measurement of fetal fibronectin in cervical and vaginal secretions, 38
Febrile
morbidity, puerperal, diagnostic imaging in, 207
perioperative patients, blood cultures in evaluation of, 261
Fecundity
rates (*see* Pregnancy, rates)
Feeding
breast, and HIV transmission, 218, 221
Femoral
bone density after hormone replacement therapy, effects of plasma estradiol levels on, 422
vein, common, duplex ultrasound in pregnancy and puerperium, 205
Fertility
adrenal hyperplasia due to 21-hydroxylase deficiency and, late-onset, 455
after laparoscopic treatment of ectopic pregnancy, 523
postpartum, return monitored by enzyme immunoassay for salivary progesterone, 386
prediction in men with normal sperm concentration, relevance of adenosine triphosphate in semen on, 440
Fertilization
in vitro
comparison to gamete intrafallopian transfer and intrauterine insemination with superovulation, 468
in infertility, unexplained, 469
results, multicenter study, 471
in unstimulated cycles, 474
α-Fetoprotein
levels, second trimester, 142
in Down's syndrome, 138
Fetus
adrenal cells, regulation of corticotropin responsiveness in, 7
anemia, cordocentesis in prediction of, 131
blood
endothelin-1 in, relation to asphyxia, 6
gases related to computer analysis data of fetal heart rate patterns in small for gestation fetuses, 146
sampling in prenatal diagnosis of cytomegalovirus infection, 125
volume changes, acute response of umbilical artery pulsatility index to (in sheep), 141
breathing movements and prostaglandin E concentrations in, effects of glycemia on (in sheep), 12

cells isolated from maternal blood by flow cytometry, prenatal diagnosis with, 199
circulation (*see* Circulation, fetal-placental)
cytomegalovirus infection, prenatal diagnosis of, 124
effects of angiotensin converting enzyme inhibitors in pregnancy on, 198
fibronectin in cervical and vaginal secretions as predictor of preterm delivery, 36
growth (*see* Growth, fetal)
heart
function in intrauterine growth retardation, 107
hemodynamics, reproducibility of ultrasonic measurement of, 158
rate (*see* Heart, rate, fetal)
hemodynamics (*see* Hemodynamics, fetal)
hemolytic disease, cordocentesis in (*see* Cordocentesis, in fetal hemolytic disease)
hydrops (*see* Hydrops, fetalis)
large for gestational age at term, sonographic diagnosis of, 173
loss and lupus anticoagulants and anticardiolipin antibodies, 53
metabolism, effect of birth-related events on (in sheep), 29
monitoring (*see* Monitoring, fetal)
outcome after invasive cervical cancer in pregnancy, 306
-pelvic index in estimation of fetal-pelvic disproportion, 174
small for gestation, fetal blood gases related to data from computer analysis of fetal heart rate patterns in, 146
surgery for cleft lip, 236
tachycardia, supraventricular, and hydrops fetalis, 237
toxicity from maternal indomethacin, in twins, 135
transfusion (*see* Transfusion, intrauterine)
transplantation of fetal liver stem cells into, in-utero, 235
uropathy, clinical outcome of, 238
well-being, umbilical artery resistance index as screening test for, 148
Fever (*see* Febrile)
Fibronectin
fetal, in cervical and vaginal secretions, as predictor of preterm delivery, 36
Fibrosis
cystic fibrosis gene transfer to airway epithelium, in vivo, 240
Fistula
vesicovaginal, after hysterectomy, early repair of, 256
Flap
Boari, in iatrogenic ureteral injury after gynecological surgery, 256
Flow
cytometry (*see* Cytometry, flow)
velocity waveforms, Doppler
fetal and umbilical, between 10-16 weeks' gestation, 159
in high risk pregnancies, 153
regurgitant, during pregnancy, 22
umbilical, after hydralazine or labetalol in hypertensive pregnancy, 16
umbilical, and maternal angiotensin sensitivity, 160
Fluconazole
in vaginitis, candidal, 375
Fluid
amniotic (*see* Amniotic, fluid)
collections, pelvic, ultrasound-guided drainage of, 367
Fluorescent
treponemal antibody absorption test for syphilis, 231
Fluoride
osteoporosis and, postmenopausal, xxviii-xxix
Fluoxetine
in late luteal phase dysphoric disorder, 532
Flushes
hot, causes of, xxxvi
Flutamide
in hirsutism, 398
Folic acid
supplementation in prevention of neural tube defects, 193
Follicle
aspiration, ultrasound-guided, for ovulation induction in polycystic ovary syndrome, 451
recruitment, multiple, and intrauterine insemination outcomes compared by age and diagnosis, 463
Forceps
delivery, long-term effects of, 163
Forskolin
effect on corticotropin responsiveness in fetal adrenal cells, 7
Fragile X syndrome
DNA analysis in, 188
Frozen section

accuracy in diagnosis of ovarian neoplasms, 336

Fusobacterium nucleatum
infection, amniotic fluid, and preterm labor, 66

G

Gallstones
oral contraceptives and non-contraceptive estrogens and, 484

Gamete intrafallopian transfer
comparison to in vitro fertilization and intrauterine insemination combined with superovulation, 468
hysteroscopic, 475
in infertility, unexplained, 469

Gas(es)
blood, fetal, related to computer analysis data of fetal heart rate patterns in small for gestation fetuses, 146
respiratory, relationships between uterine and umbilical veins in pregnancy, 20

Gastric
emptying in postpartum period, 204

Gene
cystic fibrosis, in vivo transfer to airway epithelium, 240

Genetic
aspects of prenatal diagnosis of cystic kidney disease, 190

Genitourinary
prolapse
repair, stress incontinence after, 274
urodynamic tests in, 271

Gentamicin
/clindamycin in pelvic inflammatory disease, 370
in intra-amniotic infection, 57

Gestation (*see* Pregnancy)

Gestodene
in oral contraceptives, 491

GIFT (*see* Gamete intrafallopian transfer)

Gittes suspension
transvaginal ultrasound and urodynamic evaluation after, 276

Globulins
total, effect of Norplant implants on, 500

Gloving
double, effect on frequency of glove perforations, 259

Glucocorticoid
prenatal, respiratory disease in very low birth weight infant after, 219

Glucose
tolerance after long-term oral contraceptive use, 483

Glycemia
effects on breathing movements and prostaglandin E concentrations in fetus (in sheep), 12

Gonadotropin
chorionic, human
levels in Down's syndrome, 138
luteal phase support with, in hMG-stimulated cycles, 454
serum β-, as early predictor of pathologic pregnancy, 509
serum β-, serial, in screening for ectopic pregnancy, 520
menopausal, human, for ovulation induction
luteal support with hCG and, 454
in polycystic ovary syndrome, 452
in women with non-responsive ovaries, 449
-releasing hormone
agonist goserelin (*see* Goserelin)
agonist with cyclical hormone replacement therapy for dysfunctional uterine bleeding, 402
analogue in endometrial cancer, 320
therapy, low-dose, for ovulation induction in polycystic ovary syndrome, 450

Gonococcal
cervical infections, nonoxynol-9 in prevention of, 358

Gonorrhea
cefixime vs. ceftriaxone in, 369
trends in 1980s, 357

Goserelin
depot, with cyclic hormone replacement therapy for dysfunctional uterine bleeding, 402
in endometrial cancer, 320
implant in endometriosis, cholesterol fractions and apolipoproteins during, 406

Granulomatous
disease and vulvar carcinoma, 352

Granulosa
cell growth, in vitro ovarian, effect of immunoglobulin on, 388

Grid
mammography, in ultrasound of breast masses, 588

Growth
factor, epidermal, receptor content in breast cancer, 594

fetal
in hypertensive pregnancies, effect of maternal hemodynamics on, 98
retardation (*see* Growth, retardation, intrauterine)
hormone for ovulation induction, 449
retardation, intrauterine
aspirin in prevention of, low-dose, 40
autoantibodies during third trimester and, 94
Doppler scan in screening for, 155
heart function in, fetal, 107
heart rate variation in, fetal, numeric analysis of, 130
respiratory gas relationshpis between uterine and umbilical veins in, 20
ventricular dimension and, maternal left, 122
Gyne
T 380 Slimline and Gyne T 380 IUDs, comparison of, 496
Gynecologic
problems, and congenital coagulopathies, 84
surgery iatrogenic injury during
bladder, early repair of, 255
ureter, 256
ureter, early repair of, 255
Gynecologist
role in breast disease diagnosis and management, 537

H

hCG (*see* Gonadotropin, chorionic, human)
Head
growth after maternal cocaine use, 227
Heart
(*See also* Cardiac; Cardiovascular)
function, fetal, in intrauterine growth retardation, 107
rate
fetal (*see below*)
in hyperthyroid pregnancy, 102
rate, fetal
after hydralazine or labetalol in hypertensive pregnancy, 16
in intrauterine growth retardation, numeric analysis of, 130
in labor (*see below*)
patterns in small for gestation fetuses, computer analysis, relation to fetal blood gases, 146
rate, fetal, in labor
computer analysis of, 149
early, computer analysis of, 144
pseudosinusoidal patterns, 136
sinusoidal patterns, 145
Height
adolescent, and
diethylstilbestrol-associated clear cell vaginal adenocarcinoma, 351
Hematoma
perineal, due to congenital coagulopathies, 84
Hemodynamic
stress responses to cesarean delivery in preeclampsia, effect of anesthesia on, 180
Hemodynamics
fetal
cardiac, reproducibility of ultrasonic measurement of, 158
during hydralazine or labetalol therapy in maternal hypertension, 16
maternal
central, in untreated preeclampsia, 86
effect on fetal growth in hypertensive pregnancies, 98
during hydralazine or labetalol therapy in maternal hypertension, 16
in pregnancies complicated by hyperthyroidism, 101
Hemolytic
disease, fetal, cordocentesis in (*see* Cordocentesis, in fetal hemolytic disease)
Hemophilia
A, obstetric and gynecological problems in, 84
Hemorrhage
(*See also* Bleeding)
intracranial, neonatal, after immune thrombocytopenic purpura in pregnancy, 81
intraventricular, in preterm infant, effect of cesarean section on, 168
during labor in Ehlers-Danlos syndrome patient, effect of prophylactic DDAVP on, 108
periventricular, in very low birth weight infants, incidence and outcome, 228
postpartum, due to congenital coagulopathies, 84
tentorial subdural, in newborn, 224
Hemorrhagic
problems in obstetrics and gynecology patients with congenital coagulopathies, 84
Hemostasis

menstrual, in essential menorrhagia, effects of mefenamic acid on, 401
Hepatitis
B virus infection, perinatal, maternal transmission of, 211
Hepatocellular
adenomas (*see* Adenomas, hepatocellular)
Herpes
simplex infection of placenta, 128
Hibiscrub
optimum duration of surgical scrub-time with, 258
Hirsutism
androgen blockade vs. androgen suppression in, 396
flutamide in, 398
Histologic
dating of secretory endometrium, error in, 434
differences between colposcopic-directed biopsy and loop excision of transformation zone, 303
Histology
endometrial, after 8 years of continuous estrogen/progestogen therapy, 428
HIV
blood donations screened for, evaluation by culture and DNA amplification of pooled cells, 77
infection
high risk for first-born twins, 50
perinatal, early detection of IgA antibodies in, 229
in pregnancy, zidovudine in, 75
replication during first weeks of life, 213
transmission, female to male, 378
transmission, male to female, 378, 379
transmission, mother-to-child
late in pregnancy, 78
postnatal, 221
risk factors for, 217
from seronegative or indeterminate mothers, 85
in twins or siblings, 103
-2, lack of evidence of vertical transmission, 225
hMG (*see* Gonadotropin, menopausal, human)
Home
uterine activity monitoring (*see* Monitoring, uterine activity, home)
Hormone
adrenocorticotropic (*see* Corticotropin)
circulating, in long-term follow-up after wedge resected polycystic ovary syndrome, 395
corticotropin-releasing, in preterm labor, 3, 191
gonadotropin-releasing (*see* Gonadotropin, -releasing hormone)
growth, for ovulation induction, 449
luteinizing (*see* Luteinizing hormone)
replacement therapy, postmenopausal (*See also* Estrogen, replacement therapy, postmenopausal)
androgen addition to, xxvii-xxviii
breast cancer and, xxx-xxxiv
calcium supplementation in, xxviii-xxix
continuous, treatment of breakthrough bleeding with, xxi-xxii
continuous vs. sequential, xx-xxi
cyclical, with depot goserelin for dysfunctional uterine bleeding, 402
in elderly, xxix-xxx
levonorgestrel-releasing IUD as method for, 430
in osteoporosis prevention, 416
in prevention of central distribution of body fat after menopause, 414
what agent or route of administration is best? xix-xx
steroid, receptors, effect on prognosis in operable breast cancer, 580
therapy in early breast cancer, 582
thyrotropin-releasing, prenatal, respiratory disease in very low birth weight infant after, 219
Hospital
teaching status, influence on cesarean birth rate, 175
Hospitalization
for pelvic inflammatory disease, 361
Hot flushes
causes of, xxxvi
Human immunodeficiency virus (*see* HIV)
Hybridization
in situ DNA, in herpes simplex infection of placenta, 128
Hydatidiform mole
flow cytometric study of, 346
risk factors for, 330
Hydralazine
in hypertensive pregnancy
continuous infusion, 54
hemodynamic effects of, 16
Hydrocephalus
in very low birth weight infants, 228
Hydrocortisone
effect on fertility in women with late-onset adrenal hyperplasia due to 21-hydroxylase deficiency, 455
Hydronephrosis
in pregnancy, ultrasound of, 58

Hydrops
  fetalis
    nonimmune, due to parvovirus B19, intrauterine transfusion in, 239
    tachycardia and, fetal supraventricular, 237
  placental, flow cytometric study in, 346
Hydrotubation
  sonographic, vs. hysterosalpingography, 436
21-Hydroxylase
  deficiency causing late-onset adrenal hyperplasia, effect on fertility, 455
Hyperbaric oxygen
  in carbon monoxide intoxication in pregnancy, 27
Hyperkeratosis
  on Pap smears, 294
Hyperplasia
  adrenal, late-onset, due to 21-hydroxylase deficiency, effect on fertility, 455
  lactotroph, causing functional hyperprolactinemia, 393
Hyperprolactinemia
  functional, due to lactotroph hyperplasia, 393
  idiopathic, clinical history and outcome of, 391
  long-term effects of time, medical treatment and pregnancy in, 392
Hypertension
  during pregnancy
    calcium supplementation in, 35
    fetal growth and, effect on maternal hemodynamics on, 98
    hydralazine in (*see* Hydralazine, in hypertensive pregnancy)
    labetalol in, 16
    mild, management of, 92
    prorenin and, 23
    proteinuric, respiratory function in, 80
    in renal allograft recipients, and perinatal outcome, 114
    renovascular, 41
    third trimester, and autoantibodies, 94
  pulmonary, primary, in newborn after indomethacin in preterm labor, 44
Hypertensive
  disorders of pregnancy
    aspirin in prevention of, low-dose, 47
    calcium supplementation in prevention of, 42
    placental bed spiral arteries in, 104
Hyperthyroidism
  in pregnancy, and maternal hemodynamics, 101
Hypertriglyceridemia
  -induced pancreatitis during pregnancy, 79
Hypoplasia
  pulmonary, fetal and neonatal, after angiotensin converting enzyme inhibitors in pregnancy, 198
Hysterectomy
  abdominal
    for menorrhagia, 249
    total, adverse urinary symptoms after, 289
  effect on anorectal and urethrovesical physiology, 252
  iatrogenic injury to ureter or bladder during, early repair of, 256
  outcomes, self-reported long-term, 251
  ovarian cancer after, 324, 325
  progesterone after, xxvii
  vaginal, oophorectomy at, 254
Hysterosalpingography
  ultrasound and, color Doppler, 438
  vs. sonographic hydrotubation, 436
Hysteroscopy
  gamete intrafallopian transfer by, 475

I

Iatrogenic
  injury
    to bladder during gynecologic surgery, early repair of, 255
    to ureter during gynecologic surgery, 256
    to ureter during gynecologic surgery, early repair of, 255
    to ureter during obstetric surgery, 256
Ig (*see* Immunoglobulin)
Imaging
  diagnostic, in puerperal febrile morbidity, 207
  magnetic resonance (*see* Magnetic resonance imaging)
Immune
  therapy in early breast cancer, 582
  thrombocytopenic purpura, in pregnancy, management of, 81
Immunoassay
  enzyme (*see* Enzyme, immunoassay)
Immunodeficiency
  disease, severe fetal, in-utero transplantation of fetal liver stem cells in, 235
  syndrome, acquired (*see* AIDS)
  virus, human (*see* HIV)
Immunoglobulin

A antibody serological assay for early diagnosis of perinatal HIV infection, 229
effect on ovarian granulosa cell growth in vitro, 388
IV
for miscarriage, recurrent, 508
in toxic shock syndrome, 381
Immunohistochemical
studies
of fetal fibronectin, 38
of herpes simplex infection of placenta, 129
in simultaneous carcinoma of endometrium and ovary, 344
Immunosuppression
lymphocyte-initiated, in pregnancy, 73
Implant
collagen, para-urethral, for stress incontinence, 283
Norplant, effect on liver, lipid, and carbohydrate metabolism, 500
Incontinence
urinary
prevalence and consequences of, 263
prevalence, incidence and correlates of, in middle-aged women, 264
stress (*see below*)
urodynamic assessment in, 269
urodynamic assessment in, vs. lateral urethrocystography, 268
urinary, stress
bladder neck suspension for (*see* Bladder, neck suspension)
collagen implant for, para-urethral, 283
colporrhaphy for, anterior, 25-year experience, 284
endosonography in, transvaginal, 272
Kegel exercise for (*see* Kegal exercise)
after prazosin, 265
after vaginal repair, prediction of, 274
Indomethacin
in labor, preterm
effect on maternal corticotropin-releasing hormone, 191
fetal toxicity in twin gestation, 135
vs. ritodrine, 44
Infant
HIV transmission from mother to (*see* HIV, transmission, mother-to-child)
mortality (*see* Mortality, infant)
preterm
at age 3 months, maternal employment effects on, 209
intraventricular hemorrhage in, effect of cesarean section on, 168
Infarction
myocardial, and oral contraceptives, 489
Infection
labor and, 60
laparotomy wound, midline, effects of electrocautery on, 259
after surgical management of vaginal vault prolapse, 255
Infertility
assisted conception for, expectations of, 472
endometriosis with, buserelin for, 459
hysterosalpingography in
ultrasound and, color Doppler, 438
vs. sonographic hydrotubation, 436
nontubal, transvaginal peritoneal oocyte and sperm transfer for, 476
as risk factor for ectopic pregnancy, 517
salpingitis isthmica nodosa in, 439
unexplained, treatment of, 469
Inflammatory
disease, pelvic (*see* Pelvis, inflammatory disease)
Inhibin
concentrations during menstrual cycle, 383
Insemination
donor, therapeutic, 445
intraperitoneal
after superovulation, 470
in unexplained infertility, 469
intrauterine
in infertility, unexplained, 469
multiple follicular recruitment and, outcomes compared by age and diagnosis, 463
pregnancy rates after, effect of controlled ovarian hyperstimulation on, 464
slow release vs. bolus, and cervical mucus hostility, 444
superovulation with, 470
superovulation with, comparison to in vitro fertilization and gamete intrafallopian transfer, 468
two regimens in controlled ovarian hyperstimulation cycles, 462
vs. timed intercourse, 446
Inspiratory
effort and breathlessness in pregnancy, 13
Instrumental
deliveries and epidural analgesia in labor, 183
Intelligence
scores after vacuum or forceps delivery, 163
Intercourse

natural, after superovulation, 470
timed, vs. intrauterine insemination, 446
Interferon-α
in papillomavirus infection, 297
Intoxication
carbon monoxide, in pregnancy, hyperbaric oxygen in, 27
Intracranial
hemorrhage, neonatal, after immune thrombocytopenic purpura in pregnancy, 81
Intraepithelial
neoplasia
cervical (*see* Cervix, neoplasia, intraepithelial)
vaginal, grade 3, laser vaporization of, 348
Intrafallopian
transfer, gamete (*see* Gamete intrafallopian transfer)
Intrapartum
chemoprophylaxis for group B streptococcus, 82
Intraperitoneal
chromic phosphate in early ovarian carcinoma, 340
insemination (*see* Insemination, intraperitoneal)
Intratubal
methotrexate for ectopic pregnancy, 528
Intrauterine
device (*see* IUD)
growth retardation (*see* Growth, retardation, intrauterine)
insemination (*see* Insemination, intrauterine)
transfusion (*see* Transfusion, intrauterine)
transplantation of fetal liver stem cells into fetuses, 235
Intraventricular
hemorrhage in preterm infant, effect of cesarean section on, 168
In vitro fertilization (*see* Fertilization, in vitro)
Irradiation (*see* Radiotherapy)
IUD
copper
Gyne T 380 Slimline vs. Gyne T 380, 496
pregnancy after, planned, 501
levonorgestrel-releasing
as hormone replacement therapy, 430
pregnancy after, planned, 501
occult, ultrasound-guided retrieval in early pregnancy, 499
pelvic inflammatory disease and, 497
as risk factor for ectopic pregnancy, 517
use, prolonged, 494
IVF (*see* Fertilization, in vitro)

J

Juvenile
rheumatoid arthritis and pregnancy, 95

K

Kaolin clotting time
in detection of lupus anticoagulants, 507
Karyotypic
abnormalities and omphalocele contents, 196
Kegel exercise
for stress incontinence
in elderly, 279
long-term effect of, 281
performance after brief verbal instruction, 280
Kelly-Kennedy-type colporrhaphy technique
anterior, 25-year experience, 285
Kidney
allograft recipients, perinatal outcome in, 114
disease, cystic, prenatal diagnosis of, 190
dysfunction, fetal and neonatal, after angiotensin converting enzyme inhibitors in pregnancy, 198
Killer cell
natural, activity in pregnancy, effect of RU 486 on, 14

L

Labetalol
in hypertensive pregnancy, hemodynamic effects of, 16
Labor
active management of
controlled trial, 171
effect on incidence of cesarean section for dystocia, 170
analgesia during (*see* Analgesia, epidural, in labor)
desmopressin in, in prevention of hemorrhage in Ehlers-Danlos syndrome patient, 108
heart rate in, fetal (*see* Heart, rate, fetal, in labor)
induction vs. serial antenatal monitoring in post-term pregnancy, 34
infection and, 60

oligohydramnios in, prophylactic amnioinfusion for, 126
oxytocin secretion in, 10
preterm
amniotic fluid infection and, 66
clindamycin in, 45
corticotropin-releasing hormone in, 3, 191
detection with home uterine activity monitoring, 152
indomethacin in (*see* Indomethacin, in labor, preterm)
ritodrine in, 44
Lactational
amenorrrhea method for family planning, 479
Lactobacillus
acidophilus-containing yogurt in prevention of candidal vaginitis, 373
Lactotroph
hyperplasia causing functional hyperprolactinemia, 393
Laparoscopy
ectopic pregnancy treatment by
fertility after, 523
outpatient, with local methotrexate injection, 526
electrocautery via, ovarian (*see* Electrocautery, ovarian)
lysis of adhesions by, after laser photocoagulation of polycystic ovaries, pregnancy rates after, 453
ovarian cyst management by, 246
tuboplasty via, distal, 457
Laparotomy
second-look, in stage I ovarian epithelial carcinoma, 339
staging, in uterine adenosarcoma, 321
wound infection, midline, effect of electrocautery on (in rat), 259
Large for gestational age fetus
at term, sonographic diagnosis of, 173
Laser
cervical excision conization, thermal injury zones in, 302
photocoagulation of polycystic ovaries, laparoscopic lysis of adhesions after, effect on pregnancy rates, 453
vaporization of grade 3 vaginal intraepithelial neoplasia, 348
Leiomyosarcoma
uterus, cisplatin in, 322
Leuprorelin
in endometrial cancer, 320
Levonorgestrel
-releasing IUD (*see* IUD, levonorgestrel-releasing)
Life-style
osteoporosis and, postmenopausal, xxix
Limb
deficiencies
chorionic villus sampling and, 186
after cocaine use, maternal, physiatric management of, 185
Lip
cleft, fetal surgery for, 236
Lipid
metabolism, effect of Norplant implants on, 500
peroxide/vitamin E imbalance in preeclampsia, 48
values, effects of postmenopausal estrogen therapy on, 425
Lipopolysaccharide
-stimulated decidua as source of tumor necrosis factor, 26
Lipoprotein
apheresis for hypertriglyceridemia-induced pancreatitis during pregnancy, 79
metabolism, effects of desogestrel and gestodene in oral contraceptives on, 491
Litigation
breast cancer malpractice, 539
causes of, 538
Liver
cell adenomas (*see* Adenomas, hepatocellular)
metabolism, effect of Norplant implant on, 500
stem cells, fetal, in-utero transplantation into fetuses, 235
Loop excision (*see* Electrosurgical, loop excision)
Low birth weight infant
cerebral palsy in, 214
very
effect of aspirin in prevention of hypertensive pregnancy on, 47
improvement of outcome for, 220
periventricular hemorrhage and hydrocephalus in, 228
respiratory disease after prenatal thyrotropin-releasing hormone and glucocorticoid in, 219
Lumpectomy
adequacy of margins, 570
breast tumor recurrence after, ipsilateral, 589
in invasive breast cancer, 600
Lung (*see* Pulmonary)
Lupus
anticoagulant
detection methods, 507

fetal loss and, 94
during third trimester pregnancy, 94
erythematosus, systemic, miscarriage and thrombosis, 507
Luteal phase
defect in habitual abortion, 505
dysphoric disorder, late, fluoxetine in, 532
support with hCG, effect on fecundity rate in hMG-stimulated cycles, 454
Luteinizing hormone
-releasing hormone agonist for ovulation induction in polycystic ovary syndrome, 452
-timed intercourse vs. intrauterine insemination, 446
Lymphadenectomy
in ovarian cancer, morbidity and mortality of, 341
Lymphatic
involvement, retroperitoneal, with ovarian tumors, 337
Lymphocyte
-initiated immunosuppression in pregnancy, 73
Lysis
of adhesions, laparoscopic, after laser photocoagulation of polycystic ovaries, pregnancy rates after, 453

M

Macroscopic
cysts in breast, natural history of, 541
Magnesium
oral, for premenstrual mood changes, 532
Magnetic resonance imaging
in cerebral palsy, 212
in puerperal febrile morbidity, 207
Magnetic resonance spectroscopy
phosphorus, in prediction of outcome after birth asphyxia, 123
Malpractice
litigation, breast cancer, 539
causes of, 538
Mammography
after cyst aspiration, 543
in cystosarcoma phyllodes, 549
grid in ultrasound of breast masses, 588
-guided fine-needle aspiration of nonpalpable lesions, 554
of palpable and impalpable lesions, prevalence of carcinoma in, 563
of papillary neoplasms, benign, 543
patients, self-referred, 558
prognostic factors and survival, 560
regular, 559
screening, noncompliance, reasons for, 557
use
effects of ethnicity, socioeconomic status, and psychological barriers on, 565
effects of race and ethnicity on, 566
in relatives of women with breast cancer, 593
in women less than 35 years of age, 562
Manchester procedure
prediction of stress incontinence after, 274
Marijuana
use in pregnancy, two-year follow-up, 227
Mastalgia
drug treatments for, 540
Mastectomy
for cancer
invasive, 600
primary, nonmetastatic, 601
immediate reconstruction after, selection criteria for, 570
timing, optimal, 581
vs. breast conservation, 574
Maternal
angiotensin sensitivity and fetal Doppler umbilical artery flow waveforms, 160
antibody status and outcome of congenital cytomegalovirus infection, 119
blood (*see* Blood, maternal)
corticotropin-releasing hormone level increase in preterm labor, 3, 191
employment effects on family and preterm infants at age 3 months, 209
α-fetoprotein levels, serum, at second trimester screening, 142
hemodynamics (*see* Hemodynamics, maternal)
impact of anaerobic coverage for intra-amniotic infection, 57
outcome after invasive cervical cancer in pregnancy, 306
serologic tests for syphilis, 230
transmission
of hepatitis B virus infection, 211
of HIV (*see* HIV, transmission, mother-to-child)
ventricular dimension, left, in fetal growth retarded pregnancies, 122
Meconium
analysis, drug screening of newborns by, 203

Medroxyprogesterone
  acetate, depot-
    breast cancer and, 567
    cervical cancer and, 502
    endometrial cancer and, 310
Mefenamic acid
  effects on menstrual hemostasis in essential menorrhagia, 401
Membrane
  rupture (*see* Rupture of membranes)
Mengert's index
  in fetal-pelvic disproportion, 174
Menopausal
  gonadotropin, human (*see* Gonadotropin, menopausal, human)
Menopause
  body fat distribution after, central, postmenopausal hormone replacement therapy in prevention of, 414
  early, in long-term survivors of adolescent cancer, 410
  management, controversial issues in, xix-xliii
  transition, normal, 409-410
  what is normal about it? xxxvi-xxxviii
Menorrhagia
  danazol vs. norethisterone in, 400
  endometrial resection for, 398
    vs. abdominal hysterectomy, 249
  essential, effects of mefenamic acid on menstrual hemostasis in, 401
  in von Willebrand's disease, 84
Menstrual
  cycle, inhibin concentrations during, 383
  hemostasis in essential menorrhagia, effects of mefenamic acid on, 401
  symptoms and endometriosis, 460
Mental
  retardation
    fragile X syndrome of, DNA analysis in, 188
    syndrome, X-linked, associated with α thalassemia, 195
Metabolism
  carbohydrate (*see* Carbohydrate, metabolism)
  fetal, effect of birth-related events on (in sheep), 29
  lipid, effect of Norplant implants on, 500
  lipoprotein, effects of desogestrel and gestodene in oral contraceptives on, 491
  liver, effect of Norplant implants on, 500
  oral contraceptives and, long-term, 483
Metastases
  from cystosarcoma phyllodes of breast, 548
    prediction of, 546
  ovarian, in stage IB cervical carcinoma, 332
Methotrexate
  in gestational trophoblastic tumors, 347
  injection, local, in outpatient laparoscopic ectopic pregnancy management, 526
  transvaginal intratubal, for ectopic pregnancy, 528
  for trophoblast persisting after surgery for ectopic pregnancy, 524
Metronidazole
  in vaginosis, bacterial
    comparison of different regimens, 376
    vs. clindamycin cream, 377
Microbial
  invasion of amniotic cavity (*see* Amniotic, cavity, microbial invasion of)
Mifepristone (*see* RU 486)
Miscarriage
  (*See also* Abortion, spontaneous)
  in lupus erythematosus, systemic, 507
  multiple, IV immunoglobulin for, 508
Mitral
  valvotomy, percutaneous balloon, during pregnancy, 100
Model
  silicone breast, training health professionals in breast examination with, 587
Mole
  hydatidiform (*see* Hydatidiform mole)
Molecular
  pathology in diagnosis of herpes simplex infection of placenta, 128
Monitoring
  antenatal (*see* fetal *below*)
  fetal
    in perinatal sepsis, 157
    serial, vs. labor induction in post-term pregnancy, 34
  salivary progesterone, enzyme immunoassay, in return of postpartum fertility, 386
  uterine activity, home
    in detection of preterm labor, 152
    randomized controlled trials of, 156
Monoclonal
  antibody FDC-6 measurement of fetal fibronectin in cervical and vaginal secretions, 38
Mononuclear

cells, maternal antihepatitis Be positive, causing perinatal hepatitis B infection, 211
Mood
changes, premenstrual, oral magnesium for, 532
Morbidity
febrile puerperal, diagnostic imaging in, 207
of ovarian cancer operations, 341
Morphine
metabolites in newborn, meconium analysis for, 203
Mortality
infant
in cesarean section, 164
college-educated parents and, 33
twin, in U.S., 133
of ovarian cancer operations, 341
perinatal, and aspirin in prevention of hypertensive pregnancy, 47
Mosaicism
diagnosis in chorionic villus sampling, follow-up and pregnancy outcome after, 137
MRI (*see* Magnetic resonance imaging)
Mucinous
ovarian tumors with pseudomyxoma peritonei, 335
Mucus
cervical (*see* Cervix, mucus)
sperm, interaction in clomiphene citrate cycles, 443
Multiple sclerosis
relapse during pregnancy, 96
Muscle
pelvic, exercise (*see* Kegel exercise)
Myocardial
infarction and oral contraceptives, 489
Myometrium
invasion from uterine adenosarcoma, 321
platelet-activating factor binding sites in, role in uterine contraction, 9

N

Nafarelin
in endometriosis, 403
Natural killer cell
activity in pregnancy, effect of RU 486 on, 14
Nd-YAG
laser photocoagulation of polycystic ovaries, laparoscopic lysis of adhesions after, 453
Necrosis
tumor necrosis factor, decidua as source of, 26
Needle
biopsy
core, stereotactic, of nonpalpable breast lesions, 555, 556
fine- (*see* Aspiration, fine-needle)
colpo-needle suspension for stress incontinence, 288
Neonate (*see* Newborn)
Neoplasm (*see* Tumor)
Nephrostomy
temporary percutaneous, for iatrogenic injury to ureter during surgery, 257
Neural tube
defects, prevention of, 193
Neurodevelopmental
outcome of periventricular hemorrhage and hydrocephalus in very low birth weight infants, 228
Neuroendocrine
stress responses to cesarean delivery in preeclampsia, effect of anesthesia on, 180
Neurological
impairment due to congenital cytomegalovirus infection, 232
Nevi
dysplastic, vulvar, 351
Newborn
drug screening by meconium analysis, 203
effects of angiotensin converting enzyme inhibitors in pregnancy on, 198
hemorrhage in
intracranial, after immune thrombocytopenic purpura in pregnancy, 81
tentorial subdural, 224
HIV replication in, during first weeks of life, 213
hypertension in, primary pulmonary, after indomethacin in preterm labor, 44
infections and group B streptococcus, 82
limb deficiencies after prenatal cocaine exposure, physiatric management of, 185
outcome after amniotic fluid infection and preterm labor, 66
serologic tests for syphilis, 230
Nipple
Paget's disease of, 578
Nitric oxide
attenuation of vasoconstrictor effects of thromboxane and endothelin in fetal-placental circulation by, 18

Nitroprusside
  in preeclampsia, 90
Nonoxynol-9
  in prevention of gonococcal and chlamydial cervical infections, 358
Norethisterone
  in menorrhagia, 400
Norfloxacin
  in urinary tract infection, 290
Norplant
  capsules, planned pregnancy after, 501
  implants, effect on liver, lipid, and carbohydrate metabolism, 500
  II rods, planned pregnancy after, 501
Novak
  curette vs. Pipelle endometrial sampling device, 313
Nulliparas
  effect of active management of labor on incidence of cesarean section for dystocia in, 170
Numeric
  analysis of heart rate variation in intrauterine growth-retarded fetuses, 130
Nurse
  improving clinical breast examination by, 587
Nylidrin
  in preterm labor, 191

O

Obesity
  breast carcinoma prognosis and, 598
  endometrial cancer and, 310
Obstetric
  performance, effect of gestational age on, 61
  problems and congenital coagulopathies, 84
  surgery, iatrogenic injury to ureter during, 256
Office visits
  for pelvic inflammatory disease, 361
Oligohydramnios
  fetal and neonatal, after angiotensin converting enzyme inhibitors in pregnancy, 198
  in labor, prophylactic amnioinfusion for, 126
Omphalocele
  contents and karyotypic abnormalities, 196
Oocyte
  transvaginal peritoneal oocyte and sperm transfer for nontubal infertility, 476
Oophorectomy
  at hysterectomy, vaginal, 254
  in prevention of ovarian cancer, 325
  videolaseroscopy for, 248
Oral
  contraception (*see* Contraception, oral)
Organon combined contraceptive vaginal ring, 503
Osteoporosis
  postmenopausal
    prevention of, 416
    treatment with calcitriol or calcium, 418
Ovaries
  ablation in early breast cancer, 582
  cancer (*see* Cancer, ovaries)
  carcinoma (*see* Carcinoma, ovaries)
  cyst (*see* Cyst, ovaries)
  electrocautery for ovulation induction in polycystic ovary syndrome, 452
  granulosa cell growth in vitro, effect of immunoglobulins on, 388
  hyperstimulation, controlled
    ectopic pregnancy and, 518
    intrauterine insemination after, pregnancy rates after, 464
    intrauterine insemination after, two regimens, 462
  metastases in stage IB cervical carcinoma, 332
  non-responsive, and ovulation induction with GH/gonadotropin, 229
  polycystic (*see* Polycystic, ovarian syndrome)
  stromal tissue, increased steroid production by, in postmenopausal women with endometrial cancer, 311
  syndrome
    postmenopausal palpable, 329
    resistant, and immunoglobulins, 388
  tubo-ovarian abscess drainage, percutaneous, 368
  tumors
    borderline, DNA cytophotometry and prognosis in, 331
    borderline, risk factors for, 345
    borderline, treatment impact, 333
    frozen section diagnosis in, accuracy of, 336
    of low malignant potential, retroperitoneal lymphatic involvement in, 337
    of low malignant potential, stage III, cisplatin in, 307

mucinous, with pseudomyxoma peritonei, 335
Ovulation
cycles
clomiphene and spontaneous, cervical mucus score and in vitro sperm interaction in, 443
gonadotropin-stimulated, human menopausal, effect of luteal phase support with hCG, 454
unstimulated, in vitro fertilization in, 474
induction in polycystic ovary syndrome
follicular aspiration for, ultrasound-guided, 451
gonadotropin for, 452
gonadotropin for, low-dose, 450
induction in women with non-responsive ovaries, GH/gonadotropin for, 449
superovulation (*see* Superovulation)
Oxygen
hyperbaric, in carbon monoxide intoxication in pregnancy, 27
Oxygenation
at birth, effect on fetal metabolism (in sheep), 29
Oxytocin
secretion in labor, 10

P

Paget's disease
of nipple, 578
Palsy
cerebral (*see* Cerebral palsy)
Pancreatitis
hypertriglyceridemia-induced, during pregnancy, 79
Papanicolaou smear
borderline results, long-term follow-up, 294
cytobrush for, during pregnancy, 293
endocervical glandular atypia in, 295
hyperkeratosis on, 294
Papilloma
breast, mammography of, 543
Papillomavirus
-associated minor cervical dysplasia, management of, 300
infection
after borderline Pap smear, 294
polymerase chain reaction-detected, 296
Wellferon in, 297
vulvar carcinoma and, 352
Paracetamol
absorption technique for gastric emptying in postpartum period, 204
Paraffin
-embedded sections, DNA from, in linkage analysis in familial retinoblastoma, 187
Para-urethral
collagen implantation for stress incontinence, 283
Parents
college-educated, and infant mortality, 33
Parturition (*see* Labor)
Parvovirus
B19 infection causing nonimmune hydrops fetalis, intrauterine transfusion in, 239
Pathology
molecular, in diagnosis of herpes simplex infection of placenta, 128
Pelvimetry
x-ray vs. CT, 178
Pelvis
abscesses, ultrasound-guided transvaginal drainage of, 367
fetal-pelvic index in estimation of fetal-pelvic disproportion, 174
fluids collections, ultrasound-guided transvaginal drainage of, 367
inflammatory disease
acute, long-term sequelae of, 366
clindamycin/gentamicin vs. cefoxitin/doxycycline in, 370
findings during inpatient treatment, 365
IUDs and, 497
self-reported, in U.S., 364
trends in hospitalizations and office visits, 361
muscle exercise (*see* Kegel exercise)
Penicillin
/erythromycin, intrapartum, for group B streptococcus, 83
Percutaneous
balloon mitral valvotomy during pregnancy, 100
drainage of tubo-ovarian abscesses, 368
Pereyra bladder neck suspension
modified, for stress incontinence, outcome of, 273
Perimenopausal woman
how to treat, xxiv-xxxvi
Perinatal
care and cerebral palsy in low birth weight infants, 214
hepatitis B virus infection, maternal transmission of, 211

HIV infection
IgA antibody detection in, early 229
in siblings and twins, 103
impact of anaerobic coverage for intra-amniotic infection, 57
mortality and aspirin in prevention of hypertensive pregnancy, 47
outcome in renal transplant recipients, 114
sepsis, fetal monitoring in, 157
Perineal
hematoma due to congenital coagulopathies, 84
Perioperative patients
fever evaluation in, blood cultures in, 261
Peritoneal
(*See also* Intraperitoneal)
oocyte and sperm transfer, transvaginal, for nontubal infertility, 476
Periventricular
hemorrhage in very low birth weight infants, incidence and outcome, 228
Pethidine
in labor, computerized analysis of fetal heart rate after, 149
Phenylpropanolamine
for stress incontinence, in elderly, 279
Phosphate
intraperitoneal chromic, in early ovarian carcinoma, 340
Phosphorus
magnetic resonance spectroscopy in prediction of birth asphyxia outcome, 123
Photocoagulation
laser, of polycystic ovaries, laparoscopic lysis of adhesions after, effect on pregnancy rates, 453
Phyllodes
tumor (*see* Cystosarcoma, phyllodes of breast)
Physiatric
management of limb deficiencies after prenatal cocaine exposure, 185
Physical
examination of palpable breast cysts after aspiration, 543
Physicians
improving clinical breast examination by, 587
Pipelle
endometrial sampling device vs. Novak curette, 313
Pituitary
enlargement with suprasellar extension in functional hyperprolactinemia due to lactatroph hyperplasia, 393
Placenta
accreta, sonography in, 71
bed spiral arteries in hypertensive disorders of pregnancy, 104
blood flow and combined ventricular output in fetus, 25
circulation (*see* Circulation, fetal-placental)
herpes simplex virus infection of, 128
hydropic, flow cytometric study of, 346
-mediated treatment of fetal supraventricular tachycardia and hydrops fetalis, 237
uteroplacental blood flow resistance in second trimester, Doppler studies of, 155
Platelet
-activating factor binding sites in myometrium, role in uterine contraction, 9
Platinum
based chemotherapy in stage I ovarian epithelial carcinoma, 339
CIS- (*see* Cisplatin)
Pneumonia
varicella, in pregnancy, acyclovir for, 113
Pneumothorax
after aspiration of breast, fine-needle, 553
Polychemotherapy
in breast cancer, early 582
Polycystic
ovarian syndrome
breast cancer and, 569
clomiphene/dexamethasone in, 448
laser photocoagulation in, laparoscopic lysis of adhesions after, effect on pregnancy rates, 453
ovulation induction in (*see* Ovulation, induction in polycystic ovary syndrome)
wedge resection in, long-term follow-up, 395
Polydrug
/cocaine use in pregnancy, two-year follow-up, 226
Polymerase chain reaction
amplification of pooled cells from screened blood donations for HIV-1, 77
for DNA from paraffin-embedded sections in familial retinoblastoma, 187
for HIV replication during first weeks of life, 214

papillomavirus infection detected by, 296
Polyps
endometrial, postmenopausal bleeding from, after tamoxifen therapy, 314
Postmenopausal
bleeding from endometrial polyps due to tamoxifen, 314
bone loss (*see* Bone, loss, postmenopausal)
estrogen therapy (*see* Estrogen, replacement therapy, postmenopausal)
hormone replacement therapy (*see* Hormone, replacement therapy, postmenopausal)
osteoporosis (*see* Osteoporosis, postmenopausal)
palpable ovary syndrome, 329
progestogen (*see* Progestogen, /estrogen replacement therapy, postmenopausal)
women
adnexal cysts in, simple, 245
asymptomatic, ultrasound screening for ovarian cancer in, 326
endometrial cancer in, and increased steroid production by ovarian stromal tissue, 311
tamoxifen effects on cardiovascular risk factors in, 583
Postnatal
HIV transmission from mother to infant, 221
Postpartum
(*See also* Puerperium)
fertility return monitored by enzyme immunoassay for salivary progesterone, 386
flare in juvenile rheumatoid arthritis symptoms, 96
hemorrhage due to congenital coagulopathies, 84
multiple sclerosis relapse, 96
period, gastric emptying in, 204
thyroid dysfunction, T-cell etiology for, 73
Prazosin
stress incontinence due to, 265
Prednisolone
/aspirin for recurrent aborters with antiphospholipid antibody, 511
Preeclampsia
albumin infusions in, 64
cesarean section in, and anesthesia, 180
endomyocardial ultrastructural findings in, 39
lipid peroxide/vitamin E imbalance in, 48
nitroprusside in, 90
severe, in second trimester, 111
tromboxane/prostacyclin imbalance in, 48
untreated, central hemodynamics in, 86
uteroplacental Doppler scan in screening for, second trimester, 155
Pregnancy
angiotensin converting enzyme inhibitors in, fetal and neonatal effects of, 198
antiepileptic drug concentrations during, plasma, 55
antiphospholipid antibodies and, 514
breathlessness and inspiratory effort in, 13
calcium supplementation in, 35
carbon monoxide intoxication in, hyperbaric oxygen in, 27
cervical cancer in, invasive, maternal and fetal outcome after, 306
chlamydial tests in, rapid, comparison of three, 372
cocaine use during (*see* Cocaine, use during pregnancy)
cytobrush during, efficacy and safety of, 293
Doppler regurgitant flow velocities during, 22
drug use in, two-year follow-up, 226
early
flow velocity waveforms in, fetal and umbilical, 159
occult IUD retrieval in, ultrasound-guided, 499
termination, Mifepristone or vacuum aspiration in, 512
ectopic
laparoscopic treatment (*see* Laparoscopy, ectopic pregnancy treatment by)
methotrexate in, transvaginal intratubal, 528
ovarian hyperstimulation and, controlled, 518
risk factors in, 517
screening for, endovaginal color flow imaging in, 522
screening for, single serum progesterone measurement vs. serial serum hCG for, 520
surgery for, methotrexate for persistent trophoblast after, 524
treatment of, nonsurgical, inclusion criteria for, 519

femoral vein in, common duplex ultrasound of, 205
high risk, Doppler flow velocity waveforms in, 153
HIV infection in, zidovudine for, 75
HIV transmission from mother to child in (*see* HIV, transmission, mother-to-child)
in hyperprolactinemic women, long-term effects of, 392
hypertension during (*see* Hypertension, during pregnancy)
hypertensive disorders of (*see* Hypertensive, disorders of pregnancy)
hyperthyroidism in, and maternal hemodynamics, 101
immunosuppression in, lymphocyte-initiated, 73
multiple, prenatal diagnosis in, 132
multiple sclerosis relapse during, 96
natural killer cell activity in, effect of RU 486 on, 14
outcome
  Ebstein's anomaly and, 97
  after mosaicism diagnosis in chorionic villus sampling, 137
ovarian tumors and, borderline, 346
pancreatitis during, hypertriglyceridemia-induced, 79
pathologic, early predictors of, 509
planned, after use of Norplant capsules, Norplant II rods, or IUDs, 501
penumonia in, varicella, acyclovir for, 113
post-term, labor induction vs. serial antenatal monitoring in, 34
prorenin and, 23
rates
  after intrauterine insemination, effect of controlled ovarian hyperstimulation on, 464
  after intrauterine insemination and multiple follicular recruitment, 463
  after laparoscopic lysis of adhesions due to laser photocoagulation of polycystic ovaries, 453
  luteal phase support with hCG during hMG-stimulated cycles and, 454
  in superovulated women after intrauterine insemination, intraperitoneal insemination, or natural intercourse, 470
respiratory gas relationships between uterine and umbilical veins in, 20
rheumatoid arthritis and, juvenile, 95
second trimester
  amniotic fluid estriol, dehydroepiandrosterone sulphate, and human chorionic gonadotropin levels in Down's syndrome, 138
  α-fetoprotein levels at, maternal serum, 142
  preeclampsia in, severe, 111
  uteroplacental blood flow resistance in, Doppler studies of, 155
shunts and, cerebrospinal fluid, 68
streptococci in, group B, rapid screening test for, 52
third trimester, autoantibodies in, 94
thrombocytopenic purpura in, immune, management of, 81
tubal, salpingitis isthmica nodasa in, 439
twin, fetal toxicity from maternal indomethacin in, 135
ureter in, sonographic visualization of, 58
valvotomy during, percutaneous balloon mitral, 100
vasopressin during, adrenocorticotropin and cortisol responses to (in baboon), 5
Premenstrual syndrome
  symptoms
    cyclical, spontaneous anovulation causing disappearance of, 529
    epidemiology of, 530
    mood-related, oral magnesium for, 532
Prenatal
  cocaine exposure (*see* Cocaine, use during pregnancy)
  diagnosis
    of cystic kidney disease, 190
    of cytomegalovirus infection, 124
    with fetal cells isolated from maternal blood by flow cytometry, 199
    in multiple gestation, 132
  echography positive for obstructive uropathy, predictive value of, 238
  monitoring (*see* Monitoring, fetal)
  social support to prevent preterm birth, 51
  thyrotropin-releasing hormone and glucocorticoid, respiratory disease in very low birth weight infant after, 219
Preterm
  birth (*see* Delivery, preterm)
  delivery (*see* Delivery, preterm)
  infant (*see* Infant, preterm)
  labor (*see* Labor, preterm)
  rupture of membranes, erythromycin therapy in, 31
Primrose oil

evening, in mastalgia, 540
Procainamide
in fetal supraventricular tachycardia and hydrops fetalis, 237
Progesterone
/estrogen replacement therapy
breast cancer and, xxxiii-xxxiv
does progesterone subtract from cardiovascular benefit of estrogen? xxii-xxvii
after hysterectomy, xxvii
receptor measurement in prognosis of operable breast cancer, 580
salivary
enzyme immunoassay monitoring, in return of postpartum fertility, 386
in luteal phase defect in habitual abortion, 505
serum
as early predictor of pathologic pregnancy, 509
single measurement in screening for ectopic pregnancy, 520
Progestogen
/estrogen
contraceptive vaginal ring, 503
replacement therapy, postmenopausal, continuous, endometrial histology and bleeding patterns 8 years after, 428
replacement therapy, postmenopausal, endometrial cancer and, 427
Prorenin
diabetes mellitus, pregnancy, and hypertension, 23
Prostacyclin
aspirin effects on, controlled-release, 17
/thromboxane imbalance in preeclampsia, 48
Prostaglandin
E concentrations, fetal, effect of glycemia on (in sheep), 12
Proteins
total, effect of Norplant implants on, 500
Pruritus
after sufentanil, 183
Pseudomyxoma
peritonei and mucinous ovarian tumors, 335
Psychological
adjustment after breast conservation vs. mastectomy, 574
barriers, influence on use of mammography, 565
factors in spontaneous abortion, 506
function in postmenopausal women, effect of estrogen on, 411
p24 antigen
for HIV replication during first weeks of life, 214
Puerperium
(*See also* Postpartum)
febrile morbidity in, diagnostic imaging in, 207
femoral vein in, common, duplex ultrasound of, 205
Pulmonary
disease, chronic, in very low birth weight infant after prenatal thyrotropin-releasing hormone and glucocorticoid, 219
hypertension, primary, in newborn after indomethacin in preterm labor, 44
hypoplasia, fetal and neonatal, after angiotensin converting enzyme inhibitors in pregnancy, 198
Purpura
thrombocytopenic, immune, in pregnancy, management of, 81
Pyrrolidone carboxylic acid
for premenstrual mood changes, 532

Q

Quality of life
after breast conservation vs. mastectomy, 574
QUIDEL
EIA test for group B streptococci in pregnancy, 52

R

Race
breast cancer screening behaviors and attitudes and, 566
infant mortality and college-educated parents, 33
pelvic inflammatory disease and, self-reported, 364
preterm delivery and, 65
Radiophosphorus
intraperitoneal, in early ovarian carcinoma, 340
Radiotherapy
of breast cancer
early-stage, node-positive, 575
intraductal, 571
primary, nonmetastatic, 601
stage I or II, underutilization of, 573

cervical carcinoma recurrence after, cervicovaginal cytology in detection of, 308
of endometrial carcinoma, 318
of ovarian tumors, borderline, 334
Reagin
test, rapid plasma, for syphilis, 231
Reconstruction
breast, immediate, selection criteria for, 570
Regurgitant
flow velocities, Doppler, during pregnancy, 22
Relatives
of women with breast cancer, breast cancer screening among, 593
Renal (*see* Kidney)
Renin
system, greater, 23
Renovascular
hypertension during pregnancy, 41
Respiratory
disease in very low birth weight infants after prenatal thyrotropin-releasing hormone and glucocorticoid, 219
function in severe gestational proteinuric hypertension, 80
gas relationships between uterine and umbilical veins in pregnancy, 20
Retardation
growth (*see* Growth, retardation, intrauterine)
mental (*see* Mental, retardation)
Retinoblastoma
familial, DNA from paraffin-embedded sections in linkage analysis in, 187
Retroperitoneal
lymphatic involvement with ovarian tumors, 337
Rheumatoid
arthritis, juvenile, and pregnancy, 95
Ritodrine
in preterm labor, 44
RPR test
for syphilis, 231
RU 486
effect on natural killer cell activity in pregnancy, 14
in termination of early pregnancy, 513
Runners
amenorrheic, total body bone density in, 387
Rupture of membranes
preterm premature, erythromycin therapy in, 31
at term, spontaneous, microbial invasion in amniotic cavity in, 60
Russell's viper venom time
dilute, in detection of lupus anticoagulants, 507

S

Salivary
progesterone (*see* Progesterone, salivary)
Salpingitis
isthmica nodasa in infertility and tubal diseases, 439
as risk factor for ectopic pregnancy, 517
Sarcoma
uterus, cisplatin in, 322
Sclerosis
multiple, relapse during pregnancy, 96
Scrub-time
surgical, optimum duration of, 258
Self-examination
breast, in relatives of women with breast cancer, 593
Self-referred
mammography patients, 558
Semen
adenosine triphosphate in, and fertility prediction, 440
Sensorineural
deafness due to congenital cytomegalovirus infection, 232
Sepsis
perinatal, fetal monitoring in, 157
Serological test
HIV-IgA, in early diagnosis of perinatal HIV infection, 229
maternal vs. newborn, for syphilis, 230
Sexually
transmitted diseases
barrier contraceptives and, 360
threat of, response of American women to, 533
Shock
toxic shock syndrome, IV immunoglobulin in, 381
Shoulder
dystocia (*see* Dystocia)
Shunt
cerebrospinal fluid, and pregnancy, 68
Siblings
perinatally exposed, HIV-1 infection in, 103
Silicone
breast models, training health professionals in breast examination with, 587
Small for gestation
fetuses, relation of fetal blood gases and computer analysis of fetal heart rate patterns in, 146

Smear
  Papanicolaou (*see* Papanicolaou smear)
Smoking
  cervical cancer and, 305
  menopause transition and, 409
  oral contraceptives and myocardial infarction, 489
  osteoporosis and, postmenopausal, xxix
  papillomavirus infection and cervical cancer, 297
  during pregnancy, two-year follow-up, 227
Social
  support, antenatal, in prevention of preterm birth, 51
Socioeconomic
  status and mammography use, 565
Sonography (*see* Ultrasound)
Spectroscopy
  magnetic resonance, phosphorus, in prediction of outcome after birth asphyxia, 123
Sperm
  concentration, normal, relevance of adenosine triphosphate in semen in fertility prediction in men with, 440
  fresh vs. frozen, in therapeutic donor insemination, 445
  mucus interaction in clomiphene cycles, 443
  transvaginal peritoneal oocyte and sperm transfer for nontubal infertility, 476
Spiral arteries
  placental bed, in hypertensive disorders of pregnancy, 104
Spironolactone
  in hirsutism, 397
Sponge
  contraceptive, and sexually transmitted diseases, 361
Squamous
  differentiation in endometrial carcinoma, 317
ST
  segment depression during cesarean section under regional anesthesia, 169
Stamey suspension
  transvaginal ultrasound and urodynamic evaluation after, 276
  urethrovesical position and mobility after, 278
Staphylococcus
  saprophyticus urinary tract infection, norfloxacin in, 291
Stem cells
  fetal liver, in-utero transplantation into fetuses, 235
Stents
  ureteral, for iatrogenic ureteral injury during surgery, 257
Stereotactic
  needle-core biopsy of nonpalpable breast lesions, 555, 556
Sterilization
  tubal
    ovarian cancer after, 324
    as risk factor for ectopic pregnancy, 517
Steroid
  hormone receptors, effect on prognosis in operable breast cancer, 580
  production increase by ovarian stromal tissue of postmenopausal women with endometrial cancer, 311
Stones
  gallstones after oral contraceptives and non-contraceptive estrogens, 484
Streptococci
  group B
    neonatal infections and, 82
    in pregnancy, rapid screening test for, 52
Streptococcus
  pyogenes toxin causing toxic shock syndrome, IV immunoglobulin in, 381
Stress
  incontinence (*see* Incontinence, urinary, stress)
Stroke
  postmenopausal estrogen therapy and, 423
  volume and hyperthyroid pregnancy, 102
Stromal
  overgrowth as predictor of metastatic potential of breast cystosarcoma phyllodes, 547
  tissue, ovarian, increased steroid production by, in postmenopausal women with endometrial cancer, 311
Subdural
  hemorrhage, tentorial, in newborn, 224
Subfertile
  males, ejaculatory duct obstruction in, 441
Suburban setting
  cocaine use in, maternal, 223
Sufentanil
  /bupivacaine epidural analgesia during labor, and instrumental deliveries, 183

Superovulation
comparison of intrauterine insemination, intraperitoneal insemination, and natural intercourse after, 470
in infertility, unexplained, 469
with intrauterine insemination, comparison to in vitro fertilization and gamete intrafallopian transfer, 468
Support
antenatal social, in prevention of preterm birth, 51
Supraventricular
tachycardia, fetal, and hydrops fetalis, 237
Surecell chlamydial EIA
vs. Clearview, 372
Surgery
fetal, for cleft lip, 236
gynecologic (*see* Gynecologic, surgery)
obstetric, iatrogenic injury to ureter during, 256
scrub-time, optimum duration of, 258
Syntocinon
in labor, computerized analysis of fetal heart rate after, 149
Syphilis
serologic tests for, maternal vs. newborn, 230
trends in 1980s, 357
vulvar carcinoma and, 352

T

Tachycardia
supraventricular, fetal, and hydrops fetalis, 237
Tamoxifen
in breast cancer
contralateral primary tumors after, 598
early, 582
postmenopausal bleeding from endometrial polyps due to, 314
in postmenopausal women, effects on cardiovascular risk factors, 583
Taxol
in ovarian cancer, epithelial, 344
T cell
etiology for postpartum thyroid dysfunction, 73
Teaching
status, hospital, influence on cesarean birth rate, 175
Tentorial
subdural hemorrhage, in newborn, 224
Testosterone
/estradiol implants in prevention of postmenopausal bone loss, 422
Testpack chlamydial EIA
vs. Clearview and Surecell, 372
T_4
index, free, in hyperthyroid pregnancy, 102
Thalassemia
α-, and X-linked mental retardation syndrome, 195
major, fetal, in-utero transplantation of fetal liver stem cells in, 235
Thermal
injury zones in loop electrical vs. laser cervical excisional conization, 302
Thrombocytopenic purpura
immune, in pregnancy, management of, 81
Thromboembolism
venous, and oral contraceptives, 490
Thromboplastin
time, partial, in detection of lupus anticoagulants, 507
Thrombosis
lupus erythematosus and miscarriage, 507
venous, and estrogen replacement therapy, 426
Thromboxane
A_2, effects of controlled-release aspirin on, 17
in fetal-placental circulation, effect of nitric oxide on vasoconstrictor effects of, 18
/prostacyclin imbalance in preeclampsia, 48
release and action, effect on endothelin-1-induced vasoconstriction, 59
Thyroid
dysfunction, postpartum, T-cell etiology for, 73
Thyrotropin
-releasing hormone, prenatal, respiratory disease in very low birth weight infant after, 219
Thyroxine
index, free, in hyperthyroid pregnancy, 102
Tissue
sections, paraffin-embedded, DNA from, in linkage analysis in familial retinoblastoma, 187
Tobacco (*see* Smoking)
Tomography, computed (*see* Computed tomography)
Toxic

shock syndrome, IV immunoglobulin in, 381
Toxicity
fetal, of indomethacin for preterm labor, in twins, 135
Transcervical
ultrasound, endoluminal catheter-assisted, of embryo, 201
Transfer
gamete intrafallopian (*see* Gamete intrafallopian transfer)
gene, cystic fibrosis, in vivo, to airway epithelium, 240
transvaginal peritoneal oocyte and sperm, for nontubal infertility, 476
Transformation zone
histological differences between colposcopic-directed biopsy and loop excision of, 303
Transfusion
intrauterine
in hemolytic disease, fetal, 121
in hydrops fetalis due to parvovirus B19, 239
Transplantation
in-utero, of fetal liver stem cells into fetuses, 235
kidney, perinatal outcome in recipients of, 114
Transvaginal
intratubal methotrexate for ectopic pregnancy, 528
peritoneal oocyte and sperm transfer for nontubal infertility, 476
ultrasound (*see* Ultrasound, transvaginal)
Treponemal
antibody absorption test, fluorescent, for syphilis, 231
Triglyceride
levels
effect of Norplant implants on, 500
after oral contraceptives, long-term, 483
Trophoblast
persistent, after surgery for ectopic pregnancy, methotrexate for, 524
Trophoblastic disease
gestational
high-risk, EMA/CO regimen in, 347
risk factors for, 330
Tubal
diseases, salpingitis isthmica nodosa in, 439
gamaete intrafallopian transfer (*see* Gamete intrafallopian transfer)
intratubal methotrexate for ectopic pregnancy, 528
sterilization (*see* Sterilization, tubal)
Tubo-ovarian
abscess, percutaneous drainage of, 368
Tuboplasty
laparoscopic distal, 457
Tumor
breast (*see* Breast, tumor)
cervix (*see* Cervix, neoplasia), intraepithelial)
necrosis factor, decidua as source of, 26
ovaries (*see* Ovaries, tumors)
phyllodes (*see* Cystosarcoma, phyllodes of breast)
trophoblastic (*see* Trophoblastic disease, gestational)
vagina (*see* Vagina, neoplasia)
Turner syndrome
estrogen replacement therapy in, 389
Twins
fetal toxicity from maternal indomethacin in, 135
first-born, high risk for HIV-1 infection for, 50
infant mortality, in U.S., 133
perinatally exposed, HIV-1 infection in, 103

U

Ultrasound
of adnexal cysts, simple, in postmenopausal women, 245
breast
of cystosarcoma phyllodes, 549
of occult masses, 588
in women less than 35 years of age, 562
diagnosis of large for gestational age fetus at term, 173
Doppler
color, endovaginal, in screening for ectopic pregnancy, 522
color, and hysterosalpingography, 438
flow velocity waveforms (*see* Flow, velocity waveforms, Doppler)
of hemodynamic effects of hydralazine or labetalol in hypertensive pregnancy, 16
of umbilical artery as screening test for fetal well-being, 148
of uteroplacental blood flow resistance in second trimester, 155
duplex
of femoral vein, common, in pregnancy and puerperium, 205
in renovascular hypertension during pregnancy, 42

of embryo, endoluminal catheter-assisted transcervical, 201
-guided retrieval of occult IUD in early pregnancy, 499
hydrotubation vs. hysterosalpingography, 436
measurement
of fetal cardiac hemodynamics, reproducibility of, 158
in fetal-pelvic disproportion, 174
of omphalocele contents related to karyotypic abnormalities, 196
of ovarian cysts, 247
in placenta accreta, 71
in postmenopausal palpable ovary syndrome, 330
in prenatal diagnosis of cystic kidney disease, 190
in puerperal febrile morbidity, 207
in tentorial subdural hemorrhage diagnosis, in newborn, 224
transvaginal
-guided drainage of pelvic abscesses and fluid collections, 367
-guided drainage of tubo-ovarian abscesses, 368
-guided follicular aspiration for ovulation induction in polycystic ovary syndrome, 451
in incontinence, stress, 272
in ovarian cancer screening, in asymptomatic postmenopausal women, 326
in ovarian cancer screening, familial, 327
after suspension operations, 276
of ureter in pregnancy, 58
after urinary tract infections, recurrent, 267
Ultrastructural
findings, endomyocardial, in preeclampsia, 39
Umbilical
artery
flow velocity waveforms (*see under* Flow, velocity waveforms)
pulsatility index, acute response to fetal blood volume changes (in sheep), 141
resistance index as screening test for fetal well-being, 148
cord occlusion at birth, and fetal metabolism (in sheep), 29
Ureaplasma urealyticum
infection, amniotic fluid, and preterm labor, 66
Ureter
injury, iatrogenic, after gynecologic/obstetric surgery, 256
early repair of, 255
in pregnancy, sonographic visualization of, 58
Ureteroileocystostomy
for iatrogenic injury to ureter during gynecologic/obstetric surgery, 257
Ureteroneocystostomy
for iatrogenic injury to ureter during gynecologic/obstetric surgery, 257
Urethra
para-urethral collagen implantation for stress incontinence, 283
Urethrocystography
lateral
modified, in prediction of stress incontinence after vaginal repair, 274
vs. urodynamic assessment in incontinence, 268
Urethrovesical
junction position and mobility after suspension operations, 278
physiology, effect of hysterectomy on, 252
Urinary
incontinence (*see* Incontinence, urinary)
symptoms, adverse, after total abdominal hysterectomy, 289
tract infections
after ovarian cancer operations, 342
norfloxacin in, 290
recurrent, urologic investigation in, 267
Urodynamic
assessment
in genitourinary prolapse, 271
in incontinence, 269
in incontinence, vs. lateral urethrocystography, 268
after suspension operations, 276
Urography
excretory, after recurrent urinary tract infections, 267
Urologic
investigation in recurrent urinary tract infections, 267
Uropathy
fetal, clinical outcome of, 238
Uterus
(*See also* Intrauterine)
activity monitoring, home (*see* Monitoring, uterine activity, home)
adenosarcoma, study of, 321
bleeding (*see* Bleeding, uterine)
carcinoma, papillary serous, 319

contraction, role of platelet-activiting factor binding sites in myometrium in, 9
-placental blood flow resistance in second trimester, Doppler studies of, 155
sarcoma, cisplatin in, 322
venous drainage of, 20
Uveitis
anterior, during pregnancy, in juvenile rheumatoid arthritis patients, 96

V

Vacuum
aspiration in termination of early pregnancy, 512
delivery, long-term effects of, 163
Vagina
(*See also* Transvaginal)
adenocarcinoma, diethylstilbestrol-associated clear cell, risk factors for, 350
carcinoma, invasive, upper vaginectomy in, 349
cytology in detection of recurrent cervical carcinoma after radiotherapy, 308
hysterectomy via, and oophorectomy, 254
neoplasia, grade 3 intraepithelial
laser vaporization of, 348
vaginectomy in, upper, 349
repair, prediction of stress incontinence after, 274
ring, estrogen/progestogen contraceptive, 503
secretions, fetal fibronectin in, as predictor of preterm delivery, 36
vault prolapse, surgical management of, 254
Vaginectomy
upper, in invasive vaginal carcinoma, 349
Vaginitis
candidal
treatment of, 375
yogurt in prevention of, 373
Vaginosis
bacterial
clindamycin cream vs. oral metronidazole, 377
clindamycin in preterm labor and, 45
metronidazole regimens in, 376
Valvotomy
mitral, percutaneous balloon, during pregnancy, 100
Vaporization
laser, of grade 3 vaginal intraepithelial neoplasia, 348
Varicella
pneumonia in pregnancy, acyclovir for, 113
Vascular
cardiovascular (*see* Cardiovascular)
renovascular hypertension during pregnancy, 41
resistance, systemic
in preeclampsia, 89
total peripheral, in hyperthyroid pregnancy, 102
Vasoconstriction
endothelin-1-induced, effect of thromboxane release and action on, 59
Vasoconstrictor
effects of thromboxane and endothelin in fetal-placental circulation, attenuation by nitric oxide, 18
Vasodilation
verapamil, effect on respiratory function in severe gestational proteinuric hypertension, 80
Vasography
in ejaculatory duct obstruction in subfertile males, 442
Vasopressin
during pregnancy, adrenocorticotropin and cortisol responses to (in baboon), 5
Vein
femoral, common, duplex ultrasound in pregnancy and puerperium, 205
Venous
drainage of uterus, 20
thromboembolism and oral contraceptives, 490
thrombosis and estrogen replacement therapy, 426
Ventilation
at birth, effect on fetal metabolism (in sheep), 29
Ventricle
dimension, left maternal, and fetal growth retardation, 122
function, hyperdynamic left, in preeclampsia, 90
intraventricular hemorrhage in preterm infant, effect of cesarean section on, 168
output, combined fetal, and placental blood flow, 25
perinventricular hemorrhage in very low birth weight infants, incidence and outcome, 228

supraventricular tachycardia, fetal, and hydrops fetalis, 237
Verapamil
effect on respiratory function in severe gestational proteinuric hypertension, 80
Vertebral
bone density after hormone replacement therapy, effects of plasma estradiol levels on, 422
Vesicovaginal
fistula after hysterectomy, early repair of, 256
Videolaseroscopy
for oophorectomy, 248
Villus
chorionic (*see* Chorionic, villus)
Vincristine
in gestational trophoblastic tumors, 347
Virus
cytomegalovirus (*see* Cytomegalovirus)
hepatitis B virus infection, perinatal, maternal transmission of, 211
herpes simplex virus infection of placenta, 128
immunodeficiency, human (*see* HIV)
papillomavirus (*see* Papillomavirus)
parvovirus B19 infection causing nonimmune hydrops fetalis, intrauterine transfusion in, 239
Visits
office, for pelvic inflammatory disease, 361
Vitamin
D and postmenopausal osteoporosis, xxviii
E/lipid peroxide imbalance in preeclampsia, 48
supplementation in prevention of neural tube defects, 193
Voiding
difficulties after surgical management of vaginal vault prolapse, 255
Volume
expansion, effect on respiratory function in severe gestational proteinuric hypertension, 80
von Willebrand's disease
obstetric and gynecological problems in, 84
Vulva
carcinoma (*see* Carcinoma, vulva)
nevi, dysplastic, 351

W

Weight
adolescent, and diethylstilbestrol-associated clear cell vaginal adenocarcinoma, 351
birth
infant mortality in cesarean section and, 164
low (*see* Low birth weight infant)
shoulder dystocia and cesarean section, 127
Well-being
fetal, umbilical artery resistance index as screening test for, 148
Wellferon
in papillomavirus infection, 297
White
blood cell count, amniotic fluid, 109
Wolff-Parkinson-White syndrome
pregnancy outcome and, 98
Wound
infection, midline laparotomy, effect of electrocautery on (in rat), 259

X

X-linked
mental retardation syndrome associated with α thalassemia, 195
X-ray
pelvic measurement, Colcher-Sussman, 175
pelvimetry vs. CT pelvimetry, 178

Y

Yogurt
in prevention of candidal vaginitis, 373

Z

Zacharin procedure
for vaginal vault prolapse, 254
Zidovudine
in HIV infection in pregnancy, 75

Author Index

A

Aaby P, 225
Aartsen E, 342
Abdeen N, 557
Abell KB, 138
Abner AL, 575
Abrams P, 283
Abuzeid MI, 472
Abuzeid MIM, 468
Achard JM, 79
Adamson GD, 445
Adashek JA, 171
Addison WA, 365
Advani H, 317
Adzick NS, 236
Ahlgren M, 517
Ajzen SA, 58
Aksu T, 453
Alford CA, 119
Allen GJ, 58
Alnaser HMI, 452
Alperstein P, 373
Altieri LA, 522
Alvarez F, 494, 496, 501
Amos CI, 50
Anders GJPA, 137
Andersen RN, 521
Anderson GD, 168
Anderson RJ, 228
Anderson RL, 132
Anderson S, 589
Andersson I, 543
Andersson K, 430
Andronikou AD, 436
Ang MS, 182
Angeid-Backman E, 543
Anthony J, 80, 104
Anton H, 268
Anyaegbunam A, 71
Aral SO, 364
Arduini D, 107
Arheart KL, 168
Arps H, 331
Askergren J, 598
Asperilla MO, 113
Atanasoff P, 295
Atrash HK, 164
Atri M, 528
Austin DF, 410
Averette HE, 325
Avila C, 60, 109
Awobuluyi M, 336
Ayres NA, 135

B

Bäckström T, 529
Bada HS, 168
Badell A, 185
Badenoch DF, 255
Badger GJ, 434
Baggish MS, 302
Bagshawe KD, 347
Bairnsfather LE, 448
Baka JJ, 207
Baker JR Jr, 14
Balbi L, 64
Baldwin W, 533
Balen A, 476
Ballard PL, 219
Ballard RA, 219
Barash F, 302
Barden E, 503
Bargon J, 240
Barkovich AJ, 212
Barreto J, 344
Barrett JM, 293
Barrett-Connor E, 412, 426
Barry W, 381
Barton JR, 39
Basili S, 507
Bassett LW, 554, 562, 563
Bastert G, 268
Battaglia FC, 20
Baumann R, 398
Bawdon R, 57
Bayani N, 94
Bazin B, 40
Bazubagira A, 221
Beaufils M, 40
Becerra JW, 164
Beck RP, 284
Beeby AR, 158
Beecham J, 322
Beecham JB, 307
Beekhuis JR, 137
Beex LVAM, 594
Begent RHJ, 347
Behnke E, 10, 60
Belfort MA, 80
Belinson JL, 319
Belizán JM, 42
Bell DA, 295
Bell SG, 13
Bembi B, 238
Benedetti TJ, 98, 101
Benedetto C, 64
Bengtsson G, 524
Ben-Hur H, 351
Bennett A, 251
Bennett B, 259
Benraad TJ, 594
Benussi G, 238
Beral V, 323, 481
Berchuck A, 340
Bergel E, 42
Berkowitz RL, 124, 173
Berkowitz RS, 346
Berkus MD, 127
Bernardi S, 96
Bernardus RE, 471
Bernstein MR, 346
Bertollini R, 96
Bertrand F, 186
Besinger RE, 44
Beute BJ, 585
Bewley S, 155
Bhan V, 327
Bhatia NN, 271
Biancalana V, 188
Bianchi C, 459
Bianchi S, 459
Biggar RJ, 50
Billaud L, 455
Birmann B, 486
Björses U-M, 505
Blake PR, 320
Blamey RW, 578
Blandy JP, 255
Blankenberg F, 539
Blessing JA, 322
Blickstein I, 351
Blumenfeld D, 271
Blumenfeld S, 188
Bocciolone L, 330, 459
Bohlin A-B, 78
Boike GM, 325
Bolaji II, 386
Bolas NM, 123
Boll TJ, 119
Boltz NL, 445
Bonavita MS, 507
Bonduelle M, 400
Bonfiglio T, 307
Bongard FS, 261
Booth M, 323
Borella P, 532
Borenstein MT, 373
Bornstein BA, 571
Borstad E, 274
Boué J, 188
Boulos R, 229
Bounds W, 503
Bourne TH, 327
Bowes WA Jr, 145
Boyer P, 75
Boylan P, 170
Boys RJ, 22
Bozzetti P, 20
Brache V, 494, 496, 501
Bracken M, 219
Bradle P, 228
Brady M, 203
Brady MF, 321
Braga SLN, 100
Braly PS, 245
Brambilla DJ, 409
Brateng D, 41
Brateng DA, 98
Breart G, 40
Breed ASPM, 137
Bret P, 528
Brewer AS, 18, 59
Brewer WH, 588
Brideau N-A, 405
Brienza RS, 487
Brink CA, 279
Britt WJ, 119
Brockman DE, 18, 59

Bromberg K, 230
Brooks M, 302
Brown B, 173
Brown E, 295
Brown JM, 97
Brown WA, 532
Bruhat MA, 457, 523
Bruskewitz R, 273
Bryce RL, 51
Bryman I, 524
Buchberger W, 549
Bukovsky I, 256
Bump RC, 280
Bundy BN, 307, 317, 332
Burgio KL, 264
Burke BJ, 556
Burke TW, 353
Burns WN, 462
Buscaglia M, 20
Busch MP, 77
Buster JE, 521
Butz A, 229
Buyalos RP, 509
Buytaert Ph, 537
Byrd EW, 7
Byrn F, 434
Byrne DL, 303
Byrne J, 410

C

Cahill DJ, 468, 472
Calder AA, 400
Caldwell E, 128
Cameron L, 583
Campbell AA, 533
Campbell HS, 587
Campbell S, 155, 327, 476
Campbell WG Jr, 23
Campodonico L, 42
Canavese C, 64
Candiani GB, 459
Canick J, 138
Canis M, 457, 523
Cao L, 213
Capitant C, 40
Cardenosa G, 543
Carey MP, 278
Carlson KC, 98
Carlson KL, 101
Carmichael JA, 300, 338
Carmina E, 396
Caroline DF, 207
Carr BR, 7
Carriaga M, 576
Cartier MS, 522
Caruso R, 108
Casal D, 36
Caselli D, 103
Casola G, 367, 368
Casper RF, 463
Caspi E, 256, 288
Cassell GH, 60
Cates W Jr, 364
Cathomas G, 124
Cavanagh D, 348, 349
Cavioni V, 392
Cedermark B, 598
Cefalo RC, 81
Cenaiko DF, 13
Cerami A, 26
Cetin I, 20
Cha SS, 339
Chappatte OA, 303
Chapron C, 523
Chasnoff IJ, 226
Chastang C, 27
Chen J-H, 360, 497
Chiari S, 345
Child AG, 92
Chiumello G, 389
Cho AMW, 204
Christiaens GCML, 401
Christiansen C, 414
Christiansen OB, 508
Chu J, 427
Chutivongse S, 358
Chvapil M, 259
Chvapil TA, 259
Claes H, 269
Clark GM, 581
Clarke RJ, 17
Clarke-Pearson DL, 340
Clatterbaugh HE, 223
Cobin RH, 73
Cohen HS, 228
Cohn-Cedermark G, 548
Coker AL, 480
Colditz GA, 423, 544
Cole DD, 600
Cole P, 350
Coleman CN, 575
Coleman P, 180
Collins A, 136
Collins WP, 327
Colliver D, 503
Come SE, 575
Connelly RR, 410
Connolly JL, 544, 575
Conway WF, 588
Cook CM, 160
Cook RL, 81
Cooper D, 155
Cooperberg PL, 58
Coppens M, 537
Corbett G, 258
Corley D, 314
Corwin M, 152
Coste J, 506, 518
Cottington E, 65
Cotton DB, 54
Coulam CB, 433, 438
Coutinho E, 494
Covino JM, 369
Cowell CA, 463
Cowell JK, 187
Crandall BF, 201
Crary WG, 411
Creasman WT, 332
Creasy RK, 219
Creighton SM, 254
Cristo M, 411
Critchley JAJH, 204
Crona N, 395
Crook D, 483
Croquette M-F, 188
Crosignani PG, 392, 469
Cross MA, 571
Crum CP, 352
Crystal AM, 249
Crystal RG, 240
Cuckle HS, 138
Curtis MT, 314
Cusack TJ, 228
Czajkowski J, 78
Czernobilsky B, 351

D

Dabis F, 221
Daffos F, 124
D'Agostino HB, 367, 368
Dahlgren E, 395
Dahrouge D, 366
Dalemans W, 240
Daling JR, 427, 485
Danon YL, 163
Darney P, 501
Datta S, 167
Daunter B, 308
D'Avanzo B, 484
Davenport D, 108
Davey DA, 104
David M, 53
Davidson AJ, 360
Davies TF, 73
Davis JC Jr, 85
Davis R, 296
Davison JM, 114
Dawes G, 148
Dawes GS, 144, 149
Dax J, 57
Day D, 157
Day NE, 560
de Cagny B, 79
DeCesare SL, 349
DeCherney AH, 246
Degendorfer P, 306
de Haan J, 141
De Jaegher K, 269
de Kretser DM, 383
Delgado G, 332
Deligdisch L, 36
DeLozier-Blanchet C, 188
de Martino M, 103
Dembo AJ, 333
de Meijer AJ, 342
DeMets DL, 583
Demopoulos R, 336
Demopoulos RI, 301, 335
De Muylder X, 269
Densem JW, 138
deParedes E, 600

DePriest PD, 326
Derome P, 393
Deutsch M, 589
Develioglu O, 453
Devlieger H, 183
Devor M, 426
Dgani R, 351
Dias F, 225
Diaz J, 494, 496
Diaz MM, 494
Diaz S, 494, 496, 501
Dick IM, 416
Dictor M, 78
Diepeveen DA, 153
Dietel M, 331
DiMaio T, 336
DiMarzo SJ, 464
DiMattina M, 509
Diokno AC, 279
Dische MR, 36
Ditkoff EC, 411
Dixon AR, 578
Dockter M, 199
Dodin S, 405
Dogliani M, 64
Doherty MG, 311
Dolk H, 186
Donaldson ES, 326
Donnelly JE, 97
Donta ST, 381
Doswell L, 403
D'Ottavio G, 238
Doubilet P, 25
Douglas JM, 360
Douglas JM Jr, 369
Dovey S, 418
Dowden RV, 570
Dowlatshahi K, 555
Drexhage H, 388
Drogendijk AC, 263
Duddy MJ, 205
Duff P, 259
Duffy SW, 560
Duggin GG, 92
Duliège A-M, 50
Dunlop W, 158
Dunnihoo DR, 448
Dupuy M, 393
Duse M, 103
Dwyer PL, 265, 278

E

Eadie MJ, 55
Easterling TR, 41, 98, 101
Eble BE, 77
Eckert LO, 182
Eckford SD, 283
Eddowes HA, 468, 472
Edge SB, 600
Edge V, 196
Egley CC, 145
Ehret JM, 369
Ehrnst A, 78
Eidelman A, 256
Ekholm U-B, 529
Eklund GW, 543
El-Harazy E, 73
Elias S, 199
Elkharrat D, 27
Ellis IO, 578
El Mahgoub S, 494
El Medjadji M, 94
Elston CW, 578
Emanuel D, 124
Emerson DS, 522
Engel BT, 264
Engstrom PF, 559
Enomoto K, 580
Epstein F, 68
Eschenbach DA, 66
Estape RE, 325
Esteves CA, 100
Estle L, 121
Ettinger B, 420
Evans J, 470

F

Facchinetti F, 532
Fagerberg G, 560
Fahy U, 472
Fahy UM, 468
Fairbank J, 249
Falcone T, 528
Falk Rj, 509
Fantl JA, 280
Farley TMM, 497
Fasoli M, 330
Faundes A, 494
Fears TR, 410
Fedele L, 459
Feigal D Jr, 426
Feldberg E, 351
Feldesman MR, 245
Feldman S, 455
Felker RE, 522
Felton S, 50
Ferenczy A, 304
Fernandez H, 506, 518, 519
Ferrante FM, 167
Ferriero DM, 212
Ferris DG, 372
Ferro D, 507
Fetter B, 321
Feyzi J, 583
Fianchino O, 64
Fick GH, 530
Field SK, 13
Fieschi C, 96
Filly RA, 196
Finan MA, 349
Fiorica JV, 348, 349
Fioroni L, 532
Firtion G, 213
Fischer WE, 92
Fisher B, 589
Fisher C, 546
Fisher ER, 589
FitzGerald GA, 17
Fitzgerald M, 249
Flaherty SP, 446
Flamigni C, 475
Fleming CF, 472
Fletcher SW, 587
Fliegner JR, 82
Forbes CD, 84
Ford WCL, 472
Forest J-C, 405
Forestier F, 124
Forss M, 312
Fottrell PF, 386
Fournier A, 79
Fourquet A, 571
Fowble BL, 571
Fowden AL, 12
Fowler CG, 255, 320
Fowler KB, 119
Fowler MG, 133
Fox HE, 75
Fox SA, 565
Frable WJ, 550, 552
France K, 373
Franceschi S, 309, 323, 484
Francis MM, 474
Francoual C, 213
Franke U, 331
Frankenfield-Chernicoff M, 223
Frankowski R, 170
Franks S, 450
Fraser C, 460
Free K, 308
Freedman LS, 576
Freier C, 226
French JI, 45, 157
Friedman AC, 207
Frierson HF Jr, 600
Frimodt-Møller C, 281
Frydman R, 519
Fuchs A-R, 10
Fujita S, 211
Fukayama M, 240
Fundarò C, 103
Fyles AW, 333

G

Gabiano C, 103
Gad A, 560
Gadir AA, 444, 452
Gagnon S, 304
Gahnem F, 23
Gail MH, 410
Gajdos P, 27
Gal D, 315
Galaid EI, 361
Gale R, 163
Galea MH, 578
Gall S, 152
Gallagher CJ, 320
Galli L, 103

Gallion HH, 326
Gammon MD, 569
Gannon MJ, 249
Ganz PA, 574
Garite TJ, 36
Garland SM, 82
Garner JB, 51
Garnett T, 422
Gateley CA, 540, 553
Gause S, 203
Gauthier R, 53
Gelman RS, 575
Genant HK, 420
Genazzani AR, 532
Gentile A, 484
Gershenson DM, 353
Gershman KA, 357
Getachew MM, 196
Geurts-Moespot A, 594
Geuze HJ, 401
Giacomelli A, 103
Giacomelli GJ, 175
Gibbons RJ, 195
Gibson M, 434
Giglio L, 238
Gilgenkrantz S, 188
Gillis GL, 279
Gilstrap LC III, 57
Gin T, 204
Giovangrandi Y, 124
Giuliano AE, 554, 563
Given HF, 258
Glandon GL, 175
Glas U, 598
Glassman LM, 509
Gliedman J, 317
Gloeb DJ, 75
Godfrey BM, 446
Godfrey RS, 570
Godsland IF, 483
Goedert JJ, 50
Goff BA, 295
Golan A, 256
Goland RS, 3, 5
Golbus MS, 132
Gold RH, 562, 563
Goldberg JD, 132, 196
Goldenberg SL, 58
Goldfien A, 530
Goldman ML, 41
Goldstein DP, 346
Goldstein M, 575
Goldstein RB, 196
Gonzalez L, 42
Goodacre BW, 367
Goodman RL, 571
Gore SM, 575
Gosink BB, 245
Gotfredsen A, 414
Goto S, 511
Gottschau A, 225
Granato PA, 52
Grandilli AM, 507
Grant A, 117
Grant EG, 201
Grant SS, 121, 131
Grasso MG, 96
Gray LA, 522
Gray M, 152
Green CE, 425
Green LM, 298
Green M, 376
Greene JW Jr, 39
Greenhalf JO, 249
Greer IA, 84
Gregory L, 470
Greven KM, 318
Griffith DR, 226
Griffith-Jones MD, 289
Grimes DA, 156
Grischke E-M, 268
Gröntoft O, 560
Groshen S, 596
Gross I, 219
Grunnet N, 508
Guarneri MP, 389
Guggino WB, 240
Guo J, 48
Gürgan T, 453
Gurioli L, 64
Gutin B, 387

H

Haan G, 471
Haarbo J, 414
Hagay Z, 109
Haglund A, 375
Hakala T, 312
Halabi S, 566
Halimi J-M, 23
Hallak M, 135, 237
Halsey N, 229
Hamilton-Fairley D, 450
Hammami M, 94
Hammarbäck S, 529
Hammers LW, 522
Hammill H, 75
Hanaoka S, 109
Handsfield HH, 369
Handwerker SM, 68
Hanigan WC, 228
Hannah ME, 34
Hannah WJ, 34
Hansen GC, 201
Hansen KA, 14
Hansen U, 439
Hanssens M, 198
Harada T, 451
Harboun C, 27
Harding R, 12
Harker CP, 368
Harnish DG, 296
Harper A, 16
Harris JR, 571, 575
Harris MM, 416
Harrison JK, 100
Harrison MR, 236
Harvey CJ, 168
Hasaart THM, 141
Hasegawa I, 511
Haspels AA, 401
Haverkamp A, 157
Hawkins RE, 546
Hayes CW, 588
Heads A, 158
Heaton J, 267
Hebert SA, 464
Heilbron D, 77
Heim K, 549
Heintz APM, 342
Heitz D, 188
Hellman J, 34
Henderson NK, 416
Henderson-Smart D, 92
Hendry WF, 441
Hennekens CH, 423
Henrion R, 213
Henson DE, 576
Herbert SH, 318
Herbold D, 317
Herndon JL, 593
Hertz J, 439
Heuvel JJTM, 594
Hewson S, 34
Hiett AK, 39
Higgs DR, 195
Hill GB, 365
Hillier SL, 66
Hilsenbeck S, 581
Hilton E, 373
Hines SE, 85
Hirata Y, 6
Hirschowitz L, 294
Hitimana D-G, 221
Hjalmar M-L, 598
Hobbins JC, 109
Hoek A, 388
Hoekstra JW, 276
Hoffman MS, 348, 349
Hoffman-Tretin JC, 71
Hofmeyr GJ, 436
Hogan PE, 318
Hogan WM, 314
Hogue CJR, 33, 164
Hohmann SF, 175
Holden L, 347
Holimon JL, 293
Hollander IN, 272
Hollanders JMG, 471
Holloway RW, 293
Holma P, 501
Holmes FF, 410
Holmes GF, 410
Holt EM, 249
Holt VL, 485
Homburg R, 449
Homesley H, 322
Hong MK, 425
Hook EW III, 369
Hope PL, 123
Hope-Stone HF, 320
Hopper KD, 556
Horan M, 209

Horbay GLA, 463
Horowitz LF, 301
Horvath JS, 92
Hoskins WJ, 328, 329
Houston AB, 169
How H, 152
Huang C-C, 224
Hudgins L, 381
Huff RW, 127
Hughes AO, 294
Hughes LE, 540
Huhta JC, 237
Huisman TWA, 159
Hulka BS, 480
Hull MGR, 468, 472
Hunter GC, 259
Hunter S, 22, 158
Hurt WG, 280
Hutter RVP, 585
Hutton N, 229

I

Iino H, 580
Ikeda DM, 543
Imperiale TF, 47
Infante-Rivard C, 53
Insunza A, 60
Irwin KL, 324
Isenberg HD, 373
Isozaki-Fukuda Y, 6
Ives NK, 123
Iwamoto HS, 29

J

Jackson GL, 566
Jackson R, 503
Jackson VP, 558
Jacobs HS, 449
Jain M, 298
Jalbert P, 188
Jamison SB, 167
Jannet D, 94
Janson PO, 395
Jars-Guincestre MC, 27
Järvinen H, 312
Jarvis GJ, 289
Jeffrey JF, 338
Jenkins BJ, 255
Jennings J, 148
JO , 249
Jobe WE, 556
Job-Spira J, 506
Job-Spira N, 518
Joensuu H, 592
Johansson B, 78
Johansson S, 395
Johnson CA, 294
Johnson CC, 487
Johnson JD, 272
Johnson JP, 85
Johnson JV, 462
Johnson P, 136
Johnson TRB, 44
Johnston DA, 182
Johnston JM, 9
Jokich PM, 555
Jones L, 36
Jordan VC, 583
Judson FN, 360

K

Kaban LB, 236
Kaelber A, 108
Kahn H, 407
Kahn MA, 335
Kaku T, 321
Kalisher L, 585
Kanazawa K, 511
Kaplan KM, 593
Karita E, 221
Karlan BY, 328
Kasumi F, 580
Katz VL, 81
Kayne HL, 152
Keefe D, 10
Keenan JA, 454
Keirse MJNC, 198
Keith RE, 35
Kelley JL III, 353
Kelly MJ, 273
Kennedy JF, 464
Kenney A, 303
Kern KA, 538
Kessel SS, 133
Keyes WG, 44
Khalife S, 528
Khayam-Bashi H, 77
Kiddy D, 450
Kiely JL, 133
Kienhuis CBM, 594
Kil PJM, 276
Killam WP, 142
Kimme-Smith C, 201
Kimura M, 580
King E, 559
Kinne DW, 596, 598
Kirby CA, 446
Kirk ME, 338
Kirkman RJE, 503
Kirschner MA, 398
Kirshon B, 54, 80
Kisnisci HA, 453
Kitchen WH, 220
Klaisle C, 501
Kleerekoper M, 487
Klein SR, 261
Klein TA, 14
Kleinman JC, 33, 133
Kline RL, 229
Klinger K, 199
Kluskens LF, 555
Knielsen K, 273
Knight KB, 35
Knutsson F, 395
Kobayashi Y, 6
Koch TK, 212
Koenders PG, 594
Koenigsberg M, 71
Kojima T, 6
Korach JM, 27
Korda AR, 92
Koren G, 306
Korones SB, 168
Korson R, 434
Koyama H, 580
Kratzert KJ, 68
Krepart GV, 338
Kretz C, 188
Krivine A, 213
Krohn MA, 66
Kryscio RJ, 326
Kujas M, 393
Kumagai SG, 259
Kurki T, 191
Kurman R, 317
Kurtz J, 571
Kuske R, 571
Kuttenn F, 455
Kvinesdal BB, 225
Kwok S, 77

L

Laatikainen T, 191
Labbok MH, 479
Lacarra M, 501
Lagasse LD, 328
Lage JM, 346
Lalau JD, 79
Lambert JS, 75
Lamensdorf H, 272
Lanciano RM, 318
Lander CM, 55
Lanes SF, 486
Langdon G, 18, 59
Langer O, 127
Langer R, 256, 288
Laor A, 163
Lapinski R, 173
LaPolla JP, 348
Lappöhn RE, 391
Laragh JH, 23
Lasry J-CM, 579
Latourette HB, 410
Latrous H, 94
Lau GSN, 204
Lauritsen JG, 508
Lauritzen E, 225
La Vecchia C, 309, 323, 330, 345, 484, 596
Layfield LJ, 554
Lazovich D, 573
Lazzarin A, 379
Leach GE, 273
Leake JF, 337
Leather A, 422
Leather AT, 428
Lebon P, 213

Lechat MF, 186
Lecocq J-P, 240
Lee JJ, 574
Lee KR, 319, 434
Lee NC, 324, 481
Leerentveld RAL, 471
Legarth J, 512
Lehtovirta P, 312
Lelaidier C, 519
Lelong F, 94
Lemay A, 405
Lenton EA, 383
Lentz SS, 339
Lepage P, 221
Lerman C, 559
Lesser ML, 598
Leventhal H, 583
Levi F, 309
Levin W, 333
Levine AB, 173
Lev-Toaff AS, 207
Lew JKL, 204
Li JY, 393
Lichtman S, 387
Liese BS, 294
Lietz H, 331
Lilley S, 169
Lin MC, 245
Lin S, 587
Lindblom B, 524
Lindgren S, 78
Lindstedt G, 395
Linell F, 543
Ling FW, 313, 521
Lishner M, 306
Lisse IM, 225
Little BB, 57
Liu T-H, 563
Livengood C III, 365
Livingston EG, 75
Livolsi VA, 314
Lloyd RP, 433
Lobo RA, 396, 411, 474
Lockwood CJ, 36, 173
Lockwood GM, 398
Loke DFM, 500
London SJ, 544
Longaker MT, 236
López-Zeno JA, 171
Lorenzetti LA, 294
Love EJ, 530
Love RR, 583
Loveland-Cherry CJ, 209
Lovin JD, 556
Lowe GDO, 84
Lu L, 167
Lugo-Miro VI, 376
Lundberg P-A, 395
Lundy RO, 566
Luthold WW, 398
Lynch L, 124

M

Maberry MC, 57
McAllister JM, 7
Macarthy PO, 509
Macaso TM, 474
McCall JB, 550
McCann MF, 480
MacCarter G, 5
McCarthy T, 494, 501
Maccolini A, 475
McCormack WM, 369
McCormick B, 571
McCormick S, 284
McDermott A, 468, 472
McGregor JA, 45, 157
McGuire WL, 581
McHugo JM, 205
Mackenzie EFD, 294
McKinlay SM, 409
McKinna JA, 546
McKnight B, 427, 485
McLaughlin J, 296
McLintic AJ, 169
McMahon JT, 201
McNamara HM, 289
McNeese M, 571
MacNeily AE, 58
Macri CJ, 126
Maddox PR, 553
Madvig P, 420
Mage G, 457
Maggi R, 345
Maggioni P, 392
Magill HL, 168
Magos AL, 398
Mahajan DK, 448
Maheux R, 405
Mahmood TA, 460
Maier D, 514
Maiman M, 336
Major FJ, 321, 332
Makowski EL, 20
Mamounas EP, 589
Manchul LA, 333
Mandel J-L, 188
Mangili G, 330
Mangioni C, 345
Manhes H, 457, 523
Mann J, 489, 490
Mann V, 296
Manogue K, 26
Mansel RE, 540, 553
Manson JE, 423
Mantell BS, 320
Mantingh A, 137
Manzarbeitia C, 407
Marcondes JAM, 398
Marconi AM, 20
Margolese R, 589
Margolese RG, 579
Mark SD, 346
Markman M, 344
Marslew U, 414
Martin WH, 372
Mashiach S, 163
Mason JI, 7
Massobrio M, 64
Mathiesen O, 508
Matias-Guiu X, 344
Mattei AM, 392
Matthews CD, 446
Matthews KA, 264
Mattos CER, 494
Mattson L-Å, 395
Mattsson A, 598
Mattsson L-Å, 430
Maygarden SJ, 550, 552
Mayo G, 17
Mazor M, 26, 60, 109
Mazur L, 376
Mazzoni PL, 103
Mecklin J-P, 312
Medlin JF, 229
Meehan FP, 386
Meigs JW, 410
Meirik O, 497
Meisel R, 124
Melega C, 475
Mercer B, 111
Mercer BM, 31
Merchant L, 109
Meriwether C, 377
Meyer WR, 522
Meyers CM, 199
Michelsen JW, 512
Miers M, 540
Millard SP, 101
Miller A, 321
Miller AB, 298
Miller C, 407
Miller E, 232
Miller RC, 81, 142, 329
Miller TC, 228
Milliez J, 94
Mills C, 476
Mills MS, 468, 472
Milne MA, 249
Milner R, 34
Minkoff H, 75
Minnani SL, 398
Mio Y, 451
Mishell DR Jr, 494, 501
Mitri FF, 436
Mitsuda T, 211
Mittal K, 336
Miura S, 580
Moe RE, 573
Moghissi KS, 454
Moise KJ Jr, 135
Mølbak K, 225
Møller M, 281
Monga M, 338
Montiel F, 60
Moorcraft J, 123
Moore D, 485
Mora S, 389
Morales A, 267
Moretti ML, 31

Morgan AM, 228
Morgan MA, 174
Morgan PL, 313
Morgan TM, 587
Morimoto T, 580
Moriniere Ph, 79
Morris M, 353
Morrotti R, 60
Morton MJ, 122
Mosher WD, 364
Mou SM, 152
Moulden M, 144, 149
Mourisse P, 183
Mouritsen L, 281
Mowafi RS, 452
Mowszowicz I, 393, 455
Moya FR, 219
Msellati P, 221
Muharib NS, 444
Muijsers GJJM, 141
Mulder EJH, 130
Müller E, 549
Mulvihill JJ, 410
Muntz HG, 295
Murata PJ, 565
Murnaghan GA, 16
Murphy EL, 77
Murphy KW, 136
Murphy M, 489, 490
Murray J, 226
Musicco M, 379
Myatt L, 18, 59
Myers MH, 410
Myerson M, 387

N

Naaktgeboren N, 471
Nagamani M, 311
Naides SJ, 239
Nair P, 85
Nappi RE, 532
Narod SA, 298
Nash JD, 329
Nayagam M, 303
Nazir M, 237
Neerhof MG, 237
Negri E, 309, 323, 330, 345, 484, 596
Neijt JP, 342
Nethersell A, 297
Neuman M, 256
Neven P, 269
Newcomb PA, 583
Newlands ES, 347
Newnham JP, 153
Nezhat C, 248
Nezhat F, 248
Ngai JH, 570
Nickel JC, 267
Nicolaides KH, 146
Nicolle LE, 290
Nicolosi A, 379
Niebyl JR, 44
Nieman LK, 14
Niermeyer MF, 190
Niruthisard S, 358
Nissen SE, 39
Nizzoli G, 389
Noel Y, 302
Nomura Y, 580
Noorduin H, 183
Nordenskjöld F, 517
Nordstrom L, 284
Nores J, 109
Noumoff JS, 314
Novotny DB, 552

O

Oberlé I, 188
Obiakor I, 336
O'Connor WN, 39
O'Dea MR-A, 153
Odén A, 395
Odlind V, 496, 501
O'Dwyer EM, 386
Oh TE, 204
Okuda KJ, 402
Oleske DM, 175
Olive DL, 462
Oliver RTD, 320
Olsson S-E, 496, 501
O'Malley VP, 258
Omura GA, 307
Onadim Z, 187
Ono A, 6
Opsahl MS, 14
Oram DH, 320
Orr JW Jr, 293
Orr PF, 293
Ory HW, 481
Ozzi F, 96
O'Shaughnessy M, 258
Osser S, 375
Østensen M, 95
Ostergaard H, 449
Ostrea EM Jr, 203
O'Sullivan MJ, 75
Ouwerkerk R, 123
Oyarzun E, 10, 26, 60

P

Padberg B-C, 331
Padbury J, 219
Paduano L, 238
Palinkas LA, 412
Pampiglione J, 476
Paniel BJ, 94
Panzarella T, 306
Parazzini F, 309, 323, 330, 345, 459, 484, 596
Pardi G, 20
Pareschi A, 475
Paris J, 40
Parisi VM, 182
Parke AL, 514
Parker SH, 556
Parkinson B, 554
Parra M, 10, 60
Parrish K, 170
Pasolini D, 389
Pass RF, 119
Patel V, 152
Pater JL, 338
Paterson C, 61
Patrick SL, 3
Pattinson R, 148
Paul MS, 122
Paul RH, 126
Paulson RJ, 474
Pavez M, 494, 496, 501
Pavirani A, 240
Pavlik EJ, 326
Peaceman AM, 171, 182
Pearlstein TB, 532
Peckham CS, 217, 232
Pedersen RG, 491
Pee D, 410
Peillon F, 393
Pellerito JS, 522
Pello LC, 144, 149
Peratoner L, 238
Perbeck L, 598
Pérez A, 479
Perkins HA, 77
Perpinyal S, 436
Perrella RR, 201
Perricaudet M, 240
Perry R, 237
Pesanti EL, 381
Peters AJ, 433, 438
Peters GN, 566
Petersen KR, 491
Peterson HB, 324, 481
Petosa MT, 52
Petrulis AS, 47
Phillips OP, 199
Phippard AF, 92
Pierson RN Jr, 387
Pijnenborg R, 104
Pilgrim CA, 587
Plappert T, 25
Plotkin D, 539
Podratz KC, 339
Polinsky ML, 574
Polk DH, 219
Porcu MC, 64
Posner JG, 409
Possati G, 475
Poulsen A-G, 225
Pouly JL, 457, 523
Powell DE, 326
Prak FM, 471
Prat J, 344
Pretorius DH, 245
Prevost RR, 31
Price JO, 199
Price P, 17
Price RI, 416
Prince RL, 416

Pringle JF, 333
Pringle SD, 169
Prior A, 252
Pryor JP, 441
Puls LE, 326
Pushkin S, 271

Q

Quedens-Case C, 522
Queenan JT, 479
Quinn TC, 229
Quintarelli C, 507
Quintero R, 109

R

Rabin A, 71
Rackley CE, 425
Radda GK, 123
Radecki PD, 207
Rader JS, 337
Radford DJ, 97
Radici E, 459
Raffle AE, 294
Ragavendra N, 201
Rainey WE, 7
Rajagopalan B, 123
Raju KS, 303
Ralph MM, 12
Raman S, 178
Ramanathan J, 180
Ramcharan S, 530
Ramos AIO, 100
Ramos IM, 522
Ramsay MEB, 232
Ramsdell J, 426
Randall JM, 443
Raphael JC, 27
Rappaport WD, 259
Ratnam SS, 500
Raux-Demay M-C, 455
Rawlings GA, 333
Rawls W, 296
Rawstron SA, 230
Ray RM, 502
Raymundo AL, 203
Read NW, 252
Reagan K, 425
Recht A, 571, 575
Recio FO, 315
Redman C, 148
Redman CWG, 144, 149
Redman S, 251
Redmond C, 589
Rees A, 104
Rehpenning W, 331
Reichart CA, 369
Reid KP, 153
Reiter AA, 135
Rekers H, 263
Renvall M, 426
Restelli C, 345
Reuss A, 190
Reynolds HE, 558
Rhodes P, 481, 598
Ribbert LSM, 130, 146
Rice LW, 295
Richart RM, 304
Richley D, 22
Ries L, 576
Rifka SM, 509
Rimer BK, 559
Ringborg U, 598
Riphagen F, 263
Rivard G-E, 53
Rizzo G, 107
Roberts DJ, 346
Roberts WS, 348, 349
Robertson DM, 383
Robinson B, 85
Robson SC, 22
Rochelson B, 108
Roddy RE, 358
Rohan T, 296
Rolfs RT, 357, 361
Roman SH, 73
Romero R, 10, 26, 60, 109
Romm PA, 425
Rosales RF, 259
Rosen PP, 596, 598
Rosenberg DC, 464
Rosenberg MJ, 360, 497
Rosendahl I, 548
Rosenfeld MA, 240
Rosenshein NB, 337
Rosenthal ER, 240
Rosenzweig BA, 271
Rosevear SK, 144, 149
Roskamp D, 273
Rosner B, 423
Rotstein S, 598
Rountree R, 170
Rousseau F, 188
Rowe J, 314
Rowe PJ, 440, 497
Rowley D, 33
Royston P, 327
Rubattu S, 23
Ruble RA, 294
Rud T, 274
Rudolph AM, 29
Ruff A, 229
Rumore GJ, 570
Russell V, 136
Rustin GJS, 347
Rutqvist LE, 548, 598
Rybo G, 430

S

Saarikoski S, 297
Safrin S, 366
Saginur R, 290
Sagle M, 450
Sahakian V, 239
St John Sutton MG, 25
Saliola M, 507
Salminen-Lappalainen K, 191
Samojlik E, 398
Samuel D, 178
Samueloff A, 127
Sances G, 532
Sanchez RB, 367
Sanson-Fisher RW, 251
Saracco A, 379
Sarinoglu C, 111
Sauer MV, 474
Saunders N, 61
Savvas M, 422, 428
Sawaragi I, 6
Sawaragi S, 6
Sawicki JE, 570
Schachter J, 366
Schag CAC, 574
Scharosch LL, 239
Schenken RS, 462
Schmitt C, 377
Schmucker BC, 101
Schmucker BS, 98
Schnack Peen UB, 512
Schnitt SJ, 544, 575
Schoemaker J, 388
Schoendorf KC, 33
Schofield JB, 546
Schofield MJ, 251
Schreinemachers LMH, 276
Schrimmer DB, 126
Schröcksnadel H, 549
Schröder S, 331
Schultz DJ, 571
Schultz LR, 487
Schulz KF, 156
Schutzman DL, 223
Schwartz DA, 128
Schwartz M, 407
Scoutt LM, 522
Sealey JE, 23
Seeds JW, 142
Seidman DS, 163
Sekizuka N, 511
Selwyn B, 170
Senie RT, 598
Senyei AE, 36
Seo K, 45
Seracchioli R, 475
Severini V, 392
Sevin B-U, 332
Shah KD, 36
Sharp GB, 350
Shaver DC, 168
Shaw RW, 444, 452
Sheinbaum KA, 185
Shelley WE, 338
Shen E-Y, 224
Shermer RW, 552
Sheth SS, 254
Shield PW, 308
Shier RM, 296
Shimizu H, 211
Shook D, 199
Shoupe D, 494

Shulman LP, 199
Sibai B, 180
Sibai BM, 31, 111
Sightler SE, 325
Silfen SL, 248
Silfverswärd C, 548
Silva EG, 353
Silver B, 575
Silver M, 12
Silverberg KM, 462
Silverberg SG, 321
Simm J, 333
Simonon A, 221
Simpson JL, 199
Singer J, 223
Singer S, 486
Singh K, 500
Singh KB, 448
Sipes SL, 121, 131
Sivin I, 494, 496, 501
Sixma JJ, 401
Skibsted L, 439
Skjeldestad FE, 499
Skoog L, 598
Skouby SO, 491
Skrede M, 274
Slevin ML, 320
Sluijmer AV, 391
Small A, 593
Smans AJ, 276
Smego RA Jr, 113
Smith ARB, 252
Smith D, 296, 368
Smith M, 416
Smith WC, 522
Smyth J, 123
Snijders RJM, 130, 146
Sninsky J, 77
Sobel JD, 377
Socol ML, 171
Soetens M, 183
Soliani A, 469
Solin LJ, 571
Sommell A, 598
Sondag-Thull D, 221
Sonnendecker EWW, 136
Sönnerborg A, 78
Sood AK, 305
Soper JT, 340
Sousa JEMR, 100
South MC, 560
Spears GFS, 418
Speizer FE, 423
Sperling L, 439
Sperling RS, 75
Spitalier J-M, 571
Stadberg E, 430
Stagnaro-Green A, 73
Stagno S, 119
Stampfer MJ, 423
Stanley FJ, 51, 214
Stanley K, 252
Stanton SL, 254
Stark RI, 5
Steer C, 476
Stegner H-E, 331
Steiger P, 420
Stein JA, 565
Stenman U-H, 505
Stergachis A, 485
Stern J, 494, 496, 501
Sterns EE, 541
Stevens A-M, 221
Stevens M, 203
Stevenson DK, 163
Stewart PA, 159
Stier LE, 240
Stolz W, 268
Stone AB, 532
Stovall TG, 313, 521, 522
Strandness DE, 41
Strasser K, 549
Stratford-Perricaudet L, 240
Stratta P, 64
Stratton P, 75
Strong LC, 410
Stuart CA, 311
Studd J, 422
Studd JWW, 428
Stuenkel CA, 245
Sturgeon JFG, 333
Sturgiss SN, 114
Subak LL, 445
Sumdin G, 78
Sunderji SG, 152
Sundin G, 78
Suresh K, 178
Sutcliffe SB, 306
Sutherland JC, 259
Sutton GP, 307, 332
Sviggum O, 499
Sweet RL, 366
Syrjänen K, 297
Syrjänen S, 297

T

Tabar L, 560
Takakuwa K, 511
Tallon DF, 386
Tan S-J, 574
Tan S-L, 476
Tanaka K, 511
Tanikawa M, 451
Tao L-C, 493
Tashiro H, 580
Taylor B, 367
Taylor KJW, 522
Teele JS, 265
Teitel DF, 29
Templeton A, 443
Templeton AA, 460
ten Bokkel Huinink WW, 342
Terado H, 451
Terakawa N, 451
Tessler FN, 201
Testa G, 392
Thalabard J-C, 455
Tharapel A, 199
Theeuwes AGM, 276
Theise N, 407
Theuer CP, 261
Theve T, 598
Thevenin F, 494
Thian S, 12
Thiedemann C, 331
Thigpen JT, 322
Thomas DB, 502, 573
Thomas EJ, 402
Thomas GM, 333
Thomas NM, 402
Thomas NWM, 255
Thomas-McCauley T, 228
Thompson DW, 298
Thompson WD, 569
Thomson J, 418
Thomson L, 460
Thorburn J, 169, 524
Thornton KL, 246
Thorogood M, 489, 490
Thorp JA, 182
Thouvenez V, 519
Thung SN, 36, 407
Thurman AE, 272
Thurnau GR, 174
Tiller DJ, 92
Tiltman A, 104
Tilyard MW, 418
Tishler S, 575
Toaff ME, 207
Toda T, 451
Todros T, 64
Toikkanen S, 592
Tominaga T, 580
Tommerup N, 188
Tornos C, 353
Touraine J-L, 235
Tovo P-A, 103
Trainer TD, 434
Trapnell BC, 240
Trichopoulos D, 323
Trimble EL, 328
Trimbos JB, 342
Trock B, 559
Trudinger BJ, 160
Truwit CL, 212
Tulandi T, 528
Tulppala M, 505
Turnbull AC, 398
Tuveng JM, 499
Tyson VJ, 509
Tzonou A, 323

U

Ugol JH, 157
Urman B, 453
Uzan S, 40

V

Vaes L, 183

Vaira D, 221
Valesini G, 507
Valkenburg H, 263
Vamvakas EC, 301
Van Aken H, 183
Van Assche A, 104
Van Assche AF, 183
Van Assche FA, 198
van Belle G, 427
Van de Perre P, 221
van der Burg MEL, 342
Van Der Hagen C, 188
van der Meijden APM, 276
Vandermeulen E, 183
van Eijkeren MA, 401
Van Goethem C, 221
van Huisseling H, 141
Vankelecom F, 198
van Lent M, 342
van Lindert ACM, 342
Van Lith JMM, 137
van Nagell JR Jr, 326
van Oosterom AT, 342
van Sonnenberg E, 367
vanSonnenberg E, 368
Van Steenberge A, 183
van Vliet-Bleeker I, 388
van Weissenbruch MM, 388
Varney RR, 368
Veille J-C, 122
Venesmaa P, 341
Vercruysse L, 104
Verdon MS, 369
Vermorken JB, 342
Vernon SW, 566
Vertommen JD, 183
Vessey M, 489, 490
Vicini FA, 575
Viegas OAC, 500
Vilcoq JR, 571
Villanueva B, 464
Villar J, 42
Vincens M, 393
Vink PE, 85
Violi F, 507
Virji SK, 65
Visser GHA, 130, 146
Visser W, 86
Voelckel M-A, 188
Voet R, 317
Vogel VG, 566
Voigt LF, 427
von Fournier D, 268
von Lutterotti N, 23
Vosters R, 137
Vyas GN, 77

W

Wachtel SS, 199
Wagner D, 145
Wahlström T, 505
Wajchenberg BL, 398
Wald NJ, 138
Walker AM, 486
Walker JJ, 84, 400
Walker S, 470
Wall C, 298
Wall RE, 157
Wallenburg HCS, 86
Wallenstein S, 73
Walsh SW, 48
Walters DE, 469
Walters WAW, 251
Walton LA, 480
Wang J, 387
Wang Y, 48
Wardlaw SL, 5
Wardle PG, 472
Warnes GM, 446
Warren MP, 387
Warren WB, 3, 5
Wasserstrum N, 54, 90
Watson H, 450
Watson N, 422
Wattiez A, 457, 523
Watts DH, 66, 75
Weatherall DJ, 195
Webb PG, 416
Weber G, 389
Weinberg GB, 593
Weiner CP, 121, 131, 239
Weiser EB, 329
Weiss NS, 324, 427, 485
Wells C, 470
Wells TJ, 279
Wenstrom KD, 121, 131
West C, 449
Westeel PF, 79
Weström L, 375
Wharton JT, 353
Whitby DJ, 236
White E, 573
Whitehead MI, 327
Whitelaw WA, 13
Wickerham DL, 589
Widness JA, 121, 131
Wieand HS, 339
Wiebe DA, 583
Wilhelm MC, 600
Wilkie AOM, 195
Wilking N, 598
Willaert J, 183
Willemse PHB, 342
Willett WC, 423
William A, 34
Williamson RA, 121, 131, 239
Wilson D, 514
Wilson J, 98, 267
Wiltshaw E, 546
Wingo PA, 481
Wisoff JH, 68
Witt BR, 526
Witzke DB, 259
Wladimiroff JW, 159, 190
Wolberg WH, 601
Wolf GC, 526
Wolf SI, 245
Wolfe R, 279
Wolmark N, 589
Wong J, 554
Wong SP, 168
Woodruff JD, 337
Woodward AJ, 383
Word RA, 9
Wright RG, 308
Wright TC Jr, 304
Wyman JF, 280
Wynn V, 483

Y

Yakes WF, 556
Yamada K, 511
Yamamoto H, 580
Yarali H, 453
Yaremko ML, 555
Ylikorkala O, 191, 341, 505
Yliskoski M, 297
Yokota S, 211
Yoneyama K, 240
Yordan E, 322
Yordan EL, 307
Yoshimura K, 240
Young BK, 68
Young PE, 464
Youngblut JM, 209
Ysrael C, 562
Ysrael M, 562
Yu H, 296
Yuen PM, 204

Z

Zaccardi MJ, 41
Zaidi AA, 361
Zaino R, 332
Zaino RJ, 317
Zamurovic D, 315
Zelles GW, 570
Zemlickis D, 306
Zhang J, 48
Zhu Y-p, 9